Breast Cancer: A Woman-Centered Approach

Breast Cancer: A Woman-Centered Approach

Edited by Ava Santiago

hayle
medical

New York

Hayle Medical,
750 Third Avenue, 9ᵗʰ Floor,
New York, NY 10017, USA

Visit us on the World Wide Web at:
www.haylemedical.com

ISBN: 978-1-63241-690-2

Cataloging-in-Publication Data

Breast cancer : a woman-centered approach / edited by Ava Santiago.
p. cm.
Includes bibliographical references and index.
ISBN 978-1-63241-690-2
1. Breast--Cancer. 2. Breast--Tumors. 3. Breast--Cancer--Etiology. 4. Breast--Cancer--Treatment.
5. Cancer in women. I. Santiago, Ava.
RC280.B8 B73 2019
616.994 49--dc23

Contents

Preface

This book aims to highlight the current researches and provides a platform to further the scope of innovations in this area. This book is a product of the combined efforts of many researchers and scientists, after going through thorough studies and analysis from different parts of the world. The objective of this book is to provide the readers with the latest information of the field.

The cancer of the breast or breast cancer develops in the cells of the lining of milk ducts or in the lobules that supply the ducts with milk. The most noticeable symptom of breast cancer is a lump in breast tissue. Some of the other signs of breast cancer are a change in breast shape and size, dimpling of the skin, fluid secretion from the nipple, red or scaly patch of skin and a newly inverted nipple. When the cancer spreads, swollen lymph nodes, yellow skin and shortness of breath may be witnessed. The tumor can be removed usually through a surgery, after which a breast reconstruction surgery can be done to improve the aesthetic appearance of the operated area. Women with breast cancer experience and cope with the illness in different ways. Premenopausal women might have to confront the issue of the early onset of menopause. Women can reduce the risk of breast cancer by adhering to a healthy lifestyle with increased physical activity, reducing alcohol use, maintaining a healthy weight and breast-feeding. The book aims to shed light on some of the unexplored aspects of breast cancer with a woman-centered approach. It presents researches and studies performed by experts across the globe on the clinical assessment and management of breast cancer. It attempts to assist those with a goal of delving into this field.

I would like to express my sincere thanks to the authors for their dedicated efforts in the completion of this book. I acknowledge the efforts of the publisher for providing constant support. Lastly, I would like to thank my family for their support in all academic endeavors.

Editor

Assessing brain volume changes in older women with breast cancer receiving adjuvant chemotherapy: a brain magnetic resonance imaging pilot study

Bihong T. Chen[1*], Sean K. Sethi[2], Taihao Jin[1], Sunita K. Patel[3], Ningrong Ye[1], Can-Lan Sun[4], Russell C. Rockne[5] ,
E. Mark Haacke[2,6], James C. Root[7], Andrew J. Saykin[8], Tim A. Ahles[7], Andrei I. Holodny[9], Neal Prakash[10],
Joanne Mortimer[11], James Waisman[11], Yuan Yuan[11], George Somlo[11], Daneng Li[11], Richard Yang[4], Heidi Tan[4],
Vani Katheria[4], Rachel Morrison[4] and Arti Hurria[4,11]

Abstract

Background: Cognitive decline is among the most feared treatment-related outcomes of older adults with cancer. The majority of older patients with breast cancer self-report cognitive problems during and after chemotherapy. Prior neuroimaging research has been performed mostly in younger patients with cancer. The purpose of this study was to evaluate longitudinal changes in brain volumes and cognition in older women with breast cancer receiving adjuvant chemotherapy.

Methods: Women aged ≥ 60 years with stage I–III breast cancer receiving adjuvant chemotherapy and age-matched and sex-matched healthy controls were enrolled. All participants underwent neuropsychological testing with the US National Institutes of Health (NIH) Toolbox for Cognition and brain magnetic resonance imaging (MRI) prior to chemotherapy, and again around one month after the last infusion of chemotherapy. Brain volumes were measured using Neuroreader™ software. Longitudinal changes in brain volumes and neuropsychological scores were analyzed utilizing linear mixed models.

Results: A total of 16 patients with breast cancer (mean age 67.0, SD 5.39 years) and 14 age-matched and sex-matched healthy controls (mean age 67.8, SD 5.24 years) were included: 7 patients received docetaxel and cyclophosphamide (TC) and 9 received chemotherapy regimens other than TC (non-TC). There were no significant differences in segmented brain volumes between the healthy control group and the chemotherapy group pre-chemotherapy ($p > 0.05$). Exploratory hypothesis generating analyses focusing on the effect of the chemotherapy regimen demonstrated that the TC group had greater volume reduction in the temporal lobe (change = − 0.26) compared to the non-TC group (change = 0.04, p for interaction = 0.02) and healthy controls (change = 0.08, p for interaction = 0.004). Similarly, the TC group had a decrease in oral reading recognition scores (change = − 6.94) compared to the non-TC group (change = − 1.21, p for interaction = 0.07) and healthy controls (change = 0.09, p for interaction = 0.02).

(Continued on next page)

* Correspondence: Bechen@coh.org
[1]Department of Diagnostic Radiology, City of Hope National Medical Center, Duarte, CA 91010, USA
Full list of author information is available at the end of the article

(Continued from previous page)

Conclusions: There were no significant differences in segmented brain volumes between the healthy control group and the chemotherapy group; however, exploratory analyses demonstrated a reduction in both temporal lobe volume and oral reading recognition scores among patients on the TC regimen. These results suggest that different chemotherapy regimens may have differential effects on brain volume and cognition. Future, larger studies focusing on older adults with cancer on different treatment regimens are needed to confirm these findings.

Keywords: Brain MRI, Brain volume, Chemotherapy, Cancer-related cognitive impairment, Breast cancer

Background

Cognitive decline is among the most feared symptoms in older adults undergoing treatment for cancer [1, 2]. As cancer incidence increases with age [3] and cognitive changes frequently occur following cancer systemic therapy, it is imperative to understand who is most at risk and what is the neuroanatomical basis underlying these changes. The majority of patients with breast cancer self-report cognitive problems during and after chemotherapy [4]; however, neuropsychological testing has yielded widely varying results. Different studies have reported that 13–70% of patients receiving chemotherapy demonstrate objective changes, with memory, processing speed, and executive function being the most commonly affected domains [5]. The discrepancy between patient-reported symptoms and objective results from neuropsychological testing, the wide range of results within neuropsychological testing, and the recent emphasis on individualized care all highlight the critical need to identify individuals who are especially at risk for post-therapeutic cognitive decline [6, 7]. The disparity between subjective, patient-reported cognitive problems and objective identification of cognitive problems highlights the need to better understand the neural correlates of cognitive decline.

Brain magnetic resonance imaging (MRI) can be used to identify risk factors and imaging-based biomarkers for adverse cognitive outcomes of chemotherapy treatment in patients with cancer. Adjuvant chemotherapy for breast cancer is associated with changes in structural MRI including an overall decrease of gray matter density. However, these studies have been primarily performed in younger cohorts of patients with a mean age (SD) ranging from 46.3 (6.1) to 52.9 (8.6) years [8–10]. Older adults may be at increased risk for cognitive decline. For example, a longitudinal study of individuals aged 46–86 years demonstrated that aging is associated with a reduction in brain volume, estimated at 0.5–1.5% per year in all brain structures [11] and the loss in brain volume was associated with cognitive decline [12]. However, there is a gap in knowledge regarding whether chemotherapy is associated with accelerated loss of brain volume in older adults with breast cancer.

This is a pilot longitudinal study to evaluate the association between changes in brain volume and cognition in older women with breast cancer after receiving adjuvant chemotherapy. The overall goal of the study was to evaluate the longitudinal volume measurements of brain structures that were highly associated with cognition—total gray matter, frontal lobe, and temporal lobe—among older adults with breast cancer [13]. We hypothesized that the volumes of the total gray matter, the frontal lobe, and the temporal lobe would be reduced in older women with breast cancer from pre to post-adjuvant chemotherapy and that these changes would be accompanied by decreased performance in neuropsychological testing. Recent literature shows that different chemotherapy regimens may exert different neurotoxicity profiles [14]. Thus, we performed an exploratory hypothesis-generating analysis to examine how different chemotherapy regimens affected brain volumes in our study cohort.

Methods

The present study is a frequency matched case-control study. Cases were women aged ≥ 60 years with stage I–III breast cancer. The inclusion criteria for cases were: (1) stage I–III breast cancer in patients scheduled to receive adjuvant chemotherapy; (2) able to provide informed consent; (3) age 60 years and older; (4) of any performance status; and (5) no history of neurological or psychiatric disorders or stroke. The exclusion criteria for cases were: (1) metastatic disease or (2) MRI exclusion criteria such as claustrophobia, cardiac pacemaker, and orbital metal implants. Age-matched and sex-matched healthy controls with no history of cancer or chemotherapy exposure were recruited from the community with the same inclusion and exclusion criteria except the healthy controls did not have a cancer diagnosis. This research protocol was approved by the Institutional

Review Board at City of Hope National Center. Written informed consent was obtained from all study participants.

The pre-chemotherapy assessment, including a brain MRI scan and neuropsychological testing with the US National Institutes for Health (NIH) Toolbox for Cognition, was performed after surgery but before the start of adjuvant therapy (time point 1, baseline). The follow-up assessment for chemotherapy-treated patients was conducted around one month after the last infusion of chemotherapy (time point 2). The healthy control group underwent the same assessments at matched intervals.

Brain MRI scans and brain volume measurements
Imaging parameters
All brain MRI scans were performed on the same 3T VERIO Siemens scanner (Siemens, Erlangen, Germany). Sagittal T1-weighted three-dimensional (3D) magnetization prepared rapid gradient echo (MPRAGE) imaging data were acquired with the following parameters: echo time (TE) = 2.94 ms, repetition time (TR) = 1900 ms, fractional anisotrophy (FA) = 9°, bandwidth = 170 Hz/pixel, imaging matrix = 256 × 176 pixels, with a voxel size of $1 \times 1 \times 1$ mm^3 in the axial, coronal, and sagittal planes.

Brain volume measurement
Brain volumes were measured using the cloud-based Neuroreader™ software (Horsens, Denmark, https://brainreader.net/) [15–18]. This software is a commercially available and it can be used for automated volumetric measurement of segmented brain structures from 3D T1-weighted MPRAGE data. The brain volume segmentation of the imaging data was repeated three times to ensure accuracy of the automated segmentations. The output of this data analysis was carefully examined by the team for consistency. No significant inconsistency was noted during data analysis. The segmented brain structures included total gray matter, total white matter, frontal lobe, temporal lobe, parietal lobe, and occipital lobe. The volumes of bilateral lobes were combined as an overall lobe in statistical analysis.

Neuropsychological testing
All study participants completed neuropsychological testing using the NIH Toolbox for Cognition [19]. The NIH Toolbox (http://www.healthmeasures.net/explore-measurement-systems/nih-toolbox) uses a computerized format with national standardization. The cognition battery consists of seven measures that target the subdomains of executive function, episodic memory, language, processing speed, working memory, and attention. This battery generates three composite scores and seven individual scores.

Demographic and disease characteristics
The participants' demographic characteristics, including age, education, race, and ethnicity, were obtained through a self-reported questionnaire. Disease stage and treatment information (the chemotherapy regimen) were obtained through medical record abstraction. The chemotherapy toxicity risk scores (as defined by the Cancer and Aging Research Group) were calculated utilizing results from the medical records and the geriatric assessment questionnaire [20, 21]. Details of the questionnaire included in this assessment have been previously published [22]. Treatment duration was calculated as days between the first infusion and last infusion of chemotherapy.

Statistical analysis
All participants were female. The healthy controls were frequency matched to the patients with breast cancer in terms of age distribution. Unconditional logistic regression was used to compare the patients with breast cancer and healthy controls in terms of ethnicity and education. All healthy controls were white, thus the Fisher's exact test was used to compare the race/ethnicity distribution between the patients and the healthy controls.

Statistical analysis was performed on the volume measurements from brain segmentation output using the Neuroreader™ image processing pipeline. For chemotherapy patients and healthy controls, the mean and standard deviations were presented for total white matter, total gray matter, and lobar volumes. All brain volumes were controlled using measured total intracranial volume (mTIV) and expressed as mTIV ratios. Changes were calculated as mTIV ratios at time point 2 minus mTIV ratios at time point 1. Percent changes were calculated as changes divided by mTIV ratios at time point 1. Linear mixed modeling, taking into consideration the correlation of repeated measurements within subjects, was used for longitudinal brain volume analysis [23]. Within-subject correlation was accounted for using a compound symmetry covariance structure. Time points (1 and 2) and group (patients receiving chemotherapy versus healthy controls) were both considered categorical fixed effects in the model. The interaction term of the group indicator with time point was included in the model to examine whether the changes in brain volume in the chemotherapy patient group differed significantly from those of the healthy control group. Using this linear mixed effect model with a compound symmetry covariance structure to account for correlation between repeated measurements, we examined: (1) whether there were any differences in segmented brain volumes between the chemotherapy group and the healthy control group at time point 1 and time point 2;

(2) whether there were any significant changes from time point 1 to time point 2 within the chemotherapy group and the healthy control group; and (3) whether the brain volume changes differed by group (*p* for interaction). All statistical tests were two-sided. Since the main hypothesis for this study focused on total gray matter, frontal lobe, and temporal lobe, a conservative Bonferroni method was used to correct for multiple testing, with *p* values <0.01 considered statistically significant. The Bonferroni method was not applied to the statistical tests involving the neuropsychological data or any other analyses. Data were analyzed using SAS 9.3 (SAS Institute, Cary, NC, USA).

Results

The demographic data for all study participants are summarized in Table 1. The participants consisted of 16 consecutive eligible patients with breast cancer (mean age 67, SD 5.39 years) and 14 age-matched and sex-matched healthy controls (mean age 67.8, SD 5.24 years). A total of 15 healthy controls were initially enrolled; however, one healthy control did not have the sagittal T1-weighted 3D MPRAGE sequence included in the brain MRI scan and hence was not included in the final analysis. There were no significant differences between the chemotherapy group and the healthy control group in terms of age or overall education (*p* = 0.51). All study participants were female and were right-handed. The chemotherapy group included 11 (68.8%) white women and 5 (31.2%) black women, while all healthy controls (*n* = 14) were white women (*p* = 0.04). There was no difference in ethnicity between groups. There were 5 (31.3%) patients with stage I, 8 (50.0%) patients with stage II, and 3 (18.7%) patients with stage III breast

Table 1 Demographic data of the study participants

Variable	Chemotherapy group (*n* = 16)		Healthy controls (*n* = 14)	
	Number	Percent	Number	Percent
Age, years				
Mean (SD)	67.0 (5.39)	N/A	67.8 (5.24)	N/A
Range	60–82	N/A	60–78	N/A
Race				
White	11	68.8%	14	100%
Black	5	31.2%	0	0.0%
Ethnicity				
Hispanic or Latina	2	12.5%	2	14.3%
Non-Hispanic	14	87.5%	12	85.7%
Education				
High school	4	25.0%	1	7.1%
Some college or junior college	6 + 2	50.0%	4 + 4	57.1%
College degree	3	18.8%	3	21.4%
Post college	1	6.2%	2	14.4%
Stage				
I	5	31.3%	N/A	N/A
II	8	50.0%	N/A	N/A
III	3	18.7%	N/A	N/A
Regimen				
TC	7	43.75%	N/A	N/A
TCPH	1	6.25%	N/A	N/A
Paclitaxel/trastuzumab	4	25.0%	N/A	N/A
Docetaxel/cyclophosphamide/PH	1	6.25%	N/A	N/A
Carboplatin/paclitaxel	1	6.25%	N/A	N/A
ddAC – paclitaxel	1	6.25%	N/A	N/A
TAC	1	6.25%	N/A	N/A

Abbreviations: TC docetaxel and cyclophosphamide, *TCPH* docetaxel, carboplatin, pertuzumab, trastuzumab, *Docetaxel/cyclophosphamide/PH* docetaxel, cyclophosphamide, pertuzumab, trastuzumab, *ddAC - Paclitaxel* dose-dense doxorubicin and cyclophosphamide followed by paclitaxel, *TAC* docetaxel, doxorubicin, and cyclophosphamide, *N/A* not applicable

cancer. Out of the 16 patients, 7 (43.8%) received docetaxel and cyclophosphamide (TC regimen) and 9 (56.2%) received a chemotherapy regimen other than TC: 4 (25.0%) received paclitaxel and trastuzumab, and the remaining 5 patients (each 6.25%) received different chemotherapy regimens as noted in Table 1. The median duration of the chemotherapy treatment was 63 days (range 42–112 days). The median time between treatment completion and the time point 2 MRI was 22 days (range 1–42 days). The median time interval between treatment completion and neurocogitive testing was 22 days (range 1–98 days).

Table 2 presents the summary of the brain volume measurements normalized by mTIV of total gray matter, total white matter, and lobar structures at time point 1 and time point 2 for both the chemotherapy group and healthy control group. The volumes of bilateral lobes were combined as an overall lobe in statistical analysis. Representative images from brain segmentation output are shown in Fig. 1. There were no significant differences between the chemotherapy group and the healthy control group ($p > 0.05$) in total gray matter, total white matter, the segmented lobar brain structures at time point 1 (baseline) or at time point 2.

Table 3 presents the longitudinal brain volume changes within each of the two groups from time point 1 to time point 2 and compares the changes between the two groups (group by time interaction). In the chemotherapy group, there were non-significant volume reductions over time in total gray matter (change = – 2.05, $p = 0.02$), significant volume reductions in the frontal lobe (change = – 0.33, $p = 0.003$), and non-significant volume increase in total white matter (change = 1.65, $p = 0.06$) from time point 1 to time point 2. However, non-significant volume reductions over time in total gray matter (change = – 0.99, $p = 0.27$) and in the frontal lobe (change = – 0.27, $p = 0.02$), and non-significant volume increase in total white matter (change = 0.90, $p = 0.32$)

were also observed in the healthy control group, thus the volume changes between the two groups were not significantly different. A non-significant reduction was observed in the temporal lobe in the chemotherapy group (change = – 0.09, $p = 0.16$) and no significant reduction was observed for the healthy control group (change = 0.08, $p = 0.25$). There was a weak group-by-time interaction in the temporal lobe (p for interaction = 0.08). There were no significant reductions in the parietal lobe, the occipital lobe, or in total white matter in either the chemotherapy group or the healthy control group.

Further exploratory analyses of the chemotherapy group revealed that the temporal lobe reduction occurred mainly among patients who received the TC regimen (docetaxel and cyclophosphamide) (change = – 0.26, $p = 0.006$) (Table 4). Compared to the healthy control group, the TC group had significant volume reduction in the temporal lobe (p for interaction = 0.004) (Fig. 2). The TC group had a reduction in temporal lobe volume of 2.4% from time point 1 to time point 2, while the non-TC group and healthy control group did not have a reduction. Sensitivity analysis by excluding one or two patients at a time in the TC group did not change the findings. The TC group also demonstrated significant total gray matter reduction over time (change = – 3.99, $p = 0.002$), although the reduction was not statistically significantly different from that in the non-TC group (change = – 0.56, p for interaction = 0.04) or the healthy control group (change = – 0.99, p for interaction = 0.05). There were no differences between the TC group and non-TC group in age, education, race/ethnicity, or cancer stages. There were also no significant differences between the TC group and non-TC group in the chemotherapy toxicity risk score and measures of physical function including activities of daily living measured by the Medical Outcome Study (MOS) Physical Health scale and the Instrumental Activities of Daily Living (IADL) scale. Furthermore, there were no significant differences in brain volume at baseline

Table 2 Measured total intracranial volume (mTIV) and brain volume measurements normalized by mTIV (mTIV ratio)

	Chemotherapy group (n = 16)				Healthy control group (n = 14)			
	Time point 1		Time point 2		Time point 1		Time point 2	
	Mean	SD	Mean	SD	Mean	SD	Mean	SD
mTIV (ml)	1718.46	114.77	1707.12	110.23	1734.76	130.92	1714.87	119.83
Volume (mTIV ratio)								
Total white matter	26.75	3.15	28.40	4.77	27.94	3.33	28.84	2.57
Total gray matter	31.70	3.39	29.64	4.21	31.24	3.81	30.26	4.62
Frontal lobe	20.23	1.86	19.89	1.66	20.17	1.52	19.90	1.70
Parietal lobe	10.70	0.79	10.63	0.81	10.78	0.81	10.70	0.90
Occipital lobe	5.29	0.51	5.30	0.59	5.48	0.48	5.46	0.53
Temporal lobe	11.05	0.71	10.96	0.72	11.30	0.82	11.38	0.82

SD standard deviation

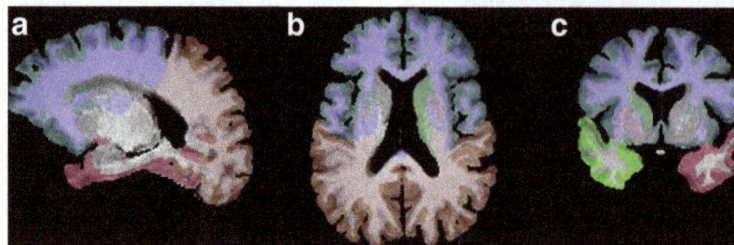

Fig. 1 Representative images of segmented brain volumes in a study participant. This set of images shows segmented brain structures in sagittal, axial, and coronal planes (**a**, **b**, **c**)

between the two groups. However, the patients in the TC group had a shorter chemotherapy duration (an average of 60 days), than the non-TC group (average of 86 days, $p = 0.003$).

Table 5 summarizes all neuropsychological testing scores with the NIH Toolbox for Cognition in both the chemotherapy group and the healthy control group at time point 1 and time point 2. There were no significant differences in the neuropsychological scores between the chemotherapy group and the healthy control group at time point 1. For most of the domains, there were no significant changes over time in either the chemotherapy group or the healthy control group. The healthy control group demonstrated higher scores at time point 2 compared to time point 1, possibly due to practice effect (Table 5). However, for the chemotherapy group as a whole, most of the time point 2 scores did not increase as expected from practice effect. On the contrary, the chemotherapy group had a decrease in the oral reading recognition scores (change = – 3.71) compared to healthy controls (change = 0.09, p for interaction = 0.11). Further subgroup analysis showed that the reduction in oral reading recognition scores was only observed in the patients who received the TC regimen (change = – 6.94) compared to the healthy control group (change = 0.09, p for interaction = 0.02) (Table 6 and Fig. 2). There was no significant correlation between the volume reduction in the temporal lobe or total gray matter and decreases in the oral reading recognition score.

Among patients who received chemotherapy, the Spearman's correlation coefficient was 0.27 ($p = 0.31$); among the patients who received the TC regimen, the Spearman's correlation coefficient was 0.17 ($p = 0.70$).

Discussion

To the best of our knowledge, the current study is one of few prospective longitudinal studies examining changes in brain volume on brain MRI and neurocognitive function among older adults with breast cancer receiving chemotherapy. There were no significant differences in the segmented brain volumes between the healthy control group and the chemotherapy group; however, exploratory analyses demonstrated temporal lobe volume reduction in the chemotherapy subgroup of patients who received the TC regimen. Patients who received the TC regimen also had a decreased score on the oral reading recognition test.

Several of our findings are in general accord with prior structural neuroimaging studies of chemotherapy and cognition in patients with breast cancer. Most reported neuroimaging studies of cancer-related cognitive impairment were cross-sectional in design and were conducted in breast cancer survivors. These prior studies reported reduced gray matter volume [24], smaller total brain volume and gray matter volume [25], and decreased gray matter density [26]. In a cross-sectional study of breast cancer survivors treated with chemotherapy, Inagaki and colleagues showed significant differences in regional

Table 3 Longitudinal volume changes (in measured total intracranial volume (mTIV) ratio) within the chemotherapy group and the healthy control group

	Chemotherapy group ($n = 16$)		Healthy control group ($n = 14$)		p comparing groups*
	changes in mTIV ratio (SD)	p value	changes in mTIV ratio (SD)	p value	
Total white matter	1.65 (3.63)	0.06	0.90 (2.91)	0.32	0.54
Total gray matter	−2.05 (3.38)	0.02	−0.99 (3.18)	0.27	0.38
Frontal lobe	−0.33 (0.39)	0.003	−0.27 (0.44)	0.02	0.68
Temporal lobe	−0.09 (0.31)	0.16	0.08 (0.16)	0.25	0.08
Parietal lobe	−0.07 (0.27)	0.27	−0.08 (0.22)	0.23	0.89
Occipital lobe	0.01 (0.18)	0.77	−0.02 (0.14)	0.65	0.60

*p values from comparison of volume changes between the two groups (group-by-time interaction)

Table 4 Comparison of longitudinal volume changes in the chemotherapy subgroups and the healthy control (HC) group

	Non-TC ($n = 9$)	TC ($n = 7$)	HC ($n = 14$)	TC vs. non-TC, p	Non-TC vs. HC, p	TC vs. HC, p
Total white matter	0.04	3.25	0.90	0.46	0.67	0.24
Total gray matter	−0.56	−3.99*	−0.99	0.04	0.75	0.05
Frontal lobe	−0.34	−0.32	−0.27	0.91	0.68	0.80
Temporal lobe	0.04	−0.26*	0.08	0.02	0.70	0.004
Parietal lobe	−0.13	0.01	−0.08	0.26	0.64	0.42
Occipital lobe	0.04	−0.03	−0.02	0.40	0.38	0.92

The TC subgroup ($n = 7$) included the patients on the docetaxel and cyclophosphamide chemotherapy regimen. The non-TC subgroup ($n = 9$) included the patients on a chemotherapy regimen other than the TC regimen. *$p < 0.01$

brain volume between the chemotherapy and non-chemotherapy groups after 1 year using a different imaging analysis method [27]. However, these differences in regional brain volume were not noted in a 3-year interval in the same study. A long-term survivorship study confirmed the late effects (more than 9 years) of adjuvant chemotherapy with gray matter reduction in the posterior parts of the brain in breast cancer survivors exposed to chemotherapy [24].

There are few other longitudinally designed studies of brain structural alterations in patients with breast cancer receiving adjuvant chemotherapy [9, 10, 28, 29]. McDonald and colleagues conducted a longitudinally designed study with a similar number of chemotherapy patients and healthy controls (17 patients with breast cancer on chemotherapy, 12 patients with breast cancer no chemotherapy, and 18 healthy controls), but in a younger age group at baseline: 50.6 (6.5) to 52.7 (7.2) mean years of age (SD). Their study showed acute reduction in gray matter density one month after completion of chemotherapy with a similar timeframe as our study. Their study also showed a partial recovery at 1-year follow-up assessment [9]. Additional longitudinal brain structural MRI studies presented further evidence of a similar pattern of gray matter alterations [10, 28]. Both cross-sectional and

longitudinal studies have clearly identified a decrease in gray matter in the chemotherapy group compared to the non-chemotherapy cancer control group or healthy controls [13]. However, the gray matter reduction in the chemotherapy group observed in our study was not more than the reduction in the healthy control group. This lack of a significant difference could be due to our modest sample size and not having enough power to detect a modest change.

Our study showed frontal lobe volume reduction in the healthy control group as well as in the chemotherapy group. This result was not entirely surprising since our study cohort was older, ranging from 60 to 82 years of age, and older adults may experience some brain volume loss over time. Our study results were generally in line with volumetric studies of healthy aging, in which gradual gray matter atrophy has been shown as part of the normal aging process in several brain areas, especially in the frontal and temporal lobes [30, 31]. We identified frontal lobe volume loss in the healthy control group over a short interval of 2–5 months, which we had not anticipated; however, in review of the literature, a prior study showed extensive cortical reduction in the prefrontal cortex and temporal lobe after just 1 year in healthy elderly participants at 60–91 years of age,

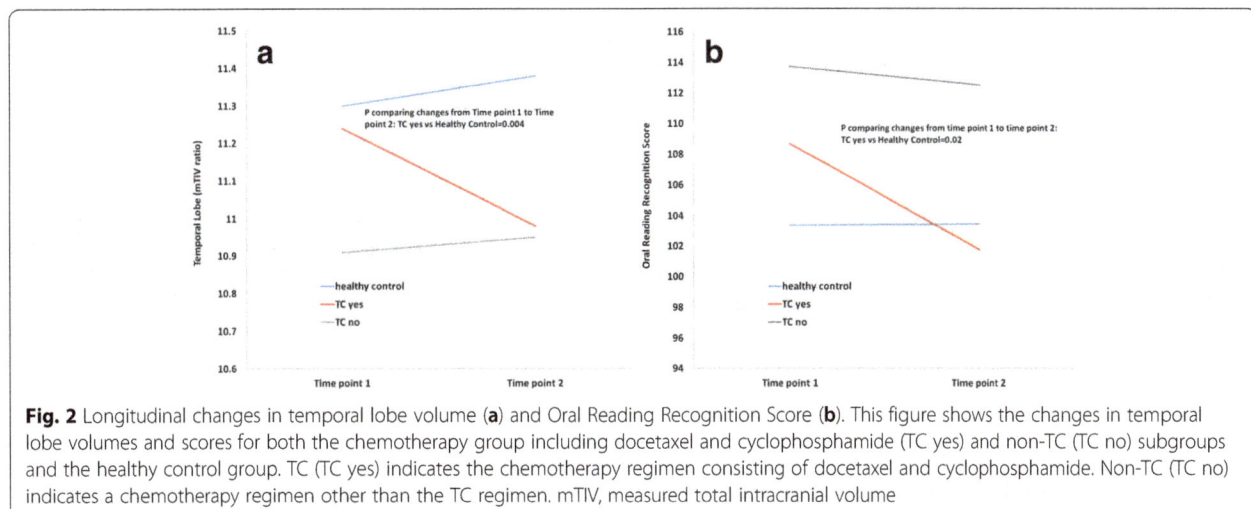

Fig. 2 Longitudinal changes in temporal lobe volume (**a**) and Oral Reading Recognition Score (**b**). This figure shows the changes in temporal lobe volumes and scores for both the chemotherapy group including docetaxel and cyclophosphamide (TC yes) and non-TC (TC no) subgroups and the healthy control group. TC (TC yes) indicates the chemotherapy regimen consisting of docetaxel and cyclophosphamide. Non-TC (TC no) indicates a chemotherapy regimen other than the TC regimen. mTIV, measured total intracranial volume

Table 5 Summary of neuropsychological testing data with NIH Toolbox for Cognition (score and SD)

NIH Toolbox score	Time point 1		Time point 2		Change over time		
	Chemotherapy group	Healthy controls	Chemotherapy group	Healthy controls	Chemotherapy group	Healthy controls	p^{**}
Crystallized composite	110.87 (16.12)	107.38 (15.57)	110.56 (11.82)	107.05 (18.53)	−0.31 (7.21)	−0.33 (6.44)	1.00
Fluid composite	99.69 (14.43)	99.22 (10.65)	100.23 (14.62)	105.08 (15.85)	0.54 (11.66)	5.86 (11.84)	0.23
Total composite	105.10 (19.11)	101.48 (15.02)	104.14 (15.05)	105.11 (20.37)	−0.95 (10.00)	3.63 (8.78)	0.20
Dimensional change card sort	100.66 (11.83)	101.78 (12.62)	101.70 (7.06)	106.91 (9.64)	1.04 (8.37)	5.13 (12.26)	0.29
Flanker Inhibitory control	95.78 (10.97)	96.92 (9.12)	92.50 (9.25)	99.74 (6.11)	−3.27 (12.33)	2.81 (6.77)	0.11
Working memory	101.45 (16.31)	100.18 (16.35)	107.01 (10.64)	105.00 (17.00)	5.57 (10.19)	4.83 (14.10)	0.87
Oral reading recognition	**111.52 (11.95)**	**103.37 (12.51)**	**107.80 (12.33)**	**103.45 (14.00)**	**−3.71 (5.74)***	**0.09 (6.91)**	**0.11**
Processing speed	91.29 (14.08)	96.84 (14.06)	91.14 (17.05)	95.39 (16.45)	−0.14 (14.94)	−1.44 (14.94)	0.81
Episodic memory	111.73 (20.06)	103.49 (15.26)	109.70 (21.33)	110.29 (25.05)	−2.02 (12.24)	6.80 (21.18)	0.17
Picture vocabulary	107.06 (14.94)	109.13 (16.63)	110.30 (8.88)	107.66 (16.52)	3.23 (9.94)	−1.47 (6.30)	0.14

$^*p = 0.02$
$^{**}p$ comparing change over time between chemotherapy group and healthy control group. Bold numbers indicate key findings

indicating accelerated brain atrophy with increasing age [32]. A study combining analyses of 56 longitudinal studies on the aging brain showed rapid brain volume loss after 60 years of age [33]. Furthermore, prior research has pointed out that some conditions, such as hypertension, subclinical depression, and preclinical neurodegenerative disease, may accelerate brain volume loss [34, 35]. These potentially confounding variables were not controlled for in the healthy control group in our study. Celle et al. reported significant blood pressure-related decreases in gray matter volume in the left superior and middle frontal gyrus [34]. There were also reports of depressive symptoms at a subclinical level in late life being associated with decreased volumes in the frontal and temporal lobes [35]. We did not have detailed blood pressure measurements or information to evaluate for any subclinical depression or preclinical

neurodegenerative disease in the healthy controls in our study.

Although when examined as a whole, our study did not show a significant difference in volume changes in the temporal lobe between the chemotherapy group and the healthy control group, we did observe a significant volume reduction in the temporal lobe in patients who received the docetaxel and cyclophosphamide (TC) regimen compared to the healthy control group. Accompanying this reduction in temporal lobe volume, patients in the TC group also had reductions in oral reading recognition scores in neuropsychological testing. Other than length of the chemotherapy treatment, there were no differences between the TC and non-TC groups in terms of disease stage, age, physical functions and chemotherapy toxicity risk score. Furthermore, at baseline, there was no significant difference in temporal lobe

Table 6 Comparison of longitudinal changes in neuropsychological scores in the chemotherapy subgroup and the healthy control (HC) group

	Non-TC ($n = 9$)	TC ($n = 7$)	HC ($n = 14$)	Non-TC vs. HC, p	Non-TC vs. TC, p	TC vs. HC, p
Crystallized composite	−0.17	−0.49	−0.33	0.96	0.92	0.96
Fluid composite	−4.23	6.67	5.86	0.04	0.06	0.88
Total composite	−2.94	1.58	3.63	0.12	0.35	0.64
Dimensional change card sort	−1.99	4.94	5.13	0.11	0.19	0.97
Flanker inhibitory control	−5.29	−0.69	2.82	0.07	0.38	0.46
Working memory	5.31	5.90	4.83	0.93	0.93	0.85
Oral reading recognition	**−1.22**	**−6.94**	**0.09**	**0.62**	**0.07**	**0.02**
Processing speed	−6.17	7.59	−1.45	0.45	0.07	0.18
Episodic memory	−4.85	1.62	6.80	0.12	0.46	0.52
Picture vocabulary	−0.05	7.46	−1.48	0.68	0.08	0.02
Picture vocabulary	−0.05	7.46	−1.48	0.68	0.08	0.02

The TC subgroup ($n = 7$) included the patients on the docetaxel and cyclophosphamide chemotherapy regimen. The non-TC subgroup ($n = 9$) included the patients on a chemotherapy regimen other than the TC regimen. Bold numbers indicate key findings

volume between the two groups. Our study results point to a potential treatment-specific loss of temporal lobe volume and decrease in neuropsychological testing score specifically in patients treated with the TC regimen.

The temporal lobe has been shown to be one of the brain structures affected in patients with breast cancer treated with chemotherapy [27]. Brain structures in the medial temporal lobe, such as the parahippocampal gyrus, have been shown to have reduction in volume in patients treated with chemotherapy [27]. The oral reading recognition test in the NIH Toolbox for Cognition assesses reading decoding and it measures the participant's ability to pronounce single words or letters on the computer screen [36]. The TC regimen consisted of docetaxel and cyclophosphamide and it is usually given every 21 days for four cycles. Since a taxane was also included in all of the non-TC regimens, docetaxel was less likely to be implicated. On the other hand, cyclophosphamide (which was only included in some of the non-TC regimens) is known to cross the blood-brain barrier resulting in direct neurotoxicity [37], which might have played a role in the reduction of oral reading recognition scores in the TC group. However, our explanation is mostly based on speculation and the definitive mechanisms responsible for reduction in temporal lobe volume and oral reading recognition scores in the subgroup of patients treated with the TC regimen cannot be extrapolated from this pilot study. Furthermore, we acknowledge that the oral reading recognition test is viewed as a "hold" test to estimate baseline intelligence and therefore it is possible our finding of reduced scores on this measure reflects the effects of regression to the mean rather than chemotherapy-related impact. Nevertheless, this novel finding has provided a direction for our future studies with larger cohorts to understand how different chemotherapy regimens affect brain volume and cognition in older women with breast cancer.

There were differences between our study and the published literature. For example, we did not observe a greater brain volume reduction in total gray matter and the frontal lobe in the chemotherapy group as compared to the healthy control group [13]. There are several possible reasons for the discrepancy between our data and the prior studies, including differences in study methodology (i.e. participant demographics and imaging analysis methodology), and the older age of our study participants (ranging from 60 to 82 years) than those in the reported studies. The effect of chemotherapy on brain volumes is largely unknown within a short interval (2–5 months) in this older population. Additionally, we used Neuroreader™ software for brain segmentation while the previous studies used other methods such as voxel-wise analysis [38]. In addition, Neuroreader™ reports the actual

volumes of brain structures based on anatomical boundaries of specific brain structures. Therefore, it is possible that there might be significant alterations in the voxel-wise probability, which are not detected in segmented brain volumes. The heterogeneity of chemotherapy regimens for the chemotherapy group may also play a role in the varying brain volume changes, as neurotoxicity related to chemotherapy treatment may differ depending on the therapy given.

There are several limitations to this study. First of all, a modest number of participants were evaluated in this pilot study pre and post chemotherapy over a short time course of 2–5 months. Second, the majority of our participants were non-Hispanic white women, thus limiting the generalizability of our findings to other races. Third, some comorbidities such as high blood pressure and subclinical depression, which may be associated with brain volume loss in the healthy population, were not collected in this study. In addition, our study lacked a non-chemotherapy breast cancer control group, which may have helped to assess the effect of breast cancer as a source of brain structural changes. Furthermore, different methods such as voxel-based morphometry (VBM) may be utilized to assess the changes in brain volume associated with chemotherapy. It is conceivable that there might be alterations in the voxel-wise gray or white matter probability obtained with the VBM method that was not detected in our study. Last, although we did observe a larger reduction in the temporal lobe in the TC treated patients, we should caution against drawing any definitive conclusions, given the limitations of working with such a small sample size and the possibility of exaggerated effect size.

Despite these limitations, there are strengths in this study utilizing brain MRI to evaluate brain volume changes among patients receiving chemotherapy. Our study is unique in its focus on older women with breast cancer receiving different adjuvant chemotherapy regimens. Older patients with cancer are potentially vulnerable for cognitive decline, possibly from accelerated aging. However, few studies have taken advantage of utilizing the non-invasive brain MRI to study neuro-correlates of cancer-related cognitive impairment in the older population. In addition, the availability of the healthy control group in our study enabled us to compare volume changes and to identify volume reduction beyond what is expected in healthy aging.

Conclusions

We observed no significant differences in the segmented brain volumes between patients receiving chemotherapy and the healthy control group; however, exploratory analyses demonstrated a treatment-specific reduction in both temporal lobe volume and oral reading recognition scores in the subgroup of older patients who received a regimen consisting of docetaxel and cyclophosphamide. Further studies should be conducted to examine the effect of specific chemotherapies on brain structure. Additional longitudinal studies with a larger sample size and longer follow-up intervals are needed to understand the mechanism and to validate the results from this pilot study.

Abbreviations
ddAC - Paclitaxel: Dose-dense doxorubicin and cyclophosphamide followed by paclitaxel; Docetaxel/cyclophosphamide/PH: Docetaxel, cyclophosphamide, pertuzumab, trastuzumab; MPRAGE: Magnetization prepared rapid gradient echo; MRI: Magnetic resonance imaging; mTIV: Measured total intracranial volume; NIH: National Institutes of Health; TAC: Docetaxel, doxorubicin, and cyclophosphamide; TC: Docetaxel and cyclophosphamide; TCPH: Docetaxel, carboplatin, pertuzumab, trastuzumab

Acknowledgements
The authors would like to acknowledge Jamila Ahdidan, Ph.D. for her technical support in using the Neuroreader™ software. The preliminary data were presented as a poster at NIH/NIA U13 "Models and Studies of Aging" conference in Washington D.C. from 21 to 23 September 2016.

Funding
This study was funded by NIH/NIA grants R03 AG045090 (BTC) and R01 AG037037 (AH).

Authors' contributions
BTC, SKP and AH contributed to the concept, design, and conduct of the study. BTC prepared the manuscript. SKS and EMH contributed to neuroimaging data analysis. SKS, TJ, NY, CS, RCR, EMH, JCR, AHo, AJS, TAA, NP, and RM contributed to interpretation and description of the data. CS performed statistical analysis. JM, JW, YY, GS, DL, RY, HT, and VK contributed to study accrual and procedures. All authors approved the final manuscript.

Competing interests
AH reports research funding from Celgene, Novartis, and GSK, and has served as a consultant for MJH Healthcare Holdings, LLC, Pierian Biosciences, Sanofi, Boehringer Ingelheim Pharmaceuticals, and Carevive, outside the submitted work. All other authors declare that they have no competing interests.

Author details
[1]Department of Diagnostic Radiology, City of Hope National Medical Center, Duarte, CA 91010, USA. [2]The MRI Institute for Biomedical Research, Magnetic Resonance Innovations, Inc., Detroit, MI, USA. [3]Department of Population Science, City of Hope National Medical Center, Duarte, CA 91010, USA. [4]Center for Cancer and Aging, City of Hope National Medical Center, Duarte, CA 91010, USA. [5]Division of Mathematical Oncology, City of Hope National Medical Center, Duarte, CA 91010, USA. [6]Department of Biomedical Engineering, Wayne State University, Detroit, MI 48202, USA. [7]Neurocognitive Research Lab, Memorial Sloan Kettering Cancer Center, 641 Lexington Avenue, 7th Floor, New York, NY 10022, USA. [8]Center for Neuroimaging, Indiana University School of Medicine, 355 West 16th Street, Indianapolis, IN 46202, USA. [9]Department of Radiology, Memorial Sloan-Kettering Cancer Center, 641 Lexington Avenue, 7th Floor, New York, NY 10022, USA. [10]Division of Neurology, City of Hope National Medical Center, Duarte, CA 91010, USA. [11]Department of Medical Oncology, City of Hope National Medical Center, Duarte, CA 91010, USA.

References
1. Fried TR, Bradley EH, Towle VR, Allore H. Understanding the treatment preferences of seriously ill patients. N Engl J Med. 2002;346(14):1061–6.
2. Mandelblatt JS, Jacobsen PB, Ahles T. Cognitive effects of cancer systemic therapy: implications for the care of older patients and survivors. J Clin Oncol. 2014;32(24):2617–26.
3. Edwards BK, Howe HL, Ries LA, Thun MJ, Rosenberg HM, Yancik R, Wingo PA, Jemal A, Feigal EG. Annual report to the nation on the status of cancer, 1973-1999, featuring implications of age and aging on U.S. cancer burden. Cancer. 2002;94(10):2766–92.
4. Kohli S, Griggs JJ, Roscoe JA, Jean-Pierre P, Bole C, Mustian KM, Hill R, Smith K, Gross H, Morrow GR. Self-reported cognitive impairment in patients with cancer. J Oncol Pract. 2007;3(2):54–9.
5. Wefel JS, Vardy J, Ahles T, Schagen SB. International Cognition and Cancer Task Force recommendations to harmonise studies of cognitive function in patients with cancer. Lancet Oncol. 2011;12(7):703–8.
6. Hurria A, Wong FL, Villaluna D, Bhatia S, Chung CT, Mortimer J, Hurvitz S, Naeim A. Role of age and health in treatment recommendations for older adults with breast cancer: the perspective of oncologists and primary care providers. J Clin Oncol. 2008;26(33):5386–92.
7. Kornblith AB, Kemeny M, Peterson BL, Wheeler J, Crawford J, Bartlett N, Fleming G, Graziano S, Muss H, Cohen HJ, et al. Survey of oncologists' perceptions of barriers to accrual of older patients with breast carcinoma to clinical trials. Cancer. 2002;95(5):989–96.
8. McDonald BC, Conroy SK, Ahles TA, West JD, Saykin AJ. Alterations in brain activation during working memory processing associated with breast cancer and treatment: a prospective functional magnetic resonance imaging study. J Clin Oncol. 2012;30(20):2500–8.
9. McDonald BC, Conroy SK, Ahles TA, West JD, Saykin AJ. Gray matter reduction associated with systemic chemotherapy for breast cancer: a prospective MRI study. Breast Cancer Res Treat. 2010;123(3):819–28.
10. McDonald BC, Conroy SK, Smith DJ, West JD, Saykin AJ. Frontal gray matter reduction after breast cancer chemotherapy and association with executive symptoms: a replication and extension study. Brain Behav Immun. 2013; 30(Suppl):S117–25.
11. Narvacan K, Treit S, Camicioli R, Martin W, Beaulieu C. Evolution of deep gray matter volume across the human lifespan. Hum Brain Mapp. 2017; https://doi.org/10.1002/hbm.23604.
12. Squarzoni P, Tamashiro-Duran J, Souza Duran FL, Santos LC, Vallada HP, Menezes PR, Scazufca M, Filho GB, Alves TC. Relationship between regional brain volumes and cognitive performance in the healthy aging: an MRI study using voxel-based morphometry. J Alzheimers Dis. 2012;31(1):45–58.
13. Simo M, Rifa-Ros X, Rodriguez-Fornells A, Bruna J. Chemobrain: a systematic review of structural and functional neuroimaging studies. Neurosci Biobehav Rev. 2013;37(8):1311–21.
14. Kesler SR, Blayney DW. Neurotoxic effects of anthracycline- vs nonanthracycline-based chemotherapy on cognition in breast cancer survivors. JAMA Oncol. 2016;2(2):185–92.
15. Ahdidan J, Raji CA, DeYoe EA, Mathis J, Noe KO, Rimestad J, Kjeldsen TK, Mosegaard J, Becker JT, Lopez O. Quantitative neuroimaging software for clinical Assessment of hippocampal volumes on MR imaging. J Alzheimers Dis. 2015;49(3):723–32.
16. Tanpitukpongse TP, Mazurowski MA, Ikhena J, Petrella JR. Predictive utility of marketed volumetric software tools in subjects at risk for Alzheimer disease: do regions outside the hippocampus matter? AJNR Am J Neuroradiol. 2017; 38(3):546–52.
17. Bredesen DE, Amos EC, Canick J, Ackerley M, Raji C, Fiala M, Ahdidan J. Reversal of cognitive decline in Alzheimer's disease. Aging (Albany NY). 2016;8(6):1250–8.
18. Raji CA, Merrill DA, Barrio JR, Omalu B, Small GW. Progressive focal gray matter volume loss in a former high school football player: a possible

magnetic Resonance imaging volumetric signature for chronic traumatic encephalopathy. Am J Geriatr Psychiatry. 2016;24(10):784–90.

19. Weintraub S, Dikmen SS, Heaton RK, Tulsky DS, Zelazo PD, Bauer PJ, Carlozzi NE, Slotkin J, Blitz D, Wallner-Allen K, et al. Cognition assessment using the NIH Toolbox. Neurology. 2013;80(11 Suppl 3):S54–64.

20. Hurria A, Togawa K, Mohile SG, Owusu C, Klepin HD, Gross CP, Lichtman SM, Gajra A, Bhatia S, Katheria V, et al. Predicting chemotherapy toxicity in older adults with cancer: a prospective multicenter study. J Clin Oncol. 2011;29(25):3457–65.

21. Hurria A, Mohile S, Gajra A, Klepin H, Muss H, Chapman A, Feng T, Smith D, Sun CL, De Glas N, et al. Validation of a prediction tool for chemotherapy toxicity in older adults with cancer. J Clin Oncol. 2016;34(20):2366–71.

22. Hurria A, Gupta S, Zauderer M, Zuckerman EL, Cohen HJ, Muss H, Rodin M, Panageas KS, Holland JC, Saltz L, et al. Developing a cancer-specific geriatric assessment: a feasibility study. Cancer. 2005;104(9):1998–2005.

23. Laird NM, Ware JH. Random-effects models for longitudinal data. Biometrics. 1982;38(4):963–74.

24. de Ruiter MB, Reneman L, Boogerd W, Veltman DJ, Caan M, Douaud G, Lavini C, Linn SC, Boven E, van Dam FS, et al. Late effects of high-dose adjuvant chemotherapy on white and gray matter in breast cancer survivors: converging results from multimodal magnetic resonance imaging. Hum Brain Mapp. 2012;33(12):2971–83.

25. Koppelmans V, de Ruiter MB, van der Lijn F, Boogerd W, Seynaeve C, van der Lugt A, Vrooman H, Niessen WJ, Breteler MM, Schagen SB. Global and focal brain volume in long-term breast cancer survivors exposed to adjuvant chemotherapy. Breast Cancer Res Treat. 2012;132(3):1099–106.

26. Conroy SK, McDonald BC, Smith DJ, Moser LR, West JD, Kamendulis LM, Klaunig JE, Champion VL, Unverzagt FW, Saykin AJ. Alterations in brain structure and function in breast cancer survivors: effect of post-chemotherapy interval and relation to oxidative DNA damage. Breast Cancer Res Treat. 2013;137(2):493–502.

27. Inagaki M, Yoshikawa E, Matsuoka Y, Sugawara Y, Nakano T, Akechi T, Wada N, Imoto S, Murakami K, Uchitomi Y. Smaller regional volumes of brain gray and white matter demonstrated in breast cancer survivors exposed to adjuvant chemotherapy. Cancer. 2007;109(1):146–56.

28. Lepage C, Smith AM, Moreau J, Barlow-Krelina E, Wallis N, Collins B, MacKenzie J, Scherling C. A prospective study of grey matter and cognitive function alterations in chemotherapy-treated breast cancer patients. Spring. 2014;3:444.

29. Menning S, de Ruiter MB, Veltman DJ, Boogerd W, Oldenburg HS, Reneman L, Schagen SB. Changes in brain white matter integrity after systemic treatment for breast cancer: a prospective longitudinal study. Brain Imaging Behav. 2017; https://doi.org/10.1007/s11682-017-9695-x.

30. Raz N, Lindenberger U, Rodrigue KM, Kennedy KM, Head D, Williamson A, Dahle C, Gerstorf D, Acker JD. Regional brain changes in aging healthy adults: general trends, individual differences and modifiers. Cereb Cortex. 2005;15(11):1676–89.

31. Resnick SM, Pham DL, Kraut MA, Zonderman AB, Davatzikos C. Longitudinal magnetic resonance imaging studies of older adults: a shrinking brain. J Neurosci. 2003;23(8):3295–301.

32. Fjell AM, Walhovd KB, Fennema-Notestine C, McEvoy LK, Hagler DJ, Holland D, Brewer JB, Dale AM. One-year brain atrophy evident in healthy aging. J Neurosci. 2009;29(48):15223–31.

33. Hedman AM, van Haren NE, Schnack HG, Kahn RS, Hulshoff Pol HE. Human brain changes across the life span: a review of 56 longitudinal magnetic resonance imaging studies. Hum Brain Mapp. 2012;33(8):1987–2002.

34. Celle S, Annweiler C, Pichot V, Bartha R, Barthelemy JC, Roche F, Beauchet O. Association between ambulatory 24-hour blood pressure levels and brain volume reduction: a cross-sectional elderly population-based study. Hypertension. 2012;60(5):1324–31.

35. Dotson VM, Davatzikos C, Kraut MA, Resnick SM. Depressive symptoms and brain volumes in older adults: a longitudinal magnetic resonance imaging study. J Psychiatry Neurosci. 2009;34(5):367–75.

36. Gershon RC, Cook KF, Mungas D, Manly JJ, Slotkin J, Beaumont JL, Weintraub S. Language measures of the NIH Toolbox Cognition Battery. J Int Neuropsychol Soc. 2014;20(6):642–51.

37. Janelsins MC, Roscoe JA, Berg MJ, Thompson BD, Gallagher MJ, Morrow GR, Heckler CE, Jean-Pierre P, Opanashuk LA, Gross RA. IGF-1 partially restores chemotherapy-induced reductions in neural cell proliferation in adult C57BL/6 mice. Cancer Investig. 2010;28(5):544–53.

38. Ashburner J, Friston KJ. Voxel-based morphometry–the methods. NeuroImage. 2000;11(6 Pt 1):805–21.

2

NOTCH3 expression is linked to breast cancer seeding and distant metastasis

Alexey A. Leontovich[1†], Mohammad Jalalirad[2†], Jeffrey L. Salisbury[3], Lisa Mills[4], Candace Haddox[2], Mark Schroeder[2], Ann Tuma[2], Maria E. Guicciardi[5], Luca Zammataro[6], Mario W. Gambino[3], Angela Amato[7], Aldo Di Leonardo[7], James McCubrey[8], Carol A. Lange[9], Minetta Liu[2], Tufia Haddad[2], Matthew Goetz[2], Judy Boughey[10], Jann Sarkaria[2], Liewei Wang[2], James N. Ingle[2], Evanthia Galanis[2,4] and Antonino B. D'Assoro[2,3*] [iD]

Abstract

Background: Development of distant metastases involves a complex multistep biological process termed the *invasion-metastasis cascade*, which includes dissemination of cancer cells from the primary tumor to secondary organs. NOTCH developmental signaling plays a critical role in promoting epithelial-to-mesenchymal transition, tumor stemness, and metastasis. Although all four NOTCH receptors show oncogenic properties, the unique role of each of these receptors in the sequential stepwise events that typify the invasion-metastasis cascade remains elusive.

Methods: We have established metastatic xenografts expressing high endogenous levels of NOTCH3 using estrogen receptor alpha-positive (ERα+) MCF-7 breast cancer cells with constitutive active Raf-1/mitogen-associated protein kinase (MAPK) signaling (vMCF-7^{Raf-1}) and MDA-MB-231 triple-negative breast cancer (TNBC) cells. The critical role of NOTCH3 in inducing an invasive phenotype and poor outcome was corroborated in unique TNBC cells resulting from a patient-derived brain metastasis (TNBC-M25) and in publicly available claudin-low breast tumor specimens collected from participants in the Molecular Taxonomy of Breast Cancer International Consortium database.

Results: In this study, we identified an association between NOTCH3 expression and development of metastases in ERα+ and TNBC models. ERα+ breast tumor xenografts with a constitutive active Raf-1/MAPK signaling developed spontaneous lung metastases through the clonal expansion of cancer cells expressing a NOTCH3 reprogramming network. Abrogation of NOTCH3 expression significantly reduced the self-renewal and invasive capacity of ex vivo breast cancer cells, restoring a luminal CD44^{low}/CD24^{high}/ERα^{high} phenotype. Forced expression of the mitotic Aurora kinase A (AURKA), which promotes breast cancer metastases, failed to restore the invasive capacity of NOTCH3-null cells, demonstrating that NOTCH3 expression is required for an invasive phenotype. Likewise, pharmacologic inhibition of NOTCH signaling also impaired TNBC cell seeding and metastatic growth. Significantly, the role of aberrant NOTCH3 expression in promoting tumor self-renewal, invasiveness, and poor outcome was corroborated in unique TNBC cells from a patient-derived brain metastasis and in publicly available claudin-low breast tumor specimens.

Conclusions: These findings demonstrate the key role of NOTCH3 oncogenic signaling in the genesis of breast cancer metastasis and provide a compelling preclinical rationale for the design of novel therapeutic strategies that will selectively target NOTCH3 to halt metastatic seeding and to improve the clinical outcomes of patients with breast cancer.

Keywords: Breast cancer, Metastasis, Chromosomal instability, Centrosome amplification, Tumor stemness

* Correspondence: dassoro.antonio@mayo.edu
†Alexey A. Leontovich and Mohammad Jalalirad contributed equally to this work.
[2]Department of Medical Oncology, Mayo Clinic College of Medicine, 200 First Street SW, Rochester, MN, USA
[3]Department of Biochemistry and Molecular Biology, Mayo Clinic College of Medicine, 200 First Street SW, Rochester, MN, USA
Full list of author information is available at the end of the article

Background

Breast cancer represents the second leading cause of cancer death among women worldwide [1]. Each year it is estimated that over 240,000 women in the United States will be diagnosed with breast cancer and that more than 40,000 will die of tumor relapse and metastatic dissemination to distant organs [2]. Although breast cancer research has been devoted largely to characterization of the molecular mechanisms responsible for tumor development, metastatic growth in secondary organs after surgical eradication of the primary tumor is responsible for poor outcomes [3]. For this reason, a better understanding of the molecular mechanisms leading to cancer cell seeding and metastatic growth is imperative to develop innovative therapies that will selectively target breast tumor metastasis-initiating cells (BT-MICs) and halt tumor progression.

Several studies have demonstrated that aberrant activation of mitogen-associated protein kinase (MAPK) oncogenic signaling induces drug resistance, development of distant metastases, and ultimately poor outcome of patients with breast cancer [4–6]. However, the molecular mechanisms by which the MAPK signaling pathway promotes cancer cells seeding and metastatic dissemination are poorly understood. It has been established that cross-talk between NOTCH and MAPK pathways in breast cancer correlates with early tumor relapse and poor overall survival [7], suggesting that NOTCH developmental signaling is a key mediator of MAPK-induced metastases. Canonical NOTCH signaling consists of four NOTCH receptors (NOTCH1–4) and their ligands (Delta-like 1, 3, and 4 and Jagged 1 and 2). All receptors are synthesized as a precursor form consisting of extracellular, transmembrane, and intracellular subunits [8]. In the most widely accepted model of NOTCH activation, ligand binding unfolds the negative regulatory region admitting the second cleavage through metalloproteinases of the ADAM family [9]. After this, γ-secretase complex performs an intramembrane cleavage releasing the NOTCH intracellular domain that translocates to the nucleus [10]. Following NOTCH activation, the hairy and enhancer of split (HES) family and the hairy-related transcription factor are expressed and in turn orchestrate the NOTCH-induced nuclear reprogramming [11, 12]. Aberrant activation of NOTCH oncogenic signaling promotes an invasive phenotype through activation of epithelial-to-mesenchymal transition (EMT) signaling [13]. Changes during EMT drive the transition from a polarized epithelial phenotype to an elongated fibroblastoid-like phenotype that typifies the morphology of highly metastatic cancer cells. These cancer cells exhibit a more invasive behavior characterized by downregulation of epithelial proteins (E-cadherin and claudin) responsible for cell adhesion

and upregulation of mesenchymal proteins (N-cadherin and vimentin) involved in cell motility [14]. Several studies have established that breast cancer cells that undergo EMT acquire a CD44^{high}/CD24^{low} cancer stemlike phenotype characterized by an increased capacity for tumor self-renewal, drug resistance, and high metastatic proclivity [15–17]. The discovery of breast tumor-initiating cells (BTICs) with a CD44^{high}/CD24^{low} phenotype has been critical to elucidating the molecular mechanisms responsible for early recurrence and onset of distant metastases in advanced breast cancer. The correlation between aberrant activation of NOTCH/HES1 stemness signaling and tumor metastases has been revealed through a series of experimental investigations [18, 19]. Although all four NOTCH receptors can increase HES1 expression, whether a specific NOTCH receptor is mainly responsible for HES1 overexpression and transcriptional activity during the early stages of metastatic dissemination has not been established [20]. Recent findings propose that NOTCH signaling may promote the early onset of distant metastases through activation of C-X-C chemokine receptor type 4, a chemokine receptor that plays a key role in fostering cancer cell seeding to secondary organs [21, 22]. Although these studies show the redundant activity of NOTCH signaling, individual NOTCH receptors are likely to regulate breast cancer cells in unique ways; hence, it is essential to delineate the functional role for specific NOTCH receptors in driving tumor progression. Importantly, the NOTCH signaling pathway represents a powerful "druggable target" for cancer stemlike cells, which are known to be resistant to conventional chemotherapy and radiation but seem especially sensitive to inhibition of key stem cell pathways [23]. Several classes of investigational pan-NOTCH inhibitors have been developed that include γ-secretase inhibitors (GSIs) and humanized monoclonal antibodies against NOTCH receptors [24, 25]. Although GSIs have numerous substrates besides NOTCH receptors, the pharmacologic activity and toxicity of GSIs in vivo appears to be due largely to NOTCH inhibition [26]. GSIs have been administered to patients in phase I clinical trials, either as single agents or in combination with standard chemotherapy, with promising results [27, 28].

In this study, we demonstrated that NOTCH3 expression is linked to cancer cell seeding and development of breast cancer metastases. Using variant estrogen receptor alpha-positive (ERα$^+$ MCF-7) breast tumor xenografts with constitutive active Raf-1/MAPK signaling (vMCF-7^{Raf-1}), we showed that metastatic cancer cells display a clonal origin and increased expression of NOTCH3 that is required to induce self-renewal, stemness, and high invasive capacity. Significantly, forced expression of the mitotic Aurora kinase A (AURKA), which promotes stemness and breast cancer metastases

[29], failed to restore the invasive capacity of NOTCH3-null vMCF-7^{Raf-1} cells, demonstrating that NOTCH3 oncogenic signaling is downstream of AURKA and is essential to inducing breast cancer cell invasiveness. The role of NOTCH3 expression in inducing a metastatic phenotype was corroborated in highly invasive MDA-MB-231 triple-negative breast cancer (TNBC) cells isolated from lung metastases. Moreover, we also demonstrated the clinical relevance of the NOTCH3 signaling pathway in promoting tumor invasiveness and poor outcome in unique patient-derived TNBC brain metastasis and publicly available claudin-low breast tumor specimens collected from participants of the Molecular Taxonomy of Breast Cancer International Consortium (METABRIC) database [30]. Taken together, these findings revealed the critical role of NOTCH3 oncogenic signaling in the genesis of breast cancer metastases and provided a compelling preclinical rationale for the design of novel therapeutic strategies that will selectively target the NOTCH3 signaling pathway to improve the clinical outcome of patients with advanced breast cancer.

Methods

Established breast cancer cell lines

The human breast cancer cell lines MCF-7 and MDA-MB-231 were obtained from the American Type Culture Collection (Mayo Clinic, Manassas, VA, USA). The MCF-7 cells overexpressing the Raf-1 oncoprotein were generated as previously described [29]. Human mammary epithelial cells (HMEC) were kindly provided by Wilma Lingle, PhD (Mayo Clinic). All cell lines were maintained in DMEM containing 5 mM glutamine, 1% penicillin/streptomycin, 20 µg/ml insulin (only for MCF-7 and their variants), and 10% FBS at 37 °C in a 5% CO_2 atmosphere.

Human breast cancer xenografts

Procedures established by the institutional animal care and use committee based on the National Institutes of Health Guidelines for the Care and Use of Laboratory Animals were followed for all experiments. Four-week-old nonovariectomized female NCR/Nu/Nu nude mice were anesthetized by exposure to 3% isoflurane, and five mice per group were given subcutaneous injections with 2×10^6 MCF-7 or vMCF-7$^{\Delta Raf-1}$ cancer cells suspended in 50 µl of 50% Matrigel (BD Biosciences, San Jose, CA, USA). Tumor localization and growth was monitored using an IVS imaging system (IVS, Coppell, TX, USA) from the ventral view 10 minutes after luciferin injection. After 12 weeks, mice were killed, and xenograft tumors were processed for histology and IHC analyses. Animals were examined every day, and body weight and primary tumor size were measured at least one or two times per week.

Consistent distress and potential pain (> 1 day) were alleviated by killing the mice. If some of the animals were losing more than 10% of their body weight or if blood was consistently observed in the urine or around the genitals of the mice, the mice were appropriately killed. When typical signs of distress, including labored breathing and inactivity, were consistently observed for > 1 day, the animals were appropriately killed. When the primary tumor was > 2 cm, the animals were killed. Animals were killed using pentobarbital (100 mg/kg intraperitoneally) followed by cervical dislocation. The Mayo Clinic Institutional Animal Care and Use Committee approved this study (A00002634-17). Breast tumor xenografts and experimental lung metastases were established as previously described [29, 31]. To reestablish cultures from 1GX explants, primary tumors and metastatic lungs were excised from killed animals, minced using sterile scissors, and transferred to complete culture medium, and fibroblast-free tumor cell lines were established by serial passages in culture.

Patient-derived TNBC cells

TNBC-M25 cells were isolated from a patient-derived brain metastasis TNBC xenograft model (EX170416) that was generated by the Breast Cancer Genome-Guided Therapy study (BEAUTY) in the Mayo Clinic (A17713) [32]. To establish cultured TNBC-M25 cells, patient-derived xenograft model EX170416 was excised from killed animals, minced using sterile scissors, and transferred to complete culture medium, and fibroblast-free TNBC-M25 cells were propagated in culture and used for this study.

Immunoblot, immunofluorescence, and fluorescence-activated cell sorting assays

Immunoblot and immunofluorescence assays were performed as previously described [29]. Antibodies employed to perform these studies were as follows: centrin (20H5 kindly provided by Dr. Salisbury's laboratory at the Mayo Clinic); ERα and pericentrin (Santa Cruz Biotechnology, Dallas, TX, USA); AURKA (Cell Signaling Technology, Danvers, MA, USA); CD44, CD24, NOTCH1, NOTCH2, and NOTCH3 (Abcam, Cambridge, MA, USA); and β-actin and α-tubulin (Sigma-Aldrich, St. Louis, MO, USA). Secondary antibodies were obtained from Molecular Probes (Eugene, OR, USA).

Gene microarray analysis

Total RNA was extracted from basal-like CD24$^{-/low}$ cells isolated by fluorescence-activated cell sorting (FACS) from vMCF-7^{Raf-1} 1GX cells as previously described [29], and mammospheres (MPS) were derived from vMCF-7^{Raf-1} 1GX-M cells using TRIzol reagent according to the manufacturer's instructions (Life Technologies,

Carlsbad, CA, USA). Total RNA (1 µg; A_{260}/A_{280} ratio of 1.8–2.2) was used to probe for global genome expression employing Affymetrix U133 Plus 2.0 chips (Affymetrix, Santa Clara, CA, USA). Gene network and functional enrichment analysis was performed employing MetaCore software (GeneGo, St. Joseph, MI, USA). Two independent sets of experiments were performed. The raw data regarding the transcriptomic analysis can be accessed in the Gene Expression Omnibus database (http://www.ncbi.nlm.nih.gov/geo/info/linking.html).

Cytogenetic and spectral karyotyping analysis

Cell harvest and metaphase slide preparation for routine cytogenetic and spectral karyotyping (SKY) analysis were performed as previously described [33]. Hybridization, wash, and detection of the human SKYPaint® probe (Applied Spectral Imaging, Carlsbad, CA, USA) were performed as recommended by the manufacturer. Image acquisition and spectral analysis of metaphase cells were achieved by using the SD200 SpectraCube™ Spectral Imaging System (Applied Spectral Imaging) mounted on a Zeiss Axioplan2 microscope (Carl Zeiss MicroImaging, Inc., Thornwood, NY, USA). Images were analyzed using HiSKY analysis software (Applied Spectral Imaging).

Mammosphere formation

Human breast cancer cells were plated in ultralow attachment 24- and 96-well culture dishes in 100 µl of MammoCult™ medium (STEMCELL Technologies, Vancouver, BC, Canada). Medium was added every 2 days for a maximum of 8 days. MPS formation was recorded after 24 days through a digital camera (Nikon Instruments, Melville, NY, USA).

Real-time apoptosis assay

MDA-MB-231 lung metastasis (LM) cells (n = 30,000) were plated in Costar 12-well plates (Corning Life Sciences, Oneonta, NY, USA) and incubated with YOYO-1 iodide. After 24 hours, cells were treated with 500 nM alisertib or 500 nM LY-411575 and incubated for additional 24 hours in the presence of YOYO-1 iodide. Apoptotic cells were quantified in real time using IncuCyte S3 (Essen BioScience, Ann Arbor, MI, USA). Experiments were performed in triplicate (± SD).

Real-time invasion assay

Cancer cell invasion capacity was assessed using 24-well plate cell culture inserts equipped with a light-tight polyethylene terephthalate membrane (8-µm pore size, Corning® FluoroBlok™ 351152; Corning Life Sciences). Cancer cells were starved overnight and labeled with 5 µM Cell Tracker Red CMTPX (C34552; Thermo Fisher Scientific, Waltham, MA, USA) for 1 hour. Inserts were placed in 24-well companion plates (353504; Corning Life

Sciences), coated with 150 µl of growth-reduced Matrigel matrix (356230; Corning Life Sciences), and incubated for 2 hours at 37 °C. Serum-free medium was used to seed 500 µl of starved cell suspension into the appropriate inserts and incubated at 37 °C for 24 hours. The cells that had migrated through the membrane were imaged and quantified by using a plate-based cell cytometer (Celigo; Nexcelom Bioscience LLC, Lawrence, MA, USA). Results are derived from three independent experiments with comparable outcomes (± SD).

Aldehyde dehydrogenase activity assay

Aldehyde dehydrogenase 1 (ALDH1) activity was detected by FACS analysis using the ALDEOFLUOR assay kit (STEMCELL Technologies) according to the manufacturer's instructions [34]. Results are derived from three independent experiments with comparable outcomes (± SD).

CRISPR-NOTCH3 breast cancer cells

Two custom small guide RNAs (sgRNAs) for NOTCH3 targeting were designed in silico via the CRISPR design tool (http://crispr.mit.edu:8079/). sgRNAs were cloned into an expression plasmid pSpcas9-T2A-GFP carrying sgRNA scaffold backbone, Cas9, and green fluorescent protein (GFP). Constructs were verified by sequencing and then transfected into the cells. GFP-positive cells were isolated by FACS followed by an expansion period to establish a polyclonal knockout cell population. To generate monoclonal cell lines from the polyclonal population, a limiting serial dilution protocol was used to seed individual cells in 96-well plates at an average density of 0.5 cells/well, and plates were kept in an incubator for 2 to 3 weeks. Genomic DNA was extracted from cells grown as monoclonal populations, and external primers were designed in the 5′-flanking region of sgRNAs (NOTCH3-F1: 5′-GCCAGAGGATTACCAGG AAGAGAA-3′ and Notch3-R1: 5′-CCCAGGGAA GGAGGGAGGAG-3′) were used for initial selection of knockout clones. Internal primers (NOTCH3-F1: 5′-GC CAGAGGATTACCAGGAAGAGAA-3′ and 5′-GCCA AGCTGGATTCTGTGTACCTA-3′) were used to verify prescreened clones, and the intensity of amplified product band was used as a marker for knockout efficiency. (The lower intensity is indicative of higher knockout efficiency.) Clone 416, which showed the most efficient NOTCH3 knockout, was selected and expanded, and NOTCH3 protein expression was assessed by immunoblot analysis.

METABRIC analysis

Claudin-low breast tumor specimens were selected from participants of the METABRIC public database. The METABRIC database (http://molonc.bccrc.ca/aparicio-lab/research/metabric/) contains clinical traits, expression, copy number variation profiles, and single-nucleotide polymorphism genotypes derived from patients with breast cancer [30].

Results

Genomic convergence is linked to clonal expansion of breast cancer metastatic cells

To investigate in vivo the role of Raf-1/MAPK oncogenic signaling in the genesis of BT-MICs, we used a variant MCF-7 cell line expressing a constitutive active Raf-1 oncoprotein (vMCF-7^{Raf-1}) that has been described previously [5, 29]. Nude mice carrying vMCF-7^{Raf-1} xenografts were killed 12 weeks after implantation to isolate putative BT-MICs from lung metastatic nodules. Although animals carrying MCF-7 xenografts did not develop lung metastases, vMCF-7^{Raf-1} xenografts gave rise to lung micrometastatic nodules (Fig. 1a). Because breast cancer progression is functionally linked to development of centrosome amplification, which represents one of the major driving forces of chromosomal instability (CIN) [35, 36], we investigated the centrosome phenotype in MCF-7, vMCF-7^{Raf-1}, and cancer cells isolated from tumor xenografts (referred to as first generation derived from xenografts [1GX]) [29]. HMEC were employed as controls because of their normal centrosome phenotype. Whereas MCF-7, MCF-7 1GX, and vMCF-7^{Raf-1} cells showed a low grade of centrosome amplification, with the majority of cells harboring two or four centrioles, centrosome amplification (more than four centrioles in a single cell) was observed in the invasive vMCF-7^{Raf-1} 1GX cells (Fig. 1b and c), in agreement with our previous findings [29]. To investigate the extent to which the degree of centrosome amplification increases during tumor progression, we also cultured metastatic cancer cells isolated from lung tissue (referred to as vMCF-7^{Raf-1} 1GX-M). Remarkably, vMCF-7^{Raf-1} 1GX-M cells showed a normal centrosome phenotype compared with their vMCF-7^{Raf-1} 1GX matching cells (Fig. 1b and c).

To establish whether loss of centrosome amplification in vMCF-7^{Raf-1} 1GX-M cells was linked to genomic convergence and restoration of a stable karyotype, we performed SKY analysis of MCF-7 and their variant vMCF-7^{Raf-1} cells. Although MCF-7 and variant vMCF-7^{Raf-1} cells exhibited different degrees of structural and numerical chromosomal abnormalities, vMCF-7^{Raf-1} 1GX-M cells showed the lowest percentage of numerical chromosomal aberrations (Table 1 and Fig. 2a and b). In view of the fact that aneuploidy in cancer cells represents the "state," whereas CIN indicates the "rate," of chromosomal aberrations [36], we investigated the percentage of cells with nonclonal chromosomal abnormalities as a measure of CIN in MCF-7 and their variant vMCF-7^{Raf-1} cells. Unique chromosomal aberrations were considered nonclonal if they were present exclusively in one or two cancer cells (Table 1). Significantly, whereas nonmetastatic MCF-7 1GX cells showed the highest degree of CIN, vMCF-7^{Raf-1} 1GX-M cells exhibited only clonal chromosomal abnormalities (Table 1 and Fig. 2c).

Metastatic cells show increased self-renewal capacity that is linked to upregulation of NOTCH3 reprogramming network

To define whether clonal metastatic cancer cells exhibited higher stemness capacity than matching parental cells, vMCF-7^{Raf-1}, vMCF-7^{Raf-1} 1GX, and vMCF-7^{Raf-1} 1GX-M cells were cultured under nonadherent conditions to test the efficiency of MPS formation that represents an excellent in vitro surrogate assay of tumor self-renewal capacity [29]. vMCF-7^{Raf-1} 1GX-M cells showed the highest number of MPS formations, demonstrating their increased ability to self-renew compared with matching parental cells (Fig. 3a and b). Because breast cancer invasiveness is functionally linked to loss or reduction of the CD24 epithelial surface marker and development of an invasive basal-like phenotype [29], we assessed CD24 expression in breast cancer cells under nonadherent conditions. Immunofluorescence analysis showed loss of CD24 expression in MPS derived from vMCF-7^{Raf-1} 1GX-M cells compared with parental cells (Additional file 1: Figure S1), demonstrating that loss of CD24 expression is linked to higher tumor self-renewal capacity and plasticity of metastatic breast cancer cells.

To identify an exclusive metastatic gene signature that typifies BT-MICs, we performed a comparative transcriptomic analysis between basal-like CD24$^{-/low}$ (isolated by FACS from vMCF-7^{Raf-1} 1GX cells [29]) and MPS derived from vMCF-7^{Raf-1} 1GX-M (harboring a CD24$^{-/low}$ phenotype) cells. Using a twofold change gene expression cutoff, global gene array analysis showed that 211 genes were differentially expressed between CD24$^{-/low}$ cells and vMCF-7^{Raf-1} 1GX-M MPS (Additional file 2: Figure S2a). Functional enrichment analysis identified 59 genes involved in nuclear reprogramming that were overexpressed in vMCF-7^{Raf-1} 1GX-M MPS (Additional file 2: Figure S2b). Significantly, Ingenuity Pathway Analysis software (IPA®; QIAGEN Bioinformatics, Redwood City, CA, USA) uncovered a noncanonical NOTCH3 network that was upregulated exclusively in vMCF-7^{Raf-1} 1GX-M MPS (Fig. 3c and d). The NOTCH3 network included nine genes (HES1, FOSB, JUN, EGR1, EGR3, MYC, TFDP2, ATF3, PGR) encoding for transcription factors that play a central role in tumor progression (Fig. 3e and Additional file 3: Figure S3). Immunofluorescence analysis showed a higher percentage of vMCF-7^{Raf-1} 1GX-M cells expressing NOTCH3 than their matching vMCF-7^{Raf-1} 1GX cells (Fig. 3f),

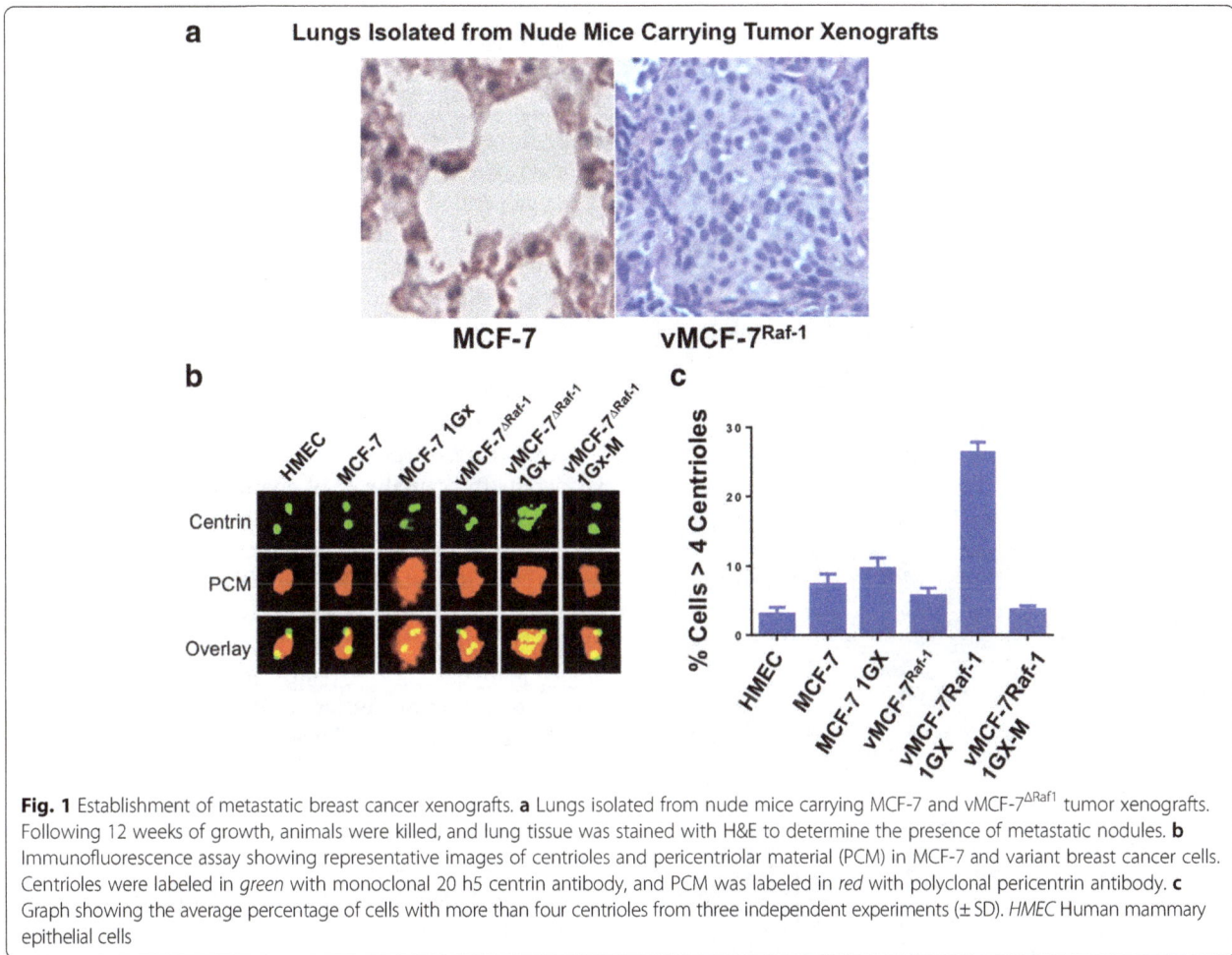

Fig. 1 Establishment of metastatic breast cancer xenografts. **a** Lungs isolated from nude mice carrying MCF-7 and vMCF-7$^{\Delta Raf1}$ tumor xenografts. Following 12 weeks of growth, animals were killed, and lung tissue was stained with H&E to determine the presence of metastatic nodules. **b** Immunofluorescence assay showing representative images of centrioles and pericentriolar material (PCM) in MCF-7 and variant breast cancer cells. Centrioles were labeled in *green* with monoclonal 20 h5 centrin antibody, and PCM was labeled in *red* with polyclonal pericentrin antibody. **c** Graph showing the average percentage of cells with more than four centrioles from three independent experiments (± SD). *HMEC* Human mammary epithelial cells

suggesting that NOTCH3-expressing cancer cells exhibited a higher capacity to promote seeding and growth to distant organs.

NOTCH3 expression is required to induce a CD44^{high}/CD24^{low}/ER^{low} breast cancer stemlike phenotype, self-renewal, and invasive capacity

Because our results indicate that NOTCH3-expressing cells originate in vMCF-7$^{\Delta Raf1}$ xenografts (Fig. 3f), we employed the CRISPR-Cas9 gene editing technology to generate unique NOTCH3-knockout breast cancer cells (vMCF-7^{Raf-1} 1GX$^{CRISPR-NOTCH3}$) and assessed their stemness and invasive properties (Additional file 4: Figure S4 and Fig. 4a and b). vMCF-7^{Raf-1} 1GX and vMCF-7^{Raf-1} 1GX$^{CRISPR-NOTCH3}$ cells were cultured under nonadherent conditions to test the efficiency of MPS formation. vMCF-7^{Raf-1} 1GX$^{CRISPR-NOTCH3}$ cells exhibited a reduction in the number and size of MPS formation compared with parental vMCF-7^{Raf-1} 1GX cells (Fig. 4c and d). To define the extent to which impairment of self-renewal capacity was linked to suppression of breast cancer stemlike phenotype, vMCF-7^{Raf-1} 1GX and vMCF-7^{Raf-1}

1GX$^{CRISPR-NOTCH3}$ MPS were stained for CD44 and CD24 breast cancer stemness markers. vMCF-7^{Raf-1} 1GX$^{CRISPR-NOTCH3}$ MPS exhibited a more differentiated CD44^{low}/CD24^{high} phenotype compared with vMCF-7^{Raf-1} 1GX MPS that showed a CD44^{high}/CD24^{low} cancer stemlike phenotype (Fig. 5a and b). Because CD44^{high}/CD24^{low} breast cancer stemlike cells also lack ERα expression [29, 37], we aimed to assess ERα expression/localization in vMCF-7^{Raf-1} 1GX and vMCF-7^{Raf-1} 1GX$^{CRISPR-NOTCH3}$ MPS. Whereas vMCF-7^{Raf-1} 1GX MPS lacked nuclear ERα expression, partial restoration of nuclear ERα expression was observed in vMCF-7^{Raf-1} 1GX$^{CRISPR-NOTCH3}$ MPS (Fig. 5a and d), corroborating the role of the NOTCH3 signaling pathway in restraining ERα expression in breast cancer cells [38]. To define the causative role of NOTCH3 expression in promoting ALDH1 activity that represents a universal functional marker of tumor stemness, chemoresistance, and metastasis [34, 39], we performed an ALDEOFLUOR assay in vMCF-7^{Raf-1} 1GX and vMCF-7^{Raf-1} 1GX$^{CRISPR-NOTCH3}$ cells. Significantly, vMCF-7^{Raf-1} 1GX$^{CRISPR-NOTCH3}$ cells showed a reduction of ALDH1 activity compared with parental vMCF-7^{Raf-1}

Table 1 Cytogenetic and SKY Analysis of Human Mammary Epithelial Cells (HMEC) and Breast Cancer Cells: Representation of Chromosomal changes detected by cytogenetic and SKY analysis in HMEC, parental and variant MCF-7 cells

Representation of Chromosomal changes detected by cytogenetic and SKY analysis in HMEC, parental and variant MCF-7 cells

1GX cells (Fig. 5e and f). Last, we aimed to investigate whether lack of NOTCH3 expression was linked to an impairment of vMCF-7^{Raf-1} 1GX cells' invasive capacity. An in vitro real-time invasion assay showed that abrogation of NOTCH3 expression significantly reduced the invasiveness of vMCF-7^{Raf-1} 1GX cells (Fig. 6a and b). These results were validated in vMCF-7^{Raf-1} 1GX cells infected with lentiviral short hairpin RNAs (lenti-shRNAs) targeting NOTCH3 messenger RNAs (mRNAs) that also showed a significant impairment of invasive capacity (Fig. 6c–f).

NOTCH3 expression is necessary to mediate AURKA-induced invasiveness of breast cancer cells

Because we have previously demonstrated in vMCF-7$^{\Delta Raf1}$ xenografts the causal role of aberrant AURKA activity in inducing the development of spontaneous lung metastases [29], we investigated whether NOTCH3 expression was necessary to mediate AURKA-induced invasive capacity of vMCF-7$^{\Delta Raf1}$ 1GX cells. vMCF-7$^{\Delta Raf1}$ 1GX and vMCF-7^{Raf-1} 1GX$^{CRISPR-NOTCH3}$ cells were infected with empty lentiviral vectors (lenti-vectors; used as control) and lenti-vectors expressing a GFP-tagged AURKA construct (Fig. 7a and b). Endogenous levels of AURKA were reduced in vMCF-7^{Raf-1} 1GX$^{CRISPR-NOTCH3}$ cells, whereas only vMCF-7$^{\Delta Raf1}$ 1GX cells expressing GFP-AURKA showed increased NOTCH3 expression (Fig. 7a–d). These results demonstrate a positive feedback loop between AURKA and NOTCH3 oncogenic pathways. To define whether NOTCH3 expression was essential to mediate AURKA-induced invasiveness of vMCF-7$^{\Delta Raf1}$ 1GX cells, we performed an in vitro real-time invasion assay. Significantly, expression of GFP-AURKA in vMCF-7$^{\Delta Raf1}$ 1GX cells enhanced their invasive capacity (Fig. 7e and f). On the contrary, expression of GFP-AURKA in vMCF-7^{Raf-1} 1GX$^{CRISPR-NOTCH3}$ cells failed to restore their invasive ability (Fig. 7e and f), demonstrating that NOTCH3 expression is required to mediate AURKA-induced breast cancer cells' aggressiveness.

Pharmacologic targeting of NOTCH signaling inhibits TNBC cell seeding and metastatic growth

To confirm in a different breast cancer model the finding that NOTCH3 expression is restricted to metastatic cells, we used CD44^{high}/CD24^{low} MDA-MB-231 TNBC cells isolated from experimental lung metastases (MDA-MB-231 LM) [37, 40]. MDA-MB-231 LM cells showed a higher percentage of cells expressing NOTCH3 than parental MDA-MB-231 cells (Fig. 8a). To assess the causal role of NOTCH3 expression in promoting the highly invasive capacity of MDA-MB-231 LM cells, we employed an in vitro real-time invasion assay. MDA-MB-231 LM cells infected with lenti-shRNAs targeting NOTCH3 significantly reduced

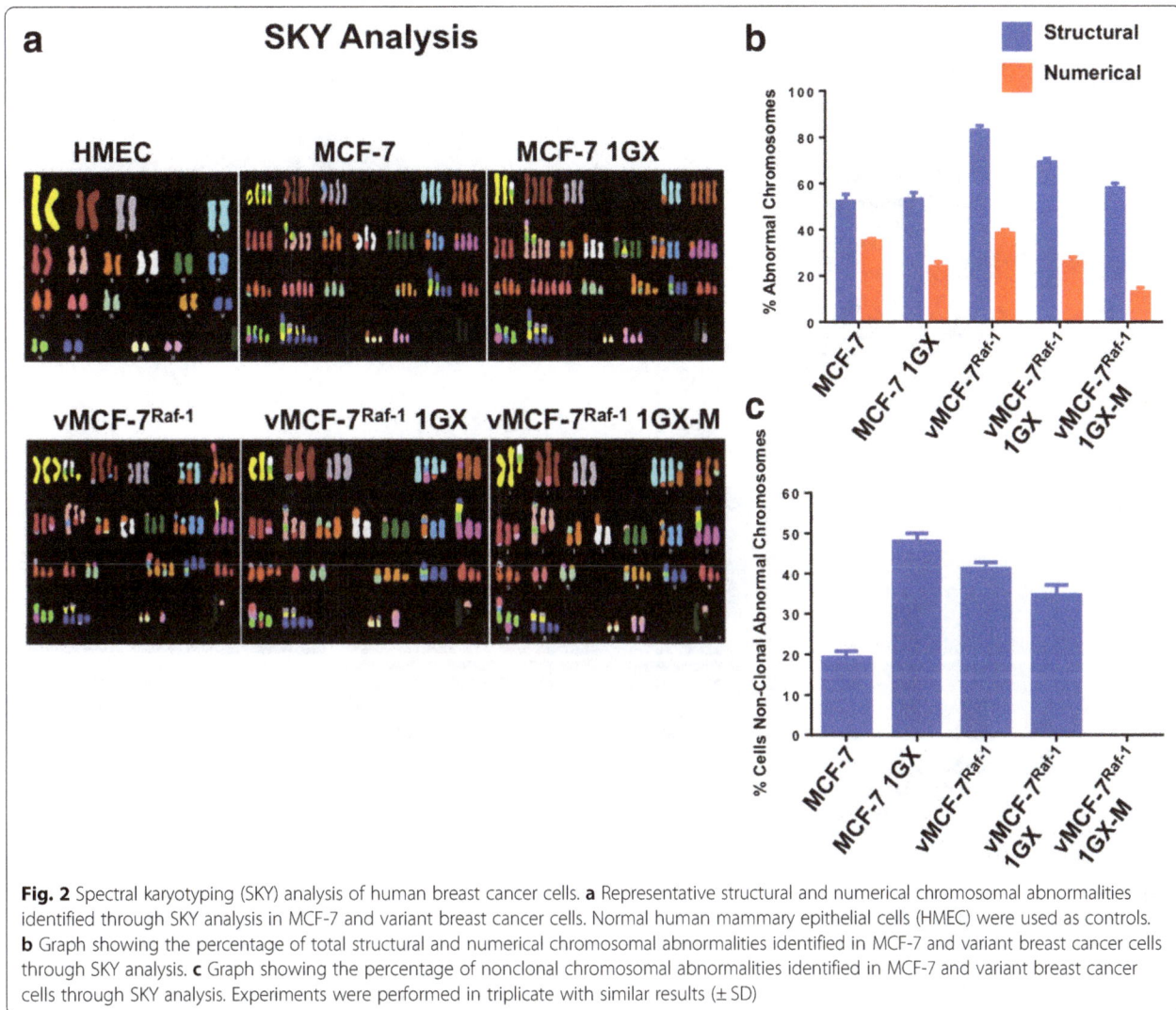

Fig. 2 Spectral karyotyping (SKY) analysis of human breast cancer cells. **a** Representative structural and numerical chromosomal abnormalities identified through SKY analysis in MCF-7 and variant breast cancer cells. Normal human mammary epithelial cells (HMEC) were used as controls. **b** Graph showing the percentage of total structural and numerical chromosomal abnormalities identified in MCF-7 and variant breast cancer cells through SKY analysis. **c** Graph showing the percentage of nonclonal chromosomal abnormalities identified in MCF-7 and variant breast cancer cells through SKY analysis. Experiments were performed in triplicate with similar results (± SD)

their invasiveness compared with MDA-MB-231 LM cells infected with scramble lenti-shRNAs used as control (Fig. 8b). Next, we aimed to establish whether pharmacologic targeting of NOTCH signaling inhibits metastatic seeding and growth of cancer cells overexpressing NOTCH3. MDA-MB-231 LM cells were treated in vitro with 500 nM of LY411575 (pan-NOTCH inhibitor), and MDA-MB-231 LM cells treated with vehicle dimethyl sulfoxide (DMSO) were used as a control. After 48-hour incubation, treated and control MDA-MB-231 LM cells were washed with PBS and cultured in drug-free medium for an additional 48 hours. Viable cells were then injected into the tail vein of immune-compromised mice to develop experimental lung metastases as previously described [29]. Whereas animals injected with DMSO-treated MDA-MB-231 LM cells developed lung metastases, animals injected with LY411575-treated MDA-MB-231 LM cells showed

impaired lung metastatic lesions (Fig. 8c). Histopathologic analysis confirmed that whereas lungs isolated from control animals exhibited metastatic lesions with several mitotic figures indicative of active proliferating cancer cells, the alveolar structure of lungs isolated from LY411575-treated animals was largely preserved (Fig. 8d). Importantly, because MDA-MB-231 LM and parental cells showed nominal levels of NOTCH1 and NOTCH2 (Additional file 5: Figure S5a and b), these results suggest that LY411575-mediated inhibition of cancer cell seeding and metastatic growth was likely associated with NOTCH3 targeting.

Genetic targeting of NOTCH3 reduces the self-renewal and invasive capacity of patient-derived brain metastasis TNBC cells

To validate in primary breast cancer cells the central role of the NOTCH3 signaling pathway in inducing a

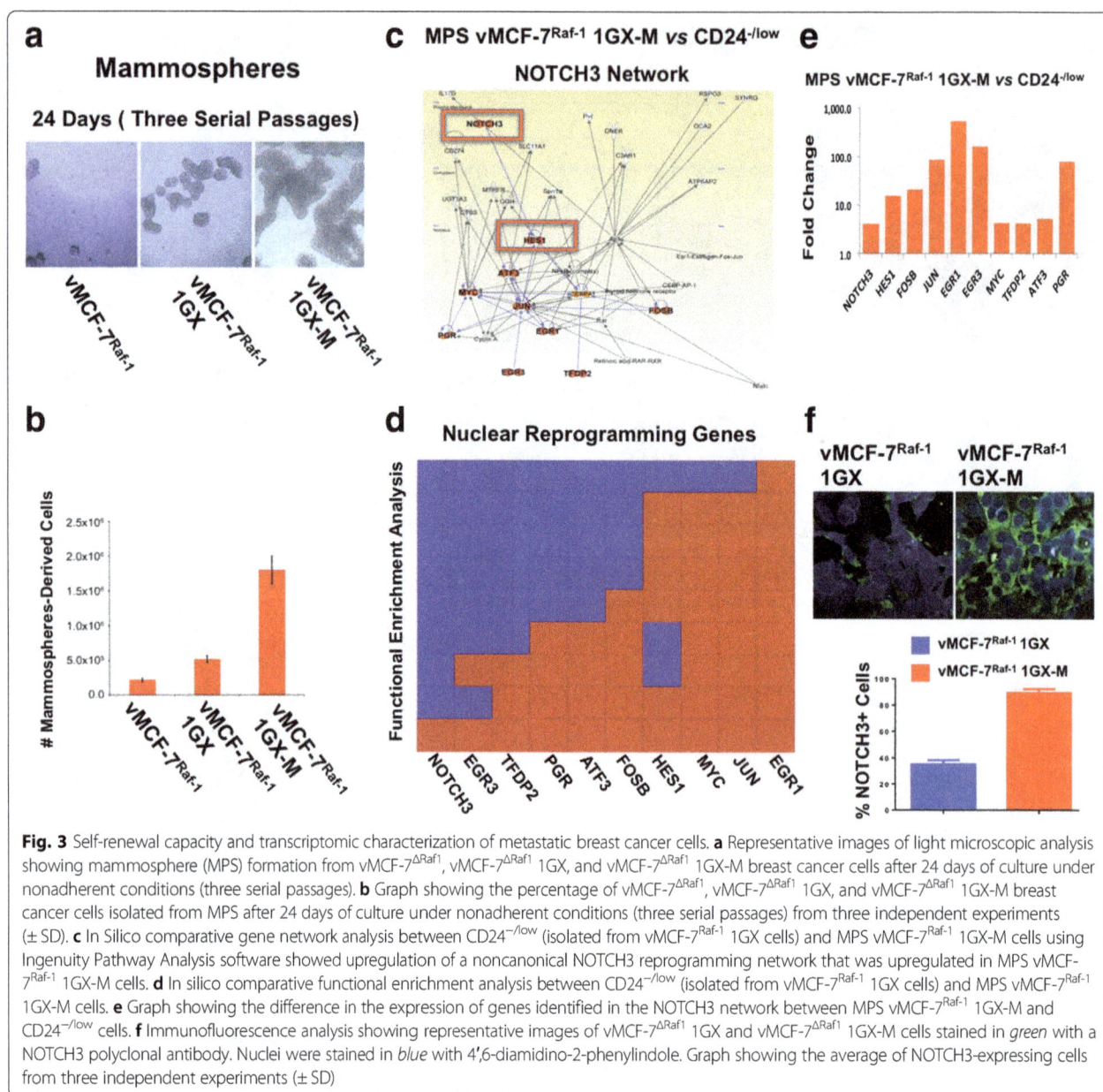

Fig. 3 Self-renewal capacity and transcriptomic characterization of metastatic breast cancer cells. **a** Representative images of light microscopic analysis showing mammosphere (MPS) formation from vMCF-7$^{\Delta Raf1}$, vMCF-7$^{\Delta Raf1}$ 1GX, and vMCF-7$^{\Delta Raf1}$ 1GX-M breast cancer cells after 24 days of culture under nonadherent conditions (three serial passages). **b** Graph showing the percentage of vMCF-7$^{\Delta Raf1}$, vMCF-7$^{\Delta Raf1}$ 1GX, and vMCF-7$^{\Delta Raf1}$ 1GX-M breast cancer cells isolated from MPS after 24 days of culture under nonadherent conditions (three serial passages) from three independent experiments (± SD). **c** In Silico comparative gene network analysis between CD24$^{-/low}$ (isolated from vMCF-7^{Raf-1} 1GX cells) and MPS vMCF-7^{Raf-1} 1GX-M cells using Ingenuity Pathway Analysis software showed upregulation of a noncanonical NOTCH3 reprogramming network that was upregulated in MPS vMCF-7^{Raf-1} 1GX-M cells. **d** In silico comparative functional enrichment analysis between CD24$^{-/low}$ (isolated from vMCF-7^{Raf-1} 1GX cells) and MPS vMCF-7^{Raf-1} 1GX-M cells. **e** Graph showing the difference in the expression of genes identified in the NOTCH3 network between MPS vMCF-7^{Raf-1} 1GX-M and CD24$^{-/low}$ cells. **f** Immunofluorescence analysis showing representative images of vMCF-7$^{\Delta Raf1}$ 1GX and vMCF-7$^{\Delta Raf1}$ 1GX-M cells stained in *green* with a NOTCH3 polyclonal antibody. Nuclei were stained in *blue* with 4′,6-diamidino-2-phenylindole. Graph showing the average of NOTCH3-expressing cells from three independent experiments (± SD)

metastatic phenotype, we developed unique TNBC cells (TNBC-M25) isolated from a patient-derived brain metastasis xenograft model that was generated by the BEAUTY trial in the Mayo Clinic [32]. TNBC-M25 cells showed increased expression of phospho-AURKA and NOTCH3 compared with MDA-MB-231 cells (Fig. 9a and b). Significantly, TNBC-M25 cells showed low levels of NOTCH1 and NOTCH2, suggesting that NOTCH3 expression plays a major role in promoting their metastatic phenotype (Additional file 6: Figure S6a and b). To define the causative role of NOTCH3 expression in inducing self-renewal capacity, TNBC-M25 cells were infected with lenti-shRNAs targeting NOTCH3 (TNBC-M25 infected with scramble lenti-shRNAs were used as a control) and were cultured under nonadherent conditions to test the efficiency of MPS formation. TNBC-M25 cells infected with lenti-shRNA NOTCH3 exhibited a significant reduction in the size of MPS formation compared with control cells (Fig. 9c and d). To investigate the extent to which impairment of self-renewal ability was linked to inhibition of invasiveness in TNBC-M25 cells with reduced NOTCH3 expression, we employed an in vitro real-time invasion assay. TNBC-M25 cells infected with lenti-shRNA NOTCH3 significantly reduced their invasive capacity compared with TNBC-M25 cells infected with scramble lenti-shRNAs used as a control (Fig. 9c and f).

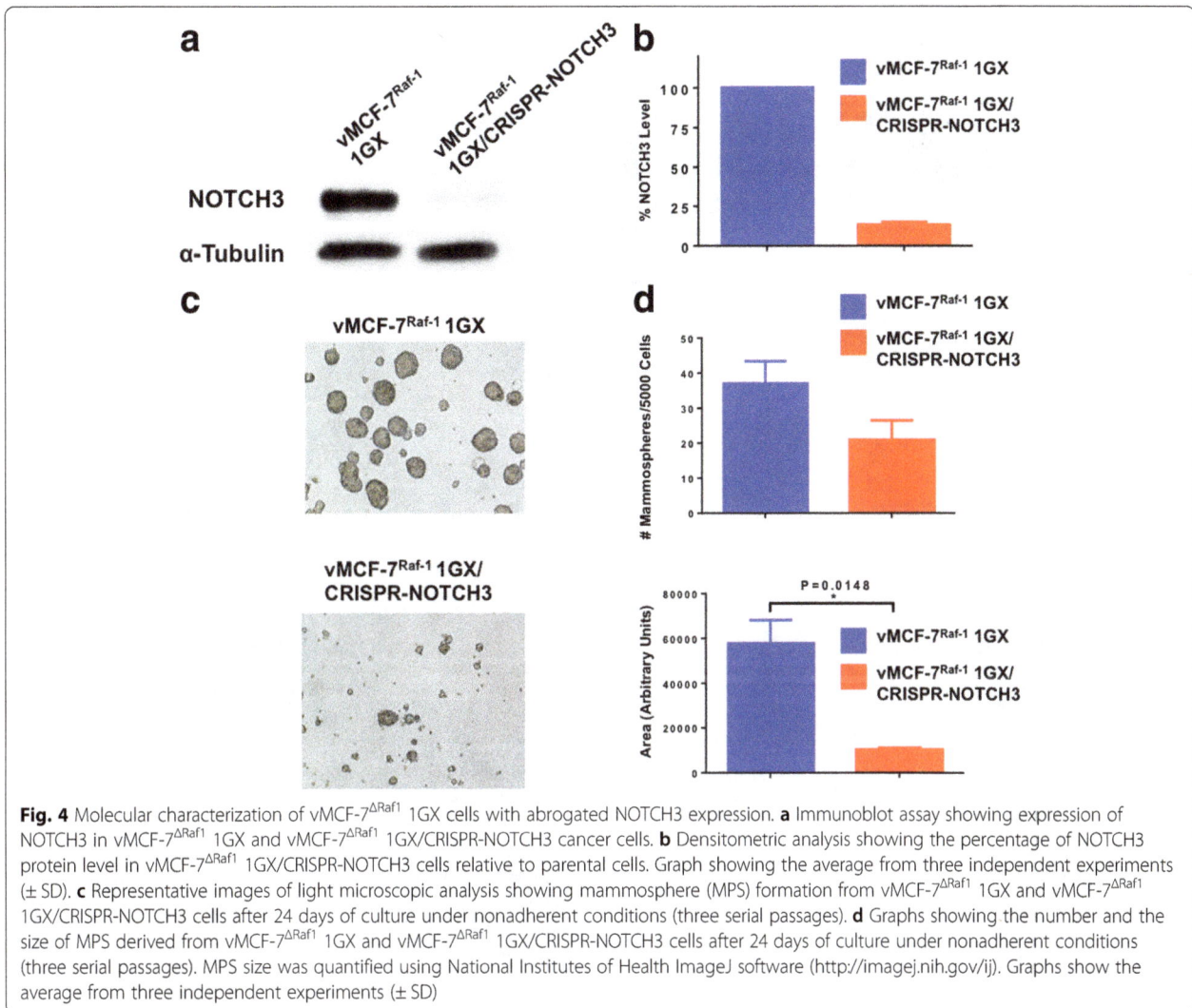

Fig. 4 Molecular characterization of vMCF-7$^{\Delta Raf1}$ 1GX cells with abrogated NOTCH3 expression. **a** Immunoblot assay showing expression of NOTCH3 in vMCF-7$^{\Delta Raf1}$ 1GX and vMCF-7$^{\Delta Raf1}$ 1GX/CRISPR-NOTCH3 cancer cells. **b** Densitometric analysis showing the percentage of NOTCH3 protein level in vMCF-7$^{\Delta Raf1}$ 1GX/CRISPR-NOTCH3 cells relative to parental cells. Graph showing the average from three independent experiments (± SD). **c** Representative images of light microscopic analysis showing mammosphere (MPS) formation from vMCF-7$^{\Delta Raf1}$ 1GX and vMCF-7$^{\Delta Raf1}$ 1GX/CRISPR-NOTCH3 cells after 24 days of culture under nonadherent conditions (three serial passages). **d** Graphs showing the number and the size of MPS derived from vMCF-7$^{\Delta Raf1}$ 1GX and vMCF-7$^{\Delta Raf1}$ 1GX/CRISPR-NOTCH3 cells after 24 days of culture under nonadherent conditions (three serial passages). MPS size was quantified using National Institutes of Health ImageJ software (http://imagej.nih.gov/ij). Graphs show the average from three independent experiments (± SD)

Aberrant NOTCH3 expression is linked to shorter overall survival of patients with breast cancer

We analyzed the genome sequencing and mRNA-sequencing data of specimens from the METABRIC study [30] to define the linkage between NOTCH3 expression and overall survival of patients with claudin-low breast tumors. The claudin-low subgroup analyzed in the METABRIC study represented a cluster of 125 patients characterized by 112 TNBC and 13 ER$^-$/PR$^-$/HER2$^+$ specimens, and the average age at diagnosis was 56.9 years. Whereas none of the 125 patients harbored any deletion or downregulation of NOTCH3, 8 of 117 cases (6 TNBC and 2 ER$^-$/PR$^-$/HER2$^+$) showed NOTCH3 alterations characterized by mRNA upregulation and/or copy number variations. Cases of death involved 6 patients with aberrant NOTCH3 expression and 46 patients without NOTCH3 alterations. Our survival analysis showed that NOTCH3 expression was significantly associated with decreased overall survival ($p =$ 0.0145). Specifically, the average of the overall survival (calculated for the whole follow-up) was 282.8 months for the cases without NOTCH3 alterations and 44.8 months for the cases with aberrant NOTCH3 expression (Fig. 10).

Discussion

Development of distant metastases involves a complex multistep biological process termed the *invasion-metastasis cascade*, which includes dissemination of cancer cells from the primary tumor to secondary organs [41]. This process is inefficient because it has been estimated that less than 1% of cancer cells will be successful in establishing clinically detectable metastatic lesions [42]. Specifically in breast cancer, BT-MICs must go through EMT, invade the extracellular matrix, intravasate and survive in the systemic circulation, extravasate at the metastatic site, and finally seed in the new microenvironment [42–44]. Importantly, each of these events is

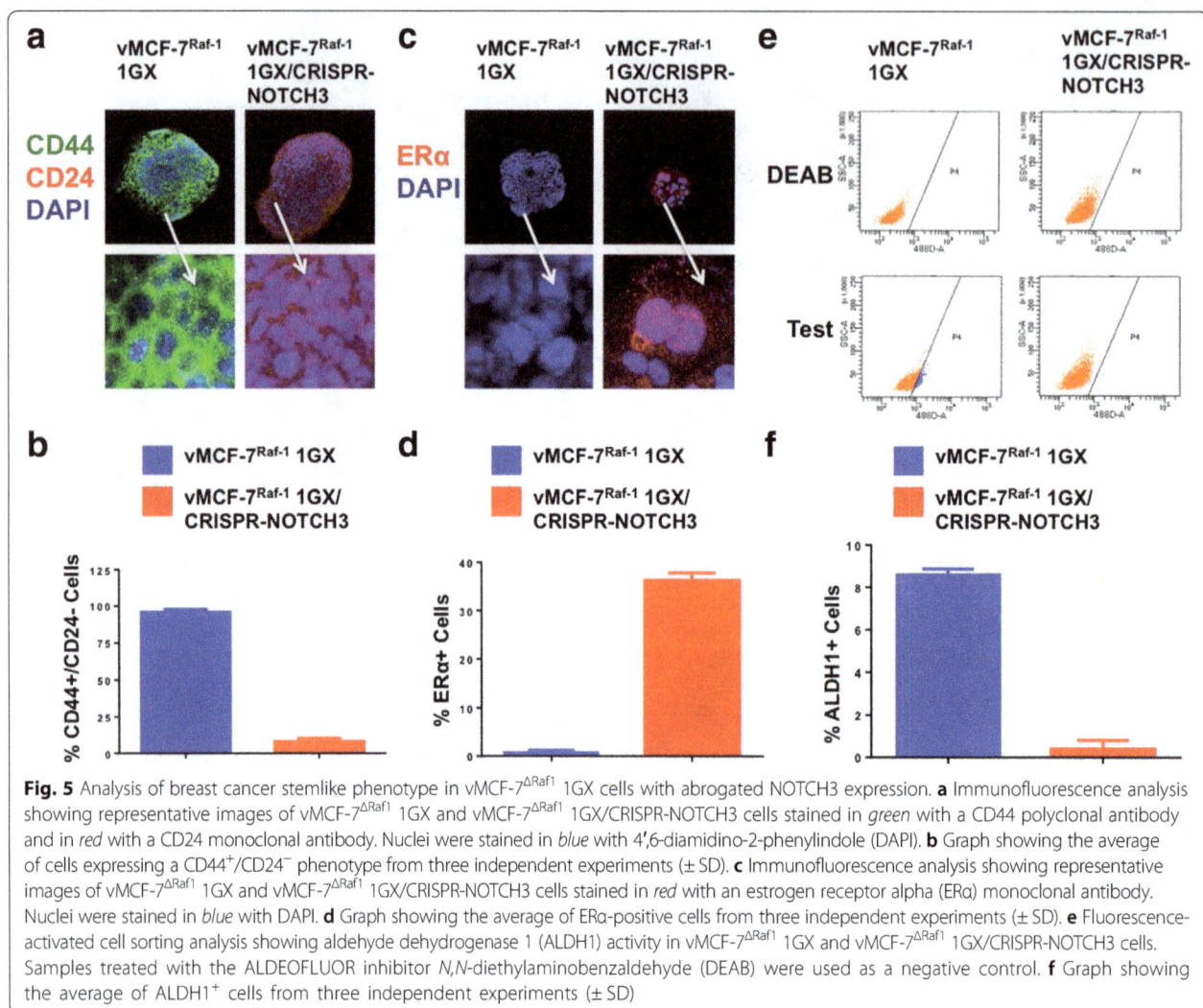

Fig. 5 Analysis of breast cancer stemlike phenotype in vMCF-7$^{\Delta Raf1}$ 1GX cells with abrogated NOTCH3 expression. **a** Immunofluorescence analysis showing representative images of vMCF-7$^{\Delta Raf1}$ 1GX and vMCF-7$^{\Delta Raf1}$ 1GX/CRISPR-NOTCH3 cells stained in *green* with a CD44 polyclonal antibody and in *red* with a CD24 monoclonal antibody. Nuclei were stained in *blue* with 4',6-diamidino-2-phenylindole (DAPI). **b** Graph showing the average of cells expressing a CD44$^+$/CD24$^-$ phenotype from three independent experiments (± SD). **c** Immunofluorescence analysis showing representative images of vMCF-7$^{\Delta Raf1}$ 1GX and vMCF-7$^{\Delta Raf1}$ 1GX/CRISPR-NOTCH3 cells stained in *red* with an estrogen receptor alpha (ERα) monoclonal antibody. Nuclei were stained in *blue* with DAPI. **d** Graph showing the average of ERα-positive cells from three independent experiments (± SD). **e** Fluorescence-activated cell sorting analysis showing aldehyde dehydrogenase 1 (ALDH1) activity in vMCF-7$^{\Delta Raf1}$ 1GX and vMCF-7$^{\Delta Raf1}$ 1GX/CRISPR-NOTCH3 cells. Samples treated with the ALDEOFLUOR inhibitor *N,N*-diethylaminobenzaldehyde (DEAB) were used as a negative control. **f** Graph showing the average of ALDH1$^+$ cells from three independent experiments (± SD)

driven by the accumulation of genetic and/or epigenetic alterations within cancer cells necessary for the clonal selection and expansion of BT-MICs that ultimately give rise to distant metastases [44]. Several lines of evidence support the hypothesis that BT-MICs might be found within subpopulations of BTICs [46]. In support of this hypothesis, it has been shown that oncogenic pathways such as MAPK, AURKA, and NOTCH that induce EMT and expansion of BTICs also promote onset of distant metastases [5, 29, 47, 48]. The characterization of the precise role of each of these oncogenic pathways in the sequential stepwise events that typify the invasion-metastasis cascade will be essential for the development of precise therapeutic strategies aimed at eradicating distant metastases.

In this study, we uncovered the linkage between NOTCH3 expression and development of distant metastases in experimental breast cancer models. First, we used luminal ER$^+$ MCF-7 and variant cells with constitutively active Raf-1/MAPK signaling (vMCF-7$^{\Delta Raf1}$) to establish in vivo the association between aberrant Raf-1/

MAPK signaling, CIN, and onset of distant metastases. In agreement with our previous studies [5, 29], only vMCF-7$^{\Delta Raf1}$ tumor xenografts developed spontaneous lung metastases, corroborating the causal role of aberrant activation of Raf-1/MAPK pathway in promoting metastatic lesions. Significantly, ex vivo cancer cells isolated from lung metastases (vMCF-7$^{\Delta Raf1}$ 1GX-M) showed a normal centrosome phenotype and clonal chromosomal aberrations compared with matching vMCF-7$^{\Delta Raf1}$ 1GX parental cells that exhibited centrosome amplification and nonclonal chromosomal aberrations resulting in CIN. These findings demonstrate in vivo that loss of centrosome amplification is linked to restoration of chromosomal stability resulting in the clonal expansion of metastatic cancer cells. Moreover, they support the genomic convergence model proposed for tumor progression in which CIN initially imposed during tumorigenesis becomes suppressed when cancer cells have acquired the suitable chromosome compositions and gene dosage that will lead to the successful

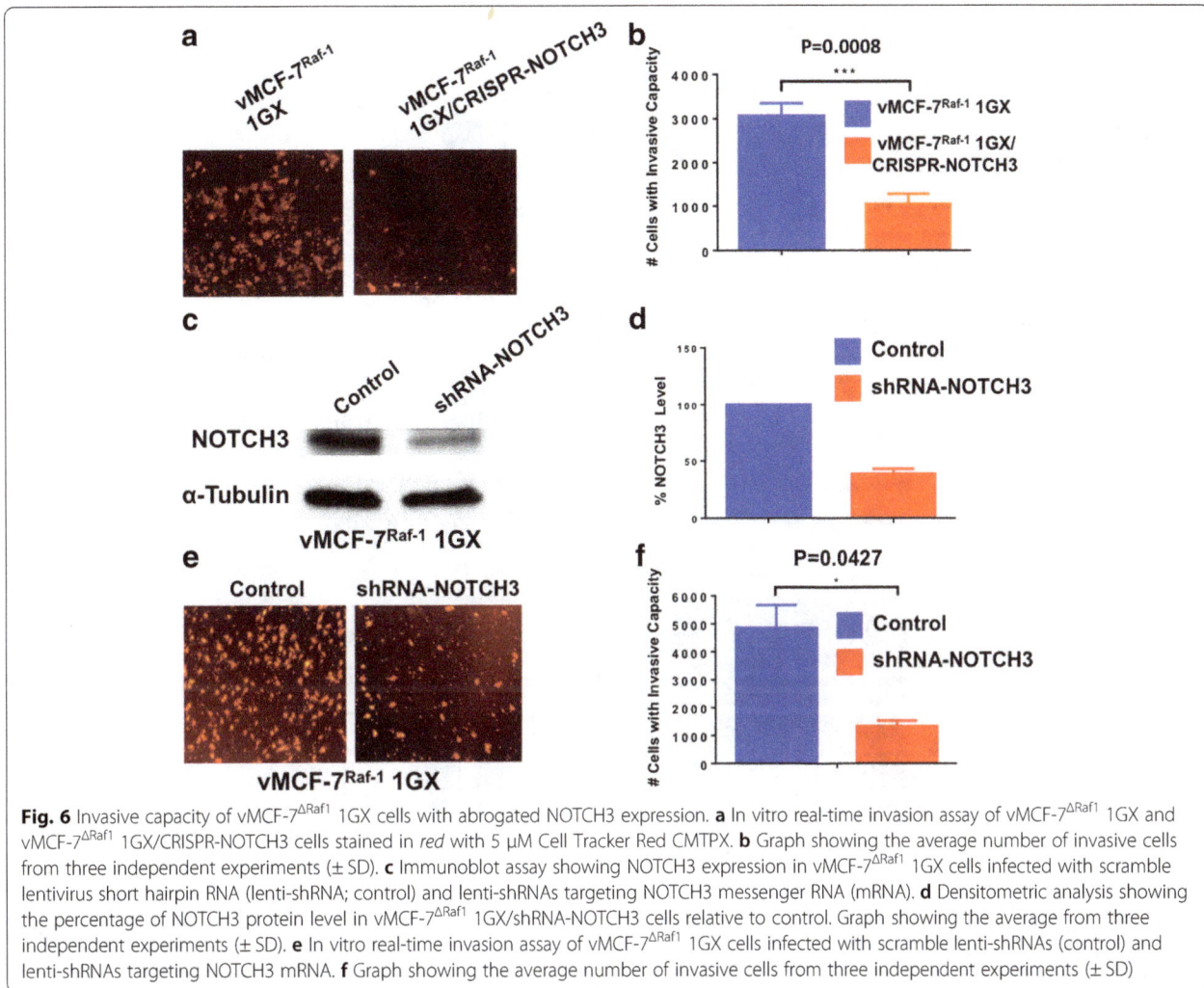

Fig. 6 Invasive capacity of vMCF-7$^{\Delta Raf1}$ 1GX cells with abrogated NOTCH3 expression. **a** In vitro real-time invasion assay of vMCF-7$^{\Delta Raf1}$ 1GX and vMCF-7$^{\Delta Raf1}$ 1GX/CRISPR-NOTCH3 cells stained in *red* with 5 μM Cell Tracker Red CMTPX. **b** Graph showing the average number of invasive cells from three independent experiments (± SD). **c** Immunoblot assay showing NOTCH3 expression in vMCF-7$^{\Delta Raf1}$ 1GX cells infected with scramble lentivirus short hairpin RNA (lenti-shRNA; control) and lenti-shRNAs targeting NOTCH3 messenger RNA (mRNA). **d** Densitometric analysis showing the percentage of NOTCH3 protein level in vMCF-7$^{\Delta Raf1}$ 1GX/shRNA-NOTCH3 cells relative to control. Graph showing the average from three independent experiments (± SD). **e** In vitro real-time invasion assay of vMCF-7$^{\Delta Raf1}$ 1GX cells infected with scramble lenti-shRNAs (control) and lenti-shRNAs targeting NOTCH3 mRNA. **f** Graph showing the average number of invasive cells from three independent experiments (± SD)

establishment of distant metastases [48]. Because it has been hypothesized that BT-MICs are late stages BTIC subclones with higher stemness capacity [45], we cultured vMCF-7$^{\Delta Raf1}$ 1GX-M and matching vMCF-7$^{\Delta Raf1}$ and vMCF-7$^{\Delta Raf1}$ 1GX parental cells under nonadherent conditions to form MPS as an in vitro surrogate assay of self-renewal capacity. vMCF-7$^{\Delta Raf1}$ 1GX-M cells showed the highest efficiency in MPS formation compared with matching parental cells. This increased self-renewal capacity was linked to loss of the CD24 epithelial marker in vMCF-7$^{\Delta Raf1}$ 1GX-M MPS. These results demonstrate that chromosomal stable vMCF-7$^{\Delta Raf1}$ 1GX-M cells have acquired higher self-renewal and CD24$^{-/low}$ basal-like plasticity that plays a critical role in EMT, cancer cell seeding, and metastatic growth to secondary organs [29]. Next, we wanted to establish whether chromosomal stability and high self-renewal capacity of vMCF-7$^{\Delta Raf1}$ 1GX-M cells was linked to an exclusive metastatic signature. To answer this question, we performed unbiased comparative transcriptomic and functional gene enrichment analyses between MPS vMCF-7$^{\Delta Raf1}$ 1GX-M (that

show CD24$^{-/low}$) and highly invasive CD24$^{-/low}$ basal-like cells isolated from matching vMCF-7$^{\Delta Raf1}$ tumor xenografts as previously demonstrated [29]. Functional gene enrichment analysis identified a noncanonical NOTCH3 reprogramming network that was upregulated in vMCF-7$^{\Delta Raf1}$ 1GX-M MPS. The NOTCH3 network comprised nine genes encoding for transcriptional factors with high oncogenic activity (HES1, FOSB, JUN, EGR1, EGR3, MYC, TFDP2, ATF3, PGR). This reprogramming network included the NOTCH downstream target HES1, suggesting that NOTCH3/HES1 stemness signaling may play a central role in promoting the survival and seeding of BT-MICs to secondary organs. Because detection of cancer cell seeding to secondary organs and onset of micrometastases is clinically challenging, expression of the NOTCH3 metastatic signature in circulating tumor cells may have promising clinical relevance in predicting early onset of distant metastases in patients with breast cancer. Importantly, the majority of vMCF-7$^{\Delta Raf1}$ 1GX-M cells were strongly positive for NOTCH3 staining by

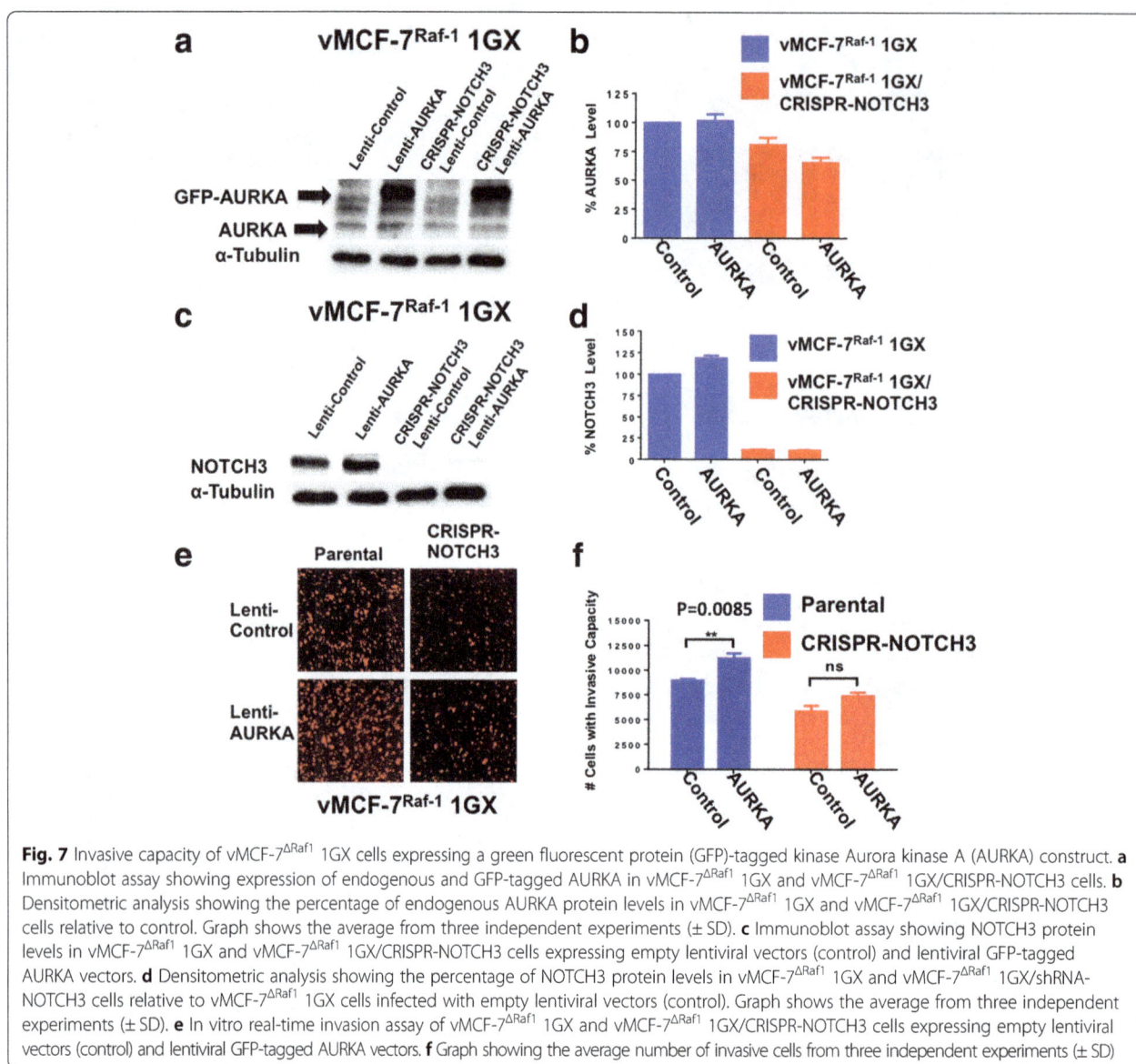

Fig. 7 Invasive capacity of vMCF-7$^{\Delta Raf1}$ 1GX cells expressing a green fluorescent protein (GFP)-tagged kinase Aurora kinase A (AURKA) construct. **a** Immunoblot assay showing expression of endogenous and GFP-tagged AURKA in vMCF-7$^{\Delta Raf1}$ 1GX and vMCF-7$^{\Delta Raf1}$ 1GX/CRISPR-NOTCH3 cells. **b** Densitometric analysis showing the percentage of endogenous AURKA protein levels in vMCF-7$^{\Delta Raf1}$ 1GX and vMCF-7$^{\Delta Raf1}$ 1GX/CRISPR-NOTCH3 cells relative to control. Graph shows the average from three independent experiments (± SD). **c** Immunoblot assay showing NOTCH3 protein levels in vMCF-7$^{\Delta Raf1}$ 1GX and vMCF-7$^{\Delta Raf1}$ 1GX/CRISPR-NOTCH3 cells expressing empty lentiviral vectors (control) and lentiviral GFP-tagged AURKA vectors. **d** Densitometric analysis showing the percentage of NOTCH3 protein levels in vMCF-7$^{\Delta Raf1}$ 1GX and vMCF-7$^{\Delta Raf1}$ 1GX/shRNA-NOTCH3 cells relative to vMCF-7$^{\Delta Raf1}$ 1GX cells infected with empty lentiviral vectors (control). Graph shows the average from three independent experiments (± SD). **e** In vitro real-time invasion assay of vMCF-7$^{\Delta Raf1}$ 1GX and vMCF-7$^{\Delta Raf1}$ 1GX/CRISPR-NOTCH3 cells expressing empty lentiviral vectors (control) and lentiviral GFP-tagged AURKA vectors. **f** Graph showing the average number of invasive cells from three independent experiments (± SD)

immunofluorescence assay, demonstrating that NOTCH3 expression was restricted to clonal metastatic breast cancer cells. vMCF-7$^{\Delta Raf1}$ 1GX xenografts exhibiting CIN showed tumor cell heterogeneity for NOTCH3 expression, indicating that NOTCH3^{high}-expressing subclones may arise from the primary tumor and promote distant metastasis owing to their higher stemness capacity, in agreement with the recent finding that metastatic clones disseminate early from primary breast tumors [49]. On the basis of these results, we developed unique NOTCH3-knockout breast cancer cells (vMCF-7^{Raf-1} 1GX$^{CRISPR-NOTCH3}$) to abrogate NOTCH3 expression and evaluate the causative role of NOTCH3 signaling in promoting stemness and invasive properties of vMCF-7$^{\Delta Raf1}$ 1GX cells. NOTCH3 expression was required to induce in vitro self-renewal capacity and a CD44^{high}/CD24^{low} breast cancer stemlike phenotype in vMCF-7$^{\Delta Raf1}$ 1GX cells. Because we and others have demonstrated that CD44^{high}/CD24^{low} BTICs also show an ERα$^{low/-}$ basal-like phenotype [29, 37, 38], we assessed ERα in MPS derived from vMCF-7^{Raf-1} 1GX$^{CRISPR-NOTCH3}$ and parental cells. Whereas MPS derived from vMCF-7^{Raf-1} 1GX cells lacked ERα expression, MPS resulting from vMCF-7^{Raf-1} 1GX$^{CRISPR-NOTCH3}$ cells exhibited restoration of ERα expression, compatible with previous studies that demonstrated the role of NOTCH3 signaling in suppressing ERα expression [38]. Because high ALDH1 activity has been linked to stemness, early onset of distant metastases, and poor prognosis in breast cancer [39], we performed an ALDEOFLUOR assay that accurately identifies highly tumorigenic cancer cells with elevated

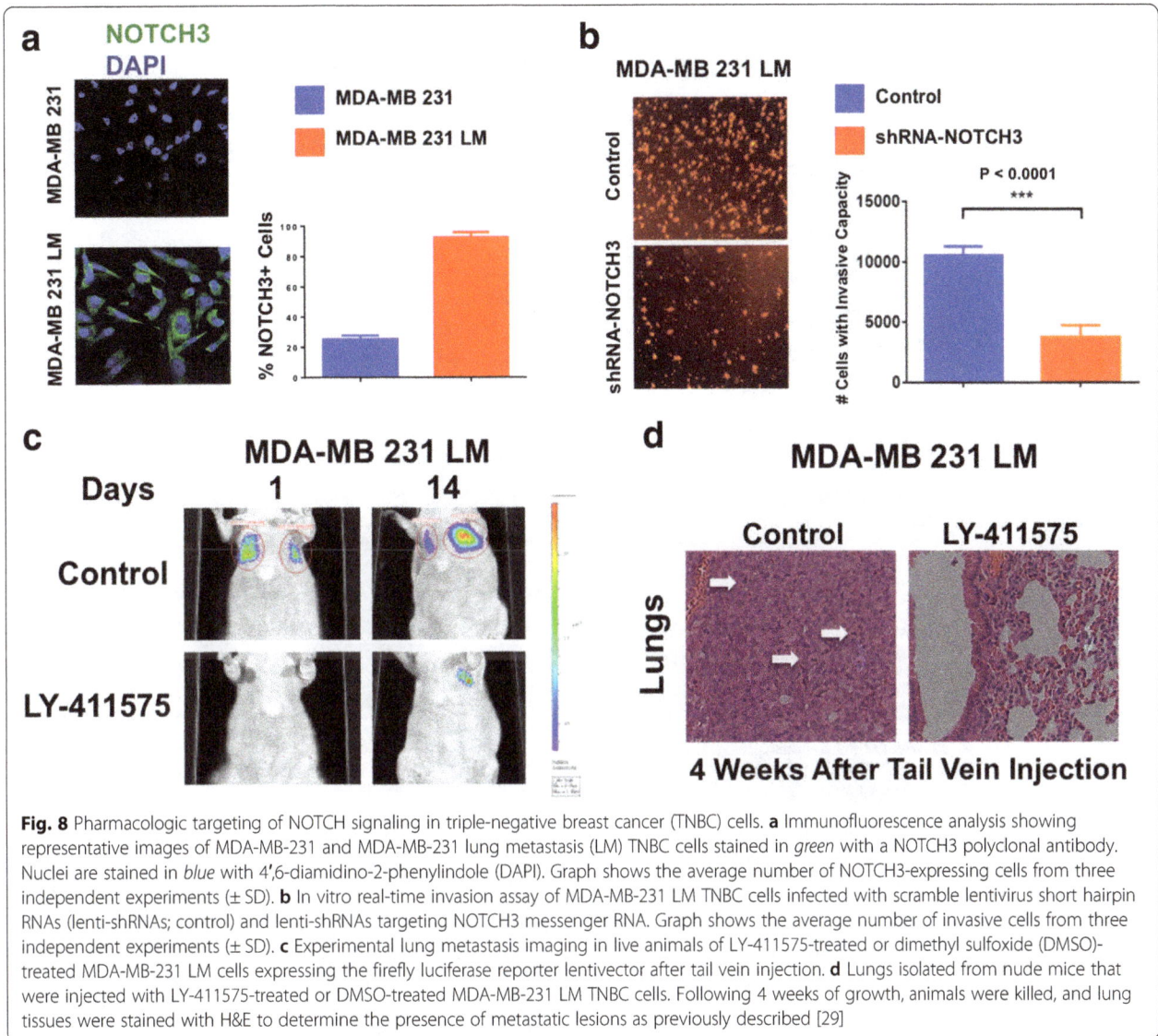

Fig. 8 Pharmacologic targeting of NOTCH signaling in triple-negative breast cancer (TNBC) cells. **a** Immunofluorescence analysis showing representative images of MDA-MB-231 and MDA-MB-231 lung metastasis (LM) TNBC cells stained in *green* with a NOTCH3 polyclonal antibody. Nuclei are stained in *blue* with 4′,6-diamidino-2-phenylindole (DAPI). Graph shows the average number of NOTCH3-expressing cells from three independent experiments (± SD). **b** In vitro real-time invasion assay of MDA-MB-231 LM TNBC cells infected with scramble lentivirus short hairpin RNAs (lenti-shRNAs; control) and lenti-shRNAs targeting NOTCH3 messenger RNA. Graph shows the average number of invasive cells from three independent experiments (± SD). **c** Experimental lung metastasis imaging in live animals of LY-411575-treated or dimethyl sulfoxide (DMSO)-treated MDA-MB-231 LM cells expressing the firefly luciferase reporter lentivector after tail vein injection. **d** Lungs isolated from nude mice that were injected with LY-411575-treated or DMSO-treated MDA-MB-231 LM TNBC cells. Following 4 weeks of growth, animals were killed, and lung tissues were stained with H&E to determine the presence of metastatic lesions as previously described [29]

ALDH1 activity. Importantly, vMCF-7^{Raf-1} 1GX$^{CRISPR-NOTCH3}$ cells showed minimal ALDH1 activity compared with parental vMCF-7^{Raf-1} 1GX cells, supporting the role of NOTCH stemness signaling in inducing ALDH1 activity and an increased metastatic behavior [50]. Next, we defined whether inhibition of self-renewal capacity and tumor stemness was functionally linked to loss of invasive capacity. An in vitro real-time invasion assay showed that abrogation of NOTCH3 expression significantly inhibited the invasive capacity of vMCF-7^{Raf-1} 1GX cells, indicating that NOTCH3 signaling pathway is necessary to promote a more aggressive phenotype. Because we have previously demonstrated the causative role of aberrant AURKA activity in driving the development of breast cancer metastases [29], we aimed to establish whether NOTCH3 expression was required to mediate AURKA-induced highly invasive capacity of vMCF-7$^{\Delta Raf1}$ 1GX cells. Forced expression of AURKA in vMCF-7$^{\Delta Raf1}$ 1GX cells increased NOTCH3 expression and their in vitro invasive capacity. Conversely, AURKA overexpression in vMCF-7^{Raf-1} 1GX$^{CRISPR-NOTCH3}$ cells failed to restore a highly invasive phenotype, demonstrating that NOTCH3 expression is required to mediate AURKA-induced high metastatic potential. Moreover, these results highlight a novel mechanistic linkage between AURKA and NOTCH3 oncogenic pathways that is critical to development of a fully metastatic phenotype in breast cancer cells. To define in a different breast cancer model whether increased expression of NOTCH3 was restricted to metastatic cancer cells, we employed MDA-MB-231 TNBC cells that exhibit a CD44^{high}/CD24^{low} basal-like phenotype and elevated endogenous MAPK activity [34, 52]. Significantly, the percentage of ex vivo MDA-MB-231 cells isolated from lung

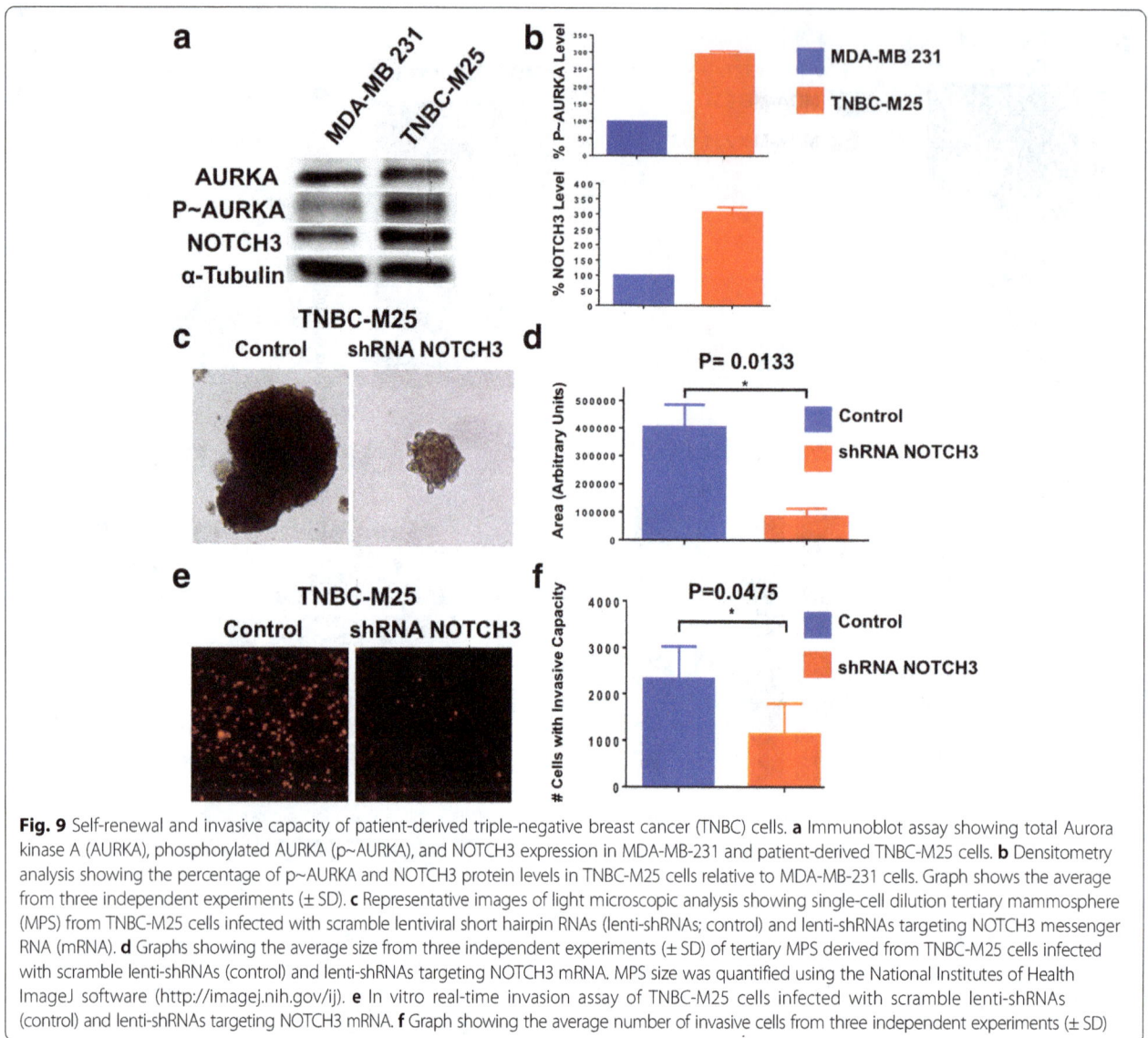

Fig. 9 Self-renewal and invasive capacity of patient-derived triple-negative breast cancer (TNBC) cells. **a** Immunoblot assay showing total Aurora kinase A (AURKA), phosphorylated AURKA (p~AURKA), and NOTCH3 expression in MDA-MB-231 and patient-derived TNBC-M25 cells. **b** Densitometry analysis showing the percentage of p~AURKA and NOTCH3 protein levels in TNBC-M25 cells relative to MDA-MB-231 cells. Graph shows the average from three independent experiments (± SD). **c** Representative images of light microscopic analysis showing single-cell dilution tertiary mammosphere (MPS) from TNBC-M25 cells infected with scramble lentiviral short hairpin RNAs (lenti-shRNAs; control) and lenti-shRNAs targeting NOTCH3 messenger RNA (mRNA). **d** Graphs showing the average size from three independent experiments (± SD) of tertiary MPS derived from TNBC-M25 cells infected with scramble lenti-shRNAs (control) and lenti-shRNAs targeting NOTCH3 mRNA. MPS size was quantified using the National Institutes of Health ImageJ software (http://imagej.nih.gov/ij). **e** In vitro real-time invasion assay of TNBC-M25 cells infected with scramble lenti-shRNAs (control) and lenti-shRNAs targeting NOTCH3 mRNA. **f** Graph showing the average number of invasive cells from three independent experiments (± SD)

metastases (MDA-MB-231 LM) expressing NOTCH3 was higher than matching MDA-MB-231 parental cells, suggesting that NOTCH3 signaling is also required for the metastatic seeding and growth of TNBC cells. These results are in agreement with a recent study that demonstrated the role of the NOTCH3 signaling pathway in promoting the growth of basal-like breast cancer cells [51–53]. Complementary to our vMCF-7^{Raf-1} model, targeting of NOTCH3 impaired the in vitro invasive capacity of MDA-MB-231 LM cells, demonstrating the key role of NOTCH3 expression in promoting the TNBC highly invasive phenotype. Next, we aimed to determine whether inhibition of NOTCH signaling decreased the metastatic capacity of MDA-MB-231 LM cells. In vitro treatment of MDA-MB-231 LM cells with the pan-NOTCH inhibitor LY-411575 resulted in the inhibition of cancer cell seeding and onset of experimental lung metastases, demonstrating

that NOTCH pharmacologic targeting interferes with late stages of the invasion-metastasis cascade in NOTCH3-expressing breast cancer cells. Importantly, MDA-MB-231 LM and matching parental cells expressed nominal levels of NOTCH1 and NOTCH2, suggesting that LY411575-mediated inhibition of cancer cell seeding and metastatic growth was primarily linked to inhibition of the NOTCH3 signaling pathway.

Owing to the limited translatability of established cancer cells, and to corroborate the central role of NOTCH3 in driving a metastatic phenotype in clinically relevant models, we established unique TNBC cells (TNBC-M25) isolated from a patient-derived brain metastasis xenograft model. TNBC-M25 cells showed high expression of phospho-AURKA and NOTCH3, whereas NOTCH1 and NOTCH2 levels were low, suggesting that the AURKA/NOTCH3 oncogenic axis plays a major role

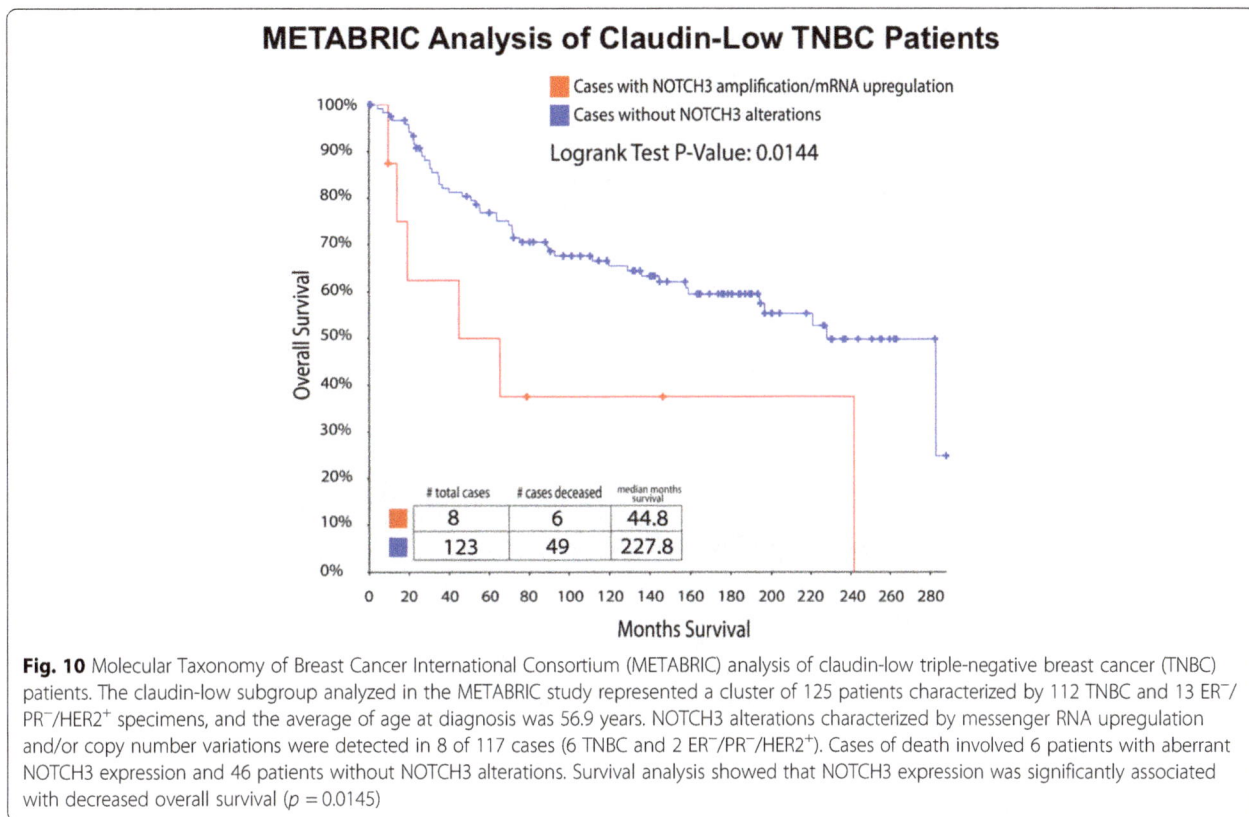

Fig. 10 Molecular Taxonomy of Breast Cancer International Consortium (METABRIC) analysis of claudin-low triple-negative breast cancer (TNBC) patients. The claudin-low subgroup analyzed in the METABRIC study represented a cluster of 125 patients characterized by 112 TNBC and 13 ER−/PR−/HER2+ specimens, and the average of age at diagnosis was 56.9 years. NOTCH3 alterations characterized by messenger RNA upregulation and/or copy number variations were detected in 8 of 117 cases (6 TNBC and 2 ER−/PR−/HER2+). Cases of death involved 6 patients with aberrant NOTCH3 expression and 46 patients without NOTCH3 alterations. Survival analysis showed that NOTCH3 expression was significantly associated with decreased overall survival ($p = 0.0145$)

in promoting their metastatic phenotype. To test this hypothesis, we reduced NOTCH3 expression by lenti-shRNAs in TNBC-M25 cells. Reduction of NOTCH3 expression impaired self-renewal capacity, resulting in a significant shrinkage of TNBC-M25 MPS, confirming the essential role of the NOTCH3 signaling pathway in promoting tumor stemness. Moreover, inhibition of NOTCH3 expression also reduced in vitro the invasiveness of TNBC-M25 cells. These results validated our findings in vMCF-7$^{\Delta Raf1}$ 1GX cells that the NOTCH3 signaling pathway is downstream of AURKA and is required to promote breast cancer cells' aggressiveness.

Finally, our findings in established and patient-derived breast cancer cells led us to analyze the correlation between aberrant expression of NOTCH3 and the overall survival of patients with claudin-low breast tumors using copy number aberrations, somatic mutations, and gene expression data derived from the METABRIC study [30]. We selected claudin-low breast tumors because they represent a molecular subtype of breast cancer with high metastatic proclivity and poor outcome originally identified by gene expression profiling [40]. The claudin-low subgroup analyzed represented a cluster of 125 patients characterized by 112 TNBC and 13 ER−/PR−/HER2+ specimens. Our analysis showed that aberrant NOTCH3 expression was significantly associated with decreased overall patient survival, supporting the pivotal role of

NOTCH3 oncogenic pathway in promoting breast cancer progression.

Conclusions

On the basis of our previous studies [5, 29, 34] and the results presented here, we propose a novel model of breast cancer progression. Primary breast tumors are comprised of heterogeneous subclones where bulk cancer cells exhibit a nontumorigenic AURKA^{low}/NOTCH3^{low} phenotype that lacks EMT, stemness activity, and invasive and metastatic capacity. Increased expression and activation of AURKA will induce EMT and the genesis of AURKA^{high}/NOTCH3^{low} BTIC subclones, and it is unlikely that these subclones will be competent to complete the invasion-metastasis cascade, owing to their limitations in high self-renewal/invasive capacity and seeding in a new microenvironment. Gain of aberrant activation of NOTCH3 oncogenic pathway among BTICs will lead to the clonal expansion of AURKA^{high}/NOTCH3^{high} BT-MICs that have acquired strong stemness properties and the capacity to successfully complete the invasion-metastasis cascade. Conversely, pharmacologic inhibition of NOTCH3 signaling inhibits AURKA^{high}/NOTCH3^{high} BT-MIC seeding to secondary organs and metastatic growth (Fig. 11). Because we identified a novel cross-talk between AURKA and NOTCH3 oncogenic pathways in

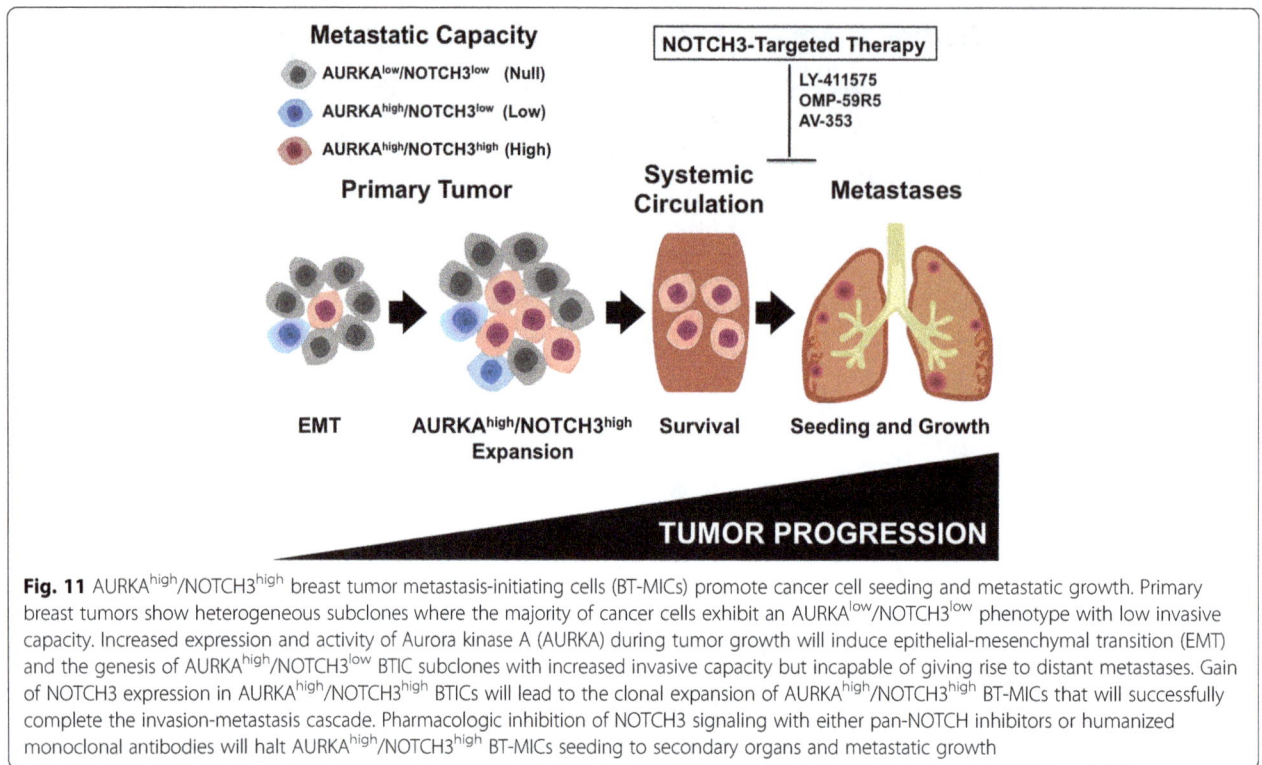

Fig. 11 AURKA[high]/NOTCH3[high] breast tumor metastasis-initiating cells (BT-MICs) promote cancer cell seeding and metastatic growth. Primary breast tumors show heterogeneous subclones where the majority of cancer cells exhibit an AURKA[low]/NOTCH3[low] phenotype with low invasive capacity. Increased expression and activity of Aurora kinase A (AURKA) during tumor growth will induce epithelial-mesenchymal transition (EMT) and the genesis of AURKA[high]/NOTCH3[low] BTIC subclones with increased invasive capacity but incapable of giving rise to distant metastases. Gain of NOTCH3 expression in AURKA[high]/NOTCH3[high] BTICs will lead to the clonal expansion of AURKA[high]/NOTCH3[high] BT-MICs that will successfully complete the invasion-metastasis cascade. Pharmacologic inhibition of NOTCH3 signaling with either pan-NOTCH inhibitors or humanized monoclonal antibodies will halt AURKA[high]/NOTCH3[high] BT-MICs seeding to secondary organs and metastatic growth

promoting breast cancer progression, we speculate that dual-targeted therapy with selective inhibitors of AURKA and NOTCH3 could also represent a novel stemness-targeted therapeutic strategy to successfully eradicate BT-MICs, particularly for the clinical management of highly aggressive TNBCs that currently lack effective U.S. Food and Drug Administration-approved targeted therapies.

Additional files

Additional file 1: Figure S1. Expression of CD24 luminal marker in MPS derived from variant vMCF-7[ΔRaf1] and vMCF-7[ΔRaf1] 1GX-M cells. **a** Immunofluorescence analysis showing representative images of vMCF-7[ΔRaf1] and vMCF-7[ΔRaf1] 1GX-M MPS stained in red with a CD24 monoclonal antibody. Nuclei were stained in blue with 4′,6-diamidino-2-phenylindole (DAPI). **b** Graph showing the average number of CD24-expressing cells from three independent experiments (± SD). (TIFF 6168 kb)

Additional file 2: Figure S2. Transcriptomic characterization of metastatic breast cancer cells. **a** Comparative global gene array analysis between CD24[−/low] (isolated by FACS sorting from vMCF-7[Raf-1] 1GX cells) and vMCF-7[Raf-1] 1GX-M MPS. **b** In silico comparative functional enrichment analysis between CD24[−/low] (isolated from vMCF-7[Raf-1] 1GX cells) and vMCF-7[Raf-1] 1GX-M MPS identified 59 genes involved in nuclear reprograming. (TIFF 6168 kb)

Additional file 3: Figure S3. Expression of genes identified in NOTCH3 metastatic network. Graphs showing the average expression values in sample replicates (from two independent experiments ± SD) for each gene represented in the NOTCH3 metastatic network. (TIFF 6168 kb)

Additional file 4: Figure S4. CRISPR-NOTCH3 breast cancer cells. **a** NOTCH3 gene knockout using CRISPR/Cas9. Lightning bolt symbols indicate the targeted gene double-stranded break (DSB) sites for different sgRNAs F1 and R2. Horizontal arrows show the PCR primers designed at

different chromosomal sites to identify deletions. **b** A PCR product of ~ 650-bp size is amplified upon a successful double-hit by SRISPR/Cas9 system. **c** Secondary screening using internal primers. Internal primers were used to screen for clones with efficient gene knockout. Clone 416 was selected for further verification by immunoblot assay (Fig. 4a). (TIFF 6168 kb)

Additional file 5: Figure S5. NOTCH1 and NOTCH2 expression in TNBC cells. **a** Immunofluorescence analysis showing representative images of MDA-MB-231 and MDA-MB-231 LM TNBC cells stained in green with NOTCH1 and NOTCH2 polyclonal antibodies. Nuclei were stained in blue with DAPI. **b** Graphs showing the average number of NOTCH1- and NOTCH2-expressing cells from three independent experiments (± SD). (TIFF 6168 kb)

Additional file 6: Figure S6. NOTCH1 and NOTCH2 expression in patient-derived TNBC cells. **a** Immunoblot assay showing NOTCH1 and NOTCH2 expression in MDA-MB-231 and patient-derived TNBC-M25 cells. **b** Densitometric analysis showing the percentage of NOTCH1 and NOTCH2 protein levels in TNBC-M25 cells relative to MDA-MB-231 cells. Graph showing the average from three independent experiments (± SD). (TIFF 6168 kb)

Acknowledgements
We acknowledge the Pathology Research Core (PRC) facility of the Mayo Clinic School of Medicine for performing IHC assays and assisting us with the interpretation of the results.

Funding
This study was supported by U.S. Army Medical Research and Materiel Command grant BC022276, Intramural RECDA, The Nan Sawyer Award, and National Cancer Institute (NCI) grant CA214893 (to ABD), NCI grant CA72836 (to JLS), the Mayo Clinic Breast Cancer Specialized Program of Research Excellence (SPORE), NCI grant CA116201 (to JNI, EG, and MEG), the Prospect Creek Foundation (to EG), the Mayo Clinic NIH Relief Fund and NCI grant CA214893 (to TH), and the Mayo Clinic Comprehensive Cancer Center.

Authors' contributions

AAL, MJ, JLS, CH, TH, MG, JNI, and ABD conceived of and designed the experiments. AAL, MJ, LM, CH, MS, LZ, MWG, AA, and ABD performed the experiments. AAL, MJ, JLS, CH, TH, MG, JS, JNI, ML, and ABD analyzed the data. MS, AT, MEG, ADL, JM, CAL, MG, JB, LW, EG, and ABD contributed reagents/materials/analysis tools. AAL, MJ, and ABD wrote the paper. All authors read and approved the final manuscript.

Competing interests

The authors declare that they have no competing interests.

Author details

[1]Department of Biomedical Statistics and Informatics, Mayo Clinic College of Medicine, 200 First Street SW, Rochester, MN, USA. [2]Department of Medical Oncology, Mayo Clinic College of Medicine, 200 First Street SW, Rochester, MN, USA. [3]Department of Biochemistry and Molecular Biology, Mayo Clinic College of Medicine, 200 First Street SW, Rochester, MN, USA. [4]Department of Molecular Medicine, Mayo Clinic College of Medicine, 200 First Street SW, Rochester, MN, USA. [5]Department of Internal Medicine, Mayo Clinic College of Medicine, 200 First Street SW, Rochester, MN, USA. [6]Department of Obstetrics, Gynecology, and Reproductive Sciences, Yale University School of Medicine, New Haven, CT, USA. [7]Department of Cellular and Developmental Biology, University of Palermo, Palermo, Italy. [8]Department of Microbiology and Immunology, Brody School of Medicine, East Carolina University, Greenville, NC, USA. [9]Department of Medicine and Pharmacology, University of Minnesota, Minneapolis, MN, USA. [10]Department of Surgery, Mayo Clinic College of Medicine, 200 First Street SW, Rochester, MN, USA.

References

1. Torre LA, Siegel RL, Ward EM, Jemal A. Global cancer incidence and mortality rates and trends—an update. Cancer Epidemiol Biomark Prev. 2016;25(1):16–27. https://doi.org/10.1158/1055-9965.EPI-15-0578
2. Siegel RL, Miller KD, Jemal A. Cancer statistics, 2017. CA Cancer J Clin. 2017; 67(1):7–30. https://doi.org/10.3322/caac.21387
3. McKee MJ, Keith K, Deal AM, Garrett AL, Wheless AA, Green RL, et al. A multidisciplinary breast cancer brain metastases clinic: the University of North Carolina experience. Oncologist. 2016;21(1):16–20.
4. Small GW, Shi YY, Higgins LS, Orlowski RZ. Mitogen-activated protein kinase phosphatase-1 is a mediator of breast cancer chemoresistance. Cancer Res. 2007;67(9):4459–66.
5. Leontovich AA, Zhang S, Quatraro C, Iankov I, Veroux PF, Gambino MW, et al. Raf-1 oncogenic signaling is linked to activation of mesenchymal to epithelial transition pathway in metastatic breast cancer cells. Int J Oncol. 2012;40:1858–64.
6. Omarini C, Bettelli S, Caprera C, Manfredini S, Caggia F, Guaitoli G, et al. Clinical and molecular predictors of long-term response in HER2 positive metastatic breast cancerpatients. Cancer Biol Ther. 2018;1-8.
7. Mittal S, Sharma A, Balaji SA, Gowda MC, Dighe RR, Kumar RV, et al. Coordinate hyperactivation of Notch1 and Ras/MAPK pathways correlates with poor patient survival: novel therapeutic strategy for aggressive breast cancers. Mol Cancer Ther. 2014;13(12):3198–209.
8. Penton AL, Leonard LD, Spinner NB. Notch signaling in human development and disease. Semin Cell Dev Biol. 2012;23(4):450–7.
9. Li H, Solomon E, Duhachek Muggy S, Sun D, Zolkiewska A. Metalloprotease-disintegrin ADAM12 expression is regulated by Notch signaling via microRNA-29. J Biol Chem. 2011;286(24):21500–10.
10. Ramakrishnan G, Davaakhuu G, Chung WC, Zhu H, Rana A, Filipovic A, et al. AKT and 14-3-3 regulate Notch4 nuclear localization. Sci Rep. 2015;5:8782.
11. Haruki N, Kawaguchi KS, Eichenberger S, Massion PP, Olson S, Gonzalez A, et al. Dominant-negative Notch3 receptor inhibits mitogen-activated protein kinase pathway and the growth of human lung cancers. Cancer Res. 2005; 65(9):3555–61.
12. Bigas A, Guiu J, Gama-Norton L. Notch and Wnt signaling in the emergence of hematopoietic stem cells. Blood Cells Mol Dis. 2013;51(4):264–70.
13. Bui QT, Im JH, Jeong SB, Kim YM, Lim SC, Kim B, et al. Essential role of Notch4/STAT3 signaling in epithelial-mesenchymal transition of tamoxifen-resistant human breast cancer. Cancer Lett. 2017;390:115–25.
14. Shao S, Zhao X, Zhang X, Luo M, Zuo X, Huang S, et al. Notch1 signaling regulates the epithelial-mesenchymal transition and invasion of breast cancer in a Slug-dependent manner. Mol Cancer. 2015;14:28.
15. Mani SA, Guo W, Liao MJ, Eaton EN, Ayyanan A, Zhou AY, et al. The epithelial mesenchymal transition generates cells with properties of stem cells. Cell. 2008;133(4):704–15.
16. Hwang-Verslues WW, Kuo WH, Chang PH, Pan CC, Wang HH, Tsai ST, et al. Multiple lineages of human breast cancer stem/progenitor cells identified by profiling with stem cell markers. PLoS One. 2009;4(12):e8377.
17. Shipitsin M, Campbell LL, Argani P, Weremowicz S, Bloushtain-Qimron N, Yao J, et al. Molecular definition of breast tumor heterogeneity. Cancer Cell. 2007;11(3):259–73.
18. Bolós V, Mira E, Martínez-Poveda B, Luxán G, Cañamero M, Martínez-A C, et al. Notch activation stimulates migration of breast cancer cells and promotes tumor growth. Breast Cancer Res. 2013;15(4):R54.
19. Zanotti S, Canalis E. Notch regulation of bone development and remodeling and related skeletal disorders. Calcif Tissue Int. 2012;90(2):69–75.
20. Liu ZH, Dai XM, Du B. Hes1: a key role in stemness, metastasis and multidrug resistance. Cancer Biol Ther. 2015;16(3):353–9.
21. Chiaramonte R, Colombo M, Bulfamante G, Falleni M, Tosi D, Garavelli S, et al. Notch pathway promotes ovarian cancer growth and migration via CXCR4/SDF1α chemokine system. Int J Biochem Cell Biol. 2015;66:134–40.
22. Mukherjee D, Zhao J. The role of chemokine receptor CXCR4 in breast cancer metastasis. Am J Cancer Res. 2013;3(1):46–57.
23. Shima H, Yamada A, Ishikawa T, Endo I. Are breast cancer stem cells the key to resolving clinical issues in breast cancer therapy? Gland Surg. 2017;6(1):82–8.
24. Fan X. γ-Secretase inhibitor-resistant glioblastoma stem cells require RBPJ to propagate. J Clin Invest. 2016;126(7):2415–8.
25. Yen WC, Fischer MM, Axelrod F, Bond C, Cain J, Cancilla B, et al. Targeting Notch signaling with a Notch2/Notch3 antagonist (tarextumab) inhibits tumor growth and decreases tumor-initiating cell frequency. Clin Cancer Res. 2015;21(9):2084–95.
26. D'Angelo RC, Ouzounova M, Davis A, Choi D, Tchuenkam SM, Kim G, et al. Notch reporter activity in breast cancer cell lines identifies a subset of cells with stem cell activity. Mol Cancer Ther. 2015;14(3):779–87.
27. Takebe N, Nguyen D, Yang SX. Targeting notch signaling pathway in cancer: clinical development advances and challenges. Pharmacol Ther. 2014;141(2):140–9.
28. Previs RA, Coleman RL, Harris AL, Sood AK. Molecular pathways: translational and therapeutic implications of the Notch signaling pathway in cancer. Clin Cancer Res. 2015;21(5):955–61.
29. D'Assoro AB, Liu T, Quatraro C, Amato A, Opyrchal M, Leontovich A, et al. The mitotic kinase Aurora-A promotes distant metastases by inducing epithelial-to-mesenchymal transition in ERα+ breast cancer cells. Oncogene. 2014;33:599–610.
30. Curtis C, Shah SP, Chin SF, Turashvili G, Rueda OM, Dunning MJ, et al. The genomic and transcriptomic architecture of 2,000 breast tumours reveals novel subgroups. Nature. 2012;486(7403):346–52.
31. Leontovich AA, Zhang S, Quatraro C, Iankov I, Veroux PF, Gambino MW, et al. Raf-1 oncogenic signaling is linked to activation of mesenchymal to epithelial transition pathway in metastatic breast cancer cells. Int J Oncol. 2012;40(6):1858–64.
32. Liu T, Yu J, Deng M, Yin Y, Zhang H, Luo K, et al. CDK4/6-dependent activation of DUB3 regulates cancer metastasis through SNAIL1. Nat Commun. 2017;8:13923.
33. Opyrchal M, Salisbury JL, Iankov I, Goetz MP, McCubrey J, Gambino MW, et al. Inhibition of Cdk2 kinase activity selectively targets the CD44+/CD24−/Low stem-like subpopulation and restores chemosensitivity of SUM149PT triple-negative breast cancer cells. Int J Oncol. 2014;45(3):1193–9.
34. Opyrchal M, Gil M, Salisbury JL, Goetz MP, Suman V, Degnim A, et al. Molecular targeting of the Aurora-A/SMAD5 oncogenic axis restores chemosensitivity in human breast cancer cells. Oncotarget. 2017;8(53): 91803–16.

35. D'Assoro AB, Barrett SL, Folk C, Negron VC, Boeneman K, Busby R, et al. Amplified centrosomes in breast cancer: a potential indicator of tumor aggressiveness. Breast Cancer Res Treat. 2002;75(1):25–34.

36. Lingle WL, Barrett SL, Negron VC, D'Assoro AB, Boeneman K, Liu W, et al. Centrosome amplification drives chromosomal instability in breast tumor development. Proc Natl Acad Sci U S A. 2002;99(4):1978–83.

37. Opyrchal M, Salisbury JL, Zhang S, McCubrey J, Hawse J, Goetz MP, et al. Aurora-A mitotic kinase induces endocrine resistance through down-regulation of ERα expression in initially ERα+ breast cancer cells. PLoS One. 2014;9(5):e96995.

38. Sansone P, Ceccarelli C, Berishaj M, Chang Q, Rajasekhar VK, Perna F, et al. Self-renewal of CD133hi cells by IL6/Notch3 signalling regulates endocrine resistance in metastatic breast cancer. Nat Commun. 2016;7:10442.

39. Tomita H, Tanaka K, Tanaka T, Hara A. Aldehyde dehydrogenase 1A1 in stem cells and cancer. Oncotarget. 2016;7(10):11018–32.

40. Iankov ID, Kurokawa CB, D'Assoro AB, Ingle JN, Domingo-Musibay E, Allen C, et al. Inhibition of the Aurora A kinase augments the anti-tumor efficacy of oncolytic measles virotherapy. Cancer Gene Ther. 2015;22(9):438–44.

41. Kwon MJ. Emerging roles of claudins in human cancer. Int J Mol Sci. 2013; 14(9):18148–80.

42. Valastyan S, Weinberg RA. Tumor metastasis: molecular insights and evolving paradigms. Cell. 2011;147(2):275–92.

43. Redig AJ, McAllister SS. Breast cancer as a systemic disease: a view of metastasis. J Intern Med. 2013;274(2):113–26.

44. Lambert AW, Pattabiraman DR, Weinberg RA. Emerging biological principles of metastasis. Cell. 2017;168(4):670–91.

45. Greaves M, Maley CC. Clonal evolution in cancer. Nature. 2012;481(7381): 306–13.

46. Baccelli I, Trumpp A. The evolving concept of cancer and metastasis stem cells. J Cell Biol. 2012;198(3):281–93.

47. Bartholomeusz C, Xie X, Pitner MK, Kondo K, Dadbin A, Lee J, Saso H, Smith PD, Dalby KN, Ueno NT. MEK inhibitor selumetinib (AZD6244; ARRY-142886) prevents lung metastasis in a triple-negative breast cancer xenograft model. Mol Cancer Ther. 2015;14(12):2773–81.

48. Takebe N, Warren RQ, Ivy SP. Breast cancer growth and metastasis: interplay between cancer stem cells, embryonic signaling pathways and epithelial-to-mesenchymal transition. Breast Cancer Res. 2011;13(3):211.

49. Chiba S, Okuda M, Mussman JG, Fukasawa K. Genomic convergence and suppression of centrosome hyperamplification in primary p53−/− cells in prolonged culture. Exp Cell Res. 2000;258(2):310–21.

50. Hosseini H, Obradović MM, Hoffmann M, Harper KL, Sosa MS, Werner-Klein M, et al. Early dissemination seeds metastasis in breast cancer. Nature. 2016; 540:552–8. https://doi.org/10.1038/nature20785

51. Mu X, Isaac C, Greco N, Huard J, Weiss K. Notch signaling is associated with ALDH activity and an aggressive metastatic phenotype in murine osteosarcoma cells. Front Oncol. 2013;3:143.

52. Hamilton SR, Fard SF, Paiwand FF, Tolg C, Veiseh M, Wang C, et al. The hyaluronan receptors CD44 and Rhamm (CD168) form complexes with ERK1,2 that sustain high basal motility in breast cancer cells. J Biol Chem. 2007;282(22):16667–80.

53. Choy L, Hagenbeek TJ, Solon M, French D, Finkle D, Shelton A, et al. Constitutive NOTCH3 signaling promotes the growth of basal breast cancers. Cancer Res. 2017;77(6):1439–52.

3

Identification and validation of single-sample breast cancer radiosensitivity gene expression predictors

Martin Sjöström[1,2*] (iD), Johan Staaf[1], Patrik Edén[3], Fredrik Wärnberg[4], Jonas Bergh[5,6], Per Malmström[1,2], Mårten Fernö[1], Emma Niméus[1,7,8†] and Irma Fredriksson[9,10†]

Abstract

Background: Adjuvant radiotherapy is the standard of care after breast-conserving surgery for primary breast cancer, despite a majority of patients being over- or under-treated. In contrast to adjuvant endocrine therapy and chemotherapy, no diagnostic tests are in clinical use that can stratify patients for adjuvant radiotherapy. This study presents the development and validation of a targeted gene expression assay to predict the risk of ipsilateral breast tumor recurrence and response to adjuvant radiotherapy after breast-conserving surgery in primary breast cancer.

Methods: Fresh-frozen primary tumors from 336 patients radically (clear margins) operated on with breast-conserving surgery with or without radiotherapy were collected. Patients were split into a discovery cohort ($N = 172$) and a validation cohort ($N = 164$). Genes predicting ipsilateral breast tumor recurrence in an Illumina HT12 v4 whole transcriptome analysis were combined with genes identified in the literature (248 genes in total) to develop a targeted radiosensitivity assay on the Nanostring nCounter platform. Single-sample predictors for ipsilateral breast tumor recurrence based on a k-top scoring pairs algorithm were trained, stratified for estrogen receptor (ER) status and radiotherapy. Two previously published profiles, the radiosensitivity signature of Speers et al., and the 10-gene signature of Eschrich et al., were also included in the targeted panel.

Results: Derived single-sample predictors were prognostic for ipsilateral breast tumor recurrence in radiotherapy-treated ER+ patients (AUC 0.67, $p = 0.01$), ER+ patients without radiotherapy (AUC = 0.89, $p = 0.02$), and radiotherapy-treated ER-patients (AUC = 0.78, $p < 0.001$). Among ER+ patients, radiotherapy had an excellent effect on tumors classified as radiosensitive ($p < 0.001$), while radiotherapy had no effect on tumors classified as radioresistant ($p = 0.36$) and there was a high risk of ipsilateral breast tumor recurrence (55% at 10 years). Our single-sample predictors developed in ER+ tumors and the radiosensitivity signature correlated with proliferation, while single-sample predictors developed in ER- tumors correlated with immune response. The 10-gene signature negatively correlated with both proliferation and immune response.

Conclusions: Our targeted single-sample predictors were prognostic for ipsilateral breast tumor recurrence and have the potential to stratify patients for adjuvant radiotherapy. The correlation of models with biology may explain the different performance in subgroups of breast cancer.

Keywords: Breast cancer, Gene expression, Radiotherapy, Radiosensitivity, Radioresistance, Ipsilateral breast tumor recurrence, Local recurrence, Nanostring, nCounter

* Correspondence: Martin.Sjostrom@med.lu.se
†Emma Niméus and Irma Fredriksson contributed equally to this work.
[1]Faculty of Medicine, Department of Clinical Sciences Lund, Oncology and Pathology, Lund University, Lund, Sweden
[2]Department of Haematology, Oncology and Radiation Physics ,Skåne University Hospital, Lund, Sweden
Full list of author information is available at the end of the article

Background

Precision medicine has been the focus of breast cancer research during recent decades. As breast cancers are detected at an earlier stage, and treatment has improved, the emphasis to avoid over treatment in addition to under-treatment has increased [1]. Currently, the majority of primary breast cancers are treated with breast-conserving surgery (BCS), and the patient is generally offered adjuvant treatment. Prognostic and treatment-predictive biomarkers based on traditional immunohistochemical analysis (IHC), or more modern molecular techniques such as gene expression profiling, are presently used to guide the use of adjuvant endocrine therapy, chemotherapy and anti-human epidermal growth factor receptor 2 (HER2)-directed therapy [2]. However, there is no diagnostic procedure to guide treatment with adjuvant radiotherapy (RT) after BCS, which is administered to a majority of patients. This is despite the knowledge that most patients who undergo BCS will remain recurrence-free without RT for at least 10 years, and around 20% will suffer a recurrence within 10 years despite RT [3]. Traditional clinicopathologic variables and IHC markers have been unable to identify patients that could be spared RT [3–5], although studies are ongoing to find patients with risk of recurrence low enough to avoid RT (e.g. the LUMINA study, NCT02653755, and the PRIMETIME study [6]).

Several attempts have been made to create gene expression-based classifiers to predict response to RT after BCS, or to estimate the risk of recurrence with or without RT [7–11]. Most recently, Speers et al. presented the radiosensitivity signature (RSS), a 51-gene random forest model to classify tumors as radioresistant or radiosensitive [12]. Tramm et al. presented a 4-gene classifier predicting the response to RT after mastectomy [13]. Torres-Roca et al. presented the radiosensitivity index (RSI), a linear model based on the rank of genes in individual samples, which has been validated in several cancer types, including breast cancer [8]. The same authors have also advanced the model by combining RSI with the linear-quadratic model for the genomic-adjusted radiation dose (GARD) [14]. In addition, genome instability is considered to sensitize cancer cells to treatment in general, and a centromere and kinetochore gene expression score was suggested to predict response to RT [15]. Taken together, promising results have been presented, but no profile or marker is yet in clinical use.

There are several reasons why gene expression profiles have not been introduced in clinical routine. First, the clinical value and cost-effectiveness has not been proven, as reported profiles lack extensive independent validation, and to date, no prospective trial or studies from existing randomized clinical trials have been presented, except in the mastectomy setting [13]. Second, few of the current profiles have been tested on technical platforms able to handle samples with low-quality RNA, such as RNA extracted from formalin-fixed paraffin-embedded (FFPE) tissue, which would greatly improve the clinical utility. Third, it has been hard to validate profiles across platforms, although attempts have been made by e.g. scaling (RSS) or rank-based models (RSI). Finally, breast cancer is a heterogeneous disease, and the response to RT and the pathways associated with radioresistance may be different in different subgroups. Indeed, this was shown when Torres-Roca et al. presented the follow-up study of RSI in estrogen receptor positive (ER+) and estrogen receptor negative (ER-) breast cancer, and only could validate previous findings in ER- tumors [16]. Interestingly, RSI was recently further shown to correlate with immune response genes, which may partly explain the subgroup-specific performance, as the immune response is more important for prognosis in ER- breast cancer [17, 18].

In this study, we aimed to address these issues and created a targeted radiosensitivity gene expression assay using the Nanostring nCounter platform, which is suitable for low quality RNA samples. Based on the targeted assay, we created single-sample predictors (SSPs) using a k-top scoring pairs (k-TSP) algorithm [19]. The SSPs were validated to be prognostic for ipsilateral breast tumor recurrence (IBTR) in samples of low RNA quality from a study cohort, and further validated in public data. The SSPs also showed potential to stratify patients for RT. In addition, the panel included the genes described for RSS and a surrogate score for RSI (referred to as the 10-gene signature, 10-GS). The previously reported signatures were prognostic for IBTR, and partially predictive of RT, but their performance was dependent on ER status. Finally, we showed that the biology behind the different models and predictors may explain this difference.

Methods

Patients and samples

Patients with invasive breast cancer radically operated on (clear margins) with BCS in three of six healthcare regions in Sweden (South, Uppsala-Örebro and Stockholm) between 1983 and 2009, and with fresh-frozen tissue available, were included ($N = 336$). Patients were excluded if they had multifocal cancer (defined as > 20 mm between tumors), neoadjuvant treatment or prior malignancy (excluding basal-cell carcinoma of the skin, in-situ cervical cancer and other curatively treated cancer at least 5 years prior to the breast cancer). First, all patients with a later IBTR were selected as cases ($N = 144$). Next, controls were selected as patients without any recurrence for at least the same time as the time to IBTR for the matched case, and were matched for RT and ER status ($N = 192$). Median follow-up time was 13.1 years in patients without IBTR (controls), and median time to IBTR was 4.4 years in patients with IBTR (cases). Systemic adjuvant treatment was not part of the inclusion criteria and was administered according to regional treatment programs at the time. The study was approved by the Ethics committee of Lund University (2010-127).

RNA extraction

RNA was extracted from approximately 30 mg of fresh-frozen tissue using commercially available extraction kits, either the Qiagen AllPrep kit, or the Qiagen RNEasy lipid tissue kit, according to the manufacturer's instructions (Qiagen, Hilden, Germany). Cancer content was confirmed microscopically and samples without cancer cells were excluded. Integrity and amount of RNA was measured; samples from one of the three biobank centers had RNA of lower quality, which most likely can be explained by degradation during the transportation process (Additional file 1: Figure S3). We chose to use the higher-quality samples from two centers as a discovery cohort ($N = 172$), and the lower-quality samples from one center as a validation cohort ($N = 164$) (Fig. 1 and Table 1). For more details, see Additional file 2.

Gene expression analysis in the discovery cohort

The discovery cohort ($N = 172$) was analyzed using Illumina HT12 v4 microarrays (Illumina, San Diego, CA, USA). The input amount was 575 ng of total RNA and RNA was hybridized on three plates. Samples were processed in a randomized order and the data have been deposited in Gene Expression Omnibus (GEO) [GEO:GSE103746].

Data analysis in the discovery cohort

All data analyses were performed using R [20] (explicitly outlined in Additional file 2). Briefly, the Illumina HT12 v4 array data was normal-exponential background corrected, quantile-normalized and log2-transformed with an offset of 16 added to avoid negative values using the limma package [21], as previously suggested [22]. The data were batch-effect corrected for hybridization plate and biobank center using the sva package [23]. Probes were filtered based on quality and a variance filter was applied to limit the number of probes to 5000. Tumors were stratified for ER and RT status creating four groups (ER+RT+, ER+RT-, ER-RT+, ER-RT-). A random forest model with double-loop cross-validation and recursive feature elimination based on the caret R package [24] was used to rank the importance of candidate genes, and select the number of genes to analyze further.

Creation of a targeted radiosensitivity gene panel

Genes included in the targeted panel were selected based on the discriminating performance of cases versus controls in the discovery cohort ($N = 155$). We further added the genes included in the previously published signatures RSI ($N = 10$), RSS ($N = 51$) and the genes described by Tramm et al. ($N = 7$) [8, 12, 13]. We also added genes associated with risk of IBTR, radioresistance or breast cancer biology identified in the literature, e.g. hormone and growth factor receptors (*ESR1*, *PGR*), human epidermal growth factor receptor 2 (*ERBB2*), proliferation genes (*MKI67* and *AURKA*), and genes related to hypoxia, apoptosis and DNA repair ($N = 15$) [25–30]. Housekeeping genes were added for purposes of normalization ($N = 13$). In total, 248 genes were selected for the targeted gene expression panel (Fig. 1). For details see Additional file 2, and Additional file 3: Table S1.

Gene expression analysis with the targeted radiosensitivity panel

Both the discovery cohort ($N = 172$) and validation cohort ($N = 164$) were analyzed in a randomized order with a custom-designed Nanostring nCounter panel (Nanostring Technologies, Seattle, WA, USA). The Nanostring probes were created with standard chemistry XT-formulation and designed and produced by the manufacturer (Nanostring). Analysis-ready probes were analyzed using the Prepstation and Digital analyzer (Nanostring), according to the manufacturer's instructions. Gene expression data have been deposited to GEO [GEO:GSE10374]. For more details, see Additional file 2.

Public datasets

Two public datasets were analyzed [11, 31]. The dataset of Servant et al. was based on anlysis using the Illumina HT12 v3 in a cohort of 343 patients who underwent BCS and were treated with RT. The dataset of van de Vijver et al. included 295 patients who underwent either BCS or modified radical mastectomy. RT was given when indicated, and gene expression was analyzed by a 25,000-gene oligonucleotide dual-channel array.

Data analysis in the targeted radiosensitivity panel

The data were quality-filtered resulting in 7 probes and 29 samples removed (4 from the discovery cohort and 25 from the validation cohort) and normalized for positive control probes and housekeeping genes (Fig. 1). SSPs to classify samples as high risk or low risk of IBTR were trained in the discovery cohort in each of the four groups (ER + RT+, ER + RT-, ER-RT+ and ER-RT-) using the switchbox R package [19]. The SSPs were based on a k-TSP algorithm that compares the relative expression of genes within a sample and creates rules in the form gene A > gene B. The default settings of the switchbox package were used, which selects the optimal number of gene pairs by cross-validation in the discovery cohort, [32] and uses the majority vote as cut point without any weighting of the pairs. The model was allowed to use all

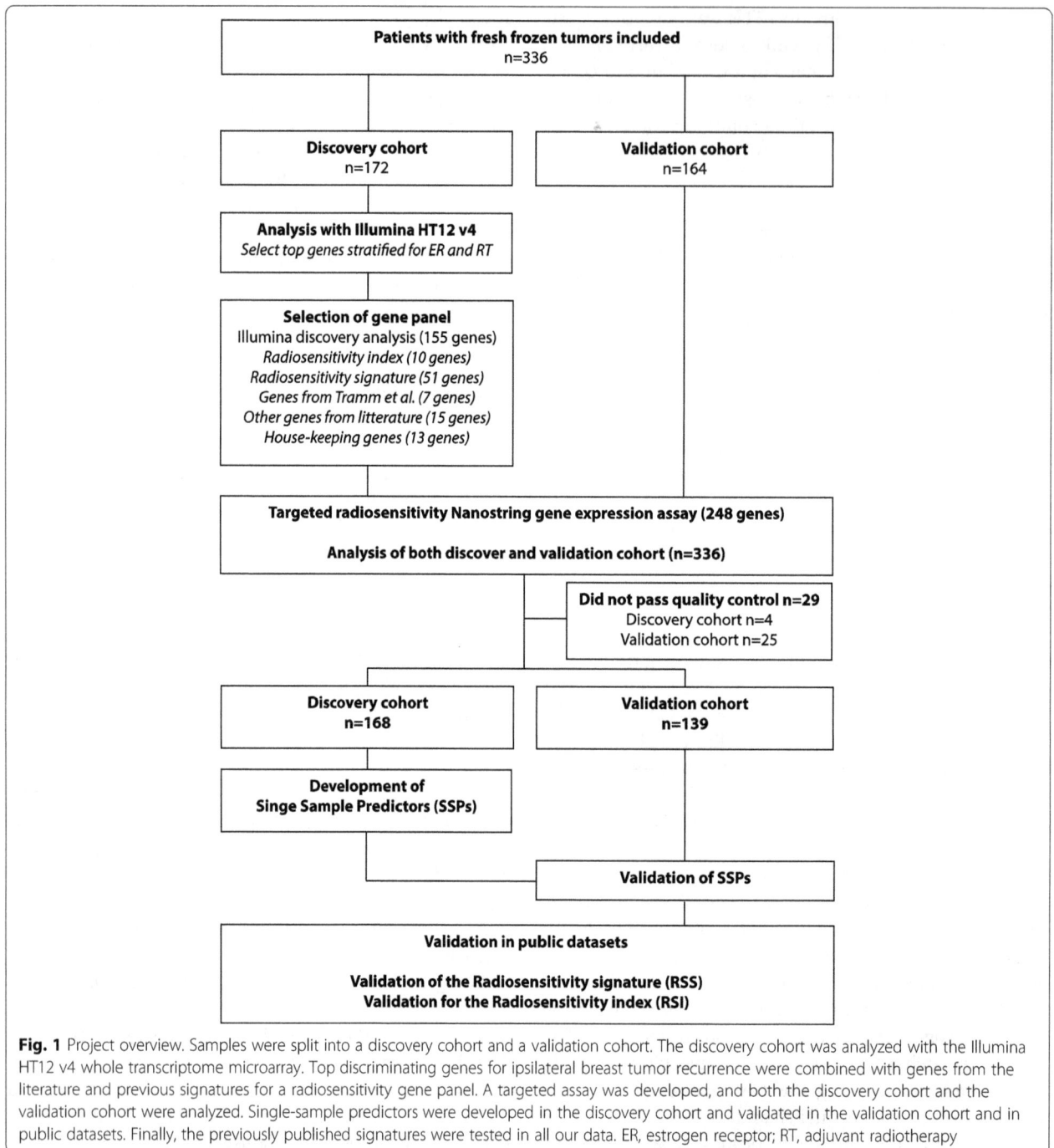

Fig. 1 Project overview. Samples were split into a discovery cohort and a validation cohort. The discovery cohort was analyzed with the Illumina HT12 v4 whole transcriptome microarray. Top discriminating genes for ipsilateral breast tumor recurrence were combined with genes from the literature and previous signatures for a radiosensitivity gene panel. A targeted assay was developed, and both the discovery cohort and the validation cohort were analyzed. Single-sample predictors were developed in the discovery cohort and validated in the validation cohort and in public datasets. Finally, the previously published signatures were tested in all our data. ER, estrogen receptor; RT, adjuvant radiotherapy

genes in the panel and minimum number of pairs to try for training was set to 100 pairs, as gene expression profiles have been shown to be more robust using higher number of genes [33]. This means that at least 200 genes were included in each SSP, and thus a combination of previously published genes and novel genes from our discovery analysis. The full set of genes and pairwise combination is presented in Additional file 4: Table S3. The locked models were then tested in the validation cohort and Kaplan-Meier curves, Cox regression models,

and log-rank p-values were calculated using the survival R package [34], and receiver operating characteristics (ROC) analysis was performed using the pROC R package [35]. Endpoint was IBTR. RSS and a surrogate score for RSI (referred to as 10-GS) were calculated as described in the original publications [8, 12]. Proliferation scores were calculated as the geometric mean of expression values for *MKI67* and *AURKA*. Immune scores were calculated as the geometric mean of genes annotated as part of the immune response (*IRF1, IGKC, STAT1,*

Table 1 Patient and tumor characteristics

	Discovery cohort	Validation cohort
Total number of patients	172	164
Analyzed with Illumina HT12 v4	172	0
Analyzed with targeted nCounter panel	172	164
Included in the final analysis	168	139
Radically operated on (clear margins)		
Yes	168 (100%)	139 (100%)
No	0	0
Extensive intraductal component (EIC)		
Yes	9	7
No	109	90
Missing	50	42
Ipsilateral breast tumor recurrence (IBTR)		
Yes	68	62
No	100	77
Tumor size mm, median (min-max)	18 (3-45)	17 (3-35)
Lymph node status		
Node negative	125 (78%)	108 (78%)
Node positive	35 (22%)	29 (22%)
Missing	8	2
Estrogen receptor (ER) status		
Positive	119 (71%)	118 (85%)
Negative	49 (29%)	21 (15%)
Histological grade		
1	16 (17%)	12 (19%)
2	46 (50%)	24 (39%)
3	30 (33%)	26 (42%)
Missing	76	77
Subtype		
Luminal A	70 (42%)	60 (43%)
Luminal B	42 (25%)	29 (21%)
Basal-like	37 (22%)	12 (9%)
Human epidermal growth factor receptor 2 (HER2)-enriched	19 (11%)	38 (27%)
Radiotherapy		
Yes	116 (69%)	119 (86%)
No	52 (31%)	20 (14%)
Chemotherapy		
Yes	34 (20%)	31 (23%)
No	133 (80%)	105 (77%)
missing	1	3
Endocrine therapy		
Yes	60 (35%)	91 (65%)

Table 1 Patient and tumor characteristics *(Continued)*

	Discovery cohort	Validation cohort
No	108 (65%)	46 (35%)
missing	0	1
Follow-up time		
Median time (range) to IBTR in cases, years	3.7 (0.7-18.7)	4.4 (0.1-22.5)
Median follow-up time (range) in controls, years	13.2 (3.0-19.6)	12.6 (1.7-26.0)

OSMR, CCL19, RelA, IRF8, FGR, TNFRSF1B, C3) in the online gene ontology tool PANTHER [36]. Correlation between the raw scores for the different models, and correlation with proliferation and immune scores were tested with Pearson correlation and linear modeling, with p-values calculated with a test for zero slope. For more details, see Additional files.

Results

Selection of genes and creation of a targeted radiosensitivity assay

The Illumina HT12 v4 microarray whole transcriptome gene expression data from the discovery cohort was analyzed stratified for ER status and RT, creating four groups (ER + RT+, ER + RT-, ER-RT+, ER-RT-). ROC analysis showed that optimal performance of the random forest models was achieved after including around 50 genes per model, with the AUC ranging from 0.67 to 0.85 depending on group, except for the ER-RT+ subgroup, where no signal was found (Additional file 5: Figure S1A and B). Based on their importance in these models, we selected 155 genes for further development of a targeted assay. To investigate the biology represented by the selected genes, hierarchical clustering was performed and correlated with known gene clusters (Additional file 2 and Additional file 6: Figure S2). Genes selected in the ER+ groups included genes correlated with proliferation, and genes selected in the ER- groups included genes correlated with immune response. However, for some clusters no correlation was found, and the genes may thus represent biological pathways more specific for radiosensitivity.

We added genes from three previously described radioresistance gene expression profiles in breast cancer to the 155 genes selected in the discovery analysis: these were the 10 genes forming the RSI, the 51 genes included in the RSS, and the 7 genes described by Tramm et al. [8, 12, 13]. We further added genes identified in the literature (Additional file 3: Table S1). Among these were genes associated with apoptosis (*BCL2*) [25], DNA-repair (*BRCA1*, *BRCA2* and survivin/*BIRC5*) [26, 27], the MET-HGF pair [28], hypoxia (*HIF1* and *HIF2*)

[29] and *WRAP53* [30]. We also added genes important for breast cancer biology or subtyping (*ER, PGR, ERBB2, MKI67, AURKA and FOXC1*). Finally, we added 13 housekeeping genes previously used by Nanostring in their targeted gene expression assays (Additional file 3: Table S1). In total, 248 genes were selected for the development of a targeted assay.

Training and validation of single-sample predictors with the targeted assay

Both the discovery cohort and the validation cohort were analyzed with the targeted Nanostring assay. SSPs were trained in the discovery cohort separately for the four groups created when stratifying for ER status and RT status (ER + RT+, ER + RT-, ER-RT+ and ER-RT-). The locked models were then applied in the validation cohort. The validation AUC was 0.67 for the SSP in ER + RT+ samples, 0.89 for the SSP in ER + RT- samples, and 0.78 for SSP in ER-RT+ samples. The ER-RT- group could not be analyzed due to too few samples ($N = 3$). The SSPs were significantly associated with IBTR in survival analysis (log-rank $p = 0.01$, $p = 0.02$ and $p < 0.001$, respectively) (Fig. 2a). Next, we tested the SSPs in two public datasets and mapped the genes to the respective platforms. Three genes were missing in the Servant et al. dataset, and 34 genes were missing in the van de Vijver dataset, and thus we used the SSPs without these gene pairs. All patients in the Servant et al. dataset were treated with RT and we could thus only test the ER + RT+ and ER-RT+ SSPs. Both SSPs were significantly predictive of IBTR (log-rank $p < 0.001$ and $p = 0.001$, respectively) with corresponding AUC values of 0.62 and 0.74 (Fig. 2b). The van de Vijver dataset also included a majority of RT-treated patients, and we therefore again tested the ER + RT+ and ER-RT+ SSPs. The ER + RT+ SSP was significantly predictive of IBTR ($p = 0.003$, AUC 0.69) but not the ER-RT + SSP ($p = 0.56$, AUC 0.50) (Fig. 2c).

Potential clinical application

The first set of analyses focused on prognostic predictors, either in RT+ patients where our SSPs may be regarded as radioresistance classifiers, or in RT- patients, in which the SSPs may be seen as a method for finding patients without the need for RT. However, the aim was to derive a classifier that can stratify patients into three groups: (1) those that could be spared RT, (2) those that benefit from and should be given RT and (3) those that are intrinsically radioresistant, and where other treatments strategies should be considered besides RT, e.g. mastectomy or more aggressive adjuvant systemic treatment. One strategy to stratify patients into the three treatment groups could be to apply our SSPs consecutively, such that we first determine which patients should be spared RT with a SSP developed in RT- patients. Patients predicted to have low risk of IBTR would be in the "No-RT" group. For the patients predicted as high risk of IBTR, the SSP developed in RT+ patients, and thus potentially testing radioresistance, could next be applied. Patients predicted as having low risk of IBTR when given RT would be in the "Give-RT" group, while patients predicted as having high risk of IBTR even with RT would be in the "More-treatment" group. To test this conceptual idea, we applied our SSPs consecutively in our validation cohort separately for ER+ and ER- tumors. For ER+ tumors, the No-RT group had no benefit from RT ($p = 0.43$), but did not have a low risk of developing IBTR (25% at 10 years) (Fig. 3a). The effect of RT was excellent in the Give-RT group ($p < 0.001$), while RT had no effect in the More-treatment group ($p = 0.36$), and the group had a substantially higher risk of IBTR than the No-RT group (55% at 10 years) (Fig. 3a). In a Cox model of the ER+ tumors including the variable of "Give RT vs No RT" and "Give more treatment", RT and the interaction term between the prediction and RT, the interaction term was significant ($HR_{interaction} = 0.12$ 95% CI 0.03–0.54, $P_{interaction} = 0.001$), further strengthening the treatment predictive potential (Additional file 7: Table S4). Among patients with ER- tumors, only two were RT-untreated, and we could thus only investigate the prognostic effect in this group. Those that were predicted as More treatment had a significantly higher rate of IBTR than the patients in the No-RT and Give-RT groups ($p < 0.001$) (Fig. 3b).

Analysis of previously published profiles in our data

The RSS described by Speers et al. was applied to our entire dataset created with the targeted assay ($N = 307$), as described in the original publication. There was an overall association with IBTR in the full dataset (log-rank $p = 0.001$, AUC of 0.59). When it was applied as stratified for ER and RT, it remained significant only in the ER + RT+ group ($p = 0.001$, AUC 0.58) (Fig. 4a). The 10-GS, based on the genes included in the RSI, was applied to the targeted dataset as described in the original publications, with the change that the cut point was set to the median value, as we have enriched for patients with later IBTR in this dataset. Overall it did not predict the development of IBTR (log-rank $p = 0.20$, AUC 0.51). However, stratified for ER and RT, it performed well in the ER-RT+ group (log-rank $p < 0.001$, AUC 0.70) (Fig. 4b). Further, high risk/radioresistance, as predicted by 10-GS, was significantly associated with fewer instances of IBTR in the ER + RT- group (log-rank $p = 0.02$, AUC 0.70 when changing the direction of analysis) (Fig. 4b).

We also tested the treatment predictive effect of RSS and 10-GS, i.e. the effect of RT in those predicted to be radioresistant or radiosensitive, respectively. Neither of the RSS groups had an effect of RT

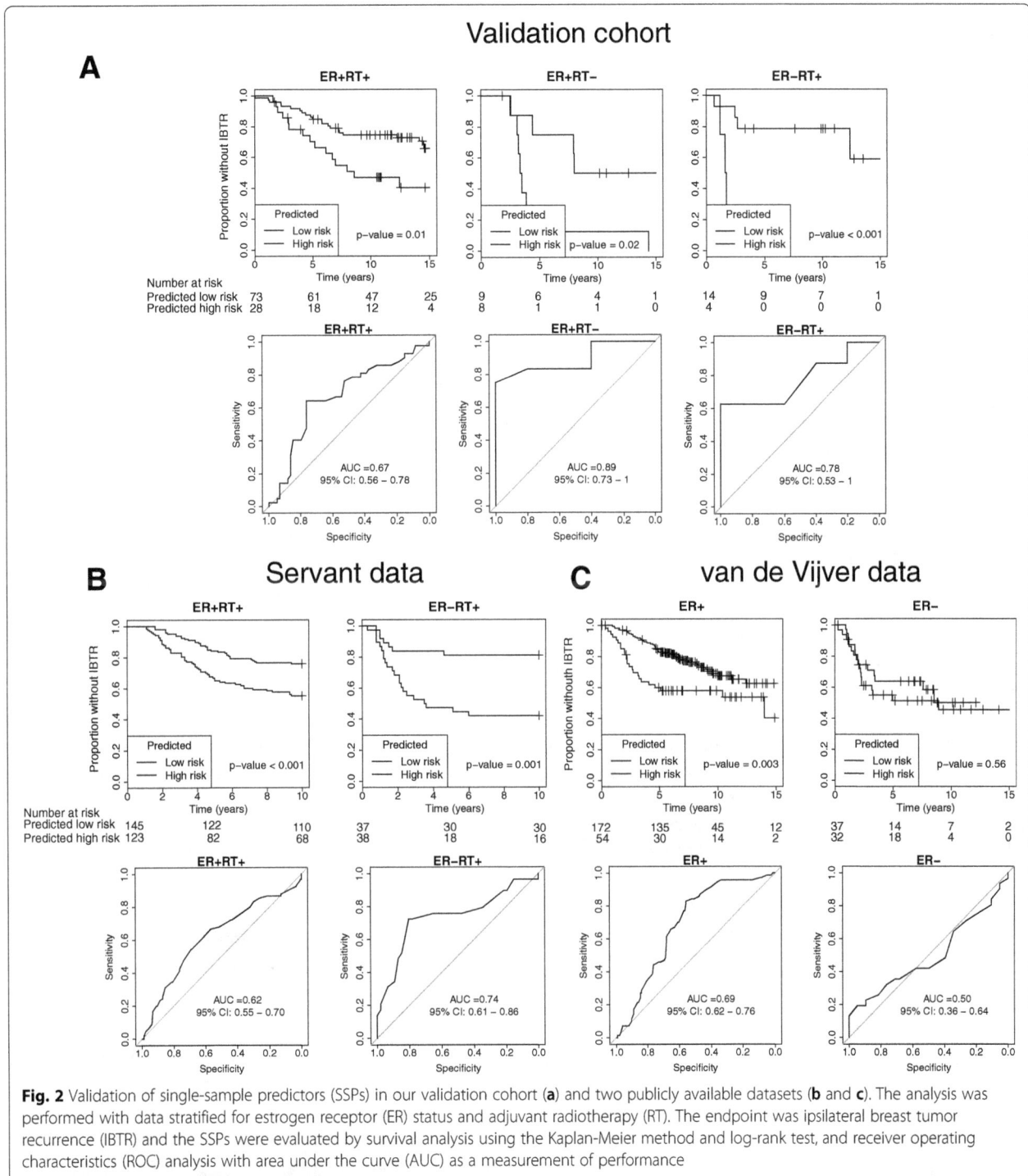

Fig. 2 Validation of single-sample predictors (SSPs) in our validation cohort (**a**) and two publicly available datasets (**b** and **c**). The analysis was performed with data stratified for estrogen receptor (ER) status and adjuvant radiotherapy (RT). The endpoint was ipsilateral breast tumor recurrence (IBTR) and the SSPs were evaluated by survival analysis using the Kaplan-Meier method and log-rank test, and receiver operating characteristics (ROC) analysis with area under the curve (AUC) as a measurement of performance

($p = 0.71$ and $p = 0.93$, respectively) (Fig. 4c). For the 10-GS, on the other hand, RT had no effect on the samples predicted to be radioresistant ($p = 0.23$), while there was an effect of RT in the samples predicted to be radiosensitive ($p = 0.06$) (Fig. 4c). A Cox regression model including RT, 10-GS and the interaction term between RT and 10-GS showed that the interaction term was significantly predictive of IBTR ($p_{interaction} = 0.03$), suggesting a treatment predictive effect of the 10-GS.

Comparison of models and association with underlying biology

To investigate similarities and differences between our newly developed SSPs and the previously published

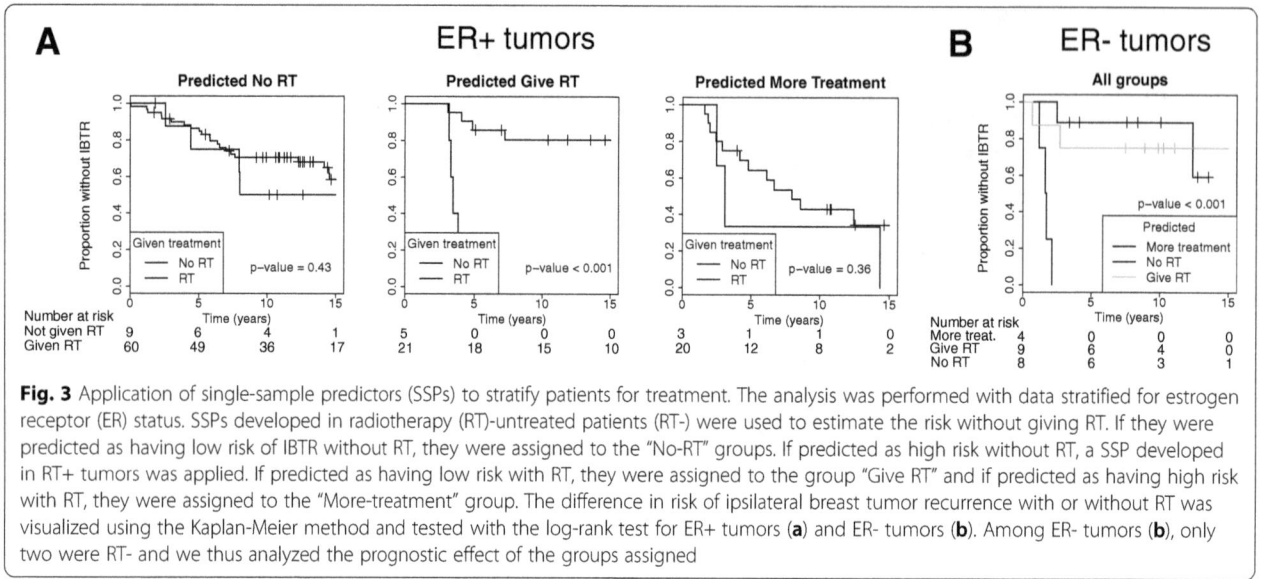

Fig. 3 Application of single-sample predictors (SSPs) to stratify patients for treatment. The analysis was performed with data stratified for estrogen receptor (ER) status. SSPs developed in radiotherapy (RT)-untreated patients (RT-) were used to estimate the risk without giving RT. If they were predicted as having low risk of IBTR without RT, they were assigned to the "No-RT" groups. If predicted as high risk without RT, a SSP developed in RT+ tumors was applied. If predicted as having low risk with RT, they were assigned to the group "Give RT" and if predicted as having high risk with RT, they were assigned to the "More-treatment" group. The difference in risk of ipsilateral breast tumor recurrence with or without RT was visualized using the Kaplan-Meier method and tested with the log-rank test for ER+ tumors (**a**) and ER- tumors (**b**). Among ER- tumors (**b**), only two were RT- and we thus analyzed the prognostic effect of the groups assigned

models, we tested correlation between the raw scores and the models (Fig. 5a-c). Overall, our SSPs were weakly positively correlated with RSS but not with 10-GS.

Cancer cell proliferation is a major biological prognostic determinant in ER+ breast cancer (also largely separating the luminal A from the luminal B subtype), while the immune response has been shown to be important for the prognosis in highly proliferating and ER- breast cancer [18]. To investigate the biology behind the models, we tested correlation between the raw model scores and proliferation and immune response, calculated as the geometric mean of the expression of genes

associated with proliferation and immune response, respectively (details in Additional file 2). Overall, our SSPs were weakly correlated with proliferation, but not immune response (Fig. 5d and g). RSS was also weakly correlated with proliferation and weakly negatively correlated with immune response (Fig. 5e and h). 10-GS, on the other hand, was more strongly negatively correlated with both proliferation and immune response (Fig. 5f and i). Further, stratified for ER and RT, the SSPs developed in ER+ tumors correlated with proliferation and weakly with immune response. Conversely, the SSPs developed in ER- tumors negatively correlated with immune response, but did not correlate with proliferation (Additional file 8: Figure S4).

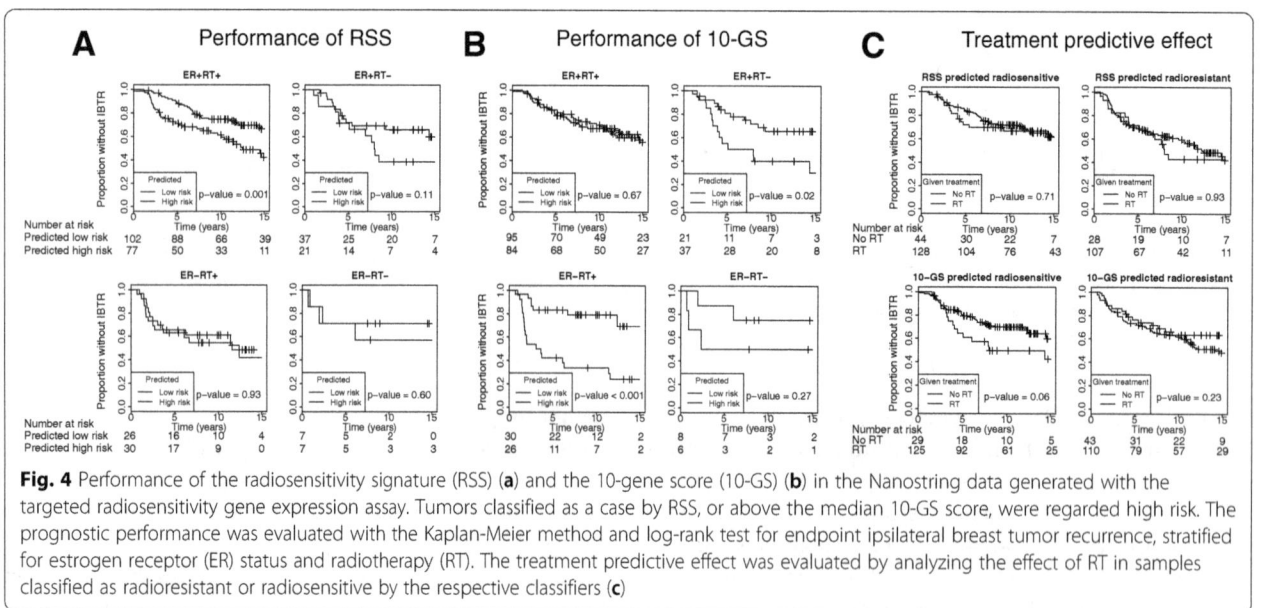

Fig. 4 Performance of the radiosensitivity signature (RSS) (**a**) and the 10-gene score (10-GS) (**b**) in the Nanostring data generated with the targeted radiosensitivity gene expression assay. Tumors classified as a case by RSS, or above the median 10-GS score, were regarded high risk. The prognostic performance was evaluated with the Kaplan-Meier method and log-rank test for endpoint ipsilateral breast tumor recurrence, stratified for estrogen receptor (ER) status and radiotherapy (RT). The treatment predictive effect was evaluated by analyzing the effect of RT in samples classified as radioresistant or radiosensitive by the respective classifiers (**c**)

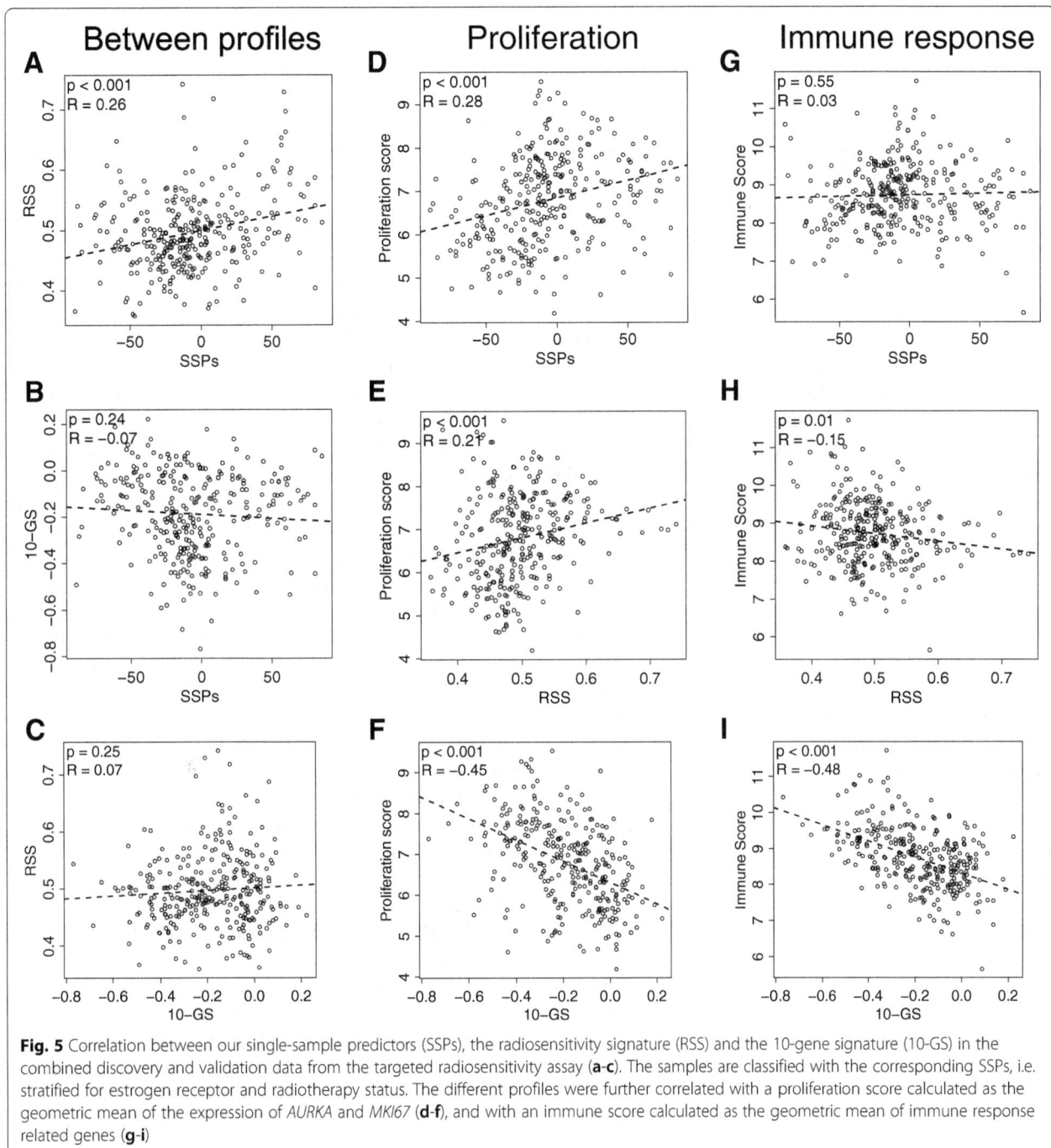

Fig. 5 Correlation between our single-sample predictors (SSPs), the radiosensitivity signature (RSS) and the 10-gene signature (10-GS) in the combined discovery and validation data from the targeted radiosensitivity assay (**a-c**). The samples are classified with the corresponding SSPs, i.e. stratified for estrogen receptor and radiotherapy status. The different profiles were further correlated with a proliferation score calculated as the geometric mean of the expression of *AURKA* and *MKI67* (**d-f**), and with an immune score calculated as the geometric mean of immune response related genes (**g-i**)

Discussion

In this study, we developed and validated single-sample predictors (SSPs) that were prognostic for IBTR using a targeted gene expression panel applicable to samples of lower RNA quality. We presented a conceptual idea of applying the SSPs to stratify patients into treatment groups with promising potential. Two previously published radiosensitivity signatures [8, 12] were also tested in our data, and their performance was found to be ER

status dependent, which may be explained by the biology behind the different models.

The treatment of primary breast cancer is highly individualized, and tests are available to guide the use of adjuvant endocrine therapy, chemotherapy and anti-HER2 treatment [37, 38]. However, no test is available to guide the use of adjuvant RT, which remains an urgent unmet clinical need. Several attempts have been made towards this aim, but no test has been introduced in clinical use.

The reasons are mainly due to lack of follow-up studies and validation, the inability to handle samples of lower RNA quality, which is typical under clinical conditions with FFPE samples, and the models being cohort dependent. We here present a novel approach that aims to overcome these problems, and move individualized RT closer to clinical use. First, we build on previous biological knowledge by including genes that have been previously described in the literature to be associated with radioresistance, in addition to our newly discovered set of genes. Our final SSP models consist of genes from these different sources, and are highly prognostic for IBTR, both in our validation data and in independent public data. In addition, the targeted assay includes genes from two previously described radiosensitivity signatures, giving us an opportunity to validate a surrogate score for these two profiles, which indeed validated our data for prognostication in certain subgroups. Importantly, the 10-GS is also treatment predictive for RT. Second, most clinical samples are handled and stored as FFPE tissue, and an assay able to process RNA extracted from FFPE samples would greatly facilitate its use in the clinical routine. Here, we have used the Nanostring nCounter platform for our targeted assay, which has shown good performance in FFPE samples and is FDA approved for such use with the ProSigna assay [39], and we validated our targeted radiosensitivity panel in samples of lower RNA quality. Although not yet directly tested in FFPE samples, our samples of lower RNA quality are similar to RNA extracted from FFPE samples in terms of the RNA integrity number (RIN) value and fragment length (data not shown). Third, we used a machine learning algorithm, (k-TSP), which relies only on the relative expression of genes within a sample, which should in theory make it both platform and cohort independent. Indeed, we validated the SSPs in data from samples that were partly degraded and in fresh-frozen tumor cohorts, without any scaling or other measure to make the data comparable.

Further, the aim of a radiosensitivity predictor in early breast cancer is to stratify patients and offer treatment only to patients in whom RT had a clinically significant effect. However, patients that do not benefit from RT after BCS may either be those that have the least aggressive tumors, and remain recurrence-free even without RT (requiring de-escalation of treatment), or those with the most aggressive and radioresistant tumors (requiring escalation of treatment). This may complicate the analysis, since those two groups of tumors most likely are not similar in their transcriptomic profiles. The strength of this study is therefore that we developed classifiers that incorporate those two different settings, for not benefitting from RT in treatment stratification, creating three groups for treatment stratification. The results were

highly significant in the validation cohort, although we acknowledge the small sample sizes, and the requirement for further validation in larger cohort studies or randomized trials.

However, although we herein showed reproducible classifiers for IBTR prognostication and RT treatment stratification, it must be noted that RT is an effective treatment, with good cost-effectiveness, and relatively mild side effects, which increases the threshold for withholding RT in patients. High predictive accuracy is required from any radiosensitivity predictor for it to be clinically useful. Although promising, the performance of our proposed SSPs and the previously published profiles show that they are not yet ready for clinical use. Validation in additional cohorts may be a next step, but further classifier development is likely needed. Indeed, our SSPs were intentionally trained with default settings using the majority of genes in the panel as a proof of concept. There is great potential to further optimize the model by e.g. reducing the number of gene pairs, weighting the gene pairs, etc. For a final clinical decision tool, one alternative may be to include additional parameters in the models, i.e. combining gene expression data with clinicopathologic variables, intrinsic subtype, and other molecular data into mixed classifiers. Indeed, combining gene expression data with additional information has already been suggested [16, 40]. However, this dataset, especially after the validation of a locked profile, is not sufficient for extensive classifier optimization or evaluation of other clinicopathologic variables.

One limitation of our study is the case-control sampling, meaning that RT was not administered in a randomized fashion. This limits the analyses that can be performed, and e.g. the proposed method of using a Cox model with an interaction term between treatment and gene expression is not feasible in this dataset [41]. Further, the cohort is enriched for patients with IBTR, and thus the Kaplan-Meier curves and HR estimates presented are not representative of the risk of recurrence in a matched population, and should only be interpreted as an indicator of how the different models perform in the specific datasets. The problem of treatment given in a non-randomized fashion is not unique to our dataset, but is a general problem in the development of a RT predictive gene expression signature. The publicly available datasets analyzed here were also non-randomized for RT, and the dataset presented by van de Vijver included patients who underwent both modified radical mastectomy and BCS, while the dataset by Servant et al. contained only patients who underwent BCS. Also, in the publicly available datasets the proportion of patients given RT differs. In the dataset of Servant et al., all patients were given RT, while this was not the case in the van de Vijver et al. cohort. This may explain the observed differences between the datasets when we validated our SSPs. Further, systemic adjuvant treatment was allowed in our study and was not specified in the inclusion criteria, which may introduce bias and make interpretation of the classifier performance difficult in relation to another cohort. Indeed, there are differences in the proportion of chemotherapy and endocrine therapy given in the discovery and validation cohorts (Table 1, Additional file 9: Table S2). However, to correct for this, we performed multivariate Cox regression adjusting for tumor characteristics (subtype, size and positive lymph nodes) and treatment (endocrine therapy and chemotherapy) for both the prognostic SSPs, and the consecutive use of SSPs to stratify patients for treatment, which did not alter the main findings (Additional file 2).

We chose to develop different models for ER+ and ER- breast cancer, as ER status is a major determinant of breast cancer biology [42]. Indeed, when we analyzed the previously reported RSS and 10-GS signatures, they did not perform uniformly for ER+ and ER- disease. To that end, we investigated the biological basis behind the models, focusing on proliferation and immune response, which have been described as the major drivers of breast cancer biology [18]. As our SSPs developed in ER+ breast cancer were correlated with proliferation, one might suspect that we found the difference between luminal A and luminal B tumors, which is defined mainly by proliferation, and that our high-risk tumors were mainly luminal B tumors. However, the rate of high-risk and low-risk predictions was similar in the luminal A and luminal B tumors. Although the performance of the SSPs were slightly higher in the luminal A tumors, the difference was not significant. Furthermore, multivariate modeling including subtype did not alter the findings (Additional file 2). RSS was also correlated with proliferation, and it was trained in a cohort with mainly ER+ tumors all treated with RT, which may explain why it could only be validated in ER + RT+ patients. More interestingly, the 10-GS could only be validated in ER-RT+ patients, and the ER + RT- tumors predicted as radioresistant actually had a lower risk of IBTR, which is consistent with the follow-up study by the original authors [16]. As the 10-GS is negatively correlated with proliferation and immune response, as was also shown recently by the original authors [17], this means that the tumors predicted as radioresistant were mainly slowly proliferating, and it therefore makes sense that ER+ tumors predicted as radioresistant have a better outcome. Further, the tumors predicted as radioresistant have a lower immune response, which may explain why ER- tumors predicted as radioresistant have a worse outcome, as the immune response is more important in highly proliferating and ER- tumors.

Conclusion

In conclusion, we developed and validated single-sample predictors based on a targeted radiosensitivity gene expression assay using the Nansotring nCounter platform. We validated our SSPs in samples of lower RNA quality, and in external data, with promising results in the treatment stratification of patients. Previously published profiles were also validated in our data, but their performance was highly dependent on the ER status of tumors. Explanations for the difference in performance may be found in the biological basis behind the different classifiers, and should be incorporated in future studies.

Additional files

Additional file 1: Figure S3. Principle component analysis (PCA) plot of the gene expression data from the targeted panel, with coloring for the biobank center from which the samples were derived. Center 1 and 3 had samples of higher quality RNA and constituted the discovery cohort. Center 2 constituted the validation cohort. (PDF 184 kb)

Additional file 2: Supplemental methods, results and discussion. (DOCX 91 kb)

Additional file 3: Table S1. Genes included in the targeted 248-gene panel. (CSV 38 kb)

Additional file 4: Table S3. Genes in the k-top scoring pairs predictors. (XLSX 24 kb)

Additional file 5: Figure S1. Selection of top discrimination genes in the Illumina discovery cohort data. Number of genes in the random forest models are plotted against performance of classifying cases and controls, as measured by cross-validated area under the curve (AUC). The analysis was stratified for estrogen receptor (ER) status and radiotherapy (RT) treatment, and with added patients from other strata, based on a biological rationale as described in the text. (ZIP 171 kb)

Additional file 6: Figure S2. Hierarchical clustering of the top discriminating genes selected in the discovery analysis. Genes are presented as rows, and samples as columns. Colors of the columns represent group after stratification for estrogen receptor (ER) status and radiotherapy (RT), with red representing tumors with later ipsilateral breast tumor recurrence (IBTR, cases). Colors of the rows shows the group in which the gene was selected. Each of the main four clusters were compared with the clusters described by Fredlund et al. and the cluster with the highest association has been marked. (PDF 1308 kb)

Additional file 7: Table S4. Univariable and multivariable Cox -models for the ER+ tumors including variables of "Give RT" vs "No RT" and "Give more treatment", radiotherapy, and the interaction term between the prediction variable and RT. (XLSX 8 kb)

Additional file 8: Figure S4. Correlation of SSP scores with proliferation and immune response. Raw SSP scores are plotted against a proliferation score and an immune score, respectively. SSP scores are calculated based on the four different models developed stratified for estrogen receptor (ER) status and radiotherapy (RT) (ER+RT+, ER+RT-, ER-RT+, ER-RT-). Pearson correlation values and p-value from a linear model with test for zero slope are plotted together with the linear model fit. (PDF 1160 kb)

Additional file 9: Table S2. Patient characteristics per cohort, estrogen receptor status and radiotherapy status. (XLSX 20 kb)

Abbreviations
10-GS: 10-Gene signature; AUC: Area under the curve; BCS: Breast-conserving surgery; CI: Confidence interval; ER: Estrogen receptor alpha; FFPE: Formalin-fixed paraffin-embedded; GEO: Gene Expression Omnibus; HER2: Human epidermal growth factor receptor 2; HR: Hazard ratio; IBTR: Ipsilateral breast tumor recurrence; k-TSP: k-top scoring pairs; PR: Progesterone receptor; ROC: Receiver operating characteristics; RSI: Radiosensitivity index; RSS: Radiosensitivity signature; RT: Adjuvant radiotherapy; SSP: Single-sample predictor

Acknowledgements

We gratefully thank Sara Baker, Carina Forsare, Kristina Lövgren and Anna-Lena Borg for excellent technical assistance. We also thank the biobanks of the South Sweden Breast Cancer Group (SSBCG), the Biobank at the Department of Oncology and Pathology Lund University biobank at Cancer Center Karolinska and the Biobank at Akademiska sjukhuset in Uppsala and Department of Pathology, Uppsala University, for collecting the samples and making them available for studies. We thank the strategic cancer research program BioCARE for providing an excellent learning environment and SCIBLU Genomics for performing the Illumina HT12 anlayses. Finally, we thank Dr. Lori J Pierce, Dr. Felix Y Feng, Dr. Corey Speers, Dr. S Laura Chang and Dr. Shuang G Zhao for assistance in calculating the RSS.

Funding

The study was made possible through support from the Swedish Breast Cancer Association (BRO), the Swedish Cancer Society (Cancerfonden), Region Skåne, Governmental Funding of Research within the Swedish National Health Service (ALF), Mrs. Berta Kamprad Foundation, Anna-Lisa and Sven-Erik Lundgren Foundation, Magnus Bergvall Foundation, the Gunnar Nilsson Cancer Foundation, the Anna and Edwin Berger Foundation, the Swedish Cancer and Allergy Foundation, Skåne County Research Foundation (FOU), Lund University Research Foundation, Skåne University Hospital Resarch Foundation, BioCARE, the King Gustaf V Jubilee Fund, The Cancer Society in Stockholm, and the Marcus and Marianne Wallenberg Foundation.

Authors' contributions

MS, FW, PM, MF, EN and IF conceived of and designed the study. MS, JS and PE performed the data analysis. FW, JB, PM, EN and IF provided the samples. FW, JB, PM, MF, EN and IF provided funding and supervision for the study. All authors analyzed and interpreted the results. All authors revised and approved the manuscript.

Competing interests

Mårten Fernö and Per Malmström declare that they receive research funding and have royalty agreements with PFS Genomics. The other authors declare no potential conflicts of interest related to the present work.

Author details

[1]Faculty of Medicine, Department of Clinical Sciences Lund, Oncology and Pathology, Lund University, Lund, Sweden. [2]Department of Haematology, Oncology and Radiation Physics ,Skåne University Hospital, Lund, Sweden. [3]Department of Theoretical Physics and Computational Biology, Lund University, Lund, Sweden. [4]Department of Surgical Sciences, Uppsala University, Uppsala, Sweden. [5]Department of Oncology and Pathology, Cancer Center Karolinska, Karolinska Institutet, Stockholm, Sweden. [6]Department of Oncology, Karolinska University Hospital, Radiumhemmet, Stockholm, Sweden. [7]Faculty of Medicine, Department of Clinical Sciences Lund, Surgery, Lund University, Lund, Sweden. [8]Department of Surgery, Skåne University Hospital, Lund, Sweden. [9]Department of Molecular Medicine and Surgery, Karolinska Institutet, Stockholm, Sweden. [10]Department of Breast- and Endocrine Surgery, Karolinska University Hospital, Stockholm, Sweden.

References

1. Hosseini A, Khoury AL, Esserman LJ. Precision surgery and avoiding over-treatment. Eur J Surg Oncol. 2017;43(5):938–43.
2. Harbeck N, Gnant M. Breast cancer. Lancet. 2017;389(10074):1134–50.
3. Darby S, McGale P, Correa C, Taylor C, Arriagada R, Clarke M, Cutter D, Davies C, Ewertz M, Godwin J, et al. Effect of radiotherapy after breast-conserving surgery on 10-year recurrence and 15-year breast cancer death: meta-analysis of individual patient data for 10,801 women in 17 randomised trials. Lancet. 2011;378(9804):1707–16.
4. Killander F, Karlsson P, Anderson H, Mattsson J, Holmberg E, Lundstedt D, Holmberg L, Malmstrom P. No breast cancer subgroup can be spared postoperative radiotherapy after breast-conserving surgery. Fifteen-year results from the Swedish Breast Cancer Group randomised trial, SweBCG 91 RT. Eur J Cancer (Oxford, England : 1990). 2016;67:57–65.
5. Sjostrom M, Lundstedt D, Hartman L, Holmberg E, Killander F, Kovacs A, Malmstrom P, Nimeus E, Werner Ronnerman E, Ferno M, et al. Response to radiotherapy after breast-conserving surgery in different breast cancer subtypes in the Swedish Breast Cancer Group 91 Radiotherapy Randomized Clinical Trial. J Clin Oncol. 2017;35(28):3222–9.
6. Kirwan CC, Coles CE, Bliss J. It's PRIMETIME. Postoperative avoidance of radiotherapy: biomarker selection of women at very low risk of local recurrence. Clin Oncol (R Coll Radiol (Great Britain)). 2016;28(9):594–6.
7. Nimeus-Malmström E, Krogh M, Malmström P, Strand C, Fredriksson I, Karlsson P, Nordenskjöld B, Stål O, Östberg G, Peterson C, et al. Gene expression profiling in primary breast cancer distinguishes patients developing local recurrence after breast-conservation surgery, with or without postoperative radiotherapy. Breast Cancer Res. 2008;10(2):R34.
8. Eschrich SA, Fulp WJ, Pawitan Y, Foekens JA, Smid M, Martens JW, Echevarria M, Kamath V, Lee JH, Harris EE, et al. Validation of a radiosensitivity molecular signature in breast cancer. Clin Cancer Res. 2012; 18(18):5134–43.
9. Kreike B, Halfwerk H, Kristel P, Glas A, Peterse H, Bartelink H, van de Vijver MJ. Gene expression profiles of primary breast carcinomas from patients at high risk for local recurrence after breast-conserving therapy. Clin Cancer Res. 2006;12(19):5705–12.
10. Nuyten DS, Kreike B, Hart AA, Chi JT, Sneddon JB, Wessels LF, Peterse HJ, Bartelink H, Brown PO, Chang HY, et al. Predicting a local recurrence after breast-conserving therapy by gene expression profiling. Breast Cancer Res. 2006;8(5):R62.
11. Servant N, Bollet MA, Halfwerk H, Bleakley K, Kreike B, Jacob L, Sie D, Kerkhoven RM, Hupe P, Hadhri R, et al. Search for a gene expression signature of breast cancer local recurrence in young women. Clin Cancer Res. 2012;18(6):1704–15.
12. Speers C, Zhao S, Liu M, Bartelink H, Pierce LJ, Feng FY. Development and validation of a novel radiosensitivity signature in human breast cancer. Clin Cancer Res. 2015;21(16):3667–77.
13. Tramm T, Mohammed H, Myhre S, Kyndi M, Alsner J, Borresen-Dale AL, Sorlie T, Frigessi A, Overgaard J. Development and validation of a gene profile predicting benefit of postmastectomy radiotherapy in patients with high-risk breast cancer: a study of gene expression in the DBCG82bc-cohort. Clin Cancer Res. 2014;20(20):5272–80.
14. Scott JG, Berglund A, Schell MJ, Mihaylov I, Fulp WJ, Yue B, Welsh E, Caudell JJ, Ahmed K, Strom TS, et al. A genome-based model for adjusting radiotherapy dose (GARD): a retrospective, cohort-based study. Lancet Oncol. 2017;18(2):202–11.
15. Zhang W, Mao JH, Zhu W, Jain AK, Liu K, Brown JB, Karpen GH. Centromere and kinetochore gene misexpression predicts cancer patient survival and response to radiotherapy and chemotherapy. Nat Commun. 2016;7:12619.
16. Torres-Roca JF, Fulp WJ, Caudell JJ, Servant N, Bollet MA, van de Vijver M, Naghavi AO, Harris EE, Eschrich SA. Integration of a radiosensitivity molecular signature Into the assessment of local recurrence risk in breast cancer. Int J Radiat Oncol Biol Phys. 2015;93(3):631–8.
17. Strom T, Harrison LB, Giuliano AR, Schell MJ, Eschrich SA, Berglund A, Fulp W, Thapa R, Coppola D, Kim S, et al. Tumour radiosensitivity is associated with immune activation in solid tumours. Eur J Cancer. 2017;84:304–14.
18. Nagalla S, Chou JW, Willingham MC, Ruiz J, Vaughn JP, Dubey P, Lash TL, Hamilton-Dutoit SJ, Bergh J, Sotiriou C, et al. Interactions between immunity, proliferation and molecular subtype in breast cancer prognosis. Genome Biol. 2013;14(4):R34.

19. Afsari B, Fertig EJ, Geman D, Marchionni L. switchBox: an R package for k-Top Scoring Pairs classifier development. Bioinformatics (Oxford, England). 2015;31(2):273–4.

20. R Core Team. R: A language and environment for statistical computing. R Foundation for Statistical Computing, Vienna, Austria. 2016. https://www.R-project.org/.

21. Ritchie ME, Phipson B, Wu D, Hu Y, Law CW, Shi W, Smyth GK. limma powers differential expression analyses for RNA-sequencing and microarray studies. Nucleic Acids Res. 2015;43(7):e47.

22. Ritchie ME, Dunning MJ, Smith ML, Shi W, Lynch AG. BeadArray expression analysis using bioconductor. PLoS Comput Biol. 2011;7(12):e1002276.

23. Leek JT, Johnson WE, Parker HS, Fertig EJ, Jaffe AE, Storey JD, Zhang Y, Torres LC: sva: Surrogate variable analysis. R package version 3.18.0. 2017.

24. Max K: Contributions from Jed Wing, Steve Weston, Andre Williams, Chris Keefer, Allan Engelhardt, Tony Cooper, Zachary Mayer, Brenton Kenkel, the R Core Team, Michael Benesty, Reynald Lescarbeau, Andrew Ziem, Luca Scrucca, Yuan Tang and Can Candan. (2016). caret: Classification and Regression Training. R package version 6.0-68. In.

25. Kyndi M, Sorensen FB, Knudsen H, Alsner J, Overgaard M, Nielsen HM, Overgaard J. Impact of BCL2 and p53 on postmastectomy radiotherapy response in high-risk breast cancer. A subgroup analysis of DBCG82 b&c. Acta oncologica (Stockholm, Sweden). 2008;47(4):608–17.

26. Nilsson MP, Hartman L, Kristoffersson U, Johannsson OT, Borg A, Henriksson K, Lanke E, Olsson H, Loman N. High risk of in-breast tumor recurrence after BRCA1/2-associated breast cancer. Breast Cancer Res Treat. 2014;147(3):571–8.

27. Vequaud E, Desplanques G, Jezequel P, Juin P, Barille-Nion S. Survivin contributes to DNA repair by homologous recombination in breast cancer cells. Breast Cancer Res Treat. 2016;155(1):53–63.

28. Veenstra C, Perez-Tenorio G, Stelling A, Karlsson E, Mirwani SM, Nordenskoljd B, Fornander T, Stal O. Met and its ligand HGF are associated with clinical outcome in breast cancer. Oncotarget. 2016;7(24):37145–59.

29. Trastour C, Benizri E, Ettore F, Ramaioli A, Chamorey E, Pouyssegur J, Berra E. HIF-1alpha and CA IX staining in invasive breast carcinomas: prognosis and treatment outcome. Int J Cancer. 2007;120(7):1451–8.

30. Garvin S, Tiefenbock K, Farnebo L, Thunell LK, Farnebo M, Roberg K. Nuclear expression of WRAP53beta is associated with a positive response to radiotherapy and improved overall survival in patients with head and neck squamous cell carcinoma. Oral Oncol. 2015;51(1):24–30.

31. van de Vijver MJ, He YD, van't Veer LJ, Dai H, Hart AA, Voskuil DW, Schreiber GJ, Peterse JL, Roberts C, Marton MJ, et al. A gene-expression signature as a predictor of survival in breast cancer. N Engl J Med. 2002;347(25):1999–2009.

32. Afsari B, Braga-Neto UM, Geman D. Rank discriminants for predicting phenotypes from RNA expression. Ann Appl Stat. 2014;8(3):1469–91.

33. Lauss M, Ringner M, Hoglund M. Prediction of stage, grade, and survival in bladder cancer using genome-wide expression data: a validation study. Clin Cancer Res. 2010;16(17):4421–33.

34. Therneau T: A package for surival analysis in S. version 2.38. 2015. http://CRANR-project.org/package=survival.

35. Robin X, Turck N, Hainard A, Tiberti N, Lisacek F, Sanchez JC, Muller M. pROC: an open-source package for R and S+ to analyze and compare ROC curves. BMC Bioinformatics. 2011;12:77.

36. Mi H, Huang X, Muruganujan A, Tang H, Mills C, Kang D, Thomas PD. PANTHER version 11: expanded annotation data from Gene Ontology and Reactome pathways, and data analysis tool enhancements. Nucleic Acids Res. 2017;45(D1):D183–d189.

37. Krop I, Ismaila N, Andre F, Bast RC, Barlow W, Collyar DE, Hammond ME, Kuderer NM, Liu MC, Mennel RG, et al. Use of biomarkers to guide decisions on adjuvant systemic therapy for women with early-stage invasive breast cancer: American Society of Clinical Oncology clinical practice guideline focused update. J Clin Oncol. 2017;35(24):2838–47.

38. Harris LN, Ismaila N, McShane LM, Andre F, Collyar DE, Gonzalez-Angulo AM, Hammond EH, Kuderer NM, Liu MC, Mennel RG, et al. Use of biomarkers to guide decisions on adjuvant systemic therapy for women with early-stage invasive breast cancer: American Society of Clinical Oncology clinical practice guideline. J Clin Oncol. 2016;34(10):1134–50.

39. Nielsen T, Wallden B, Schaper C, Ferree S, Liu S, Gao D, Barry G, Dowidar N, Maysuria M, Storhoff J. Analytical validation of the PAM50-based Prosigna Breast Cancer Prognostic Gene Signature Assay and nCounter Analysis System using formalin-fixed paraffin-embedded breast tumor specimens. BMC Cancer. 2014;14:177.

40. Kamath VP, Torres-Roca JF, Eschrich SA. Integrating biological covariates into gene expression-based predictors of radiation sensitivity. International journal of genomics. 2017;2017:6576840.

41. Tian L, Alizadeh AA, Gentles AJ, Tibshirani R. A simple method for estimating interactions between a treatment and a large number of covariates. J Am Stat Assoc. 2014;109(508):1517–32.

42. Gruvberger S, Ringner M, Chen Y, Panavally S, Saal LH, Borg A, Ferno M, Peterson C, Meltzer PS. Estrogen receptor status in breast cancer is associated with remarkably distinct gene expression patterns. Cancer Res. 2001;61(16):5979–84.

4

Syndecan-1 induction in lung microenvironment supports the establishment of breast tumor metastases

Colleen Chute[1], Xinhai Yang[1], Kristy Meyer[1], Ning Yang[1], Keelin O'Neil[1], Ildiko Kasza[6], Kevin Eliceiri[3,4,5], Caroline Alexander[3,6] and Andreas Friedl[1,2,3]*

Abstract

Background: Syndecan-1 (Sdc1), a cell surface heparan sulfate proteoglycan normally expressed primarily by epithelia and plasma cells, is aberrantly induced in stromal fibroblasts of breast carcinomas. Stromal fibroblast-derived Sdc1 participates in paracrine growth stimulation of breast carcinoma cells and orchestrates stromal extracellular matrix fiber alignment, thereby creating a migration and invasion-permissive microenvironment. Here, we specifically tested the role of stromal Sdc1 in metastasis.

Methods: The metastatic potential of the aggressive mouse mammary carcinoma cell lines, 4T1 and E0776, was tested in wild-type and genetically Sdc1-deficient host animals. Metastatic lesions were characterized by immunohistochemical analysis.

Results: After orthotopic inoculation, the lung metastatic burden was reduced in Sdc1−/− animals by 97% and more than 99%, in BALB/cJ and C57BL/6 animals, respectively. The difference in metastatic efficiency was maintained when the tumor cells were injected into the tail vein, suggesting that host Sdc1 exerts its effect during later stages of the metastatic cascade. Co-localization studies identified Sdc1 expression in stromal fibroblasts within the metastatic microenvironment and in normal airway epithelial cells but not in other cells (endothelial cells, α-smooth muscle actin positive cells, leucocytes, macrophages). The Ki67 proliferation index and the rate of apoptosis of the metastatic tumor cells were diminished in Sdc1−/− vs. Sdc1+/+ animals, and leucocyte density was indistinguishable. Sdc1-mediated metastatic efficiency was abolished when the animals were housed at a thermoneutral ambient temperature of 31 °C, suggesting that the host Sdc1 effect on metastasis requires mild cold stress.

Conclusions: In summary, Sdc1 is induced in the lung microenvironment after mammary carcinoma cell dissemination and promotes outgrowth of metastases in a temperature-dependent manner.

Keywords: Breast cancer, Proteoglycans, Extracellular matrix, Metastasis, Syndecan, Tumor microenvironment

Background

The fate of patients with breast carcinoma is determined by distant organ metastasis rather than local disease. Life-threatening metastatic disease is the end-result of a cascade of events that begins with local invasion at the primary site and includes intravasation (into blood or lymphatic vessels), survival of tumor cells in the blood stream, extravasation at the distant site and outgrowth of metastatic lesions. Recent experimental evidence suggests that the initial steps of the metastatic cascade including intravasation occur relatively early and that the later events like extravasation and outgrowth may be the rate-limiting steps [1]. Although progress has been made in uncovering the biology of some aspects of metastatic spread, little is known about the mechanisms that govern adaptation of disseminated tumor cells to the environment at the distant site and determine whether tumor

* Correspondence: afriedl@wisc.edu
[1]Department of Pathology and Laboratory Medicine, University of Wisconsin-Madison, 6051 WIMR, MC-2275, 1111 Highland Avenue, Madison, WI 53705, USA
[2]Pathology and Laboratory Medicine Service, William S. Middleton Memorial Veterans Hospital, Department of Veterans Affairs Medical Center, Madison, WI, USA
Full list of author information is available at the end of the article

cells remain dormant or actively proliferate. It is becoming increasingly clear, however, that complex reciprocal interactions between disseminated tumor cells and cells in the local microenvironment (i.e. the metastatic niche) play a crucial role [2].

Syndecan-1 (Sdc1; CD138) belongs to a four-member family of transmembrane heparan sulfate proteoglycans (HSPGs) with roles in cell signaling and adhesion [3]. Sdc1 is primarily expressed by plasma cells and epithelia, including their malignant counterparts. During development, Sdc1 expression is transiently induced in the mesenchyme and the molecule participates in paracrine epithelial-stromal interactions [4]. This mesenchymal induction is recapitulated during malignant progression, when Sdc1 expression is observed in stromal fibroblasts in a variety of carcinoma types, including carcinoma of the breast [5, 6]. Little is known about the mechanisms of Sdc1 induction in fibroblasts. Induction in mesenchymal cells has been linked to transcriptional regulation by members of the fibroblast growth factor family and extracellular matrix (ECM) constituents [7–9].

Via its heparan sulfate (HS) chains, Sdc1 engages HS-binding ligands including growth factors and many ECM molecules - a property it shares with other HSPGs [10]. Sdc1 core protein-specific binding interactions have been observed between its ectodomain and both integrin cell adhesion receptor subunits and receptor tyrosine kinases [11]. Thus, Sdc1 can act as a cell surface docking station that complexes integrins and receptor tyrosine kinases (RTKs), thereby regulating cell growth and migration. Mice globally deficient in Sdc1 have a surprisingly subtle phenotype with a slight reduction in size and weight noted as the sole abnormality [12]. When the animals are challenged, however, some defects emerge. Sdc1-knockout animals display impaired inflammatory responses, have altered vascular and endothelial cell biology and reduced tumorigenesis [12–15]. Sdc1 deficiency also affects lipid metabolism and reduces tolerance to cold temperatures [16, 17]. The molecular pathways involved in these impaired responses to external and intrinsic challenges are largely unknown.

In breast cancer, Sdc1 generally acts as a promoter of tumor growth and progression via multiple mechanisms of action. Sdc1 overexpression in human breast carcinoma correlates with a proliferative state and poor prognosis [18–20]. Mice lacking Sdc1 are relatively resistant to Wnt-induced tumorigenesis, demonstrating that Sdc1 is required for efficient tumorigenesis in this model [12]. Sdc1 modulates tumor progression not only by cell autonomous but also by cell non-autonomous mechanisms. The induction of Sdc1 expression in stromal fibroblasts triggers a reciprocal paracrine signaling loop that stimulates mammary tumor growth in vitro and in vivo [6, 21, 22]. Sdc1-expressing stromal fibroblasts also produce an altered ECM that is characterized by parallel, aligned fibronectin and collagen fibers, which is permissive to carcinoma cell migration and invasion and thus has the potential to promote carcinoma spread and metastasis [23]. Collectively, these findings indicate that Sdc1 can stimulate breast tumor progression at many levels.

The goal of the present study was to determine whether host Sdc1 plays a role in mammary carcinoma metastasis. We showed in two mouse strains that the ability of highly aggressive mouse mammary tumor cells to metastasize to the lungs is diminished in mice genetically deficient in Sdc1. The requirement of host Sdc1 for efficient metastasis is observed both after orthotopic (fat pad) and tail vein injection, which suggests that Sdc1 exerts its effect during the later steps of the metastatic cascade; likely during metastatic outgrowth. Elevating the ambient housing temperature to thermo-neutral conditions reduces metastatic efficiency in the wild-type animals to the level seen in the knockout mice suggesting that the Sdc1-dependent mechanism affecting metastasis is regulated by the thermogenic response.

Methods

Cells, tumor cell inoculations and scoring of metastases

The 4T1 mouse mammary tumor cells were obtained from American Type Culture Collection (ATCC) (CRL-2539) and were cultured in Roswell Park Memorial Institute (RPMI-1640) medium supplemented with 10% fetal bovine serum (FBS), 2 mM L-glutamine and penicillin/streptomycin at 37 °C in a humidified atmosphere containing 5% CO_2. E0771 cells were purchased from CH3 Biosystems (Amhurst, NY, USA) and cultured in RPMI-1640 medium supplemented with 10 mmol/L HEPES and 10% FBS.

For fat pad injections, mice were anesthetized with isoflurane, and 1×10^7 cells in 10 μL serum-free DMEM were injected into the exposed, intact left 4th mammary fat pad as described by Miller [24]. Tumors were allowed to grow for 30 days and then mice were humanely killed. For tail vein injections, mice were anesthetized with isoflurane and 1×10^5 tumor cells in 100 μL serum-free DMEM were injected through the tail-vein. After 15 days the mice were humanely killed.

Upon completion of in vivo studies, tissues were fixed for 12–18 h in 10% buffered formalin (Fisher Scientific, Waltham, MA, USA) and then processed and paraffin embedded. Hematoxylin and eosin (H&E)-stained slides were either scanned with an Aperio whole slide scanner (Leica Biosystems) or imaged by stitching individually acquired images in Adobe Photoshop. The image files showing sections of whole lungs were carefully examined and metastatic lesions were circled with an Intuos input device (Wacom) and analyzed using a combination of Photoshop (Adobe) and ImageJ (https://imagej.nih.gov/ij/). The number of lesions per mouse, the area of each lesion and the area of total lung tissue were recorded. Tumor burden per mouse was defined as area of lung tissue occupied by metastases divided by total area of lung.

Antibodies, reagents and histological analyses

The antibodies used for immunolabeling are listed in Table 1. Mouse tissue sections were deparaffinized and for antigen retrieval, sections were boiled with citrate buffer (pH 6.0, with 0.05% Tween 20) for 30 min. In preparation for fibroblast antibody (ER-TR7) labeling, sections of mouse tissues were incubated with proteinase K working solution (20 μg/mL in TE buffer, pH 8.0) for 15 min at 37 °C. After incubation with the primary antibody (overnight at 4 °C for CD4 and CD8; 1 h at room temperature for all others) and extensive washes, horseradish peroxidase chromogenic (Ventana) or TSA Plus fluorescence detection kits (Perkin Elmer) were applied following the manufacturers' instructions. Nuclei were counterstained with hematoxylin, 4′,6-diamidino-2-phenylindole (DAPI) or Hoechst 33,342 as appropriate. CD4 and CD8 positive T cells were visualized in mouse lung sections by manual immunolabeling using the ImmPRESS polymer detection system and diaminobenzidine (DAB) substrate.

For the analysis of immunohistochemically labeled slides, at least five images per sample were captured using a brightfield or epifluorescence microscope depending on the label. The signal was quantified using a combination of Photoshop and the National Institutes of Health (NIH) ImageJ software [25]. Lymphocyte densities were determined in the two smallest and the two largest metastases per lung. CD4+ and CD8+ lymphocyte densities were expressed as cells per 1×10^6 pixel (megapixel) on images taken at consistent magnification and resolution.

Tissue sections of breast carcinoma metastases to the lung from seven patients were analyzed by dual-labeling for Sdc1 and the mesenchymal/stromal marker vimentin. After deparaffinization and heat-induced antigen retrieval (EDTA, pH 8.5, 95–100 °C for 44 min), sections were incubated with anti-Sdc1 antibody (8 min, 37 °C). After rinsing, the UltraMap mouse HRP polymer kit (Ventana, Roche, catalog number 760–4313) was applied following the manufacturer's instructions. After denaturing and rinsing, a second round of epitope retrieval under the same conditions was applied and the sections were incubated with prediluted anti-vimentin antibody (16 min, 37 °C). After rinsing, HQ mouse polymer (Roche, 760–4814) was applied for 8 min at 37 °C followed by anti-HQ HRP solution (Roche, 760–4820; 8 min, 37 °C) and the Discovery purple detection kit (Roche 760–229).

Second harmonic generation microscopy and collagen fiber analysis

H&E-stained histology slides were placed onto an optical workstation built around a Nikon Eclipse TE300 (Nikon, Tokyo, Japan), with a Ti:Sapphire laser (Spectra-Physics-Millennium/Tsunami, Mountain View CA, USA) excitation source tuned to 890 nm, focused with a × 20 Nikon Plan Apo lens (Nikon, Tokyo, Japan), filtered with a 445 nm narrow band pass filter (TFI Technologies, Greenfield MA, USA) and back-scattered second harmonic generation (SHG) signal collected with an H7422P-40 detector (Hamamatsu, Japan) and WiscScan acquisition software developed at the Laboratory for

Table 1 Antibodies used for immunolabeling

Antigen	Dilution	Specificity	Catalog number	Company/source
CD31	1:400	Goat anti-mouse	AF3628	R&D Systems, Minneapolis, MN, USA
Ki67	1:1000	Mouse anti-human, clone MIB-1	M7240	Dako, Santa Clara, CA, USA
Ki67	1:200	Rabbit anti-mouse, clone D3B5	12,202	Cell Signaling Technology, Danvers, MA, USA
αSMA	1:500	Rabbit anti-mouse	ab5694	Abcam, Cambridge, MA, USA
F4/80	1:400	Rabbit anti-mouse	ab100790	Abcam
ER-TR7	1:200	Rat anti-mouse	ab51824	Abcam
CD45	1:200	Rabbit anti-mouse	ab10558	Abcam
CD68	1:200	Rat anti-mouse	MCA1957T	BioRad
Cleaved Caspase-3	1:200	Rabbit anti-mouse, D175	9661	Cell Signaling Technology
Sdc-1	1:200	Rat anti-mouse	NA	gift from Dr. Rapraeger
Sdc-1	1:100	Mouse anti-human, clone B-B4	MCA681H	Serotec
Vimentin	predilute	Mouse anti-human	790–2917	Ventana Medical Systems, Tucson, AZ, USA
CD4	1:200	Rabbit anti-mouse	ab221775	Abcam
CD8	1:750	Rabbit anti-mouse	ab209775	Abcam

Optical and Computational Instrumentation (LOCI), University of Wisconsin, Madison, WI, USA).

Collagen fiber angles relative to the tumor boundary were analyzed using CTFIRE and the MATLAB-based CurveAlign software developed by the LOCI (http://loci.wisc.edu/software/curvealign) [26]. Intensity of the SHG images was analyzed using the NIH ImageJ Software (as described above).

Animals

The generation of Sdc1−/− mice has been described previously [12]. Mice were housed at room temperature (20–23 °C unless otherwise specified) and maintained on a 12-h light and dark cycle with free access to water and food. For all tumor experiments, 6–8 week old female mice were used. For experiments using thermo-neutral conditions, mice were individually caged and housed at 31 °C (± 1 °C) for 2 weeks in a controlled environment prior to cell inoculation and were monitored daily.

Statistics

Data are expressed as mean +/− standard error of the mean. Statistical tests were performed using MStat, which is JAVA-based software written at the University of Wisconsin-Madison (http://mcardle.wisc.edu/mstat/) or Prism 7 software (Graphpad). The non-parametric Wilcoxon rank sum, Mann-Whitney or Kruskal-Wallis tests were used unless stated otherwise and p values less than 0.05 were deemed to be significant.

Results

Host Sdc1 is required for efficient metastasis of mammary carcinoma cells to the lungs

Both carcinoma-cell-associated and stromal Sdc1 can promote breast carcinoma growth [6, 20, 22] but the importance of this proteoglycan in breast carcinoma progression and metastatic spread is less clear. To determine the role of host Sdc1 in metastasis, we inoculated highly metastatic 4T1 mouse mammary carcinoma cells into the mammary fat pads of syngeneic BALB/cJ wild-type or genetically Sdc1-deficient mice. After 30 days, the number of metastases per mouse (Fig. 1a, b; $p = 0.004$) and the metastatic burden, defined as percent of lung tissue occupied by metastases (Fig. 1c; $p = 0.036$) were significantly reduced in Sdc1−/− compared to Sdc1+/+ animals. The average size of metastatic lesions was not significantly different between Sdc1−/− and Sdc1+/+ mice (Fig. 1d; $p = 0.11$) - presumably because of the small number of metastases in the Sdc1−/− mice and the high variability of the size of metastatic lesions in the Sdc1+/+ mice.

Since tumor behavior can be highly dependent on mouse strain variations [27] and because rate-limiting steps of metastasis may differ between carcinoma cell lines, we tested the effect of host Sdc1 in a different mouse mammary tumor metastasis model. The E0771

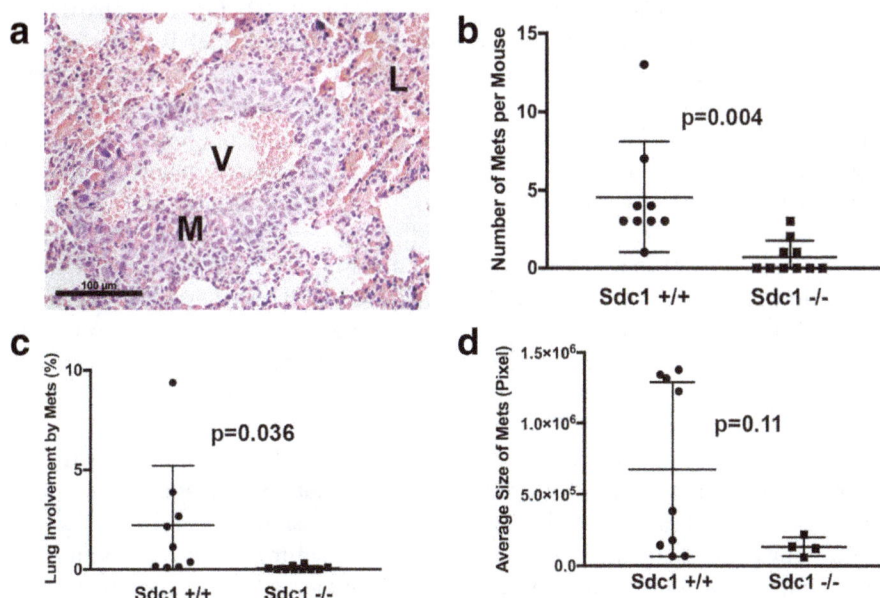

Fig. 1 Effect of host syndecan-1 (Sdc1) on metastatic efficiency of 4T1 mouse mammary carcinoma cells. The 4T1 tumor cells (1×10^7 cells in 10 μL serum-free DMEM) were injected into the exposed 4th mammary gland as described in "Methods" and mice were sacrificed after 30 days. **a** Small, early metastasis, cuffing blood vessel in lung (M, metastasis; V, vessel; L, lung parenchyma; original magnification × 400; scale bar indicates 100 μm). **b** Number of metastatic lesions per mouse. Metastases were counted on single histologic sections of both lungs. Bars indicate mean +/− standard deviation. **c** Metastatic tumor burden expressed as percent lung tissue occupied by metastatic lesions (see "Methods" for details). **d** Average area of metastatic lesions expressed in pixels as measured on histologic sections

mammary tumor cells metastasize primarily to the lungs of C57BL/6 mice, similar to 4T1 cells in BALB/cJ animals [28]. The results with C57BL/6 animals mirrored our observations in BALB/cJ mice, as the number of metastases per mouse (Additional file 1: Figure S1A, B; $p = 0.013$) and the metastatic burden (Additional file 1: Figure S1C; $p = 0.038$) were significantly reduced in Sdc1−/− compared to Sdc1+/+ animals. The average size of metastatic lesions was not significantly reduced in Sdc1−/− compared to Sdc1+/+ mice (Additional file 1: Figure S1D; $p = 0.37$). This result shows that host Sdc1 affects metastatic efficiency independent of mouse strain and cell line and implicates this proteoglycan as a regulator of metastasis.

Host Sdc1 does not significantly affect growth or microenvironmental characteristics of primary tumors

In the fat pad inoculation model, Sdc1 may affect any step of the metastatic cascade - from local invasion and intravasation, to extravasation and metastatic outgrowth. Previous work by our group and others has shown that Sdc1 is induced in stromal fibroblasts of breast carcinomas in both humans and in mice and that stromal Sdc1 can stimulate tumor growth and angiogenesis and create an invasion-permissive microenvironment [6, 21–23]. However, in this model, the average weight of mammary fat pad tumors grown in Sdc1+/+ or Sdc1−/− mice did not differ significantly (Additional file 2: Figure S2A). The absence of host Sdc1 did not affect the Ki67 proliferation index in the primary carcinoma cells, indicating that host Sdc1 does not significantly stimulate 4T1 carcinoma cell proliferation in the primary tumor site (Additional file 2: Figure S2B).

Since stromal Sdc1 has previously been shown to stimulate angiogenesis [22], we studied the tumor vasculature by labeling primary tumor sections with an antibody to the endothelial cell marker CD31. However, in this model, no difference in microvessel density was detected between tumors arising in Sdc1+/+ or Sdc1−/− mice (Additional file 2: Figure S2C). Myofibroblasts or carcinoma-associated fibroblasts (CAF) and macrophages not only stimulate tumor growth but also modulate the metastatic behavior of carcinoma cells [29, 30]. Therefore, we examined whether host Sdc1 affects these cellular constituents of the local tumor microenvironment. Alpha smooth actin (αSMA)-positive cells were arranged in a pattern similar to CD31-positive cells, suggesting that most intratumoral αSMA-positive cells are vascular smooth muscle cells or pericytes. The density of intratumoral αSMA-positive cells was similar in Sdc1+/+ and Sdc1−/− host animals (Additional file 2: Figure S2D). We were also unable to detect a difference in the density of intratumoral macrophages (Additional file 2: Figure S2E).

Given the role of stromal Sdc1 in ECM fiber assembly in vitro and in vivo, we measured the amount of collagen in the 4T1 mammary tumors by SHG imaging and collagen alignment by computer-assisted analysis of the SHG images [26, 31]. Collagen fibers were found primarily in the periphery of the tumors aggregating into a "pseudo-capsule" (Additional file 2: Figure S2F). There was no significant difference in the amount of collagen (SHG signal intensity/area; not shown) nor in the mean angles between collagen fibers and the tumor boundary when comparing Sdc1+/+ and Sdc1−/− mice (Additional file 2: Figure S2F). In summary, apart from insignificantly smaller tumor size in Sdc1−/− animals, no Sdc1-related differences were identified in the primary 4T1 mammary fat pad tumors.

Host Sdc1 is important during later stages of mammary carcinoma metastasis

Since host Sdc1-dependent differences in metastatic efficiency could not be attributed to differences in the primary tumors, we focused our attention to later stages of the metastatic cascade. After tail vein injection of tumor cells - an inoculation method that bypasses the early stages (local invasion, intravasation) of metastatic spread - host Sdc1-dependent differences in metastatic efficiency were maintained (Fig. 2). Specifically, the number of metastases (Fig. 2b), metastatic burden (Fig. 2c) and average size of metastatic lesions (Fig. 2d) were significantly reduced in Sdc1−/− mice compared to Sdc1+/+ animals ($p < 0.0001$ for all comparisons). This observation suggests that host Sdc1 is important at the distant organ site for any or all of the events occurring late during metastatic spread: extravasation, tumor cell survival, escape from dormancy or outgrowth of disseminated tumor cells; however, it does not exclude the possibility that host Sdc1 in the primary tumor also contributes to metastatic efficiency. Similarly, in the C57BL/6 model, the number of metastatic lesions (Additional file 3: Figure S3A, B; $p = 0.045$) and the metastatic burden (Additional file 3: Figure S3C; $p = 0.037$) were lower in Sdc1−/− mice, and the average size of the metastatic lesions was not significantly different (Additional file 3: Figure S3D).

Sdc1 is induced in stromal fibroblasts of mammary carcinoma lung metastasis

Sdc1 expression is induced in stromal fibroblasts of primary mammary carcinomas in mice and in humans [5, 6]. In view of our finding that host Sdc1 plays a role in the metastatic niche, we examined whether Sdc1 is induced in stromal fibroblasts in lung metastatic lesions. The stromal compartment is relatively sparse in 4T1-derived lung metastases, yet we observed co-localization between Sdc1 and fibroblasts (identified with antibodies to the fibroblast marker ER-TR7) (Fig. 3a).

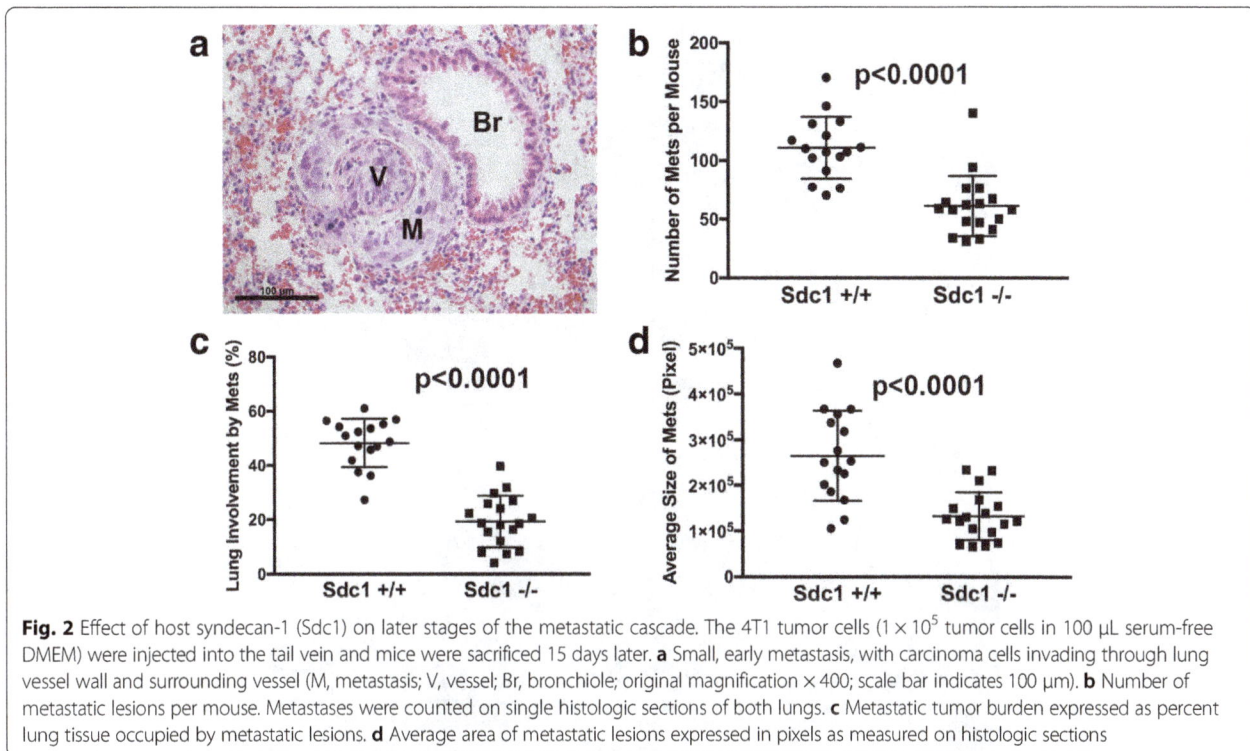

Fig. 2 Effect of host syndecan-1 (Sdc1) on later stages of the metastatic cascade. The 4T1 tumor cells (1×10^5 tumor cells in 100 μL serum-free DMEM) were injected into the tail vein and mice were sacrificed 15 days later. **a** Small, early metastasis, with carcinoma cells invading through lung vessel wall and surrounding vessel (M, metastasis; V, vessel; Br, bronchiole; original magnification × 400; scale bar indicates 100 μm). **b** Number of metastatic lesions per mouse. Metastases were counted on single histologic sections of both lungs. **c** Metastatic tumor burden expressed as percent lung tissue occupied by metastatic lesions. **d** Average area of metastatic lesions expressed in pixels as measured on histologic sections

Sdc1 was absent from (sparse) fibroblasts in normal lung tissue (Fig. 3b). Sdc1 did not co-localize with CD31-positive endothelial cells, nor with αSMA-positive cells, CD45-positive leukocytes or CD68-positive macrophages (Fig. 3c–f). Similar to the primary tumors, αSMA-positive cells were found primarily in a vascular pattern, consistent with the distribution of vascular smooth muscle cells or pericytes rather than myofibroblasts. Sdc1 is also present in airway epithelial cells (not shown). Tumor cells express Sdc1 constitutively and as allografts, independent of the mouse host genotype. Biopsy samples from a small collective of patients with breast carcinoma metastases to the lung showed a variable amount of stroma in the metastatic lesions. Stromal fibroblasts in the metastases expressed Sdc1 (Fig. 3g, h), mirroring Sdc1 induction in primary human breast carcinomas. As expected, Sdc1 was also expressed by carcinoma cells in mouse and human samples (Fig. 3c-h).

Loss of host Sdc1 decreases proliferation and apoptosis in metastatic mammary carcinoma cells but does not affect leucocyte density

As a first step towards determining the mechanism of action of Sdc1 at the lung metastatic site, we further characterized 4T1 metastatic lesions in the lungs. Inflammation is considered a driver of tumor progression and different leucocyte populations have been implicated in metastasis. Previous studies have shown that loss of Sdc1 leads to a pro-inflammatory phenotype in the endothelium and enhanced leucocyte recruitment [32, 33]. Also, neutrophils support lung colonization in several mammary tumor models [34] and certain macrophage sub-populations promote mouse mammary tumor metastasis by stimulating extravasation and growth [35, 36]. In our study, 4T1 lung metastases contained CD45-positive leucocytes primarily in the lesion periphery (Fig. 4a). Leucocyte density was indistinguishable between metastases arising in Sdc1+/+ vs. Sdc1 –/– mice, and therefore it is unlikely that an Sdc1-mediated increase or decrease in inflammation/immune cell infiltration is responsible for differences in metastatic efficiency.

Stromal Sdc1 has been shown to promote breast carcinoma cell proliferation via paracrine pathways [6, 21, 22, 37]. Therefore, Sdc1-dependent metastatic efficiency may be due to the stimulation of carcinoma cell proliferation by stromal cell-derived Sdc1. The Ki67 proliferation index in metastatic carcinoma cells was significantly ($p = 0.0002$) decreased by 86% in Sdc1–/– mice compared to their Sdc1+/+ counterparts (Fig. 4b). The proportion of apoptotic carcinoma cells - identified by active caspase 3 expression - was also lower in Sdc1–/– animals by 64% (Fig. 4c). Overall, these data are consistent with Sdc1 in the metastatic microenvironment stimulating the proliferation of carcinoma cells.

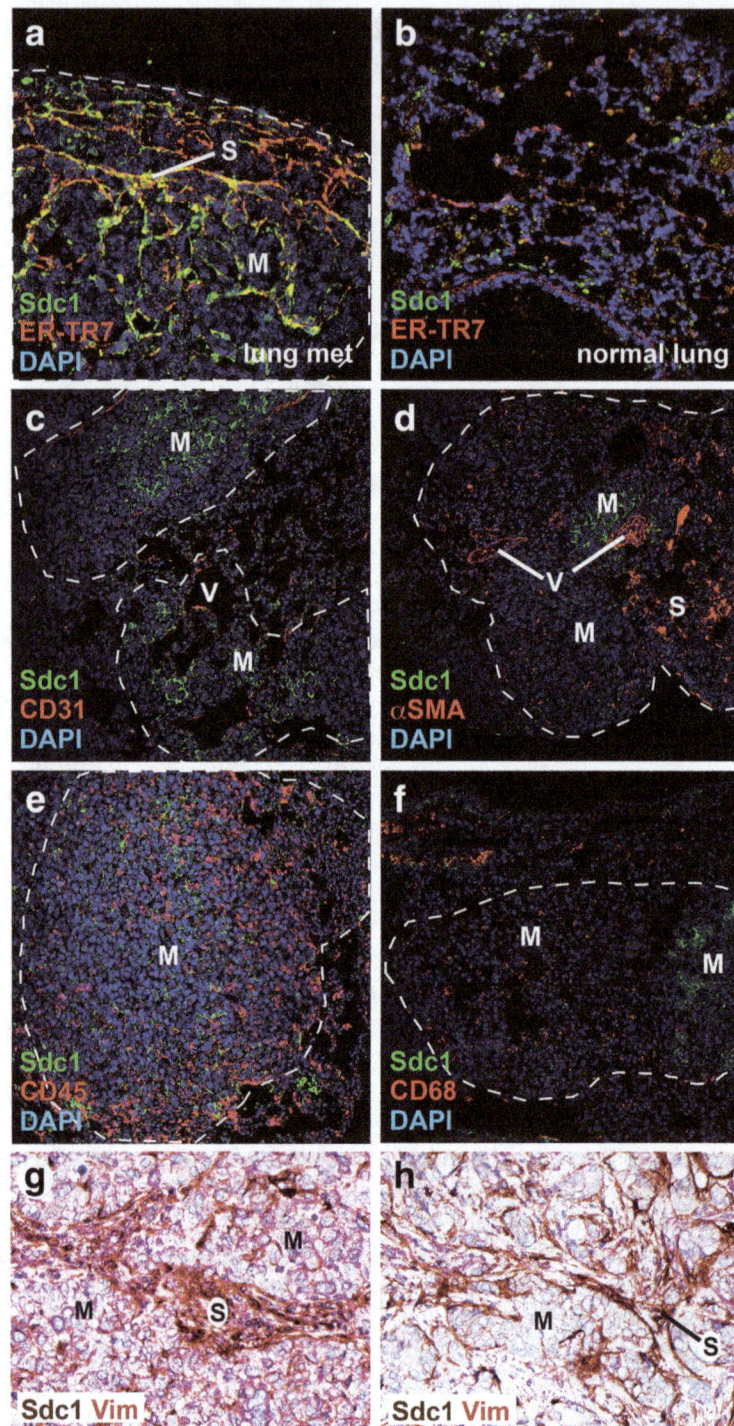

Fig. 3 Syndecan-1 (Sdc1) expression in the metastatic microenvironment. Tissue sections are from tail-vein-injected 4T1 cells in Sdc1+/+ mouse (**a-f**) or human (**g, h**) mammary carcinoma lung metastases unless stated otherwise and were labeled with antibodies to Sdc1 and cell lineage markers as indicated. **a** Sdc1 (green) and fibroblast marker ER-TR7 (red). **b** Normal lung tissue labeled for Sdc1 (green) and fibroblast marker ER-TR7 (red). **c** Sdc1 (green) and endothelial cell marker CD31 (red). **d** Sdc1 (green) and myofibroblast/smooth muscle/pericyte marker alpha smooth muscle actin (αSMA) (red). **e** Sdc1 (green) and leucocyte marker CD45 (red). **f** Sdc1 (green) and macrophage marker CD68 (red). **g** Human breast cancer metastasis to the lung labeled for Sdc1 (brown) and mesenchymal marker vimentin (Vim, magenta). Original magnification approximately × 400 for all images. Metastatic lesions are outlined with dashed lines. M, metastasis; S, stroma; V, vessel; DAPI, 4′,6-diamidino-2-phenylindole

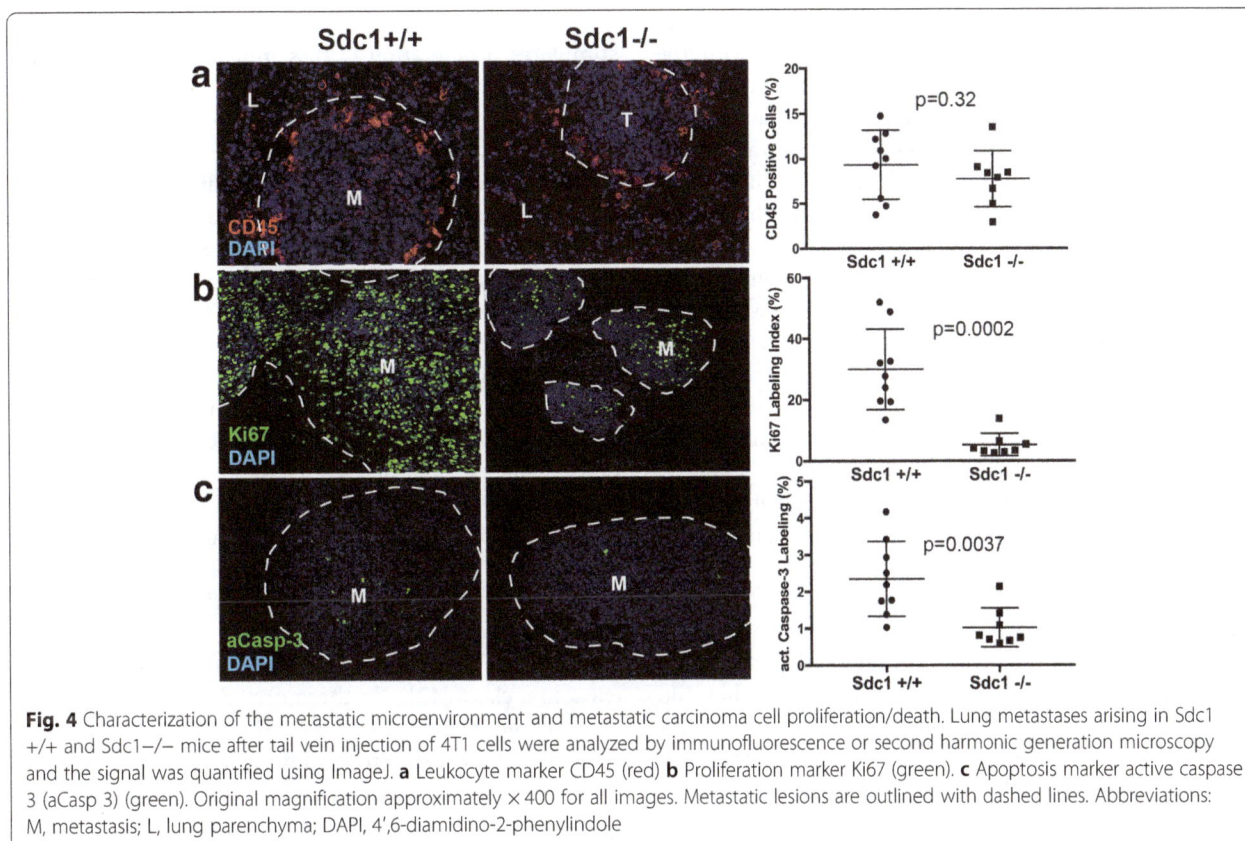

Fig. 4 Characterization of the metastatic microenvironment and metastatic carcinoma cell proliferation/death. Lung metastases arising in Sdc1 +/+ and Sdc1−/− mice after tail vein injection of 4T1 cells were analyzed by immunofluorescence or second harmonic generation microscopy and the signal was quantified using ImageJ. **a** Leukocyte marker CD45 (red) **b** Proliferation marker Ki67 (green). **c** Apoptosis marker active caspase 3 (aCasp 3) (green). Original magnification approximately × 400 for all images. Metastatic lesions are outlined with dashed lines. Abbreviations: M, metastasis; L, lung parenchyma; DAPI, 4',6-diamidino-2-phenylindole

The effect of host Sdc1 on metastatic efficiency is abolished in thermo-neutral conditions

Prior work has shown that under typical, mandated animal housing conditions (20–24 °C), Sdc1-deficient mice are susceptible to cold stress, which is linked to a reduced intradermal fat layer and results in the activation of thermogenesis and subsequent development of a β-adrenergic environment [38, 39]. These stress responses are relieved when Sdc1−/− animals are transferred to thermo-neutral (30–33 °C) temperatures. This result and the prior observation by Kokolus et al. [17] that ambient temperature influences tumorigenesis, tumor growth and metastasis, persuaded us to repeat the 4T1 fat pad injection experiment in mice subjected to higher ambient temperature; i.e., in thermo-neutral conditions. At a housing temperature of 31 °C, metastatic efficiency was indistinguishable between Sdc1+/+ and Sdc1−/− animals (Fig. 5). This suggests that the metastasis-promoting or permissive effect of host Sdc1 requires a sub-thermo-neutral environment.

Since Kokolus and coworkers had also reported correlation between housing temperature and intratumoral CD8+ T cells [17], we measured T cell numbers in our fat pad model. Abundant CD4 and CD8 T lymphocytes were identified in 4T1 lung metastases (Additional file 4: Figure S4 A and B). In larger metastases, these

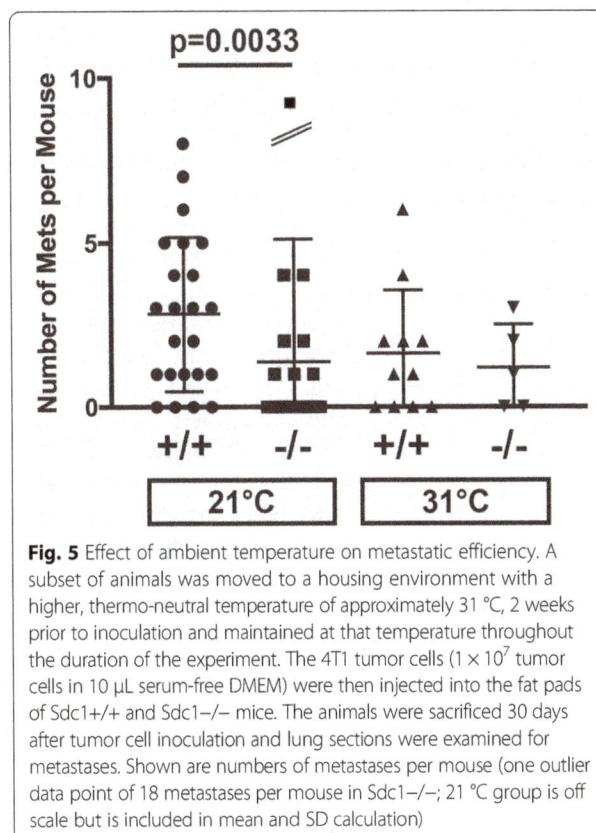

Fig. 5 Effect of ambient temperature on metastatic efficiency. A subset of animals was moved to a housing environment with a higher, thermo-neutral temperature of approximately 31 °C, 2 weeks prior to inoculation and maintained at that temperature throughout the duration of the experiment. The 4T1 tumor cells (1 × 10^7 tumor cells in 10 μL serum-free DMEM) were then injected into the fat pads of Sdc1+/+ and Sdc1−/− mice. The animals were sacrificed 30 days after tumor cell inoculation and lung sections were examined for metastases. Shown are numbers of metastases per mouse (one outlier data point of 18 metastases per mouse in Sdc1−/−; 21 °C group is off scale but is included in mean and SD calculation)

tumor-infiltrating lymphocytes were located primarily in the tumor periphery (not shown). Consistent with the findings by Kokolus et al., intratumoral CD8+ T cell numbers were increased in mice housed at 31 °C compared to 21 °C (Additional file 4: Figure S4 D). In contrast to the Kokolus study, however, we also observed elevated intratumoral CD4+ T cells in mice housed at the higher temperature of 31 °C (Additional file 4: Figure S4 C). Because of the observed effect of housing temperature on intratumoral T cells and on Sdc1-mediated metastatic efficiency, we examined a possible relationship between Sdc1 deficiency and intratumoral T cells. The Sdc1 genotype was not significantly associated with intratumoral CD4+ or CD8+ T cell numbers at either housing temperature (Additional file 4: Figure S4 E and F). In normal lung tissue, CD4+ and CD8+ cell numbers correlated with neither housing temperature nor Sdc1 status (Additional file 4: Figure S4G, H).

Discussion

Here we show that host Sdc1 is required for efficient metastasis of mammary carcinoma cells and that the HSPG acts by enhancing the outgrowth of metastatic lesions. The host Sdc1 effect is lost when the animals are placed in thermo-neutral housing conditions.

These observations describe a new pathway by which stromal cell-derived Sdc1 can drive cancer progression by stimulating proliferation of disseminated carcinoma cells at distant organ sites. This is relevant because it ascribes a role to Sdc1 at a critical transition step during the natural history of breast cancer. Local disease is typically controlled with surgical and radiation therapy. However, at the time of diagnosis, carcinoma cells may already have disseminated to distant organ sites, where they may lie dormant for many years. The mechanisms that govern escape from dormancy and outgrowth into clinically apparent metastatic lesions are unknown but are thought to rely on microenvironmental cues from the metastatic niche.

Co-localization studies identified Sdc1 expression in intratumoral fibroblasts within the metastatic niche and failed to detect Sdc1 in endothelial cells or leucocytes, pointing to metastasis-associated fibroblasts as the key cell type, regulating outgrowth. This is consistent with our understanding of stromal Sdc1 activity in primary breast carcinomas. However, airway epithelial cells also express Sdc1 and it is possible that epithelial Sdc1 is responsible for or contributes to metastatic outgrowth in the lung microenvironment. We also cannot rule out the possibility that low levels of Sdc1 expression in cell types other than stromal fibroblasts or airway epithelial cells trigger pathways that stimulate disseminated carcinoma cell proliferation.

The exact mechanism of Sdc1-stimulated metastatic outgrowth is uncertain. Judging from the decreased Ki67

proliferation index seen in Sdc1−/− mice, host Sdc1 stimulates proliferation of disseminated carcinoma cells. In 2D and in 3D co-culture models, fibroblast-derived Sdc1 promotes breast carcinoma cell proliferation via paracrine pathways [6, 21]. In these models, paracrine growth stimulation requires proteolytic cleavage of the Sdc1 core protein resulting in shedding of the Sdc1 ectodomain into the pericellular space. Prior work from several groups including ours revealed matrix metalloproteinase (MMP)14 (aka MT1-MMP) as the obligatory "sheddase" [37, 40]. Other investigators identified heparanase combined with MMP9 as a critical enzyme involved in Sdc1 shedding [41]. In our previously published in vitro model, fibroblast growth factor 2 (FGF2) and stroma-derived factor 1 (SDF-1) complete the paracrine signaling loop that begins with the induction of Sdc1 expression in stromal fibroblasts [21]. Whether or not Sdc1 shedding plays a role in the lung microenvironment in vivo is currently unknown. Sdc1 and its intracellular adapter syntenin are also key molecules in the generation of extracellular vesicles of the exosome class [42]. Furthermore, Sdc1 regulates exosome cargo composition [43]. Since exosomes participate in tumor cell-stroma interactions and exosomes have been shown to prepare the pre-metastatic niche [44], it is conceivable that host Sdc1 stimulates metastasis by modulating exosome production or loading.

Although our results point to an Sdc1 effect on metastatic outgrowth, we cannot rule out the possibility that host Sdc1 levels affect tumor cell extravasation. Götte et al. have shown that Sdc1 deficiency increases the adhesion of leucocytes to retinal endothelium [13]. Any role of endothelial Sdc1 in tumor cell extravasation is speculative at this point.

Sdc1 expression in fibroblasts also leads to the production of ECM with an aligned fiber architecture that is permissive to the directionally persistent migration and invasion of carcinoma cells [23]. ECM fiber alignment in vitro requires activation of the αvβ3 integrin [45]. Beauvais and coworkers have shown that clustering of Sdc1 on the cell surface results in the assembly of a trimeric complex that also contains an αv containing integrin and insulin-like growth factor 1 receptor (IGF1R) [11]. Ligand-independent activation of the IGF1R triggers inside-out activation of αvβ3, which could execute ECM fiber alignment. A migration and invasion-permissive microenvironment may enable carcinoma cells to escape microenvironmental niches that suppress growth of disseminated carcinoma cells. Ghajar and colleagues have described a perivascular niche in the lung that traps disseminated mammary carcinoma cells in a dormant state and ascribed a dormancy-inducing activity to endothelial-derived thrombospondin-1 [46].

The dependence of the Sdc1-induced metastasis-promoting effect on sub-thermo-neutral ambient temperatures is intriguing. Relief of cold stress does not readily explain the observation since Sdc1−/− animals in sub-thermo-neutral temperature (i.e. typical, mandated housing temperature) are the only ones in this experiment that experience significant cold stress and their metastasis rate does not change when moved to the higher ambient temperature. Kokolus and co-workers report that raising the temperature to thermo-neutral conditions increases CD8+ T-cells number and activity in the primary tumors, while decreasing T-helper cells [17]. In our study, no significant difference was identified in CD4+ or CD8+ lymphocytes between Sdc1+/+ and Sdc1−/− animals. Therefore, it is unlikely that T cells are responsible for mediating the effect of host Sdc1 on metastasis but we cannot entirely rule out differences in lymphocyte activity.

Targeting disseminated breast carcinoma cells during the long period of dormancy or preventing escape from dormancy is a promising therapeutic goal. Sdc1-mediated outgrowth of metastatic lesions may be targetable by interfering with Sdc1 core protein interactions using peptide competitors [47] or by blocking other molecules associated with the Sdc1 pathway such as integrin cell adhesion receptors or receptor tyrosine kinases like IGF1R. However, any therapeutic intervention will require a detailed understanding of the mechanism of Sdc1 action in the metastatic microenvironment.

Conclusions

In summary, we show that Sdc1 expression is induced in stromal fibroblasts in the lung metastatic microenvironment and that host Sdc1 is required for efficient outgrowth of mammary carcinoma metastases. In thermo-neutral (higher temperature of 31 °C) ambient housing conditions, Sdc1 deficiency in the host had no impact on metastasis, suggesting that the Sdc1 effect is temperature-sensitive and likely dependent on mild cold stress. These observations assign an important role to Sdc1 during the late stages of the metastatic cascade, the molecular mechanism of which requires further study.

Additional files

Additional file 1: Figure S1. Effect of host Sdc1 on metastatic efficiency of E0771 mouse mammary carcinoma cells. E0771 tumor cells (1×10^7 cells in 10 μL) were injected into the exposed 4th mammary gland as described in "Methods" and mice were killed after 30 days. (A) Metastatic lesion in lung (original magnification × 400; scale bar indicates 100 μm; M, metastasis; L, lung). (B) Number of metastatic lesions per mouse. Metastases were counted on single histologic sections of both lungs. (C) Metastatic tumor burden expressed as percent lung tissue occupied by metastatic lesions. (D) Average area of metastatic lesions expressed in pixels as measured on histologic sections. (TIF 1153 kb)

Additional file 2: Figure S2. Characterization of 4T1 primary fat pad tumors. The 4T1 tumor cells (1×10^7 cells in 10 μL) were injected into the exposed 4th mammary gland and mice were killed after 30 days. (A) Hematoxylin and eosin (H&E) stained sections of tumors in fat pad.

Carcinoma cells infiltrate adipose tissue (Ad), which contains benign mammary duct (Duct). Scatter plot graph indicates wet weights of tumors excised from Sdc1+/+ and Sdc1−/− mice. (B) Immunohistochemical (IHC) labeling for proliferation marker Ki67. Graph compares Ki67 labeling index between animal genotypes. (C) IHC labeling for endothelial cell marker CD31. Graph compares CD31-positive area between animal genotypes. (D) IHC labeling for alpha smooth muscle actin (αSMA). Graph compares number of αSMA-positive cell clusters between animal genotypes. (E) IHC labeling for macrophage marker F4/80. Graph compares density of F4/80-positive macrophages between animal genotypes. (F) Tumor border imaged by second harmonic generation (SHG) microscopy. White structures indicate fibrillar collagen. Graph compares mean collagen fiber angles relative to tumor boundary between animal genotypes. (TIF 7079 kb)

Additional file 3: Figure S3. Effect of host Sdc1 on later stages of E0771 carcinoma cell metastasis. E0771 tumor cells (1×10^5 tumor cells in 100 μL) were injected into the tail veins of C57BL/6 mice, which were killed 15 days later. (A) Metastasis growing around pulmonary vessel (magnification ×400; scale bar indicates 100 μm; V, vessel). (B) Number of metastatic lesions per mouse. Metastases were counted on single histologic sections of both lungs. (C) Metastatic tumor burden expressed as percent lung tissue involved by metastatic lesions. (D) Average area of metastatic lesions expressed in pixels as measured on histologic sections. (TIF 880 kb)

Additional file 4: Figure S4. Effect of housing temperature and host Sdc1 on T cells within lung metastases. A subset of animals was moved to a housing environment with a thermo-neutral temperature of approximately 31 °C, 2 weeks prior to inoculation and maintained at that temperature throughout the duration of the experiment. The 4T1 mouse mammary carcinoma cells were inoculated into the mammary fat pad as described. Mice were killed after 30 days and sections of lung tissue were labeled with antibodies to CD4 and CD8. CD4+ and CD8+ intratumoral and normal lung lymphocytes were counted as described in "Methods". (A, B) Photomicrographs of adjacent sections of small lung metastasis (M) next to vessel (V) labeled with antibodies to CD4 (A) and CD8 (B) (original magnification × 400). (C, D) Density of intratumoral lymphocytes in mice segregated by housing temperature expressed as number of cells per megapixel (MP) of metastasis tissue. (E, F) Density of intratumoral lymphocytes in mice segregated by housing temperature and Sdc1 genotype (same dataset as in C, D). (G, H) Density of lymphocytes in normal lung tissue at distance from any metastases. (TIF 2897 kb)

Abbreviations

αSMA: Alpha smooth muscle actin; DAPI: 4′,6-Diamidino-2-phenylindole; DMEM: Dulbecco's modified Eagle's medium; ER-TR7: Fibroblast antibody; FBS: Fetal bovine serum; H&E : Hematoxylin and eosin; HS: Heparan sulfate; HSPG: Heparan sulfate proteoglycan; IGF1R: Insulin-like growth factor 1 receptor; MMP: Matrix metalloproteinase; NIH: National Institutes of Health; RTK: Receptor tyrosine kinase; Sdc1: Syndecan-1; SHG: Second harmonic generation

Acknowledgements
This article is dedicated to the memory of Patricia Keely, Ph.D., collaborator, mentor and friend. The authors thank the University of Wisconsin Translational Research Initiatives in Pathology Laboratory, in part supported by the UW Department of Pathology and Laboratory Medicine and UWCCC grant P30 CA014520, for use of its facilities and services. We are also grateful to Dr. Alan Rapraeger for providing anti-Sdc1 antibody. The contents do not represent the views of the Dept. of Veterans Affairs or the United States Government.

Funding
This work was supported by NIH/NCI grant R01 CA107012, DOD grant W81XWH-14-1-0274, and by UWCCC Core Grant P30 CA014520, and also supported in part by award number I01 BX000137 from the Biomedical Laboratory Research and Development Service of the VA Office of Research and Development.

Authors' contributions

Concept and design - AF and CA; acquisition of data - CC, XY, KM, NY, KON and IK; analysis and interpretation - AF, CA, CC, NY, IK and KE; writing - CC and AF. All authors read and approved the final manuscript.

Competing interests

The authors declare that they have no competing interests.

Author details

[1]Department of Pathology and Laboratory Medicine, University of Wisconsin-Madison, 6051 WIMR, MC-2275, 1111 Highland Avenue, Madison, WI 53705, USA. [2]Pathology and Laboratory Medicine Service, William S. Middleton Memorial Veterans Hospital, Department of Veterans Affairs Medical Center, Madison, WI, USA. [3]University of Wisconsin Carbone Cancer Center, Madison, WI, USA. [4]Laboratory for Optical and Computational Instrumentation, University of Wisconsin-Madison, Madison, WI, USA. [5]Morgridge Institute for Research, University of Wisconsin-Madison, Madison, WI, USA. [6]Department of Oncology, University of Wisconsin-Madison, Madison, WI, USA.

References

1. Hüsemann Y, Geigl JB, Schubert F, Musiani P, Meyer M, Burghart E, et al. Systemic spread is an early step in breast cancer. Cancer Cell. 2008;13:58–68.
2. Linde N, Fluegen G, Aguirre-Ghiso JA. The relationship between dormant cancer cells and their microenvironment. Adv Cancer Res. 2016;132:45–71.
3. Beauvais DM, Rapraeger AC. Syndecans in tumor cell adhesion and signaling. Reprod Biol Endocrinol. 2004;2:3.
4. Vainio S, Jalkanen M, Bernfield M, Saxén L. Transient expression of syndecan in mesenchymal cell aggregates of the embryonic kidney. Dev Biol. 1992;152:221–32.
5. Stanley MJ, Stanley MW, Sanderson RD, Zera R. Syndecan-1 expression is induced in the stroma of infiltrating breast carcinoma. Am J Clin Pathol. 1999;112:377–83.
6. Maeda T, Alexander CM, Friedl A. Induction of syndecan-1 expression in stromal fibroblasts promotes proliferation of human breast cancer cells. Cancer Res. 2004;64:612–21.
7. Jaakkola P, Vihinen T, Määttä A, Jalkanen M. Activation of an enhancer on the syndecan-1 gene is restricted to fibroblast growth factor family members in mesenchymal cells. Mol Cell Biol. 1997;17:3210–9.
8. Määttä A, Jaakkola P, Jalkanen M. Extracellular matrix-dependent activation of syndecan-1 expression in keratinocyte growth factor-treated keratinocytes. J Biol Chem. 1999;274:9891–8.
9. Sawaguchi N, Majima T, Iwasaki N, Funakoshi T, Shimode K, Onodera T, et al. Extracellular matrix modulates expression of cell-surface proteoglycan genes in fibroblasts. Connect Tissue Res. 2006;47:141–8.
10. Choi Y, Chung H, Jung H, Couchman JR, Oh E-S. Syndecans as cell surface receptors: unique structure equates with functional diversity. Matrix Biol. 2011;30:93–9.
11. Beauvais DM, Rapraeger AC. Syndecan-1 couples the insulin-like growth factor-1 receptor to inside-out integrin activation. J Cell Sci. 2010;123:3796–807.
12. Alexander CM, Reichsman F, Hinkes MT, Lincecum J, Becker KA, Cumberledge S, et al. Syndecan-1 is required for Wnt-1-induced mammary tumorigenesis in mice. Nat Genet. 2000;25:329–32.
13. Götte M, Joussen AM, Klein C, Andre P, Wagner DD, Hinkes MT, et al. Role of syndecan-1 in leukocyte-endothelial interactions in the ocular vasculature. Invest Ophthalmol Vis Sci. 2002;43:1135–41.
14. Götte M. Syndecans in inflammation. FASEB J. 2003;17:575–91.
15. McDermott SP, Ranheim EA, Leatherberry VS, Khwaja SS, Klos KS, Alexander CM. Juvenile syndecan-1 null mice are protected from carcinogen-induced tumor development. Oncogene. 2007;26:1407–16.
16. Stanford KI, Bishop JR, Foley EM, Gonzales JC, Niesman IR, Witztum JL, et al. Syndecan-1 is the primary heparan sulfate proteoglycan mediating hepatic clearance of triglyceride-rich lipoproteins in mice. J Clin Invest. 2009;119:3236–45.
17. Kokolus KM, Capitano ML, Lee C-T, Eng JW-L, Waight JD, Hylander BL, et al. Baseline tumor growth and immune control in laboratory mice are significantly influenced by subthermoneutral housing temperature. Proc Natl Acad Sci U S A. 2013;110(50):20176–81.
18. Barbareschi M, Maisonneuve P, Aldovini D, Cangi MG, Pecciarini L, Angelo Mauri F, et al. High syndecan-1 expression in breast carcinoma is related to an aggressive phenotype and to poorer prognosis. Cancer. 2003;98:474–83.
19. Anttonen A, Kajanti M, Heikkilä P, Jalkanen M, Joensuu H. Syndecan-1 expression has prognostic significance in head and neck carcinoma. Br J Cancer. 1999;79:558–64.
20. Baba F, Swartz K, van Buren R, Eickhoff J, Zhang Y, Wolberg W, et al. Syndecan-1 and syndecan-4 are overexpressed in an estrogen receptor-negative, highly proliferative breast carcinoma subtype. Breast Cancer Res Treat. 2006;98:91–8.
21. Su G, Blaine SA, Qiao D, Friedl A. Shedding of syndecan-1 by stromal fibroblasts stimulates human breast cancer cell proliferation via FGF2 activation. J Biol Chem. 2007;282:14906–15.
22. Maeda T, Desouky J, Friedl A. Syndecan-1 expression by stromal fibroblasts promotes breast carcinoma growth in vivo and stimulates tumor angiogenesis. Oncogene. 2006;25:1408–12.
23. Yang N, Mosher R, Seo S, Beebe D, Friedl A. Syndecan-1 in breast cancer stroma fibroblasts regulates extracellular matrix fiber organization and carcinoma cell motility. Am J Pathol. 2011;178:325–35.
24. Miller FR, Medina D, Heppner GH. Preferential growth of mammary tumors in intact mammary fatpads. Cancer Res. 1981;41:3863–7.
25. Schneider CA, Rasband WS, Eliceiri KW. NIH image to ImageJ: 25 years of image analysis. Nat Methods. 2012;9:671–5.
26. Bredfeldt JS, Liu Y, Pehlke CA, Conklin MW, Szulczewski JM, Inman DR, et al. Computational segmentation of collagen fibers from second-harmonic generation images of breast cancer. J Biomed Opt. 2014;19:16007.
27. Davie SA, Maglione JE, Manner CK, Young D, Cardiff RD, MacLeod CL, et al. Effects of FVB/NJ and C57Bl/6J strain backgrounds on mammary tumor phenotype in inducible nitric oxide synthase deficient mice. Transgenic Res. 2007;16:193–201.
28. Ewens A, Mihich E, Ehrke MJ. Distant metastasis from subcutaneously grown E0771 medullary breast adenocarcinoma. Anticancer Res. 2005;25:3905–15.
29. De Wever O, Van Bockstal M, Mareel M, Hendrix A, Bracke M. Carcinoma-associated fibroblasts provide operational flexibility in metastasis. Semin Cancer Biol. 2014;25:33–46.
30. Karagiannis GS, Poutahidis T, Erdman SE, Kirsch R, Riddell RH, Diamandis EP. Cancer-associated fibroblasts drive the progression of metastasis through both paracrine and mechanical pressure on cancer tissue. Mol Cancer Res Am Assoc Cancer Res. 2012;10:1403–18.
31. Keikhosravi A, Bredfeldt JS, Sagar AK, Eliceiri KW. Second-harmonic generation imaging of cancer. Methods Cell Biol. 2014;123:531–46.
32. Voyvodic PL, Min D, Liu R, Williams E, Chitalia V, Dunn AK, et al. Loss of syndecan-1 induces a pro-inflammatory phenotype in endothelial cells with a dysregulated response to atheroprotective flow. Journal of biological chemistry. Am Soc Biochem Mol Biol. 2014;289:9547–59.
33. Teng YH-F, Aquino RS, Park PW. Molecular functions of syndecan-1 in disease. Matrix Biol. 2012;31:3–16.
34. Wculek SK, Malanchi I. Neutrophils support lung colonization of metastasis-initiating breast cancer cells. Nature. 2015;528:413–7.
35. Qian B, Deng Y, Im JH, Muschel RJ, Zou Y, Li J, et al. A distinct macrophage population mediates metastatic breast cancer cell extravasation, establishment and growth. Bereswill S, editor. PloS One. 2009;4:e6562.
36. Williams CB, Yeh ES, Soloff AC. Tumor-associated macrophages: unwitting accomplices in breast cancer malignancy. NPJ Breast Cancer. 2016;2:npjbcancer201525.
37. Su G, Blaine SA, Qiao D, Friedl A. Membrane type 1 matrix metalloproteinase-mediated stromal syndecan-1 shedding stimulates breast carcinoma cell proliferation. Cancer Res. 2008;68:9558–65.

38. Tian XY, Ganeshan K, Hong C, Nguyen KD, Qiu Y, Kim J, et al. Thermoneutral housing accelerates metabolic inflammation to potentiate atherosclerosis but not insulin resistance. Cell Metab. 2016;23:165–78.

39. Kasza I, Suh Y, Wollny D, Clark RJ, Roopra A, Colman RJ, et al. Syndecan-1 is required to maintain intradermal fat and prevent cold stress. PLoS Genet. 2014;10:e1004514.

40. Endo K, Takino T, Miyamori H, Kinsen H, Yoshizaki T, Furukawa M, et al. Cleavage of syndecan-1 by membrane type matrix metalloproteinase-1 stimulates cell migration. J Biol Chem. 2003;278:40764–70.

41. Yang Y, MacLeod V, Miao H-Q, Theus A, Zhan F, Shaughnessy JD, et al. Heparanase enhances syndecan-1 shedding: a novel mechanism for stimulation of tumor growth and metastasis. J Biol Chem. 2007;282:13326–33.

42. Baietti MF, Zhang Z, Mortier E, Melchior A, Degeest G, Geeraerts A, et al. Syndecan-syntenin-ALIX regulates the biogenesis of exosomes. Nat Cell Biol. 2012;14:677–85.

43. Parimon T, Brauer R, Schlesinger SY, Xie T, Jiang D, Ge L, et al. Syndecan-1 controls lung tumorigenesis by regulating miRNAs packaged in exosomes. Am J Pathol. 2018;188:1094–103.

44. Hoshino A, Costa-Silva B, Shen T-L, Rodrigues G, Hashimoto A, Tesic Mark M, et al. Tumour exosome integrins determine organotropic metastasis. Nature. 2015;527:329–35.

45. Yang N, Friedl A. Syndecan-1-induced ECM fiber alignment requires integrin $\alpha v \beta 3$ and syndecan-1 ectodomain and heparan sulfate chains. Cukierman E, editor. PloS one. 2016;11:e0150132.

46. Ghajar CM, Peinado H, Mori H, Matei IR, Evason KJ, Brazier H, et al. The perivascular niche regulates breast tumour dormancy. Nat Cell Biol. 2013.

47. Rapraeger AC. Synstatin: a selective inhibitor of the syndecan-1-coupled IGF1R-$\alpha v \beta 3$ integrin complex in tumorigenesis and angiogenesis. FEBS J. 2013;280:2207–15.

Nitric oxide deficiency and endothelial–mesenchymal transition of pulmonary endothelium in the progression of 4T1 metastatic breast cancer in mice

Marta Smeda[1], Anna Kieronska[1,3], Mateusz G. Adamski[1], Bartosz Proniewski[1], Magdalena Sternak[1], Tasnim Mohaissen[1], Kamil Przyborowski[1], Katarzyna Derszniak[1], Dawid Kaczor[1], Marta Stojak[1], Elzbieta Buczek[1], Agnieszka Jasztal[1], Joanna Wietrzyk[2] and Stefan Chlopicki[1,3*]

Abstract

Background: Mesenchymal transformation of pulmonary endothelial cells contributes to the formation of a metastatic microenvironment, but it is not known whether this precedes or follows early metastasis formation. In the present work, we characterize the development of nitric oxide (NO) deficiency and markers of endothelial–mesenchymal transition (EndMT) in the lung in relation to the progression of 4T1 metastatic breast cancer injected orthotopically in mice.

Methods: NO production, endothelial nitric oxide synthase (eNOS) phosphorylation status, markers of EndMT in the lung, pulmonary endothelium permeability, and platelet activation/reactivity were analyzed in relation to the progression of 4T1 breast cancer metastasis to the lung, as well as to lung tissue remodeling, 1–5 weeks after 4T1 cancer cell inoculation in Balb/c mice.

Results: Phosphorylation of eNOS and NO production in the lungs of 4T1 breast cancer-bearing mice was compromised prior to the development of pulmonary metastasis, and was associated with overexpression of Snail transcription factor in the pulmonary endothelium. These changes developed prior to the mesenchymal phenotypic switch in the lungs evidenced by a decrease in vascular endothelial-cadherin (VE-CAD) and CD31 expression, and the increase in pulmonary endothelial permeability, phenomena which coincided with early pulmonary metastasis. Increased activation of platelets was also detected prior to the early phase of metastasis and persisted to the late phase of metastasis, as evidenced by the higher percentage of unstimulated platelets binding fibrinogen without changes in von Willebrand factor and fibrinogen binding in response to ADP stimulation.

Conclusions: Decreased eNOS activity and phosphorylation resulting in a low NO production state featuring pulmonary endothelial dysfunction was an early event in breast cancer pulmonary metastasis, preceding the onset of its phenotypic switch toward a mesenchymal phenotype (EndMT) evidenced by a decrease in VE-CAD and CD31 expression. The latter coincided with development of the first metastatic nodules in the lungs. These findings suggest that early endothelial dysfunction featured by NO deficiency rather than EndMT, might represent a primary regulatory target to prevent early pulmonary metastasis.

Keywords: Breast cancer, Pulmonary endothelium dysfunction, Endothelial–mesenchymal transition

---

* Correspondence: stefan.chlopicki@jcet.eu
[1]Jagiellonian Centre for Experimental Therapeutics (JCET), Jagiellonian University, Bobrzynskiego 14 St., 30-348 Krakow, Poland
[3]Department of Pharmacology, Jagiellonian University, Medical College, Grzegorzecka 16, 31-531 Krakow, Poland
Full list of author information is available at the end of the article

Background

Breast cancer kills approximately 40,000 people worldwide each year and is a leading cause of cancer death in women [1]. Breast cancer progression is associated with inflammatory responses that promote neoplastic disease and reduce survival of patients regardless of their age, race, tumor stage, and body mass index [2]. Inflammation is both a marker and the causative factor of endothelial dysfunction and promotes cancer growth and metastasis. In particular, adhesion of metastatic cancer cells to the activated vascular endothelium and their subsequent transendothelial migration are regulated by a number of endothelium-dependent mechanisms favoring or inhibiting premetastatic micro-environment formation. Indeed, factors released from dysfunctional endothelium activate some inflammatory signaling pathways in cancer cells, promoting their invasiveness [3, 4], while endothelial vasoprotective mediators including nitric oxide (NO) inhibit adhesiveness of cancer cells to endothelial cells [5].

Decreased NO production, frequently associated with a decreased phosphorylation of eNOS [6], represents the early hallmark of endothelial dysfunction [7]. NO prevents endothelial inflammatory activation [8]. When its production or bioavailability is compromised, expression of cell-surface adhesion molecules on the endothelium surface such as vascular cell adhesion molecule 1 (VCAM-1) is increased [8]. Endothelial dysfunction can also be activated by platelet-released substances that trigger endothelial inflammation. Furthermore, proinflammatory activation of endothelial cells favors monocyte and neutrophil binding as well as platelet rosetting on the leukocyte–endothelial cell surface [9], facilitating anchoring of cancer cells to activated endothelial surface concomitantly with leukocytes forming platelet–tumor cell–leukocyte heteroaggregates [10]. Formation of such aggregates in low-resistance vascular beds, such as in the pulmonary circulation, irrevocably disturbs the laminar blood flow that could further potentiate pathological endothelial activation [11].

Endothelial dysfunction can also be manifested by increased endothelial permeability linked with disassembly of intercellular adherens junction proteins (i.e., VE-cadherin (VE-CAD)) between endothelial cells [12]. An increase in endothelial permeability is the critical event enabling cancer cells to extravasate and form metastases [13–16]. Endothelial permeability is negatively regulated by mechanisms maintaining endothelial barrier integrity, such as the Slit2–ROBO4–ROBO1 signaling pathway [17–19]. Finally, dysfunctional endothelial cells may lose their endothelium-like phenotype via TGF-β-dependent or TGF-β-independent expression of transcription factors such as Snail [20–22], which are reported to suppress endothelium-specific genes [23–25] that initiate endothelial-to-mesenchymal transition (EndMT) [26].

Since there is no comprehensive study characterizing progression of endothelial dysfunction in the metastatic organ from the very early premetastatic phase until the late metastatic phase of the disease, in the present study we aimed to characterize alterations in the phenotype of pulmonary endothelium in relation to the progression of 4T1 metastatic breast cancer injected orthotopically into mice. For that purpose, we measured NO production, eNOS phosphorylation status, markers of EndMT, endothelial permeability, as well as lung tissue remodeling and platelet activation from 1 to 5 weeks after 4T1 cancer cell inoculation into Balb/C mice. We demonstrate that early impairment of NO-dependent function in the lungs precedes the decrease in expression of endothelium-specific proteins indicating an EndMT phenotypic switch, the latter coinciding with the development of early metastatic nodules in the lungs.

Methods

Animals

Two hundred and forty female Balb/C mice, 7–11 weeks old, were purchased from Charles River Lab (Germany) and divided into healthy control mice ($n = 30$) injected orthotopically with Hank's Balanced Salt Solution (HBSS; IIET, Poland) and mice ($n = 210$) injected orthotopically with 1×10^4 4T1 murine breast cancer cells suspended in HBSS. The mice injected with 4T1 cells were euthanized (ketamine and xylazine, 100 and 10 mg/kg, respectively) in the 1st, 2nd, 3rd, 4th, and 5th week after cancer cell injection. Healthy control mice were euthanized concomitantly with mice in the 5th week of the disease. Throughout the experiment, all animals were housed 5–6 mice per cage, in a temperature-controlled environment (22–25 °C), maintained on a 12-h light/day cycle and given unlimited access to food (AIN; Zoolab, Krakow, Poland) and water. Experimental procedures involving animals were accepted by the First Local Ethical Committee on Animal Testing at Jagiellonian University (Krakow, Poland; permit no. 140/2013) and the Second Local Ethical Committee on Animal Testing in the Institute of Pharmacology, Polish Academy of Sciences (Krakow, Poland; permit no. 41/2017).

Cell culture

The mouse mammary adenocarcinoma 4T1 cells were obtained from the American Type Culture Collection (ATCC, USA) and were cultured in RPMI 1640-Glutamax medium (Sigma-Aldrich, Poland) supplemented with 10% fetal bovine serum (Gibco, Thermo Fisher Scientific, Poland), 1.0 mM sodium pyruvate (Sigma-Aldrich, Poland), and antibiotic antimycotic solution (100 units/ml penicillin and 100 µg/ml streptomycin, 25 µg/ml amphotericin B) (Sigma-Aldrich, Poland). Cells were cultured at 37 °C in a humidified atmosphere containing 5% CO_2. For inoculations, only 4T1 cells at the second passage were used. Prior to the transplantations, 4T1 cells were detached using Accu-tase solution (Sigma-Aldrich, Poland), centrifuged ($300 \times g$, 4 °C, 5 min), counted, suspended in Hank's Balanced Salt Solution (HBSS; IIET, Poland) at the appropriate concentration, and inoculated into the mammary gland of female Balb/C mice. All cell cultures were routinely tested for *Mycoplasma* contamination (MycoAlert Mycoplasma Detection Kit; Lonza).

Measurement of breast cancer primary tumor and pulmonary metastasis

Body mass was monitored throughout the experiment. To assess the primary tumor growth, the primary tumor volume was measured with calipers each week as described by Kim et al. [27]. After mice euthanasia, primary tumors, lungs, and spleens were excised, weighed, and saved for further analysis. Lungs designated for assessment of metastasis were fixed in formalin and cut into lobes, and the pulmonary metastatic nodules were counted on their surface. After assessment of pulmonary metastasis, lung lobes were paraffin-embedded, cut into 5-µm slices, and stained with hematoxylin and eosin (H&E) to visualize pulmonary metastasis. The lung cross-sections were scanned with a BX51 microscope equipped with the virtual microscopy system dotSlide (objective magnification 20×; Olympus, Japan). To visualize the reorganization of extracellular matrix in the lungs during disease progression, the lung cross-sections were stained with Unna Orcein staining for elastin fibers. Subsequently, randomly chosen visual fields for mice in each experimental group were photographed in such a way that only the lung parenchyma was visible without major pulmonary blood vessels and bronchi. The pictures were subjected to segmentation in Ilastik (developed by the Ilastik team, with partial financial support by the Heidelberg Collaboratory for Image Processing, HHMI Janelia Farm Research Campus and CellNetworks Excellence Cluster), and the relative number of pixels corresponding to elastin fibers in each experimental group was calculated using ImageJ [28].

Measurement of NO production in the lungs

Colloidal $Fe^{2+}(DETC)_2$ was used for trapping the intracellular NO with EPR detection as described by Cai et al. [29] with minor changes. Briefly, lungs perfused with ice-cold PBS were excised and cut into small pieces and placed into 0.1 ml Krebs Hepes buffer (NaCl 99 mM, KCl 4.7 mM, $CaCl_2$ 2.5 mM, $MgSO_4$ 1.2 mM, $NaHCO_3$ 25 mM, KH_2PO_4 1.03 mM, glucose 5.6 mM, HEPES 20 mM) on a 24-well plate. The buffer was bubbled for at least 30 min with argon gas on ice to remove oxygen prior to use. Then 2.25 mg of $FeSO_4 \times 7H_2O$/10 ml and 3.6 mg of DETC/10 ml were dissolved separately in argon-bubbled buffer, to obtain final concentrations 0.8 mM and 1.6 mM, respectively, mixed, and immediately added to the tissue samples (0.25 ml per well). The tissues were placed in an incubator at 37 °C and incubated for 90 min in an air atmosphere. Tissue samples were then collected, weighed, introduced into 1-ml insulin syringes, and snap-frozen in liquid nitrogen. Measurements of $Fe_2(DETC)_2$-NO signals in frozen samples were performed in a finger Dewar using an EMX Plus Bruker spectrometer with the following settings: microwave power, 10 mW; modulation amplitude, 0.8 mT; scan width, 11.5 mT; scan time, 61.44 s; number of scans, 4. The results were collected, and the amplitude of the characteristic NO triplet spectrum was analyzed using Eleana software.

Quantitative assessment of Snail expression in the pulmonary circulation

Formalin-fixed and paraffin-embedded lungs were cut into 5-µm slices. Antigen retrieval was performed according to the standard protocol. To visualize expression of Snail, the slices were incubated with primary anti-Snail antibody (ab53519; Abcam) and secondary biotinylated donkey anti-goat antibodies (705-065-147; Jackson ImmunoResearch) concomitantly with ABC vector complex. For each slice, 10 randomly chosen nonobstructed arteries were photographed with a BX51 microscope (objective 20×) equipped with the virtual microscopy system dotSlide (Olympus, Japan) and the length of Snail-positive fragment(s) within the artery was manually measured and expressed as the percentage of the entire circuit of the particular artery. At the same time, the representative images of the investigated arteries were assessed for their patency (i.e., obstruction with blood clot or cancer cells) by a blinded investigator.

Measurement of pulmonary endothelium permeability by Evans blue

Subsequent to anesthesia (100 mg/kg ketamine + 10 mg/kg xylazine, i.p.), mice were injected via the femoral vein with a solution of Evans blue (EB, 60 kDa) dye (Sigma Aldrich) at a dose of 4 ml/kg. Injected dye solution, composed of 2% EB in 0.9% saline, was left to circulate for 10 min, and then the mouse chest was surgically opened and concurrently perfused via left (systemic circulation) and right (pulmonary circulation) ventricles with PBS for 15 min. Lungs were isolated, dry weighed, and homogenized in 200 µl of 50% TCA (dissolved in distillated water). The homogenate was frozen and kept at −20 °C for EB concentration measurement. Subsequent to thawing, homogenates were centrifuged (at $10625 \times g$ for 12 min at 4 °C), and the supernatant was collected and diluted with 1:3 volumes of 95% ethanol prior to photospectrometric (Synergy 4; Bio-Tek) determination of EB concentration (fluorescence: excitation at 590 nm, emission at 645 nm, absorbance at 620 nm). Results were normalized to the tissue weight.

Western blot analysis

Lungs were perfused with PBS, excised, rinsed in saline, dried with tissue paper, weighed, cut into small pieces, and snap-frozen in liquid nitrogen; the samples were stored at − 80 °C. For western blot analysis, whole lungs were homogenized and whole lung lysates were used. Lungs were homogenized in the lysis buffer (Thermo Fisher Scientific) for protein extraction with protease and phosphatase inhibitors. Protein concentration was measured with the use of a BCA assay. Subsequently, the samples from at least six mice in each experimental group were pooled together in such a way that an equal amount of protein from each sample was dissolved in an equal volume of the lysis buffer for each mouse in the group to ensure the equal representation of each individual sample in the pooled specimen. After addition of loading buffer, samples were heated at 95 °C for 5 min and then frozen at − 80 °C. Each time, an equal amount of protein from pooled samples was loaded and run on the gel, and then transferred to a nitrocellulose membrane, blocked with 5% dry milk, and incubated with the primary antibodies directed against the following antigens: p(S1177)eNOS (ab195944; Abcam), eNOS (610,296; BD Transduction Laboratories), VEGFA (ab68334; Abcam), VEGFR2 (ab39256; Abcam), Ang-1 (ab8451; Abcam), Ang-2 (PA5-27297; Thermo Fisher Scientific), VCAM-1 (CBL1300; Merck), Slit2 (ab134166; Abcam), ROBO4 (orb101060; Biorbyt), ROBO1 (ab85312; Abcam), TGF-β1 (ab155264; Abcam), VE-CAD (sc-6458; Santa Cruz Biotechnology), CD31 (NBP1-71663H; Novus Biologicals), vWF (ab9378; Abcam), MMP-2 (ab19167; Abcam), MMP-9 (ab19016; Abcam), and MMP-14 (sab4501901; Sigma Aldrich). The appropriate horseradish peroxidase (HRP)-conjugated secondary antibodies were from Santa Cruz Biotechnology (sc-2020, sc-2004, and sc-2005). Equal protein loading was confirmed after transfer onto membranes, as measured by a stain-free technique provided by Bio-Rad [30]. Densitometric assessment of band intensity was performed using ImageJ. The results are presented as the fold change of control corresponding to healthy mice. Total protein was used as a loading control.

Measurement of platelet basal activity and ADP-induced reactivity

Blood samples were collected into a syringe containing 3.8% citrate (blood/citrate at 10:1 (v/v)) from the right heart ventricle. A blood count was performed using the animal blood counter Vet abc (Horiba Medical, France). The samples designated for flow cytometric measurements were diluted with saline and washed with Tyrode buffer. Each sample was double stained with four antibodies that included platelet-specific antigen GpIIbIIIa (CD41/61), either FITC or PE conjugated, for platelet identification and one of four platelet activation markers—PE-conjugated active form of GPIIb/IIIa and

P-selectin antibodies, FITC-conjugated fibrinogen, or von Willebrand (vWF) factor—representing platelet binding capacity. Platelets were identified based on their forward-scatter and side-scatter characteristics and were gated on the basis of the expression of platelet-specific antigen CD41/61 (see Additional file 1). Isotype control antibodies, either FITC or PE conjugated, were used to assess nonspecific binding for each individual sample. Basal and ADP-induced (20 µM) activation of circulating platelets was assessed on the basis of the measured expression/binding level of surface membrane antigens expressed as a percentage of all platelets above the isotype control fluorescent signal and the median fluorescence intensity (MFI). Flow cytometric analyses of platelet activation were performed using flow cytometry software (LSRII and FACS/Diva version 6.0, respectively; Becton Dickinson, Oxford, UK). Measurements were made on a logarithmic scale and at least 10,000 events were collected for each sample. Appropriate color compensation was determined in samples singly stained with either FITC-conjugated anti-CD41/61 or PE-conjugated anti-CD41/61.

Statistical analysis

Data were presented as mean ± SD (box) with outliers or median of the data and interquartile range (IQR) (box, from lower (25%) to upper (75%) quartile) with outliers depending on normality of the data distribution that was tested with the Shapiro–Wilk normality test, homogeneity of variances that was tested with Barlett's test, and the variable scale. Statistical significance was assessed with a one-way ANOVA or Kruskall–Wallis test followed by a post-hoc Tukey's or Dunn's multiple comparison test, respectively. Some variables nonconforming with the normal distribution and/or variance homogeneity were Box–Cox transformed and analyzed with parametric tests, otherwise they were analyzed with nonparametric inference tests. Only $P < 0.05$ was considered significant.

Results

Development of pulmonary metastasis and systemic inflammation in the orthotopic murine 4T1 breast cancer model

The first pulmonary metastatic nodules were detected in the 3rd week after breast cancer cell injection (Fig. 1d, g), while the primary tumor became detectable in the 2nd week after cancer cell inoculation (Fig. 1i). Then, both the number of pulmonary metastases and the primary tumor weight and volume increased progressively (Fig. 1). The weight of the lungs was significantly increased only in the 5th week compared to control healthy mice (Table 1), since only at that time was the presence of large metastastic foci in the lungs detected (Fig. 1f, g). The appearance of the first metastatic nodules in the lungs in the 3rd week after breast

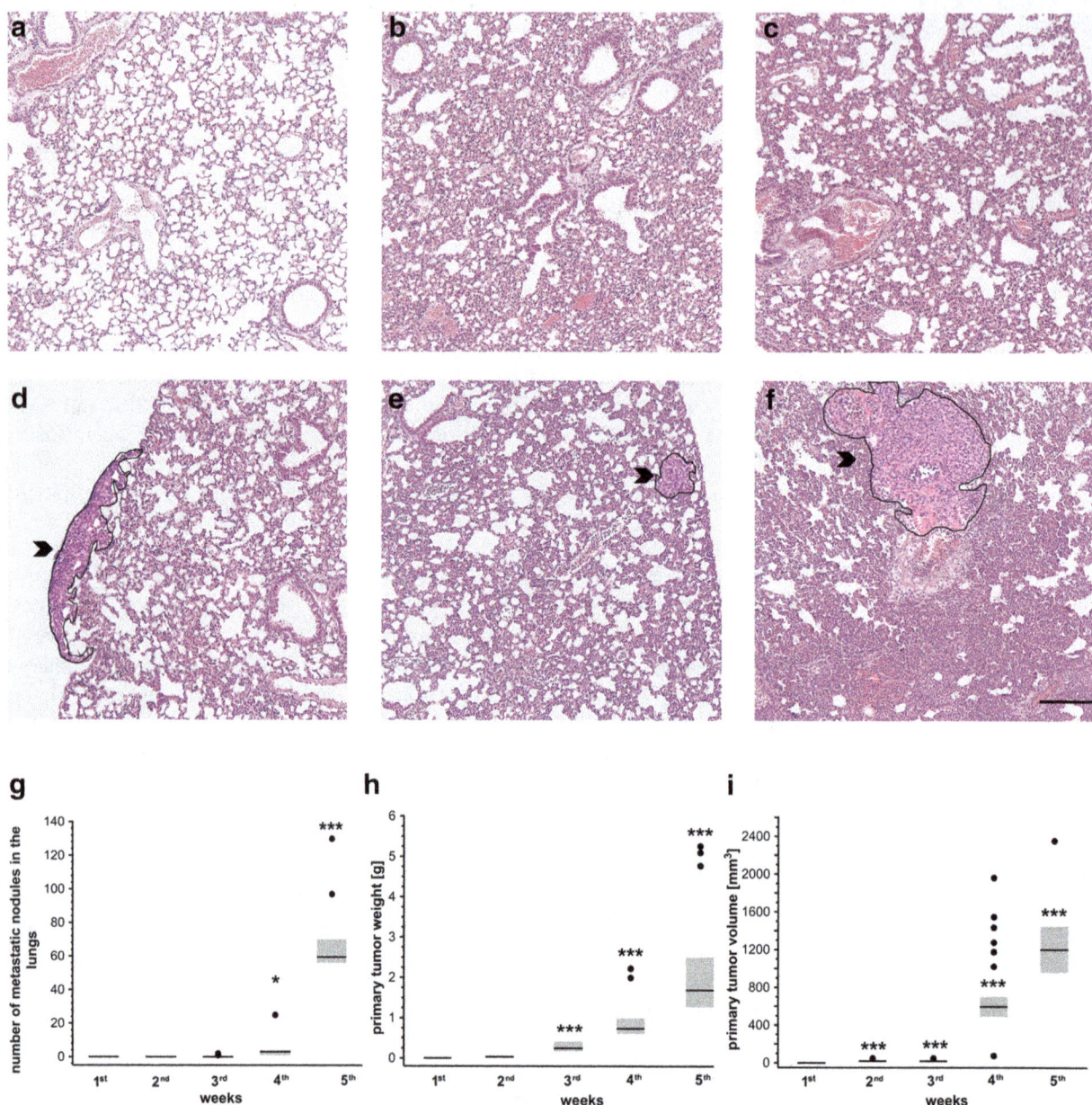

Fig. 1 Tumor growth and development of pulmonary metastasis in 4T1 breast cancer progression in mice. **a** Lung cross-section of healthy control mouse. **b–f** Mice injected orthotopically with 4T1 breast cancer cells (see Methods). Designated groups of animals sacrificed every 7 days to assess number of pulmonary metastases in 1st (**b**), 2nd (**c**), 3rd (**d**), 4th (**e**), and 5th (**f**) week after 4T1 breast cancer inoculation (black arrowheads point to metastatic nodules in lungs) on lung cross-sections stained with H&E. Scale bar represents 200 μm. **g** Number of pulmonary metastases in mice from 1st to 5th week after 4T1 cancer cell inoculation; $n = 10$ for 1st –4th week and $n = 14$ for 5th week. **h** Weight of primary tumor in consecutive weeks after 4T1 cancer cell inoculation; $n = 30$ for 1st –4th week and $n = 68$ for 5th week. (**i**) Primary tumor volume; $n = 30$ for 1st –4th week and $n = 68$ for 5th week. (g–i) Data presented as median and IQR. Black circle indicates outlier. Depending on variable scale, normality of distribution, and variance homogeneity, data analyzed with Kruskal–Wallis test followed by Dunn's multiple comparison test. Statistical significance vs mice in 1st week after 4T1 cancer cell inoculation at *$P < 0.05$ and ***$P < 0.001$

cancer cell injection correlated with the onset of systemic leukocytosis and increased spleen weight (Table 1), indicating the onset of systemic inflammation. Pulmonary metastasis was also associated with

progressive degradation of elastin fibers (Fig. 2a–g) and an increase in the expression of metalloproteinase 2, 9, and 14 (MMP-2, MMP-9, MMP-14) in the lungs 3 and 4 weeks after breast cancer cell injection,

Nitric oxide deficiency and endothelial–mesenchymal transition of pulmonary endothelium...

61

Table 1 Lung/spleen weight and blood count in the orthotopic 4T1 breast cancer model in mice

Parameter	Week after 4T1 cancer cell inoculation					
	Control	1st	2nd	3rd	4th	5th
Lung weight (g)	0.76; 0.70–0.80 (n = 30)	0.77; 0.70–0.81 (n = 29)	0.76; 0.72–0.84 (n = 30)	0.81; 0.76–0.85 (n = 29)	0.0.82; 0.77–0.91 (n = 30)	1.7; 1.3–2.22*** (n = 49)
WBC (K/µl)	4.20; 3.41–5.22 (n = 35)	4.70; 4.04–5.28 (n = 21)	5.55; 4.94–6.21 (n = 23)	17.02; 11.85–24.78*** (n = 23)	54.62; 96.18–177.10*** (n = 20)	257.30; 148.20–317.10*** (n = 36)
GRA (K/µl)	1.00; 0.80–1.20 (n = 35)	1.25; 1.10–1.40 (n = 21)	1.85; 1.35–2.40* (n = 23)	11.30; 6.95–16.10*** (n = 23)	79.00; 42.48–132.80*** (n = 20)	159.80; 89.25–220.90*** (n = 36)
LYM (K/µl)	3.10; 2.50–3.85 (n = 35)	3.25; 2.75–3.87 (n = 21)	3.40; 2.80–3.90 (n = 23)	5.65; 4.15–7.00*** (n = 23)	18.50; 9.75–24.13*** (n = 20)	46.90; 25.00–95.00*** (n = 35)
Spleen weight (g)	0.10; 0.09–0.11 (n = 20)	0.10; 0.09–0.11 (n = 30)	0.12; 0.11–0.13 (n = 30)	0.24; 0.20–0.32** (n = 30)	0.54; 0.43–0.68*** (n = 30)	0.89; 0.79–0.99*** (n = 70)

Data presented as median; interquartile range. Blood count performed to assess development of systemic inflammation whereas spleen weight recorded as an indirect marker of systemic inflammation [48]. Based on normality of distribution and variance homogeneity, data were analyzed with Kruskal–Wallis test followed by Dunn's multiple comparison test. Statistical significance vs healthy control mice at *P < 0.05, **P < 0.01 and ***P < 0.001

WBC white blood cells, *GRA* granulocytes, *LYM* lymphocytes

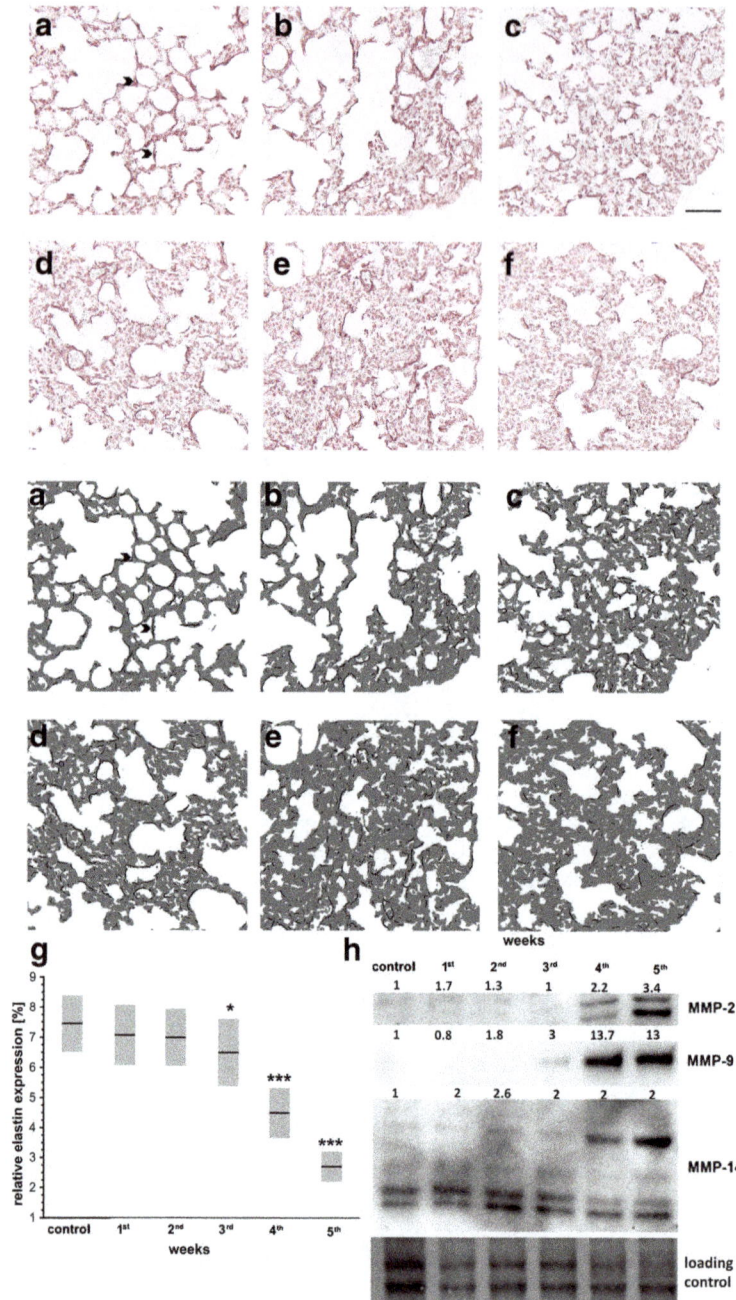

Fig. 2 Changes in pulmonary elastin and metalloproteinase expression in 4T1 breast cancer progression in mice. Paraffin-embedded lungs cut into slices to visualize elastin (see Methods). **a–f** above Representative image of (**a**) healthy control and 1st (**b**), 2nd (**c**), 3rd (**d**), 4th (**e**), and 5th (**f**) week after 4T1 cancer cell inoculation. Scale bar represents 50 μm. **a–f** below Corresponding segmentation. **g** Differences in relative elastin expression (dark gray pixels corresponding to elastin vs light gray pictures corresponding to lung tissue), shown as mean ± SD. Black circle indicates outlier; $n = 20$ for healthy control mice and mice in 1st, 2nd, and 4th week of disease; $n = 21$ for mice in 3rd week of disease; $n = 19$ for mice in 5th week of disease. Data subjected to Box–Cox transformation and analyzed by one-way AVOVA followed by Tukey's multiple comparison test due to normality of distribution and homogeneity of variances. Statistical difference vs healthy control mice at $*P < 0.05$ and $***P < 0.001$. **h** MMP-2, MMP-9, and MMP-14 expression in pooled samples ($n = 6$) (see Methods). MMP-2, higher band indicates inactive isoform while lower band indicates active isoform. MMP-14, higher band corresponds to active monomer while lower band corresponds to domains after catalytical cleavage. Results presented as fold change vs control sample corresponding to healthy mice. Total protein after transfer was used as loading control

respectively (Fig. 2h), being compatible with tissue re-modeling accompanying the advanced stage of metastasis progression.

Progressive impairment of NO production in lungs in the orthotopic murine 4T1 breast cancer model

Local NO production in the lungs was impaired already in the 1st week after 4T1 cell injection (Fig. 3a) and remained significantly compromised thereafter in 4T1 breast cancer-bearing mice. The progressive fall in NO production in mice injected with 4T1 cells corresponded with progressive decrease in eNOS phosphorylation of S1177 observed throughout the progression of the disease after 4T1 cancer cell inoculation (Fig. 3b).

Expression of endothelial–mesenchymal transition markers in pulmonary endothelium in the orthotopic murine 4T1 breast cancer model

Expression of Snail in the lungs of mice orthotopically injected with 4T1 breast cancer cells, compared with healthy control mice, was higher in the endothelial layer of small arteries as soon as 1 week after cancer cell injection and stayed elevated throughout the entire progression of the disease, except for the terminal time point 5 weeks after 4T1 breast cancer cell inoculation (Fig. 4a–g). TGF-β1 expression in the lungs was slightly

increased only in the 1st week after 4T1 breast cancer cell inoculation (Fig. 4h). The phenotypic change of pulmonary endothelium compatible with endothelial–mesenchymal transition, evidenced by downregulation of endothelium-specific proteins such as VE-CAD, CD31, vWF, or VEGFR2, seemed to be evident 3 weeks after cancer cell inoculation (Fig. 4i), concomitant with the early phase of metastasis (Fig. 1g).

Changes in pulmonary endothelial barrier function in the orthotopic murine 4T1 breast cancer model

Increased permeability of pulmonary endothelium expressed as increased deposition of Evans blue (EB) in the lungs of 4T1 breast cancer-bearing mice was found only in the 3rd week after cancer cell inoculation (Fig. 5a), indicating an evident increase in endothelial permeability at the early phase of metastasis. Then, EB leakage from the circulation into the lungs started to decrease and, finally, it was lower than in healthy control mice in the 5th week after cancer cell inoculation. Decreasing EB penetration into the lungs of mice in the 4th and 5th weeks of the disease appeared to be due to the occlusion of pulmonary vessels by cancer cells proliferating in their lumen (Fig. 5b–d), rather than due to changes in pulmonary endothelial permeability itself. Increased permeability of the pulmonary endothelium in

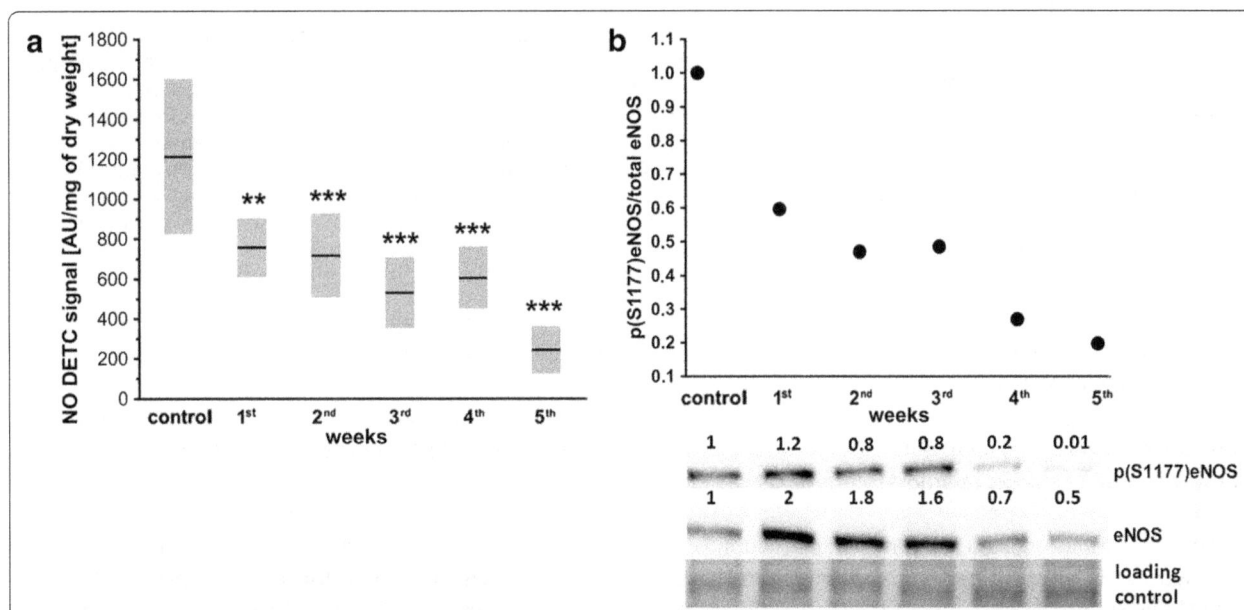

Fig. 3 Pulmonary NO production and eNOS phosphorylation in orthotopic 4T1 breast cancer model in mice. **a** NO production in lungs, presented as mean ± SD. Data were Box–Cox transformed and analyzed with one-way ANOVA followed by Tukey's multiple comparison test; $n = 10$ for control and 1st–4th week of disease; $n = 19$ for 5th week of disease. Black circle indicates outlier. Perfused lungs were excised from euthanized animals and NO production measured (see Methods). Statistical significance vs healthy control mice at **$P < 0.01$ and ***$P < 0.001$. **b** Densitometric data presenting eNOS and p(S1177)eNOS levels during progression of breast cancer used to calculate relative eNOS phosphorylation at serine 1177 (black circle) expressed as fraction of total eNOS level in lungs of control healthy mice for which an arbitrary value of 1 was ascribed. Western blot image presents fold change vs control sample corresponding to healthy mice. Total protein after transfer was used as loading control. Western blot image shows p(S1177)eNOS and eNOS levels in pooled samples in all experimental groups obtained by pooling lung homogenates from six mice in each experimental group (see Methods). AU arbitrary units, eNOS endothelial nitric oxide synthase, NO nitric oxide

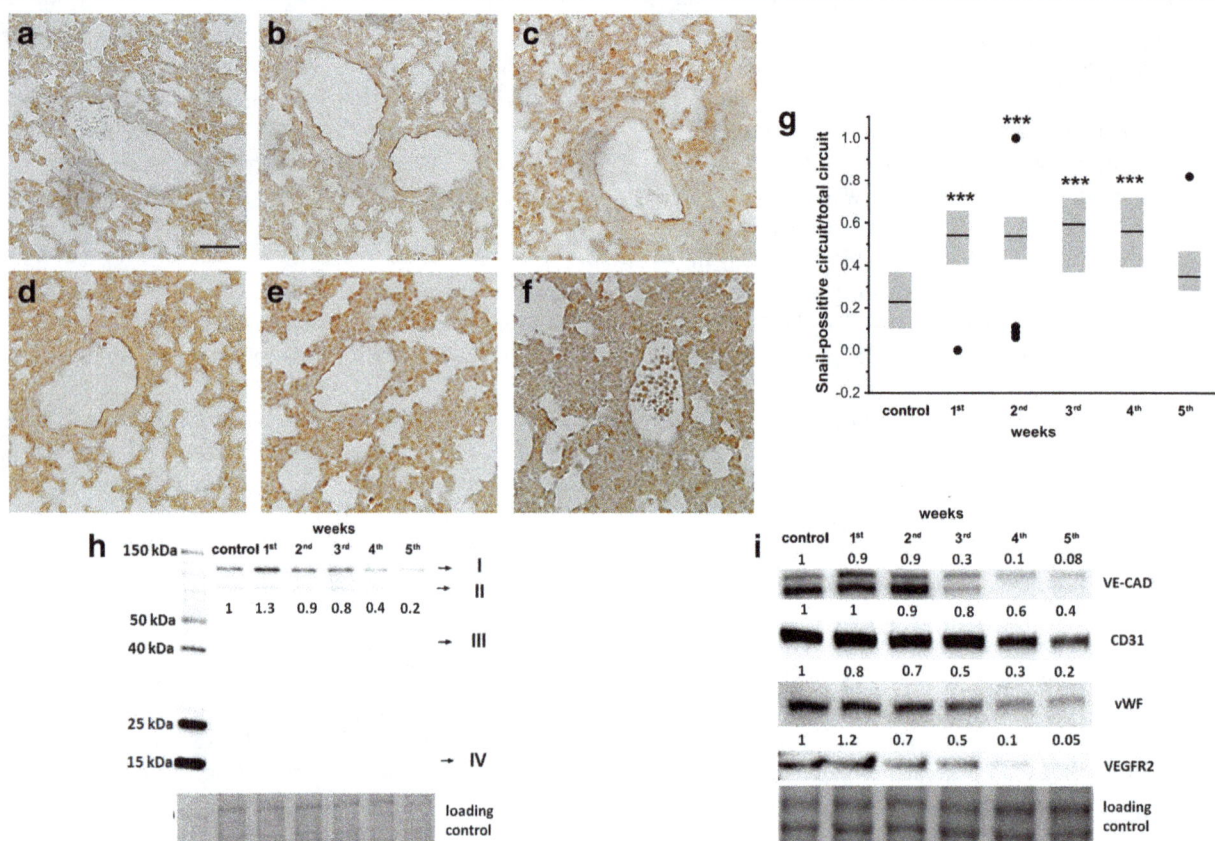

Fig. 4 Snail and EndMT-related protein expression in lungs in orthotopic murine 4T1 breast cancer model. **a–g** Expression of Snail (see Methods). Representative micrographs of arteries from control (**a**), 1st (**b**), 2nd (**c**), 3rd (**d**), 4th (**e**), and 5th (**f**) week after 4T1 cell inoculation. Scale bar represents 50 μm. **g** Quantitative expression of Snail in endothelial layer of small arteries of each group, shown as median and IQR. Black circle indicates outlier. Data analyzed with Kruskal–Wallis test followed by Dunn's multiple comparison test; $n = 61$, $n = 60$, $n = 58$, $n = 60$, $n = 60$, and $n = 59$ for control, 1st, 2nd, 3rd, 4th and 5th week. Statistical significance vs healthy control group at ***$P < 0.001$. **h, i** TGF-β1 (I, TGF-β1 and TGF-β2 heterodimers; II, TGF-β1 homodimers; III, full-length inactive TGF-β1; IV, mature TGF-β1) (**h**) and VE-CAD (vascular endothelium cadherin), CD31 (cluster of differentiation 31), vWF (von Willebrand factor), and VEGFR2 (vascular endothelial growth factor receptor 2) (**i**) levels determined by western blot analysis in pooled ($n = 6$) samples in control and 4T1 breast cancer-bearing mice from the 1st to 5th week after 4T1 cancer cell inoculation (see Methods). Results presented as fold change vs control sample corresponding to healthy mice. Total protein after transfer was used as loading control

the 3rd week after cancer cell inoculation correlated with a transient increase in VEGFA and VCAM-1 expression in the lungs (Fig. 5e).

Progressive downregulation of Slit2–ROBO4–ROBO1 pathway in the orthotopic murine 4T1 breast cancer model

Slit2 maintains endothelium integrity via interaction of its full-length or N-terminal part with endothelium-specific ROBO4 via ROBO1 [19, 31, 32]. Full-length Slit2 was undetectable in lungs homogenates of both control and 4T1 breast cancer-bearing mice, while its N-terminal fragment was found both in healthy control and breast-cancer bearing mice (Fig. 6). Upregulation of both receptors ROBO4 and ROBO1 was detected only in the 1st week after 4T1 cell injection when the level of N-terminal Slit2 binding ROBO receptors was still preserved. Starting from the 2nd week after cancer cell inoculation, the Slit2–ROBO4–

ROBO1 protective signaling pathway was gradually downregulated in the lungs of 4T1 breast cancer-bearing mice.

Changes in basal platelet activation and ADP-induced reactivity in the orthotopic murine 4T1 breast cancer model

Basal platelet activation and ADP-induced reactivity were both assessed as the percentage of platelets expressing P-selectin, active form of GPIIb/IIIa, vWF, and fibrinogen bound to platelet surface in their entire population (Fig. 7) as well as median expression of these antigens on the platelet surface (Fig. 8). The signs for activation of platelets in the early phase of metastasis and loss of reactivity to stimuli afterward were detected. The percentage of platelets expressing P-selectin and active form of GPIIb/IIIa peptide in basal condition or upon ADP stimulation were not different between healthy control and 4T1 breast cancer-bearing mice

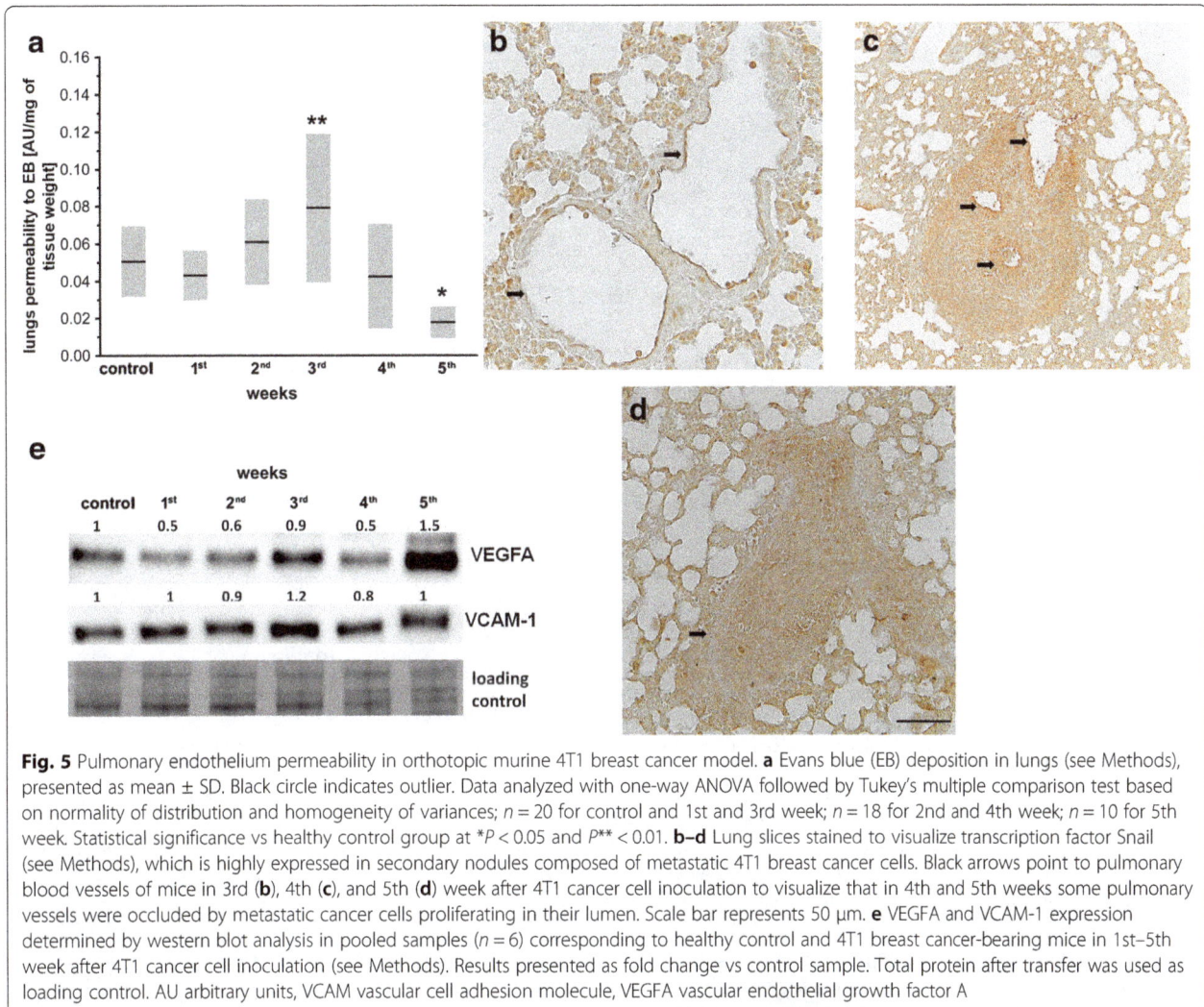

Fig. 5 Pulmonary endothelium permeability in orthotopic murine 4T1 breast cancer model. **a** Evans blue (EB) deposition in lungs (see Methods), presented as mean ± SD. Black circle indicates outlier. Data analyzed with one-way ANOVA followed by Tukey's multiple comparison test based on normality of distribution and homogeneity of variances; $n = 20$ for control and 1st and 3rd week; $n = 18$ for 2nd and 4th week; $n = 10$ for 5th week. Statistical significance vs healthy control group at $*P < 0.05$ and $P** < 0.01$. **b–d** Lung slices stained to visualize transcription factor Snail (see Methods), which is highly expressed in secondary nodules composed of metastatic 4T1 breast cancer cells. Black arrows point to pulmonary blood vessels of mice in 3rd (**b**), 4th (**c**), and 5th (**d**) week after 4T1 cancer cell inoculation to visualize that in 4th and 5th weeks some pulmonary vessels were occluded by metastatic cancer cells proliferating in their lumen. Scale bar represents 50 μm. **e** VEGFA and VCAM-1 expression determined by western blot analysis in pooled samples ($n = 6$) corresponding to healthy control and 4T1 breast cancer-bearing mice in 1st–5th week after 4T1 cancer cell inoculation (see Methods). Results presented as fold change vs control sample. Total protein after transfer was used as loading control. AU arbitrary units, VCAM vascular cell adhesion molecule, VEGFA vascular endothelial growth factor A

(Fig. 7a, b). However, fibrinogen binding in basal conditions was increased in 4T1 breast cancer-bearing mice as compared with control mice 1–3 weeks after 4T1 cancer cell inoculation, reaching significance 2 weeks after cancer cell inoculation. Similarly, vWF binding to platelets was also increased 1–3 weeks after cancer cell inoculation (not significantly). In contrast, 5 weeks after 4T1 breast cancer cell inoculation, the capacity of platelets to bind fibrinogen and vWF was significantly diminished in basal conditions as well as after ADP stimulation (Fig. 7c, d). As shown in Fig. 8, median expression of P-selectin, active form GPIIb/IIIa, vWF, and bound fibrinogen on the unstimulated platelet surface was not altered in 4T1 breast cancer-bearing mice as compared with controls. However, after ADP stimulation, platelet surface expression of vWF and fibrinogen but not P-selectin and active form of GPIIb/IIIa was increased to a lesser extent in 4T1 breast cancer-bearing mice as compared with healthy controls (Fig. 8c, d).

Discussion

This study comprehensively characterized step-by-step progression of pulmonary endothelial dysfunction during 4T1 breast cancer growth and metastasis to establish at which stage endothelial impairment and mesenchymal transformation of endothelial cells (EndMT) occurs in metastatic organs in relation to the formation of metastasis. We found that NO production in pulmonary endothelium was impaired already at the premetastatic phase of the disease concomitantly with decreased eNOS phosphorylation in the lungs (Fig. 3). However, even though the expression of Snail transcription factors in the pulmonary endothelium (Fig. 4a–g) and TGF-β1 in the lungs (Fig. 4h) (both known to be main drivers of EndMT) were increased in relation to healthy controls already in the premetastatic stage (1st week), the onset of functional phenotypic switch of pulmonary endothelium known as EndMT seemed to take place no earlier than the 3rd week after breast cancer cell inoculation

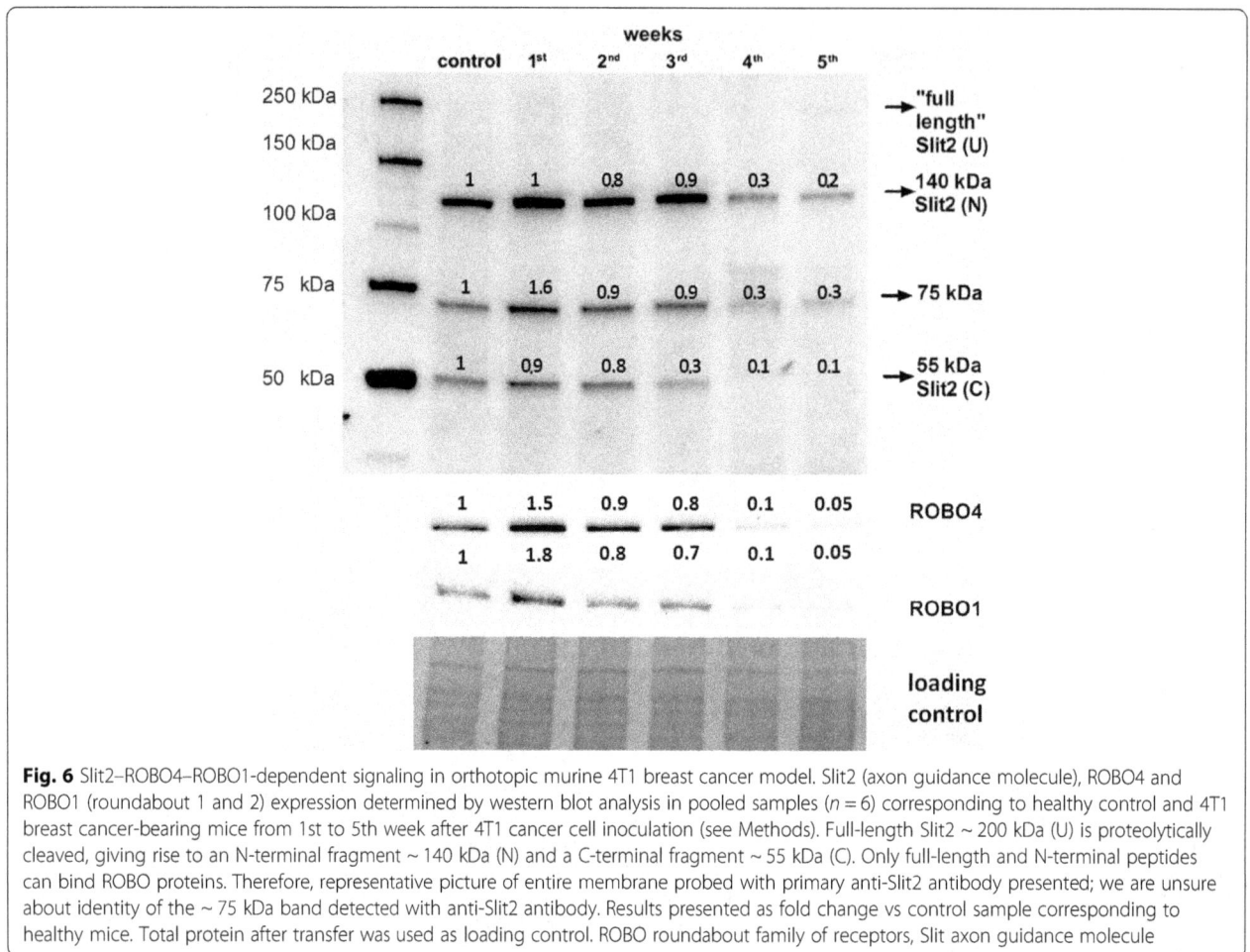

Fig. 6 Slit2–ROBO4–ROBO1-dependent signaling in orthotopic murine 4T1 breast cancer model. Slit2 (axon guidance molecule), ROBO4 and ROBO1 (roundabout 1 and 2) expression determined by western blot analysis in pooled samples (n = 6) corresponding to healthy control and 4T1 breast cancer-bearing mice from 1st to 5th week after 4T1 cancer cell inoculation (see Methods). Full-length Slit2 ~ 200 kDa (U) is proteolytically cleaved, giving rise to an N-terminal fragment ~ 140 kDa (N) and a C-terminal fragment ~ 55 kDa (C). Only full-length and N-terminal peptides can bind ROBO proteins. Therefore, representative picture of entire membrane probed with primary anti-Slit2 antibody presented; we are unsure about identity of the ~ 75 kDa band detected with anti-Slit2 antibody. Results presented as fold change vs control sample corresponding to healthy mice. Total protein after transfer was used as loading control. ROBO roundabout family of receptors, Slit axon guidance molecule

(Fig. 4i). At that stage, pulmonary endothelium became activated, as evidenced by higher VCAM-1 expression (Fig. 5e), and endothelial barrier integrity was lost, as visualized by increased deposition of EB in the lungs (Fig. 5a). Development of EndMT also seemed to coincide with progressive decrease in pulmonary elastin levels (Fig. 2a–g) and increased expression of proteolytic enzymes like metalloproteinase 2, 9, and 14 (MMP-2, MMP-9, MMP-14) in the lungs (Fig. 2h), indicating metastatic tissue remodeling at this stage. To summarize, our results identified decreased eNOS activity and phosphorylation resulting in an NO-deficiency state as an early event in breast cancer pulmonary metastasis, that occurs prior to the decrease in expression of endothelium-specific markers that indicates functional phenotypic switch of pulmonary endothelium toward a mesenchymal phenotype (EndMT), coinciding with development of the first metastatic nodules in the lungs and metastatic tissue remodeling.

Recently, it has been postulated that endothelial cells can actively augment metastatic extravasation through the shift in their phenotype known as endothelial–mesenchymal transition [26]. Moreover, in the case of the lungs, transformed endothelial cells can represent a significant source of fibroblasts [33] that can enrich the population of cancer-associated fibroblasts (CAFs) that constitute key components of tumor stroma [26]. Therefore, hampering or preventing EndMT could directly affect settlement of cancer cells in the lungs. In the present work, however, we demonstrated that the phenotypic switch of pulmonary endothelium toward mesenchymal cells (EndMT, evidenced by downregulation of VE-CAD, CD31, vWF, or VEGFR2 [34]) is a relatively late response in murine 4T1 metastatic breast cancer. It coincides with increased endothelial permeability and early metastasis but is preceded by a clear-cut NO-deficiency state, that was detected as early as 1 week after 4T1 cancer cell inoculation in the premetastatic stage, even before the primary tumor was detectable. These findings suggest that early endothelial dysfunction in the lungs, indicated by NO deficiency rather than EndMT, might represent a primary regulatory target to prevent early pulmonary metastasis. Indeed, NO was shown to inhibit heteroadhesion of cancer cells to endothelial cells [5]. Moreover, decreased NO levels in the circulation have been shown to promote EndMT [35], while eNOS stimulation had the opposite effect [36]. However, the role of NO bioavailability in

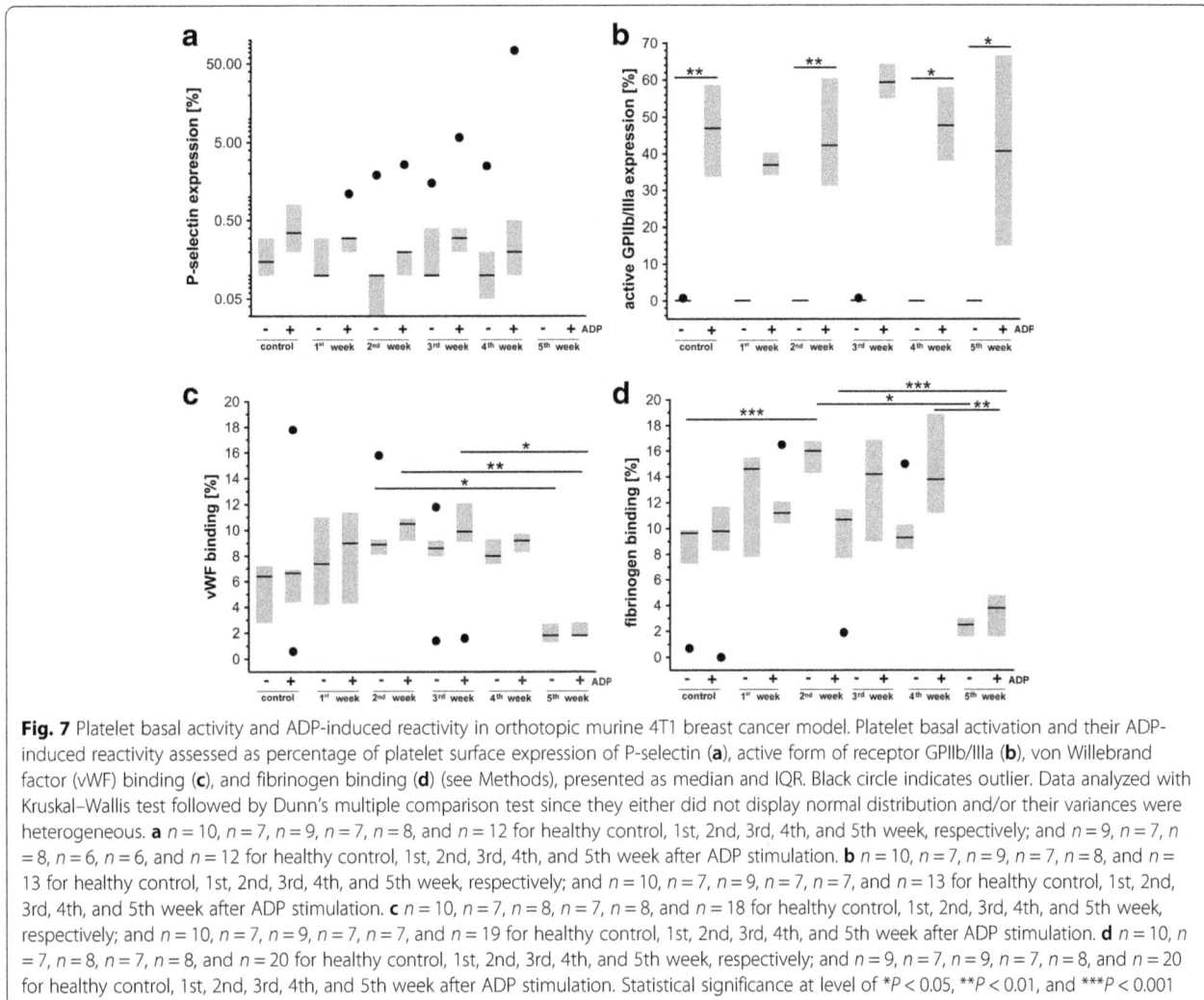

Fig. 7 Platelet basal activity and ADP-induced reactivity in orthotopic murine 4T1 breast cancer model. Platelet basal activation and their ADP-induced reactivity assessed as percentage of platelet surface expression of P-selectin (**a**), active form of receptor GPIIb/IIIa (**b**), von Willebrand factor (vWF) binding (**c**), and fibrinogen binding (**d**) (see Methods), presented as median and IQR. Black circle indicates outlier. Data analyzed with Kruskal–Wallis test followed by Dunn's multiple comparison test since they either did not display normal distribution and/or their variances were heterogeneous. **a** $n = 10$, $n = 7$, $n = 9$, $n = 7$, $n = 8$, and $n = 12$ for healthy control, 1st, 2nd, 3rd, 4th, and 5th week, respectively; and $n = 9$, $n = 7$, $n = 8$, $n = 6$, $n = 6$, and $n = 12$ for healthy control, 1st, 2nd, 3rd, 4th, and 5th week after ADP stimulation. **b** $n = 10$, $n = 7$, $n = 9$, $n = 7$, $n = 8$, and $n = 13$ for healthy control, 1st, 2nd, 3rd, 4th, and 5th week, respectively; and $n = 10$, $n = 7$, $n = 9$, $n = 7$, $n = 7$, and $n = 13$ for healthy control, 1st, 2nd, 3rd, 4th, and 5th week after ADP stimulation. **c** $n = 10$, $n = 7$, $n = 8$, $n = 7$, $n = 8$, and $n = 18$ for healthy control, 1st, 2nd, 3rd, 4th, and 5th week, respectively; and $n = 10$, $n = 7$, $n = 9$, $n = 7$, $n = 7$, and $n = 19$ for healthy control, 1st, 2nd, 3rd, 4th, and 5th week after ADP stimulation. **d** $n = 10$, $n = 7$, $n = 8$, $n = 7$, $n = 8$, and $n = 20$ for healthy control, 1st, 2nd, 3rd, 4th, and 5th week, respectively; and $n = 9$, $n = 7$, $n = 9$, $n = 7$, $n = 8$, and $n = 20$ for healthy control, 1st, 2nd, 3rd, 4th, and 5th week after ADP stimulation. Statistical significance at level of $*P < 0.05$, $**P < 0.01$, and $***P < 0.001$

regulation of progression of various cancers is complex and its antimetastatic effects seem to depend on multiple factors (i.e., disease stage [37]). Indeed, while Buczek et al. [38] showed that both local as well as systemic NO deficiency was present in the premetastatic stage of 4T1 breast cancer, increased systemic NO bioavailability at the advanced stage was associated with increased mortality of 4T1 breast cancer-bearing mice [39].

Interestingly, in spite of early NO deficiency (Fig. 3), the onset of functional EndMT in the lungs of 4T1 breast cancer-bearing mice seemed to be delayed until the 3rd week, in spite of the increased expression of Snail transcription factors in the pulmonary endothelium (Fig. 4a–g) and TGF-β1 in the lungs (Fig. 4h) known to drive mesenchymal shift of endothelial cells [22]. We are tempted to speculate that the delayed onset of EndMT could result from the activation of Slit2 and its receptors' ROBO1–ROBO4-dependent signaling in the 1st week of breast cancer progression (Fig. 6), since Slit2 was previously reported to inhibit both TGF-β [40] and

Snail [41] signaling, both involved in the triggering of mesenchymal transformation of endothelial cells [20, 22–25, 34]. When expression of Slit2 receptors started to decline progressively (2nd week of disease) (Fig. 6), a similar trend was observed in the case of VE-CAD, CD31, vWF, or VEGFR2 (Fig. 4i), indicating the onset of functional EndMT [34]. However, although this new role of Slit2-dependent signaling in inhibition of EndMT in malignant disease is emerging, mechanistic confirmation is still missing. One possibility involves Slit2-dependent inhibition of Notch signaling [42] that is known to trigger EndMT [43]. Last but not least, delayed onset of EndMT in the lungs of 4T1 breast cancer-bearing mice could also have been associated with other Slit2-independent signaling pathways, such as bFGF-dependent signaling counteracting TGF-β signaling [44].

The initiation of functional EndMT in the lungs of breast cancer-bearing mice that seemed to take place at the beginning of the metastatic phase did not coincide with the rise in TGF-β1 levels in the lungs at that time

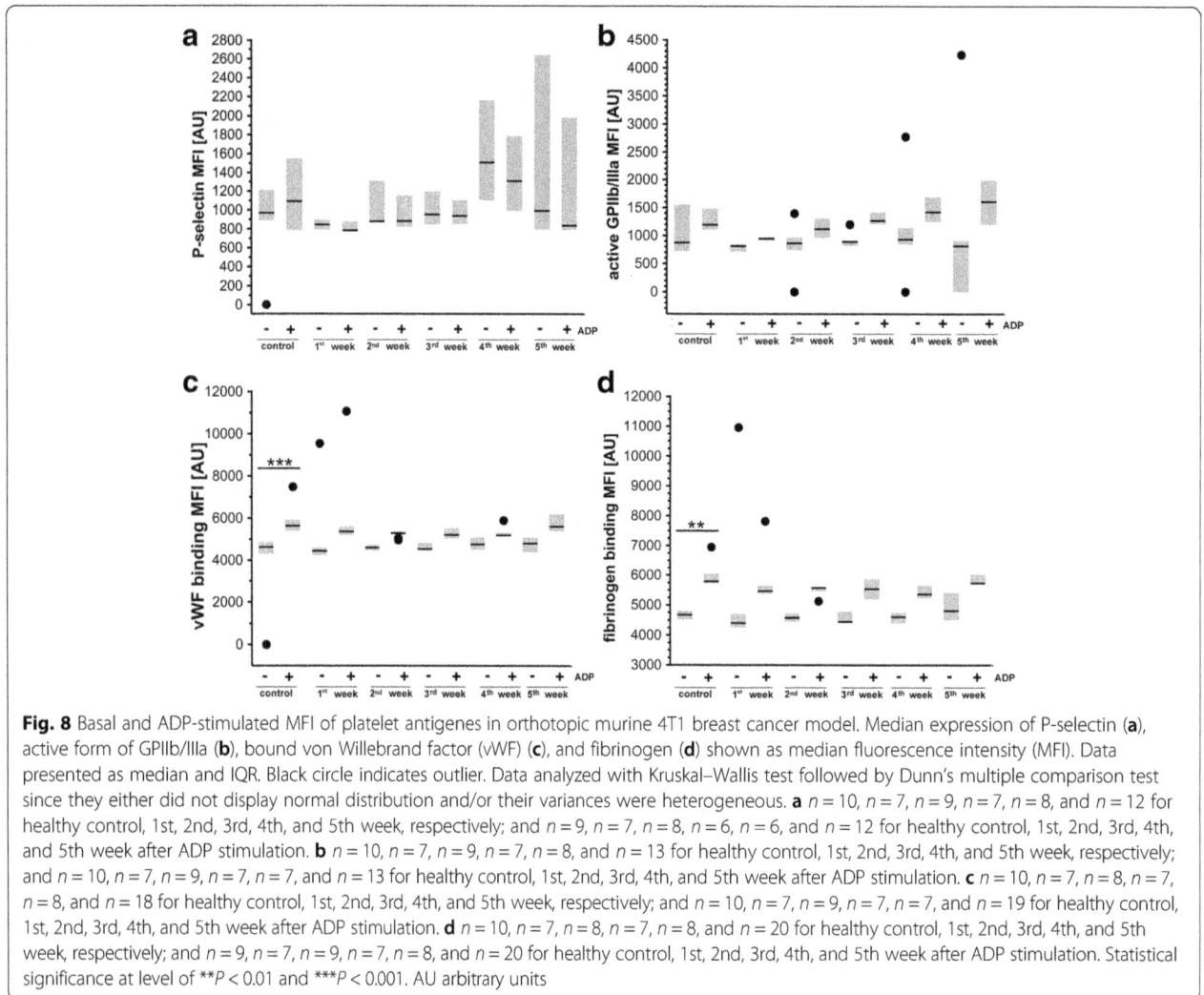

Fig. 8 Basal and ADP-stimulated MFI of platelet antigenes in orthotopic murine 4T1 breast cancer model. Median expression of P-selectin (**a**), active form of GPIIb/IIIa (**b**), bound von Willebrand factor (vWF) (**c**), and fibrinogen (**d**) shown as median fluorescence intensity (MFI). Data presented as median and IQR. Black circle indicates outlier. Data analyzed with Kruskal–Wallis test followed by Dunn's multiple comparison test since they either did not display normal distribution and/or their variances were heterogeneous. **a** $n = 10$, $n = 7$, $n = 9$, $n = 7$, $n = 8$, and $n = 12$ for healthy control, 1st, 2nd, 3rd, 4th, and 5th week, respectively; and $n = 9$, $n = 7$, $n = 8$, $n = 6$, $n = 6$, and $n = 12$ for healthy control, 1st, 2nd, 3rd, 4th, and 5th week after ADP stimulation. **b** $n = 10$, $n = 7$, $n = 9$, $n = 7$, $n = 8$, and $n = 13$ for healthy control, 1st, 2nd, 3rd, 4th, and 5th week, respectively; and $n = 10$, $n = 7$, $n = 9$, $n = 7$, $n = 7$, and $n = 13$ for healthy control, 1st, 2nd, 3rd, 4th, and 5th week after ADP stimulation. **c** $n = 10$, $n = 7$, $n = 8$, $n = 7$, $n = 8$, and $n = 18$ for healthy control, 1st, 2nd, 3rd, 4th, and 5th week, respectively; and $n = 10$, $n = 7$, $n = 9$, $n = 7$, $n = 7$, and $n = 19$ for healthy control, 1st, 2nd, 3rd, 4th, and 5th week after ADP stimulation. **d** $n = 10$, $n = 7$, $n = 8$, $n = 7$, $n = 8$, and $n = 20$ for healthy control, 1st, 2nd, 3rd, 4th, and 5th week, respectively; and $n = 9$, $n = 7$, $n = 9$, $n = 7$, $n = 8$, and $n = 20$ for healthy control, 1st, 2nd, 3rd, 4th, and 5th week after ADP stimulation. Statistical significance at level of **P < 0.01 and ***P < 0.001. AU arbitrary units

(Fig. 4h) and, therefore, must have been associated with activation of TGF-β-independent mechanisms. Recently, Krenning et al. [22] reported that EndMT could also be triggered by disturbances in shear stress and activation of mechanoreceptors such as VE-CAD, CD31, or VEGFR2 on endothelial cells. The level of VEGFA in the lungs of 4T1 breast cancer-bearing mice was transiently increased in the 3rd week of the disease (Fig. 5e) and such a local rise in VEGFA has been recently associated with oscillatory turbulent flow (Lena Claesson-Welsh, personal communication, the 2nd Nov, 2016) that could activate the mechanoreceptors on endothelial cells. Last but not least, yet another possible trigger for EndMT in pulmonary metastasis and pulmonary remodeling is hypoxia. Therefore, further investigation of signaling pathways involved in triggering EndMT of pulmonary endothelium in breast cancer progression is needed, but is beyond the scope of this work.

Effective extravasation of cancer cells could also be actively promoted by platelets. Once activated, platelets express on

their surface or release various tumor-promoting factors, protect circulating tumor cells (CTCs) from immune attack, or promote extravastation of CTCs/tumor angiogenesis [10]. In the present work, we found the signs for activation of platelets in the early phase of metastasis (Fig. 7c, d) and very early loss of their reactivity in response to ADP ex vivo (Fig. 8c, d), confirming a possible involvement of platelets in the early host response to circulating cancer cells [10, 45]. However, although activation of platelets initiates vascular inflammation associated with various diseases [15], their contribution to early pulmonary endothelial dysfunction and/or EndMT in breast cancer progression still needs to be verified.

Conclusions

This study comprehensively described progression of endothelial dysfunction in the lungs, being the primary site of metastasis in Balb/C mice bearing breast cancer. The major finding was that pulmonary endothelium dysfunction, in terms of compromised NO production and decreased eNOS phosphorylation, was an early event in breast cancer progression. It preceded the decrease in expression of endothelium-specific proteins indicating onset of the phenotypic switch of pulmonary endothelium toward the mesenchymal phenotype (EndMT) and development of first metastatic nodules in the lungs. These findings suggest that early endothelial dysfunction featured by NO deficiency in the lungs rather than EndMT might represent a primary regulatory target to prevent early pulmonary metastasis. However, further studies are needed to establish whether preventing the NO deficiency in the function of pulmonary endothelium at the premetastatic stage (i.e., by locally increasing NO bioavailability) could indeed delay or inhibit pulmonary metastasis. It also remains a matter of debate whether targeting pulmonary endothelial mesenchymal transition at the metastatic stage of a malignant disease (e.g. by inhibiting mesenchymal transformation of endothelial cells as by preventing IL-1β-dependent signaling [46, 47]) could improve disease outcomes.

Abbreviations
Ang: Angiopoetin; CD31: Cluster differentiation 31; EndMT: Endothelial-mesenchymal transition; eNOS: Endothelial nitric oxide synthase; IQR: Interquartile range; MFI: Median fluorescence intensity; MMP: Metalloproteinase; ROBO: Roundabout family of receptors; Slit: Axon guidance molecule; TGF-β: Transforming growth factor beta; VCAM: Vascular cell adhesion molecule; VE-CAD: Vascular endothelial-cadherin; VEGFA: Vascular endothelial growth factor A; VEGFR2: Vascular endothelial growth factor receptor 2; vWF: Von Willebrand factor

Funding
The study was supported by the project METENDOPHA from the National Centre for Research and Development (grant coordinated by JCET-UJ, No. STRATEGMED1/233226/11/NCBR/2015) and MINIATURA from the National Science Centre, Poland (No. K/MNT/000041).

Authors' contributions
SC conceptualized the project. JW, MSm, AK, MGA, MSte, TM, AJ, BP, KP, KD, MSto, DK, and EB performed the experiments. MSm wrote the original draft of the manuscript. SC, MGA, and BP reviewed the manuscript. MSm performed statistical analyses. SC and MSm supervised the research. All authors read and approved the final manuscript.

Competing interests
The authors declare that they have no competing interests.

Author details
[1]Jagiellonian Centre for Experimental Therapeutics (JCET), Jagiellonian University, Bobrzynskiego 14 St., 30-348 Krakow, Poland. [2]Department of Experimental Oncology, Hirszfeld Institute of Immunology and Experimental Therapy, Polish Academy of Sciences, Rudolfa Weigla 4 St., 53-114 Wroclaw, Poland. [3]Department of Pharmacology, Jagiellonian University, Medical College, Grzegorzecka 16, 31-531 Krakow, Poland.

References
1. Hutchinson L. Breast cancer: challenges, controversies, breakthroughs. Nat Rev Clin Oncol. 2010;7:669–70.
2. Pierce BL, Ballard-Barbash R, Bernstein L, Baumgartner RN, Neuhouser ML, Wener MH, et al. Elevated biomarkers of inflammation are associated with reduced survival among breast cancer patients. J Clin Oncol. 2009;27:3437–44.
3. Franses JW, Drosu NC, Gibson WJ, Chitalia VC, Edelman ER. Dysfunctional endothelial cells directly stimulate cancer inflammation and metastasis. Int J Cancer. 2013;133:1334–44.
4. Kim KJ, Kwon SH, Yun JH, Jeong HS, Kim HR, Lee EH, et al. STAT3 activation in endothelial cells is important for tumor metastasis via increased cell adhesion molecule expression. Oncogene. 2017;36:5445–59.
5. Lu Y, Yu T, Liang H, Wang J, Xie J, Shao J, et al. Nitric oxide inhibits heteroadhesion of cancer cells to endothelial cells: restraining circulating tumor cells from initiating metastatic cascade. Sci Rep. 2014;4:4344.
6. Rafikov R, Fonseca FV, Kumar S, Pardo D, Darragh C, Elms S, et al. eNOS activation and NO function: structural motifs responsible for the posttranslational control of endothelial nitric oxide synthase activity. J Endocrinol. 2011;210:271–84.
7. Sessa WC. Endothelial-derived nitric oxide as a marker for healthy endothelium. In: Groszmann RJ. Bosch J, editors. Portal Hypertension in the 21st Century. Montreal: The proceedings of a symposium sponsored by Axcan Pharma Inc and NicOX SA; 2004. p. 19–23
8. Liao JK. Linking endothelial dysfunction with endothelial cell activation. J Clin Invest. 2013;123:540–1.
9. Etulain J, Schattner M. Glycobiology of platelet-endothelial cell interactions. Glycobiology. 2014;24:1252–9.
10. Tesfamariam B. Involvement of platelets in tumor cell metastasis. Pharmacol Ther. 2016;157:112–9.
11. Gimbrone MA Jr, Nagel T, Topper JN. Biomechanical activation: an emerging paradigm in endothelial adhesion biology. J Clin Invest. 1997;99:1809–13.
12. Kumar P, Shen Q, Pivetti CD, Lee ES, Wu MH, Yuan SY. Molecular mechanisms of endothelial hyperpermeability: implications in inflammation. Expert Rev Mol Med. 2009;11:e19.
13. Ichiki T, Izumi R, Cataliotti A, Larsen AM, Sandberg SM, Burnett JC Jr. Endothelial permeability in vitro and in vivo: protective actions of ANP and omapatrilat in experimental atherosclerosis. Peptides. 2013;48:21–6.
14. London NR, Zhu W, Bozza FA, Smith MC, Greif DM, Sorensen LK, et al. Targeting Robo4-dependent slit signaling to survive the cytokine storm in sepsis and influenza. Sci Transl Med. 2010;2:23ra19.
15. Rajendran P, Rengarajan T, Thangavel J, Nishigaki Y, Sakthisekaran D, Sethi G, et al. The vascular endothelium and human diseases. Int J Biol Sci. 2013;9:1057–69.
16. Reymond N, d'Água BB, Ridley AJ. Crossing the endothelial barrier during metastasis. Nat Rev Cancer. 2013;13:858–70.
17. Jones CA, London NR, Chen H, Park KW, Sauvaget D, Stockton RA, et al. Robo4 stabilizes the vascular network by inhibiting pathologic angiogenesis and endothelial hyperpermeability. Nat Med. 2008;14:448–53.
18. Lee WL, Slutsky AS. Sepsis and endothelial permeability. N Engl J Med. 2010;363:689–91.

19. Yadav SS, Narayan G. Role of ROBO4 signalling in developmental and pathological angiogenesis. Biomed Res Int. 2014;2014:683025.

20. Wang Y, Shi J, Chai K, Ying X, Zhou BP. The role of snail in EMT and tumorigenesis. Curr Cancer Drug Targets. 2013;13:963–72.

21. Medici D. Endothelial-mesenchymal transition in regenerative medicine. Stem Cells Int. 2016;2016:6962801.

22. Krenning G, Barauna VG, Krieger JE, Harmsen MC, Moonen JR. Endothelial plasticity: shifting phenotypes through force feedback. Stem Cells Int. 2016; 2016:9762959.

23. Piera-Velazquez S, Li Z, Jimenez SA. Role of endothelial-mesenchymal transition (EndoMT) in the pathogenesis of fibrotic disorders. Am J Pathol. 2011;179:1074–80.

24. Lamouille S, Xu J, Derynck R. Molecular mechanisms of epithelial-mesenchymal transition. Nat Rev Mol Cell Biol. 2014;15:178–96.

25. Piera-Velazquez S, Mendoza FA, Jimenez SA. Endothelial to mesenchymal transition (EndoMT) in the pathogenesis of human fibrotic diseases. J Clin Med. 2016;5:E45.

26. Gasparics Á, Rosivall L, Krizbai IA, Sebe A. When the endothelium scores an own goal: endothelial cells actively augment metastatic extravasation through endothelial-mesenchymal transition. Am J Physiol Heart Circ Physiol. 2016;310:H1055–63.

27. Kim EJ, Choi MR, Park H, Kim M, Hong JE, Lee JY, et al. Dietary fat increases solid tumor growth and metastasis of 4T1 murine mammary carcinoma cells and mortality in obesity-resistant BALB/c mice. Breast Cancer Res. 2011;13:R78.

28. Schneider CA, Rasband WS, Eliceiri KW. NIH image to ImageJ: 25 years of image analysis. Nat Methods. 2012;9:671–5.

29. Cai H, Dikalov S, Griendling K, Harrison D. Detection of reactive oxygen species and nitric oxide in vascular cells and tissues. Vasc Biol Protoc. 2007;139:93–311.

30. Rivero-Gutiérrez B, Anzola A, Martínez-Augustin O, de Medina FS. Stain-free detection as loading control alternative to Ponceau and housekeeping protein immunodetection in western blotting. Anal Biochem. 2014;467:1–3.

31. Nguyen Ba-Charvet KT, Brose K, Ma L, Wang KH, Marillat V, Sotelo C, et al. Diversity and specificity of actions of Slit2 proteolytic fragments in axon guidance. J Neurosci. 2001;21(12):4281–9.

32. Chédotal A. Slits and their receptors. Adv Exp Med Biol. 2007;621:65–80.

33. Hashimoto N, Phan SH, Imaizumi K, Matsuo M, Nakashima H, Kawabe T, et al. Endothelial-mesenchymal transition in bleomycin-induced pulmonary fibrosis. Am J Respir Cell Mol Biol. 2010;43:161–72.

34. Medici D, Kalluri R. Endothelial-mesenchymal transition and its contribution to the emergence of stem cell phenotype. Semin Cancer Biol. 2012;22:379–84.

35. Charytan DM, Padera R, Helfand AM, Zeisberg M, Xu X, Liu X, et al. Increased concentration of circulating angiogenesis and nitric oxide inhibitors induces endothelial to mesenchymal transition and myocardial fibrosis in patients with chronic kidney disease. Int J Cardiol. 2014;176:99–109.

36. Guo Y, Li P, Bledsoe G, Yang ZR, Chao L, Chao J. Kallistatin inhibits TGF-β-induced endothelial-mesenchymal transition by differential regulation of microRNA-21 and eNOS expression. Exp Cell Res. 2015;337:103–10.

37. Cheng H, Wang L, Mollica M, Re AT, Wu S, Zuo L. Nitric oxide in cancer metastasis. Cancer Lett. 2014;353:1–7.

38. Buczek E, Denslow A, Mateuszuk L, Proniewski B, Wojcik T, Sitek B, et al. Alterations in NO- and PGI2-dependent function in aorta in the orthotopic murine model of metastatic 4T1 breast cancer: relationship with pulmonary endothelial dysfunction and systemic inflammation. BMC Cancer. 2018;18(1):582.

39. Smeda M, Kieronska A, Proniewski B, Jasztal A, Selmi A, Wandzel K, et al. Dual antiplatelet therapy with clopidogrel and aspirin increases mortality in 4T1 breast cancer-bearing mice by inducing vascular mimicry. Oncotarget. 2018;9:17810–24.

40. Yuen DA, Huang YW, Liu GY, Patel S, Fang F, Zhou J, et al. Recombinant N-terminal Slit2 inhibits TGF-β-induced fibroblast activation and renal fibrosis. J Am Soc Nephrol. 2016;27:2609–15.

41. Ballard MS, Zhu A, Iwai N, Stensrud M, Mapps A, Postiglione MP, et al. Mammary stem cell self-renewal is regulated by Slit2/Robo1 signaling through SNAI1 and mINSC. Cell Rep. 2015;13:290–301.

42. Li GJ, Yang Y, Yang GK, Wan J, Cui DL, Ma ZH, et al. Slit2 suppresses endothelial cell proliferation and migration by inhibiting the VEGF-notch signaling pathway. Mol Med Rep. 2017;15:1981–8.

43. Chang AC, Fu Y, Garside VC, Niessen K, Chang L, Fuller M, et al. Notch initiates the endothelial-to-mesenchymal transition in the atrioventricular canal through autocrine activation of soluble guanylyl cyclase. Dev Cell. 2011;21:288–300.

44. Xiao L, Dudley AC. Fine-tuning vascular fate during endothelial-mesenchymal transition. J Pathol. 2017;241:25–35.

45. Leblanc R, Peyruchaud O. Metastasis: new functional implications of platelets and megakaryocytes. Blood. 2016;128:24–31.

46. Nie L, Lyros O, Medda R, Jovanovic N, Schmidt JL, Otterson MF, et al. Endothelial-mesenchymal transition in normal human esophageal endothelial cells cocultured with esophageal adenocarcinoma cells: role of IL-1β and TGF-β2. Am J Physiol Cell Physiol. 2014;307:C859–77.

47. Guo B, Fu S, Zhang J, Liu B, Li Z. Targeting inflammasome/IL-1 pathways for cancer immunotherapy. Sci Rep. 2016;6:36107.

48. Murphy EA, Davis JM, Barrilleaux TL, McClellan JL, Steiner JL, Carmichael MD, et al. Benefits of exercise training on breast cancer progression and inflammation in C3(1)SV40Tag mice. Cytokine. 2011;55:274–9.

6

OSM potentiates preintravasation events, increases CTC counts, and promotes breast cancer metastasis to the lung

Ken Tawara[1], Celeste Bolin[1], Jordan Koncinsky[1], Sujatha Kadaba[1], Hunter Covert[1], Caleb Sutherland[1], Laura Bond[1], Joseph Kronz[2], Joel R. Garbow[3] and Cheryl L. Jorcyk[1*]

Abstract

Background: Systemic and chronic inflammatory conditions in patients with breast cancer have been associated with reduced patient survival and increased breast cancer aggressiveness. This paper characterizes the role of an inflammatory cytokine, oncostatin M (OSM), in the preintravasation aspects of breast cancer metastasis.

Methods: OSM expression levels in human breast cancer tissue samples were assessed using tissue microarrays, and expression patterns based on clinical stage were assessed. To determine the in vivo role of OSM in breast cancer metastasis to the lung, we used three orthotopic breast cancer mouse models, including a syngeneic 4T1.2 mouse mammary cancer model, the MDA-MB-231 human breast cancer xenograft model, and an OSM-knockout (OSM-KO) mouse model. Progression of metastatic disease was tracked by magnetic resonance imaging and bioluminescence imaging. Endpoint analysis included circulating tumor cell (CTC) counts, lung metastatic burden analysis by qPCR, and ex vivo bioluminescence imaging.

Results: Using tissue microarrays, we found that tumor cell OSM was expressed at the highest levels in ductal carcinoma in situ. This finding suggests that OSM may function during the earlier steps of breast cancer metastasis. In mice bearing MDA-MB-231-Luc2 xenograft tumors, peritumoral injection of recombinant human OSM not only increased metastases to the lung and decreased survival but also increased CTC numbers. To our knowledge, this is the first time that a gp130 family inflammatory cytokine has been shown to directly affect CTC numbers. Using a 4T1.2 syngeneic mouse model of breast cancer, we found that mice bearing 4T1.2-shOSM tumors with knocked down tumor expression of OSM had reduced CTCs, decreased lung metastatic burden, and increased survival compared with mice bearing control tumors. CTC numbers were further reduced in OSM-KO mice bearing the same tumors, demonstrating the importance of both paracrine- and autocrine-produced OSM in this process. In vitro studies further supported the hypothesis that OSM promotes preintravasation aspects of cancer metastasis, because OSM induced both 4T1.2 tumor cell detachment and migration.

Conclusions: Collectively, our findings suggest that OSM plays a crucial role in the early steps of metastatic breast cancer progression, resulting in increased CTCs and lung metastases as well as reduced survival. Therefore, early therapeutic inhibition of OSM in patients with breast cancer may prevent breast cancer metastasis.

Keywords: Oncostatin M, Breast cancer, Metastasis, Circulating tumor cells

* Correspondence: cjorcyk@boisestate.edu
[1]Department of Biological Sciences, Biomolecular Sciences Program, Boise State University, 1910 University Drive, Boise, ID 83725, USA
Full list of author information is available at the end of the article

Background

The inflammatory gp130 family of cytokines has been shown to modulate immune function [1] with important implications for tumor immunology [2]. Inflammation and inflammatory cytokines have been associated with increased breast cancer metastasis and poor survival rates [3]. Interleukin-6 (IL-6), a well-known inflammatory cytokine in the gp130 family, promotes breast cancer metastasis [4]. Other cytokines within the gp130 family also modulate inflammation. One such member, oncostatin M (OSM), has been associated with a wide variety of inflammatory disease states, such as in inflammatory bowel disease and arthritis [5, 6]. In the context of cancer, OSM has been shown to induce in vitro effects associated with cancer invasiveness and to promote breast cancer metastasis to bone in vivo [7]. In the breast tumor microenvironment, OSM is produced by breast tumor cells [8], as well as by stromal cells, including tumor-associated macrophages and neutrophils [9, 10]. After the secretion of OSM, OSM binds to and accumulates in the extracellular matrix (ECM) in an active form. This accumulated OSM may then lead to chronic local inflammation and increased tumor metastasis [11]. Specifically, it has been shown that human breast tumor cells signal neutrophils to secrete OSM, which subsequently induces tumor cell vascular endothelial growth factor (VEGF) production, cell detachment, and invasive capacity [9]. Collectively, these studies suggest that OSM functions in breast cancer progression in both an autocrine and a paracrine fashion.

OSM signaling uses two dimeric receptors. OSM binds with high affinity to the OSM receptor (OSMR), which consists of a gp130 subunit and OSMRβ, and with lower affinity to the leukemia inhibitory factor receptor (LIFR), which consists of gp130 and LIFRβ [12]. OSMR signaling initiates the JAK/STAT, mitogen-activated protein kinase (MAPK), and phosphoinositide 3-kinase/AKT pathways [13, 14], as well as the stress-activated MAPK p38 and JNK pathways [15]. Whereas OSM binding to the OSMR has been shown to promote cancer cell malignancy and reduce long-term survival in patients with breast cancer [16], LIF activation of the LIFR suppresses tumor growth and metastasis [17]. Activation of the LIFR by OSM promotes bone growth and may also suppress breast cancer metastatic phenotypes [12, 18].

As a pleiotropic cytokine, OSM appears to play an important role in promoting breast cancer metastatic potential in vitro while inhibiting breast tumor cell proliferation [19]. OSM has been shown to function in breast and various other cancer cells in culture to (1) promote an epithelial-to-mesenchymal transition (EMT) and a stem cell-like phenotype [14, 20]; (2) upregulate expression of proteases such as matrix metalloproteinases [21]; (3) promote tumor cell detachment and subsequent invasion [22, 23]; (4) induce the expression of VEGF, hypoxia inducible factor-1α, and other proangiogenic factors [24]; and (5) suppress estrogen receptor (ER)-α expression [16]. Despite increasing in vitro evidence, limited studies have addressed the role of OSM in breast cancer metastasis in vivo.

Our previous studies were the first to show the importance of OSM in breast cancer metastasis to bone. Specifically, reduced tumor cell-produced OSM expression led to a decrease in osteolytic bone metastasis in an orthotopic 4T1.2 mouse model [7]. Because it has been demonstrated that OSM functions in normal bone homeostasis [25], this work suggests an important role for OSM during postintravasation breast cancer metastasis to bone and subsequent bone destruction. Although in vitro studies suggest that OSM promotes the early steps of the metastatic cascade, no existing work differentiates between OSM's impact on pre- versus postintravasation aspects of the breast cancer metastatic cascade.

The work presented in this paper demonstrates that OSM initiates the preintravasation steps of the metastasis cascade, increases circulating tumor cell (CTC) numbers, promotes lung metastases, and decreases survival in mice. Conversely, we also show that OSM has no effect on survival in the postintravasation model that bypasses the early steps of metastasis by injecting tumor cells directly into the circulation. Collectively, our work suggests that therapeutic suppression of OSM in the tumor microenvironment not only might be an effective treatment strategy for bone metastasis but also could be used as a preventive therapeutic to mitigate overall breast cancer metastasis.

Methods

Tissue microarrays

Breast tissue from 72 patients was obtained from paraffin block archives at the Department of Pathology, Mercy Medical Center, Nampa, ID, USA. Three tissue microarrays (TMAs) of 1-mm thickness were assessed. The TMAs were stained for OSM using the Histostain kit (catalogue number 95-9843; Life Technologies, Carlsbad, CA, USA) per the manufacturer's instructions. The TMAs were deparaffinized and stained overnight with a 1:400 dilution of rabbit antihuman OSM primary antibody (catalogue number sc-129; Santa Cruz Biotechnology, Dallas, TX, USA) and for 1 hour with 1:1000 goat antirabbit IgG-alkaline phosphatase secondary antibody. TMAs stained with secondary antibody alone served as the negative control, and spleen and salivary gland served as positive controls for OSM staining. The TMAs were analyzed in multiple sets of random orders for OSM expression intensity by a pathologist and were graded as follows: 0 = no staining; 1 = light staining; 2 = medium staining; and 3 = dark staining. Grading for each patient was averaged for each cell tissue type (ductal epithelial, vessel, stroma). Additional methods are detailed in Additional file 1: Supplemental Materials and Methods.

Cell lines and culture conditions

MDA-MB-231-D3H2LN luc2 cells (Caliper Life Sciences, Waltham, MA, USA) and MDA-MB-231 human breast cancer cells (American Type Culture Collection, Manassas, VA, USA) were cultured in RPMI 1640 media supplemented with 10% FBS and 100 U/ml penicillin-streptomycin. Cells were maintained at 37 °C, 5% carbon dioxide, and 95% humidity. 4T1.2 mouse mammary cancer cells [26] were cultured in α-minimal essential medium (α-MEM) supplemented with 10% FBS, 1 mM sodium pyruvate, and 100 U/ml each of penicillin and streptomycin, and the cells were passaged for no more than 6 months. All media and supplements were obtained from HyClone Laboratories (Logan, UT, USA). All cell lines were tested for mycoplasma contamination by routine 4′,6-diamidino-2-phenylindole staining, and experiments were accomplished within ten passages after cell line thawing.

Plasmid construct design and cell transfection

To transduce MDA-MB-231-Luc2-D3H2LN cells with a tetracycline (TET)-inducible vector, the full-length OSM complementary DNA was cloned into the pLenti6.3/TO/V5-DEST vector (Life Technologies). Lentiviral transduction of the pLenti6.3/TO/V5-DEST+hOSM vector and pLenti3.3/TR vector was performed using the Vira-Power™ II Lentiviral Gateway® Expression System (K367-20; Life Technologies) in accordance with the manufacturer's instructions. Stably transduced cell lines were tested for TET induction of hOSM expression by enzyme-linked immunosorbent assay (ELISA) and Western blot analysis. To create OSM-knockdown 4T1.2 cells, OSM short hairpin RNA (shRNA) and a LacZ shRNA sequences were cloned into the pSilencer 4.1 plasmid (Life Technologies) and stably transfected into 4T1.2 cells as previously described [7]. Two viable OSM-knockdown 4T1.2 cell lines were generated using different shRNA constructs (4T1.2-shOSM1 and 4T1.2-shOSM2) [7].

ELISA

OSM produced by TET-inducible MDA-MB-231 (MDA$^{TO/OSM}$) cells was tested for in vitro activity. MDA$^{TO/OSM}$ cells were treated with 0.1 mg/ml TET for 48 hours to generate conditioned media (CM) containing OSM. The CM was then applied to parental MDA-MB-231, MDA-MB-231-Luc2, or T47D cells for 30 minutes. Respective cell lysates were then collected from treated cells using PathScan® Sandwich ELISA Lysis

Buffer (catalogue number 7018; Cell Signaling Technology, Danvers, MA, USA). The lysates were then run on a PathScan® Phospho-Stat3 (Tyr705) Sandwich ELISA in accordance with the manufacturer's instructions (catalogue number 7146; Cell Signaling Technology).

To assess OSM concentration in animal serum, whole blood was collected from (MDA$^{TO/OSM}$) tumor xenograft animals at the experimental endpoint and allowed to coagulate for 30 minutes. The coagulated blood was centrifuged at 2500 rpm for 10 minutes, and the upper layer was collected as serum. The serum was then diluted 1:3 in PBS and used in an hOSM ELISA (catalogue number DY295; R&D Systems, Minneapolis MN, USA), which was performed in accordance with the manufacturer's instructions.

Western blot analysis

OSM was induced in MDA$^{TO/OSM}$ cells for 48 hours with 0.1 mg/ml TET in 10% FBS RPMI 1640 media. The CM was collected, run on a gel, and blotted onto 0.22-μm polyvinylidene difluoride membranes (EMD Millipore, Billerica, MA, USA). Membranes were blocked using 5% nonfat dry milk diluted in PBS at pH 7.4 with 0.05% Tween 20 (NFDM-PBS-T). Antihuman OSM antibody (catalogue number sc-129; Santa Cruz Biotechnology) was used at 1:1000 dilution in 5% NFDM-PBS-T, and a secondary antirabbit horseradish peroxidase antibody (catalogue number 711-035-152; Jackson ImmunoResearch Laboratories, West Grove, PA, USA) was used at 1:5000 dilution in 5% NFDM- PBS-T.

Animals and tumor cell injections

All animal experiments were performed in accordance with the local institutional animal care and use committee (IACUCs). Six-week-old female athymic nude mice were used for the xenograft experiments, and 6-week-old female BALB/c mice were used for the syngeneic studies. All mice were obtained from the National Cancer Institute's Animal Production Facility (Frederick, MD, USA). OSM-knockout (OSM-KO) BALB/c mice were backcrossed from OSM-KO C57BL/6 mice, which were a kind gift from Dr. Peter Donovan, indirectly, through Dr. James Ihle (St. Jude's Children's Hospital, Memphis, TN, USA). Animals were backcrossed for at least ten generations, and genotyping was done at each generation to ensure the presence of the knockout allele. Nonsurgical orthotopic injections were performed as described previously with 2.0×10^6 cells diluted in 50 μl of PBS containing 10% medium for the xenograft model and with 1×10^5 cells for the syngeneic models [7]. For all animals, starting at 2 weeks postinjection, tumor length and width were measured with mechanical calipers three times per week, and tumor volume was estimated using the equation tumor volume = (length × width^2)/2. The survival endpoint was defined by the IACUC as tumor size greater than 20 mm in diameter, 10% or greater weight loss, and/or appearance of cachexia. At the experimental endpoint, animals were killed, and their organs were harvested and examined for any abnormalities. Further analysis specific to each model is described below.

For peritumoral OSM injections, either 50 μl of PBS or 1 μg of recombinant full-length human OSM (Pepro-Tech, Rocky Hill, NJ, USA) diluted in 50 μl of PBS was injected into the area surrounding the tumor three times per week until the endpoint of the experiment. When the tumors became palpable, mice were randomized into groups and began receiving peritumoral injections.

For the TET-OSM-inducible MDA-MB-231 (MDA$^{TO/OSM}$) experiments, the OSM-induced group was given 2% sucrose water containing 0.1 mg/ml TET, whereas the control mice were given just 2% sucrose water until the endpoint of the experiment. To assess blood platelet numbers, blood was collected at the endpoint into ethylenediaminetetraacetic acid (EDTA)-coated tubes (BD Biosciences, San Jose, CA, USA), and a complete blood count was performed by WestVet Veterinary Clinic (Garden City, ID, USA).

In vivo bioluminescence imaging and tumor progression

Bioluminescence imaging (BLI) of live animals was initiated at 13 days after cell injection and performed weekly. Three to five mice were scanned at one time. Ex vivo organs were also scanned using BLI. Both procedures followed our previously described protocols [27].

Detection of circulating tumor cells by Alu qPCR

The detection of human CTCs in mouse blood was performed as described previously [28]. A human DNA standard curve was prepared by adding a specified number of human MDA-MB-231 cells into mouse blood, and the DNA was then isolated for use in the qPCR reactions (Additional file 2: Figure S1). Genomic DNA was isolated from 100 μl of whole blood collected from mice at the end of the experiment. DNA was isolated using the DNeasy Blood & Tissue kit (catalogue number 69581; Qiagen, Hilden, Germany) per the manufacturer's standard instructions. DNA concentrations were normalized between each sample, and 4.5 ng of DNA was added to each 25-μl qPCR reaction. The qPCR reaction mixture was obtained from the SYBR Green GoTaq qPCR Master Mix (catalogue number TM318; Promega, Madison WI, USA), and reaction mixtures were prepared in accordance with the manufacturer's recommendations. To each reaction, 0.125 μl of 100 μM human Alu and mouse glyceraldehyde 3-phosphate dehydrogenase (*GAPDH*) primers were added. The primer

sequences are listed in Additional file 1: Table S1. Reaction conditions were as follows: 50 °C for 2 minutes, 95 °C for 3 minutes, and 40 cycles of (95 °C for 15 minutes, 60 °C for 30 minutes, and 72 °C for 30 minutes. Fluorescence measurements were taken during the annealing temperature stage (60 °C). Cycle threshold (C_t) values were determined, and the final results were normalized to mouse *GAPDH* signal levels to normalize any sample-to-sample variance in total blood volume and efficiency in total DNA purification.

Quantitative PCR

For quantitative analysis of lung metastases, lungs dissected from mice bearing mammary tumors were snap-frozen in liquid nitrogen and pulverized into a fine powder. DNA was extracted using an NaCl-Tris-EDTA buffer (100 mM NaCl, 10 mM Tris-HCl, pH 8.0, 1 mM EDTA) containing 20 μg/ml proteinase K and purified by two phenol/chloroform (1:1 vol/vol) extractions followed by ethanol precipitation. The ratio of cancer cells to normal cells was quantified by measuring the neomycin resistance gene (neo^r) DNA levels versus the vimentin DNA loading control, as described previously [29]. TaqMan PCR was performed on an Applied Biosystems 7500 real-time thermocycler (Thermo Fisher Scientific, Foster City, CA, USA). Probe and primer sequences are listed in Additional file 1: Table S1. The cycling conditions were as follows: 50 °C for 5 minutes, 95 °C for 2 minutes, then 40 cycles of 95 °C for 1 minute and 60 °C for 45 seconds. Fluorescence was measured every cycle after the annealing step, and C_t values were calculated. The data were analyzed using the $2^{-\Delta\Delta Ct}$ method [30].

In vivo magnetic resonance imaging

In vivo MRI experiments were performed using a 4.7-T small-animal magnetic resonance imaging (MRI) scanner equipped with a DirectDrive™ console (Agilent Technologies, Santa Clara, CA, USA). The instrument is built around an Oxford Instruments (Oxford, UK) magnet containing Magnex (Agilent Technologies, Yarnton, UK) actively shielded (21-cm inner diameter, ~ 30 G/cm, ~ 200 ms rise time) gradient coils driven by International Electric Company (Helsinki, Finland) gradient power amplifiers. Respiratory-gated spin-echo MRI studies were collected using a Stark Contrast (Erlangen, Germany) 2.5-cm birdcage radiofrequency coil. Prior to the imaging experiments, mice were anesthetized with isoflurane and were maintained on isoflurane/O$_2$ (1–1.5% vol/vol) throughout data collection. The animals' core body temperature was maintained at 37 ± 1 °C by circulation of warm air through the bore of the magnet. During the imaging experiments, the respiration rates for all mice were regular and ~ 2 s^{-1}.

Synchronization of MRI data collection with animal respiration was achieved with a home-built respiratory-gating unit [31], and all images were collected during postexpiratory periods. The imaging parameters were as follows: repetition time = 3 seconds; echo time = 20 milliseconds; field of view = 2.5 cm^2; data matrix = 128 × 128; slice thickness = 0.5 mm; number of averages = 4. Lung tumors were manually segmented with ImageJ software (rsbweb.nih.gov/ij; National Institutes of Health, Bethesda, MD, USA), and the number and volume of all metastatic tumors were measured and recorded on an animal-by-animal basis as described previously [32, 33].

Detection of circulating tumor cells (clonogenic assay)
Colony-forming assays were performed to detect CTCs in mouse blood. At the endpoint of the animal experiment, whole blood was collected into EDTA-coated tubes via intracardiac puncture. Red blood cells (RBCs) were lysed with RBC lysis solution (155 mM NH_4Cl, 10 mM $KHCO_3$, 0.1 mM EDTA diluted in double-distilled H_2O) for 4 minutes. The remaining cell mixture, containing white blood cells and CTCs, was spun down and washed twice with PBS. The cell pellet was then resuspended in α-MEM with 10% FBS, then plated and incubated at 37 °C for 7–10 days until colonies formed. The colonies were then fixed with 10% formalin in PBS for 15 minutes, stained with Coomassie blue, and counted.

Epithelial-to-mesenchymal transition assay
4T1.2 mouse mammary cancer cells were plated on a 6-well plate to a confluence of 30% in α-MEM with 10% FBS and 1% penicillin-streptomycin. Following a period of 24 hours to allow cells to adhere, 25 ng/ml recombinant mouse OSM (rmOSM) was added to appropriate wells. Photomicrographs were taken at a power of 100× at 24 and 48 hours to observe phenotypic EMT changes over the 2-day period.

Cell migration assay
4T1.2 cells were plated on 6-well plates to a confluency of 80% in α-MEM with 10% FBS. After the cells attached overnight, a straight scratch on the cell monolayer was made with a sterile 1000-μl polypropylene pipette tip, and loose cells and debris were washed away with three sterile PBS washes. The cells were then treated with or without 25 ng/ml rmOSM and imaged every day for 3 days on the same part of the scratch using negative phase-contrast microscopy. The images were then imported into ImageJ software, and raw unmigrated area was measured by calculating the number of pixels in the area with no migration. Relative migration intensity was

calculated as migration intensity = (day 0 unmigrated area/day n unmigrated area) – 1.

Cell detachment assay
4T1.2 mouse mammary cancer cells were plated on 24-well tissue culture dishes to a confluency of 80% in α-MEM with 10% FBS. The cells were allowed to attach overnight, and rmOSM (25 ng/ml; R&D Systems) suspended in α-MEM with 10% FBS was added to the cells. For up to 8 days, cells that were detached were collected and counted using a hemocytometer, and viable cells were detected by lack of trypan blue staining (catalogue number SV30084.01; HyClone Laboratories).

Statistical analysis
TMA mean staining values were analyzed with repeated measures in a mixed model framework using compound symmetric covariance within patients and cancer status as fixed effects. All other statistical comparisons between multiple groups were assessed by one- or two-way analysis of variance (ANOVA) using Tukey's posttest analysis. Comparisons between two groups were analyzed by Student's t test (two-tailed, unpaired). The statistical analyses were performed using Prism version 5.0b (Graph-Pad Software Inc., La Jolla, CA, USA) or SAS version 9.1.3 (SAS Institute, Cary, NC, USA) software. Survival data were analyzed using the log-rank (Mantel-Cox) test. Significance denoted as $*p < 0.05$, $**p < 0.01$, and $***p < 0.001$.

Results
High OSM expression in ductal carcinoma in situ and invasive ductal carcinoma suggests autocrine signaling
To assess breast epithelial cell expression and location of OSM in human breast tumors, TMAs containing samples from 72 patients were analyzed by IHC. Interestingly, OSM staining intensity was higher in the ductal carcinoma in situ (DCIS) tissue than in normal tissue, whereas no staining was observed using the control secondary antibody (Fig. 1a). Representative images of staining intensity are shown in Additional file 3: Figure S2. Quantification of OSM levels from all sections showed that the mean staining intensity for normal adjacent tissue (1.33) was significantly lower than that of DCIS (2.00) and invasive ductal carcinoma (IDC) (1.66) tissues, whereas metastatic tissue (1.24) was statistically similar to normal tissue (Fig. 1b and Additional file 1: Table S2). Fibroblast OSM expression in the cancerous stroma was significantly lower (0.39 mean OSM staining) than in adjacent normal stroma (0.94 mean OSM staining) ($p < 0.001$) (Additional file 1: Table S3). Additionally, OSM expression was significantly higher in patients with metastasis and those with a positive margin status than in those with a negative margin status (Additional file 1: Table S4). Similarly to stromal OSM expression, we found that endothelial cells of blood

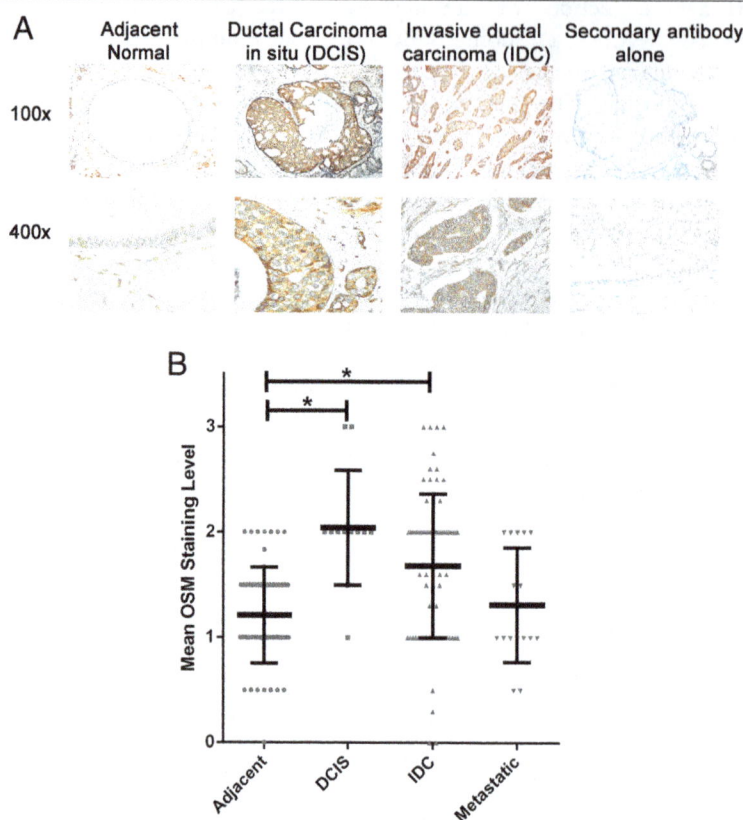

Fig. 1 Oncostatin M (OSM) is highly expressed in ductal carcinoma in situ (DCIS) and invasive ductal carcinoma (IDC). **a** To detect the presence of OSM in breast cancer tissue, histological microarrays from 72 patients with breast cancer were stained with human OSM antibody by IHC. Twelve patients had in situ DCIS, 54 patients had nonmetastatic IDC, and 16 patients had IDC with metastasis to lymph nodes (see Additional file 1). The results showed that normal adjacent tissue expresses little OSM but that OSM is highly expressed in DCIS and IDC. Secondary antibody alone did not produce any background signals. **b** Intensity quantification of OSM stained tissues. Mean staining intensity for DCIS (2.00) and IDC (1.66) tissues was significantly higher than that of normal adjacent tissue (1.33) and metastatic tissue (1.24). There was no statistically significant difference between normal and metastatic tissue. Multiple cores from the same patients were averaged. Data are expressed as mean ± SD. *$p < 0.05$ by one-way analysis of variance with Tukey's multiple comparisons test

vessels near the cancerous tissue had significantly lower OSM expression (1.22 mean OSM staining) than the blood vessel endothelium (1.66 mean OSM staining) around adjacent normal tissue ($p < 0.001$) (Additional file 1: Table S3).

On one hand, breast cancer subtype analysis of IHC staining revealed that OSM expression increased linearly with respect to HER2/Neu status in patients with IDC with increasing HER2/Neu expression (Additional file 1: Table S4). On the other hand, OSM expression levels did not change with respect to HER2/Neu in patients with metastatic disease (Additional file 1: Table S4). Additionally, OSM expression increased slightly (0.2) for every 50% increase in the expression of the ER in patients with IDC but did not change significantly in metastatic tissue. Together, these results suggest that OSM protein levels are higher in the earlier stages of breast cancer and that tumor cell-produced OSM may be important in autocrine signaling for the promotion of tumor progression. Although there is some indication

that the expression of OSM is greater in ER+ and HER2+ breast cancer tissue samples, cell lines representing these subtypes have poor tumorigenic and metastatic capacity in vivo [34]. Furthermore, significant OSM expression is present in ER− and HER2/Neu tumors. Therefore, we used metastatic in vivo models based on the MDA-MB-231-Luc2-D3H2LN cell line [35] and the highly metastatic 4T1.2 model, which are both ER−/HER2− [7, 26].

Elevated production of OSM generated from TET-inducible MDA-MB-231 (MDA$^{TO/OSM}$) cells increases metastases to lungs and decreases overall survival

In order to assess the effects of cancer cell-produced OSM in a tumor microenvironment, we developed a stably transduced triple-negative breast cancer (TNBC) MDA-MB-231-Luc2-D3H2LN cell line that secretes OSM in response to TET treatment (+TET;MDA$^{TO/OSM}$). MDA-MB-231-Luc2-D3H2LN cells have enhanced capacity to metastasize to multiple organs, including lung and bone, compared with the parental MDA-MB-231 cells, which have poor metastatic capacity via orthotopic application [35]. To compare the OSM produced by the MDA$^{TO/OSM}$ cells with recombinant human OSM (hOSM), CM from MDA$^{TO/OSM}$ cells treated with TET (0. 1 μg/ml) was collected. MDA-MB-231, MDA-MB-231-Luc, and T47D breast cancer cells were treated with either CM from MDA$^{TO/OSM}$ cells or with rhOSM (25 ng/ml) for 30 minutes. OSM signaling was assessed by measuring STAT3 activation using a pSTAT3 ELISA. For each cell line investigated, there were no significant differences in the levels of pSTAT3 induced by OSM produced from TET-induced MDA$^{TO/OSM}$ cells compared with rhOSM (Fig. 2a, left). Furthermore, the CM from MDA$^{TO/OSM}$ cells treated with TET was assessed on an hOSM immunoblot, and an expected size band (26 kDa) was detected (Fig. 2a, middle) by ELISA (Fig. 2a, right), showing an OSM concentration of 10 ng/ml in the CM.

To assess the activity of MDA$^{TO/OSM}$ cells in vivo, 1×10^6 cells were injected into the fourth mammary fat pad of female athymic nude mice. The mice were given drinking water with TET (+TET) or without TET (−TET) (0.1 mg/ml in 2% sucrose water) to induce OSM expression in the cancer cells. At the experimental endpoint, serum was then separated from whole blood, and serum OSM levels were assessed by ELISA. Tumor-bearing mice +TET had a 67-fold higher level of OSM present in their serum than −TET mice (Fig. 2b, left). Each animal's physical condition was assessed, and animals with MDA$^{TO/OSM}$ tumors +TET had significantly increased blood platelet counts (Fig. 2b, center). TET-treated mice also had a significant decrease in body weight compared with −TET mice (Fig. 2b, right; Additional file 4: Figure S3A), displaying a prominent spinal column and reduced apparent body fat, indicative of cachexia (Additional file 4: Figure S3B). It was previously reported that cachexia, elevated inflammatory factors, and kidney disease may be correlated with each other [36]. In this study, the cachexic animals had kidney abnormalities with hypoperfusion and damage to the gross morphological kidney structures (Additional file 4: Figure S3C). This correlated with +TET treatment and high levels of serum OSM in the animals (Additional file 4: Figure S3D and S3E), suggesting that high OSM levels may contribute to the development of cachexia and kidney dysfunction. Control animals without tumors treated with TET had normal body condition and normal kidney morphology (data not shown).

Additionally, in a separate experiment, animals were given TET drinking water for only 1 week so that we could assess the early effects of OSM on metastasis. Animals receiving 1 week +TET had higher levels of metastases to the lung than −TET mice, as assessed by ex vivo

imaging, (Fig. 2c). Only sporadic spine or liver metastases were detected at this early time point (data not shown), which suggests that bone and liver metastases may grow more slowly or occur as a later event. This result also suggests that a short-term elevation in the level of OSM can promote the development of metastases to the lung. To measure animal survival, mice with MDA$^{TO/OSM}$ tumors were treated with or without TET and allowed to progress to the endpoint. Mice given +TET drinking water had a mean decreased survival of 11 days compared with −TET mice (Fig. 2d). Collectively, these results demonstrated that elevated levels of tumor cell-produced OSM led to increased lung metastases, decreased survival, and deterioration in body condition indicative of cachexia.

OSM increases lung metastases and circulating tumor cell numbers in an orthotopic MDA-MB-231 model of breast cancer

To assess the paracrine effects of OSM, exogenous OSM was injected peritumorally in an orthotopic MDA-MB-231 xenograft model. In this model, 2×10^6 MDA-MB-231-Luc2-D3H2LN cells were injected into the fourth mammary fat pads of female nude mice. After the tumors were palpable (~ 3 mm), OSM (1 μg in 50 μl of PBS) or PBS alone was injected peritumorally three times per week, and mice were monitored until the endpoint criteria were met. Peritumoral injections can potentially cause supraphysiologic concentrations of OSM in the local tumor microenvironment, which may amplify any effect that OSM has on the tumor. However, in light of recent data suggesting that OSM accumulates in the acidic ECM, actual concentrations of inflammatory cytokines in the tumor microenvironment may be much higher locally than previously thought [11, 37]. Unexpectedly, tumor volume did not differ between the groups (Fig. 3a), even though OSM has been shown to reduce MDA-MB-231 cell proliferation in vitro [38]. The BLI intensities of the tumors from both groups were similar (Fig. 3b), although a few mice in each group had lower BLI intensities owing to tumor necrosis.

Mice receiving peritumoral OSM showed larger metastatic volumes in both lung and spine than mice receiving PBS, as assessed by ex vivo imaging (Fig. 3c, left). Additionally, lungs dissected from the OSM-injected group had BLI intensities that were two orders of magnitude (10^2) higher than those in the PBS-injected group (Fig. 3c, right). Similarly, spinal BLI intensity from OSM-treated mice averaged 2×10^7 photons/second, whereas control mice had a mean signal of 3×10^5 photons/second.

In patients with advanced and/or inflammatory breast cancer, high numbers of CTCs have been detected, suggesting a correlation between inflammatory factors and

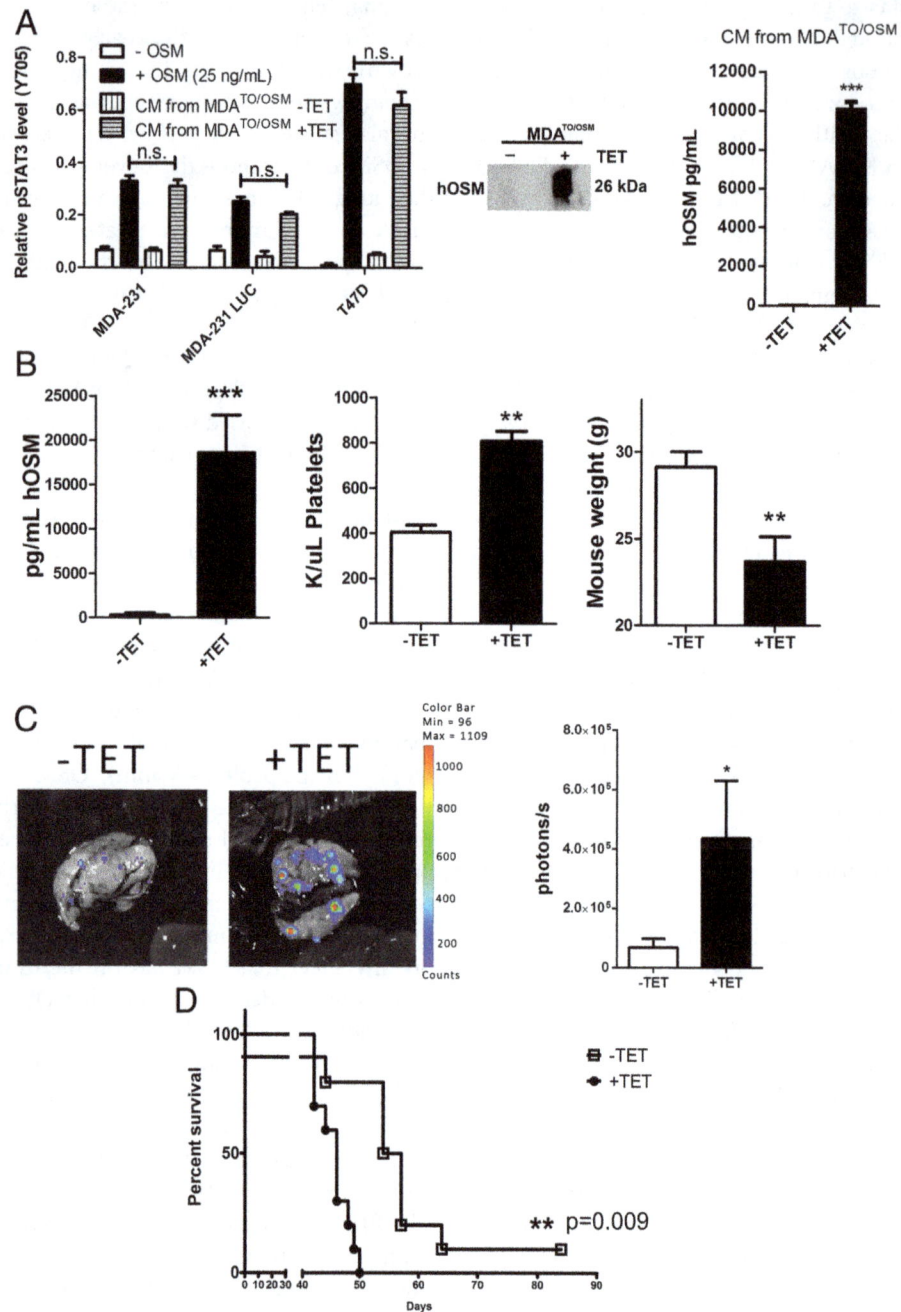

Fig. 2 (See legend on next page.)

OSM potentiates preintravasation events, increases CTC counts, and promotes breast cancer...

79

(See figure on previous page.)
Fig. 2 Oncostatin M (OSM) produced by tetracycline (TET)-inducible MDA-MB-231 (MDA$^{TO/OSM}$) cell MDA$^{TO/OSM}$) tumors increase metastasis and decrease survival. **a** MDA$^{TO/OSM}$ human breast cancer cells were treated with (+TET) or without TET (−TET), and the resultant conditioned media (CM) from the treated cells were applied to parental MDA-MB-231, MDA-MB-231-LUC, and T47D cells. *Left*: The activity of OSM accumulated in the CM was compared with commercially obtained recombinant human OSM (rhOSM) (25 ng/ml). There was no significant difference between OSM produced by MDA$^{TO/OSM}$ versus rhOSM versus its ability to induce pSTAT3. *Middle*: Western blot analysis depicting that CM produced by MDA$^{TO/OSM}$ cells stimulated with TET contain OSM. *Right*: Enzyme-linked immunosorbent assay (ELISA) analysis showed that CM from TET-treated MDA$^{TO/OSM}$ cells contain 10.1 ng/ml of hOSM. **b** *Left*: Animals with MDA$^{TO/OSM}$ tumors were given drinking water with or without TET, and whole blood was collected at the experimental endpoint. After allowing the blood to clot and serum was separated by centrifugation, the resultant serum OSM levels were measured by ELISA. Animals with MDA$^{TO/OSM}$ tumors with drinking water containing TET had 67-fold higher serum OSM levels. *Center*: Platelet counts were higher in +TET MDA$^{TO/OSM}$ tumor-bearing mice than in −TET mice. *Right*: +TET MDA$^{TO/OSM}$ tumor-bearing mice had lower body weight than −TET mice. **c** Animals with MDA$^{TO/OSM}$ tumors were given drinking water containing TET for 1 week, and their lung metastasis levels were assessed by ex vivo bioluminescence imaging. *Left*: Representative ex vivo bioluminescence image. *Right*: Average radiance analysis of the ex vivo bioluminescence imaging in photons per second per square centimeter per square radian (p/s/cm^2/sr). Animals with MDA$^{TO/OSM}$ tumors +TET had a fivefold higher bioluminescent radiance than −TET mice (−TET, $n = 3$; +TET, $n = 6$). Data are expressed as mean ± SEM. **d** Kaplan-Meier survival curve for mice with MDA$^{TO/OSM}$ tumors ± TET. Mice that did not receive TET survived, on average, 11 days longer (−TET, $n = 9$; +TET, $n = 10$). ***$p < 0.001$ by log-rank test. Data are expressed as mean ± SEM. *$p < 0.05$, **$p < 0.01$, and ***$p < 0.001$ by two-tailed t test or one-way analysis of variance with Tukey's posttest where appropriate

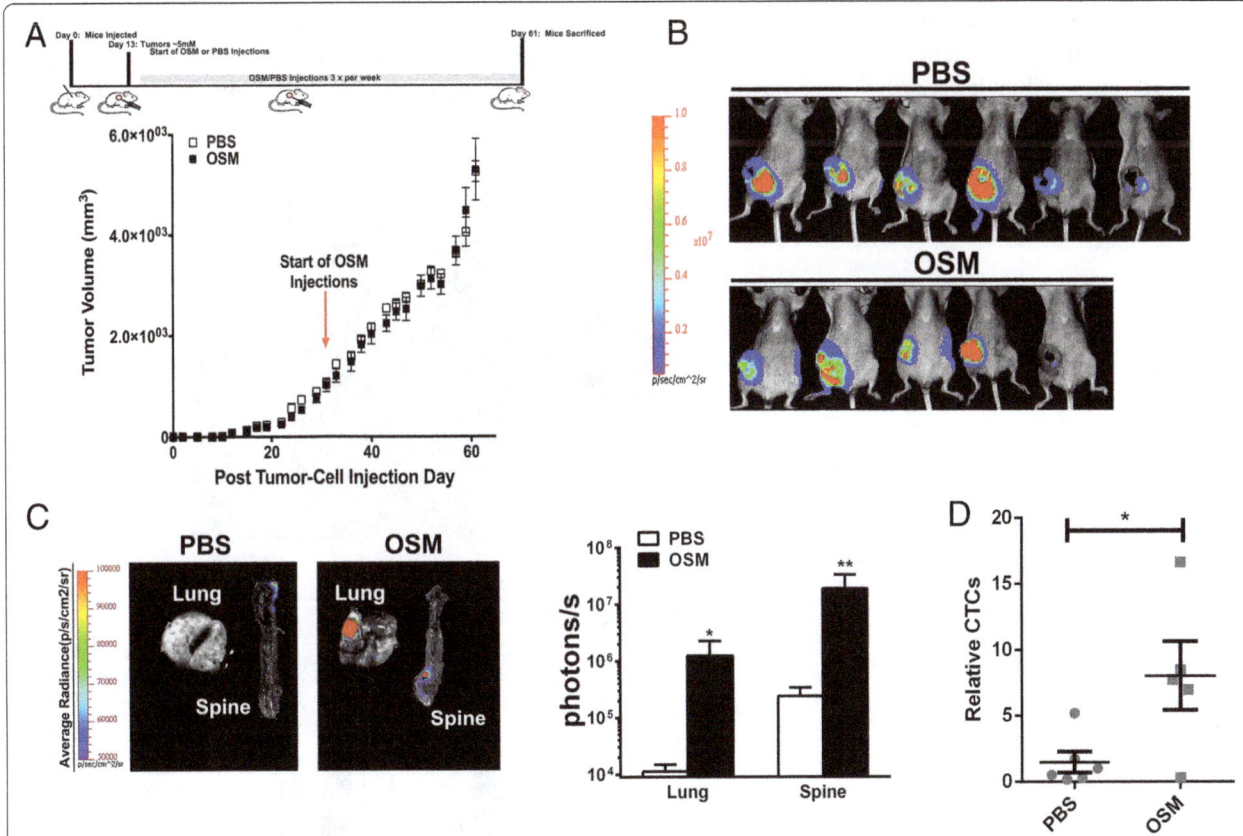

Fig. 3 Peritumoral oncostatin M (OSM) injections into mice with MDA-MB-231-D3H2LN tumors promote the development of metastases and circulating tumor cells (CTCs). **a** The timeline shows orthotopic MDA-MB-231-D3H2LN human breast tumor cell injection at day 0, peritumoral OSM or PBS injections beginning three times per week at day 13, and the final day of killing of both groups at day 61. Average tumor volume (mm^3) did not differ between the peritumorally injected OSM and PBS control groups. **b** Representative images of PBS- and OSM-injected tumor-bearing mice imaged ventrally by bioluminescence imaging (BLI). There was no statistically significant difference between the groups. **c** *Left*: Representative ex vivo BLI study of lungs and spine from mice bearing MDA-MB-231-D3H2LN Luc2 tumors that were treated with peritumoral injections of PBS or OSM. *Right*: Ex vivo BLI intensities were quantified in the lung and spine. Lungs from mice receiving peritumoral OSM injections showed a 37.9-fold higher BLI intensity than those with PBS injections, and spines from mice injected with OSM showed an approximately 25.9-fold increase over mice that received PBS injections. Data are expressed as photons/second (mean ± SEM; $n = 5$–6). **d** Human CTCs containing human Alu DNA were detected in mouse blood by qPCR. In animals that received OSM injections, there was a fourfold increase in the number of CTCs compared with controls. Data are expressed as mean ± SEM *$p < 0.05$ by two-tailed t test

the number of CTCs [39]. In our xenograft model, both human MDA-MB-231-Luc2 tumor cells and potential CTCs contained multiple copies of human Alu DNA repeat sequences. To assess CTC numbers, DNA was isolated from mouse blood, and the levels of human Alu DNA repeat sequences were determined in the blood by qPCR. The resultant C_t values were fitted to the standard curve to determine total CTC numbers in each sample (Additional file 2: Figure S1). In animals that received rhOSM injections, there was a fourfold increase in the number of CTCs per 100 μl of mouse blood compared with animals that did not receive OSM (Fig. 3d). Collectively, this suggests that increased paracrine OSM in the tumor microenvironment increases metastasis to lung and spine while also increasing CTCs.

Suppression of OSM in a syngeneic mouse model reduced lung metastases

To use an immunocompetent mouse model, we employed two highly metastatic 4T1.2 mouse mammary tumor cell lines exhibiting knockdown expression of OSM in a syngeneic, orthotopic model of breast cancer

[7]. These two independent cell lines (4T1.2-shOSM1 and 4T1.2-shOSM2), developed from two independent shRNA constructs, were shown by ELISA to secrete a 3- to 12-fold reduction in OSM, respectively, compared with control 4T1.2-LacZ cells [7]. To test the effects of OSM on mammary tumor metastasis in vivo, 1×10^5 control 4T1.2-LacZ, 4T1.2-shOSM1, and 4T1.2-shOSM2 cells were injected orthotopically into the mammary fat pads of female BALB/c mice.

The mean number of relative lung metastases was shown to be tenfold lower in mice that received 4T1.2-shOSM1 cells and fivefold lower in mice injected with 4T1.2-shOSM2 cells compared with 4T1.2-LacZ control cells (Fig. 4a). Histology performed on tissues from mice injected with parental 4T1.2 cells using an antimouse OSM antibody showed strong OSM expression in the primary mammary tumor, as well as some background expression in the normal breast connective tissue (Additional file 5: Figure S4). Specifically, very high OSM expression was seen at the leading edge of the primary mammary tumor, in closest proximity to the breast stroma.

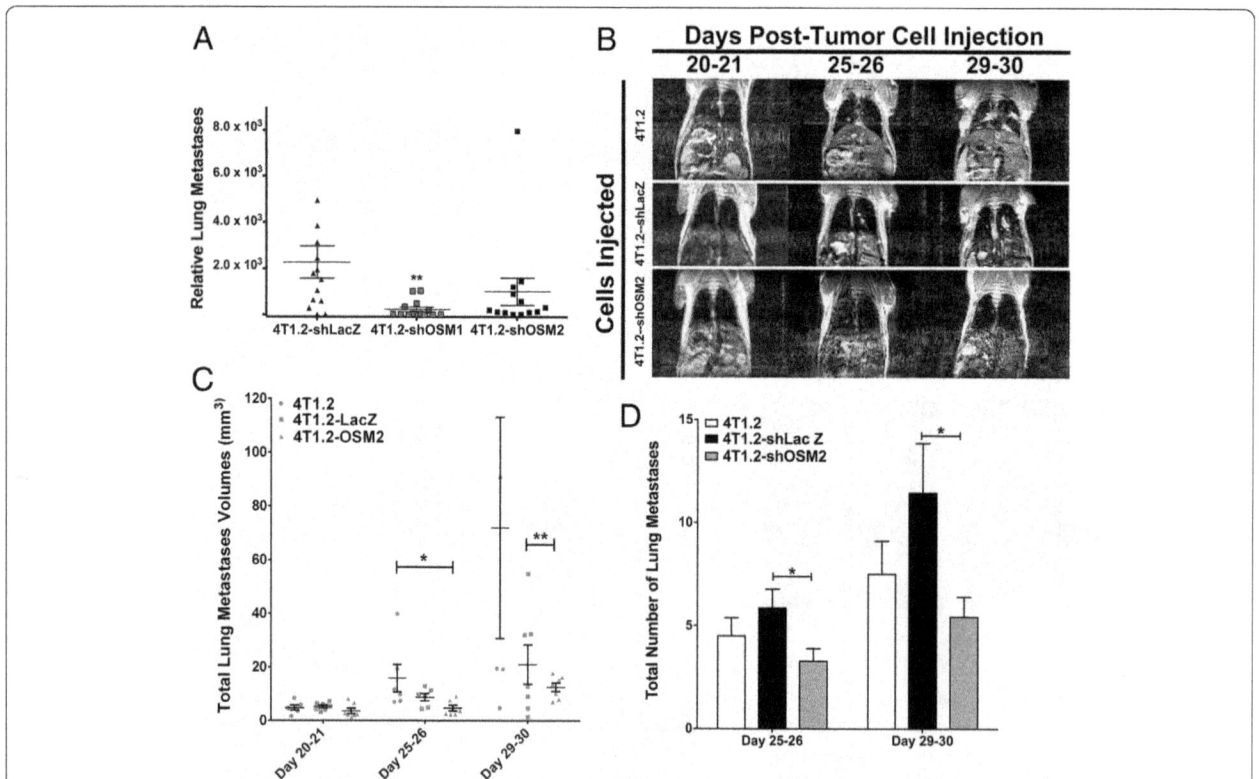

Fig. 4 Reduced oncostatin M (OSM) expression results in fewer spontaneous lung metastases and lower total volume of lung metastases by magnetic resonance imaging (MRI). **a** Lung metastasis burden was quantified by qPCR. Mice bearing mammary 4T1.2-shOSM1 or 4T1.2-shOSM2 tumors had less metastasis to the lung than mice with 4T1.2-shLacZ tumors. **b** Mice bearing 4T1.2-shOSM2 tumors had less metastatic lesions in the lung as detected by MRI at the endpoint of the experiment than mice bearing parental 4T1.2 or control 4T1.2-shLacZ tumors. MRI quantification of lung metastatic volume (**c**) and total number of lung metastases (**d**) showed significantly higher volume and number of lung metastases in the 4T1.2- or 4T1.2-shLacZ-injected mice than the 4T1.2-shOSM2-injected mice (4T1.2, $n = 6$; 4T1.2-shLacZ, $n = 7$; 4T1.2-shOSM2, $n = 7$). Data are expressed as mean ± SEM. *$p < 0.05$ and **$p < 0.01$ by one-way analysis of variance with Tukey's multiple comparisons test

MRI was used to track lung metastasis progression in vivo after injection of parental 4T1.2, control 4T1.2-shLacZ, and 4T1.2-shOSM2 cells. Mice were scanned postinjection at days 20–21, days 25–26, and just before being killed at days 29–30 (Fig. 4b). For all three cell lines, MRI studies showed essentially no detectable metastasis at days 20–21. However, at 25–26 days and 29–30 days, readily identifiable metastases were observed in lung images. The average metastasis volume was significantly decreased, by 50–80%, in 4T1.2-shOSM2 cells compared with 4T1.2-shLacZ control or parental 4T1.2 cells, respectively (Fig. 4c). There were also significant differences between the parental 4T1.2 cells and the control 4T1.2-shLacZ cells, which may be due to the potential off-target effects of shRNA activation [40–42]. This highlights the importance of using a true nontargeting shRNA control such as the 4T1.2-shLacZ cells because shRNA activation alone appears to have cell-static effects in cancer cells [40].

Further analysis revealed that the total number of metastases was also reduced by more than 50% in mice injected with 4T1.2-shOSM2 cells compared with control 4T1.2-shLacZ cells at 25–26 days and 29–30 days (Fig. 4d). Thus, in vivo MRI confirmed that OSM may be a potent inducer of the metastatic cascade that results in lung metastases originating from a primary mammary tumor. In sum, these results suggest that OSM is necessary for spontaneous mammary tumor metastasis to the lung in a syngeneic mouse model.

Suppression of OSM by shRNA increases survival from spontaneous metastasis via orthotopic injection but not via intracardiac injection in vivo

We used a tumor resection survival model to mimic surgical removal of the primary tumor in patients and to determine if suppression of tumor-produced OSM limits early metastases. Orthotopic mammary fat pad injections were performed using control 4T1.2-shLacZ cells, 4T1.2-shOSM1 cells, and 4T1.2-shOSM2 cells. Primary tumors were resected when they became palpable at day 14 (Fig. 5a), and mice were monitored until endpoint criteria were met (see the Methods section above). The mean survival time of the mice that received 4T1.2-shOSM1 and 4T1.2-shOSM2 cell injections significantly increased, by 5 and 10 days, respectively, compared with animals with 4T1.2-shLacZ tumors (Fig. 5a). These results suggest that following primary mammary tumor resection, decreased OSM expression in primary tumor cells leads to increased survival.

In order to determine if OSM affects postintravasation aspects of metastasis, we injected the mammary tumor cells directly into the circulatory system via the left ventricle of the heart. There was no statistical difference in the survival time between mice injected intracardially with 4T1.2-shLacZ versus 4T1.2-shOSM2 cells (Fig. 5b). Similarly, there was no statistical difference in lung metastatic burden in the two different tumor types as assessed by qPCR (Additional file 6: Figure S5). These results suggest that tumor cell OSM expression has little effect on the postintravasation aspects of metastasis to lung, such as extravasation and metastatic site implantation.

CTC number and metastatic burden is reduced in OSM-knockout mice compared with wild-type mice

To determine if knocking out OSM in the whole organism affects CTC numbers in the 4T1.2 mouse model, wild-type and OSM-KO BALB/c mice were orthotopically injected with either 4T1.2-shLacZ or 4T1.2-shOSM2 cells. Whole blood was collected at the endpoint, RBCs were lysed, and the remaining white blood cells containing the epithelial CTCs were examined using a clonogenic assay (Fig. 5c). Blood from control mice with no tumors had no colony formation (Additional file 7: Figure S6). Blood from OSM-KO mice injected with 4T1.2-shOSM2 cells had 15-fold fewer CTCs and 2.5-fold fewer lung metastases than wild-type mice injected with control 4T1.2-shLacZ cells (Fig. 5d, left). Additionally, OSM-KO mice bearing 4T1.2-shLacZ tumors had 10-fold fewer CTCs and 2.5-fold fewer lung metastases than wild-type mice with the same tumor type (Fig. 5d, right). In a separate in vitro assay to test the level of colony formation, there were no differences in colony numbers between the cell lines when seeded at low numbers (~ 10 cells) (Additional file 8: Figure S7), which indicates that the OSM-knockdown cells do not have reduced ability to survive and develop colonies. These results suggest that microenvironment OSM, independent of tumor cell-secreted OSM, has a large effect on tumor cell dissemination into the circulation. Furthermore, this highlights the importance of paracrine OSM in breast cancer progression and metastasis.

OSM increases preintravasation metrics of metastatic capacity in 4T1.2 cells

For tumor cells to enter the bloodstream as CTCs and subsequently metastasize, it is thought that they must first undergo EMT, followed by detachment, migration, and intravasation into the circulatory system [43]. Although OSM has been shown to increase tumor cell detachment and migration and to induce EMT in human breast cancer cell lines [16, 20–22, 44], no data have been published on murine 4T1.2 cells in relation of OSM's in vitro effects. TNBC (ER–, PR–, HER2–) 4T1.2 mouse mammary cancer cells were treated with OSM (25 ng/ml) for 24 to 48 hours. On one hand, because 4T1.2 cells are an aggressive mesenchymal mammary cancer cell type, OSM did not affect cell morphology or

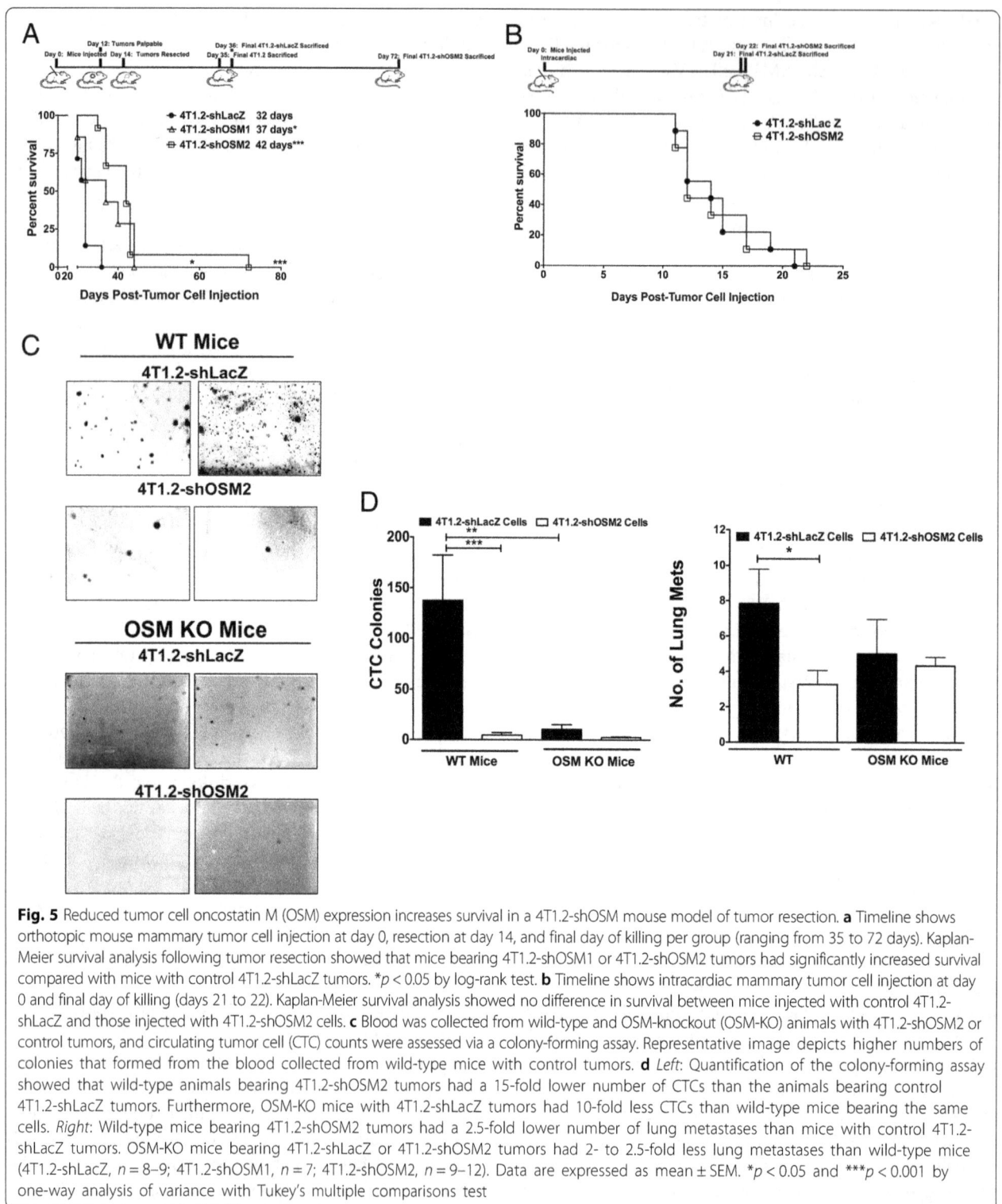

Fig. 5 Reduced tumor cell oncostatin M (OSM) expression increases survival in a 4T1.2-shOSM mouse model of tumor resection. **a** Timeline shows orthotopic mouse mammary tumor cell injection at day 0, resection at day 14, and final day of killing per group (ranging from 35 to 72 days). Kaplan-Meier survival analysis following tumor resection showed that mice bearing 4T1.2-shOSM1 or 4T1.2-shOSM2 tumors had significantly increased survival compared with mice with control 4T1.2-shLacZ tumors. *$p < 0.05$ by log-rank test. **b** Timeline shows intracardiac mammary tumor cell injection at day 0 and final day of killing (days 21 to 22). Kaplan-Meier survival analysis showed no difference in survival between mice injected with control 4T1.2-shLacZ and those injected with 4T1.2-shOSM2 cells. **c** Blood was collected from wild-type and OSM-knockout (OSM-KO) animals with 4T1.2-shOSM2 or control tumors, and circulating tumor cell (CTC) counts were assessed via a colony-forming assay. Representative image depicts higher numbers of colonies that formed from the blood collected from wild-type mice with control tumors. **d** *Left*: Quantification of the colony-forming assay showed that wild-type animals bearing 4T1.2-shOSM2 tumors had a 15-fold lower number of CTCs than the animals bearing control 4T1.2-shLacZ tumors. Furthermore, OSM-KO mice with 4T1.2-shLacZ tumors had 10-fold less CTCs than wild-type mice bearing the same cells. *Right*: Wild-type mice bearing 4T1.2-shOSM2 tumors had a 2.5-fold lower number of lung metastases than mice with control 4T1.2-shLacZ tumors. OSM-KO mice bearing 4T1.2-shLacZ or 4T1.2-shOSM2 tumors had 2- to 2.5-fold less lung metastases than wild-type mice (4T1.2-shLacZ, $n = 8$–9; 4T1.2-shOSM1, $n = 7$; 4T1.2-shOSM2, $n = 9$–12). Data are expressed as mean ± SEM. *$p < 0.05$ and ***$p < 0.001$ by one-way analysis of variance with Tukey's multiple comparisons test

produce an EMT in vitro (Fig. 6a). On the other hand, OSM significantly increased 4T1.2 mammary tumor cell migration 7-fold by day 3 in a cell migration assay (Fig. 6b) and tumor cell detachment 100-fold by day 8 (Fig. 6c). Our previous studies also demonstrated that OSM increases overall invasive potential in 4T1.2 cells [7]. These increases in migration and detachment were seen despite a 20% inhibition by OSM on 4T1.2 cell proliferation (Additional file 9: Figure S8). Together, these results suggest that OSM

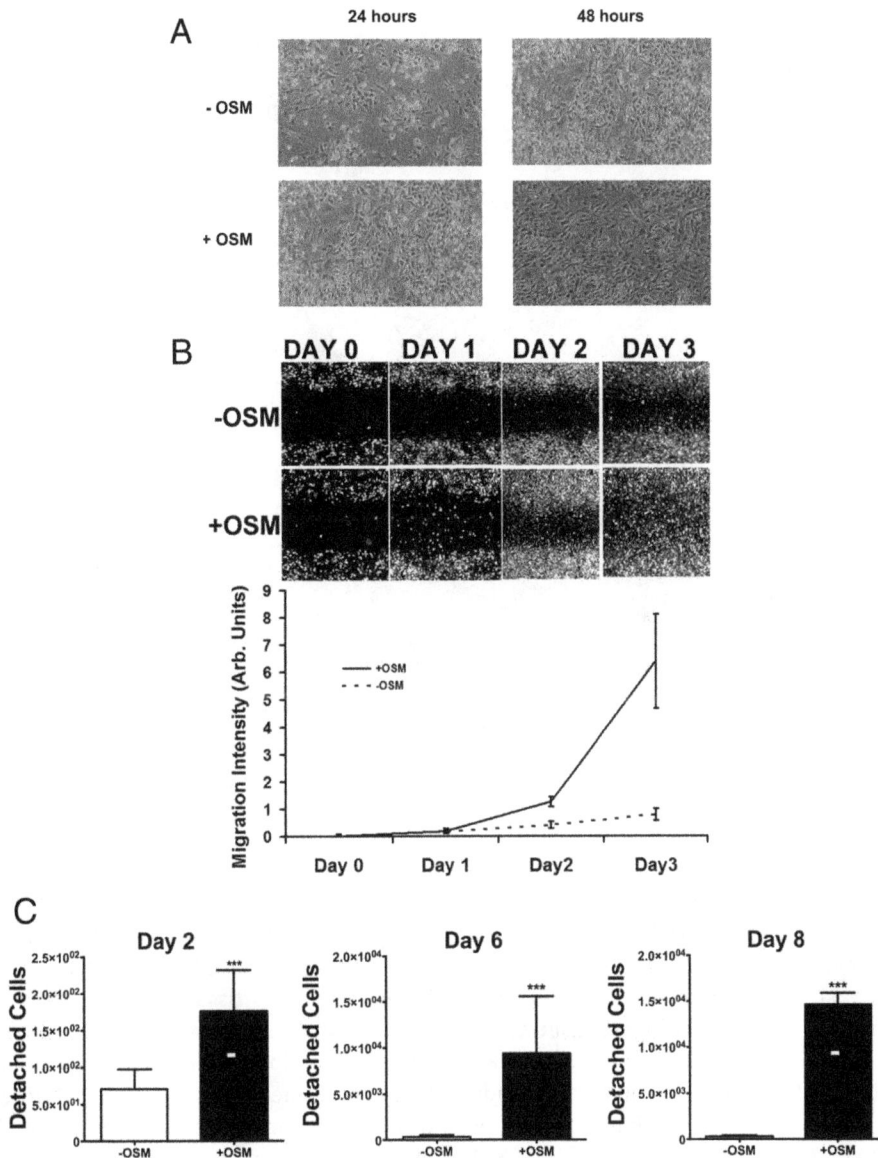

Fig. 6 Oncostatin M (OSM) promotes 4T1.2 cell detachment and migration. **a** 4T1.2 mouse mammary cancer cells were plated and treated with recombinant murine OSM (25 ng/ml) for 24 and 48 hours. No morphological changes indicative of epithelial-mesenchymal transition were detected. **b** 4T1.2 cells were grown to 80% confluence, and a uniform scratch was made. Cells treated with OSM had higher levels of migration than untreated controls (sevenfold by day 3). **c** A detachment assay was performed on 4T1.2 cells, and the number of detached cells was quantified. Cells treated with OSM had significantly higher numbers of detached cells (100-fold at day 8). Data are expressed as mean ± SEM. *$p < 0.05$ and ***$p < 0.001$ by two-tailed Student's t test

may promote tumor cell dissemination into the circulation by increasing cell migration and detachment, which may subsequently increase the number of CTCs.

Discussion

In this paper, we show that OSM, whether acting in a paracrine fashion or produced by breast tumor cells and acting in an autocrine manner, can potentiate preintravasation metastatic events, such as migration, detachment, and increased CTCs (Fig. 7). Recent studies suggest that

cells from DCIS can actually metastasize prior to their development into malignant IDC, though what triggers this early event has not been well characterized [45]. Our breast cancer IHC studies using TMAs resulted in an intriguing finding: OSM expression is highest in the epithelium of DCIS, as compared with IDC, metastatic, or adjacent normal tissue, though OSM levels in IDC are also high. When looking at the adjacent stroma, we found reduced levels of OSM in the fibroblasts and blood vessels of IDC tissues compared with normal

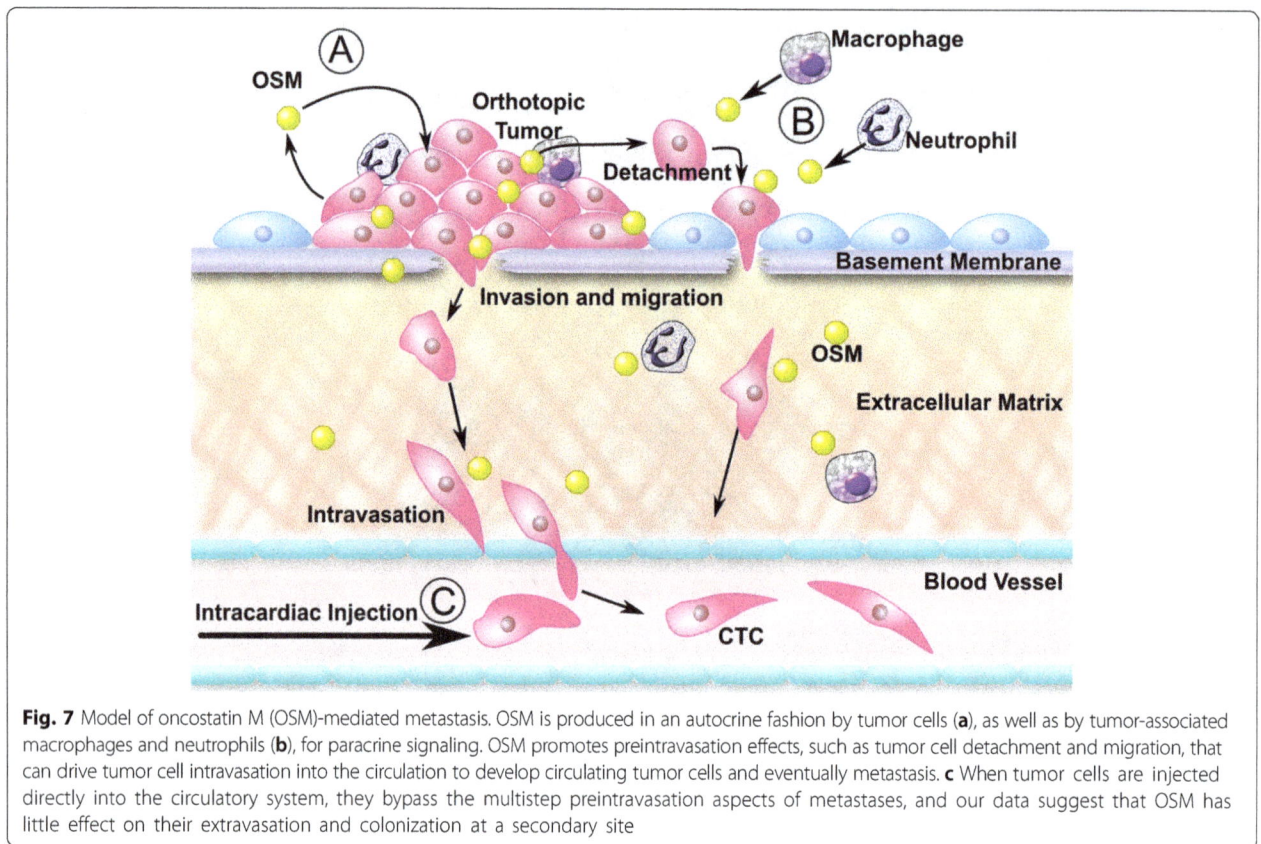

Fig. 7 Model of oncostatin M (OSM)-mediated metastasis. OSM is produced in an autocrine fashion by tumor cells (**a**), as well as by tumor-associated macrophages and neutrophils (**b**), for paracrine signaling. OSM promotes preintravasation effects, such as tumor cell detachment and migration, that can drive tumor cell intravasation into the circulation to develop circulating tumor cells and eventually metastasis. **c** When tumor cells are injected directly into the circulatory system, they bypass the multistep preintravasation aspects of metastases, and our data suggest that OSM has little effect on their extravasation and colonization at a secondary site

tissue. On one hand, this is interesting because we have previously shown that secreted OSM binds to proteins of the ECM and bioaccumulates in the tumor's acidic microenvironment [11]. On the other hand, García-Tuñón et al. observed higher levels of breast tissue OSM and OSMR in IDC than in DCIS or normal tissue [8]. Although this finding differs somewhat from our study in relation to the stage at which the highest level of OSM was seen, there is agreement that higher OSM levels were detected in cancerous tissue than in normal tissue.

In this study, three different TNBC mouse models were used: One was an immunocompetent BALB/c model using syngeneic 4T1.2 cells, and two were immunosuppressed athymic xenograft mouse models, using either MDA-MB-231-Luc2 or MDA$^{TO/OSM}$ cells. Despite the differences between the systems used in our study, our results were consistent in that suppression of OSM reduced metastasis in BALB/c mice and injection of recombinant hOSM or TET-induced hOSM expression in MDA$^{TO/OSM}$ cells increased human breast tumor metastasis in athymic mice. Although adaptive immunity is stunted in athymic mice owing to nonfunctional T cells, innate immune function is still intact [46]. Recent studies indicate that innate immunity plays a primary role in controlling progression of tumor growth and

metastatic disease [47], and innate immune cells such as macrophages home to hypoxic tumors and promote angiogenesis [10]. OSM has recently been shown to increase the tissue infiltration of both the proinflammatory M1 and the wound-healing M2 macrophages [48]. Specifically, Lauber et al. demonstrated that OSM promotes lung metastatic burden in melanoma through M2 macrophage infiltration [49]. Thus, OSM may be promoting prometastatic responses, mediated by innate immunity, in the tumor microenvironment of both athymic and BALB/c mouse models to promote metastases.

Although the traditional cause of mortality in patients with advanced cancer is metastasis to vital organs, cachexia has been shown to contribute up to 50% of cancer patient deaths [50]. Significant weight loss as a consequence of fat loss and muscle wasting, indicative of cachexia, was seen in our TET-induced OSM in MDA$^{TO/OSM}$ xenograft mouse model. TET alone does not appear to have any effect on kidney function [51]. Interestingly, TET has been shown to actually reduce tumor cell growth and aggressiveness [52], but this effect was not seen in our studies. Other studies have shown that high levels of various inflammatory cytokines, such as IL-6, potentiate loss of adipose tissue and muscle wasting [53]. Therefore, OSM may be yet another cytokine that could exacerbate cachexia in patients with breast cancer. In this study, mice with 4T1.2-shOSM1 tumors had the lowest lung metastatic burden despite the fact that 4T1.2-shOSM2 cells have lower OSM expression [7]. However, this reduced lung metastasis in 4T1.2-shOSM1 tumor-bearing mice did not translate to increased survival for 4T1.2-shOSM2 tumor-bearing mice. This supports the notion that metastatic burden may not be the only cause of increased mortality, but that elevated cytokine levels may contribute to reduced survival. Furthermore, because cytokines modulate the immune system, it is very probable that cancer cachexia is related to maladaptive immune responses [54]. Interestingly, there were also major differences between the parental 4T1.2 cells and the control 4T1.2-shLacZ cells, where the shLacZ cells had significantly reduced lung metastasis volume. This highlights the importance of using a nontargeting shRNA control cells because shRNA activation has been known to have multiple off-target effects leading to reduced cell survival, metastasis, and growth [40–42, 55].

Platelets, as an adjunct to their classical role in thrombosis, are also important in mediating inflammation and immune response [56]. We found that in the MDA$^{TO/OSM}$ mouse model, higher OSM levels were correlated with increased platelet counts and reduced animal survival. Previous studies in patients with breast cancer have shown that elevated platelet counts were associated with poor prognosis and reduced disease-free survival [57]. Platelets have also been implicated in the promotion of metastasis by acting as a reservoir for factors that induce invasion and function to protect CTCs from the immune system [58]. In our study, increased viable CTCs were detected in our mouse models when higher levels of OSM were present, which may have been due to the elevated levels of platelets in circulation.

The ability of tumor cells to intravasate into the circulation directly correlates with CTC numbers from the corresponding tumor [59]. Increased CTC numbers have been linked clinically to enhanced metastatic burden in patients and a reduced 5-year survival rate [60]. Because tumors may shed early during cancer development [61], the detection of CTCs would be an important tool in the clinic to assess the metastatic capacity of a tumor, even as early as in precancerous DCIS. Typically, CTCs are detected using cancer epithelial markers, such as cytokeratins 18/19 [62]. However, highly aggressive tumor cells that have already undergone EMT, and thus have lost their epithelial markers, may evade detection [63]. Other possibly viable markers for CTC detection include epithelial cell adhesion molecule and human mammaglobin A [62]. For our studies, the highly aggressive mesenchymal-like MDA-MB-231 cells show negative or low expression for each of these markers, making

conventional CTC detection unfeasible [63]. Thus, we employed multiple techniques that are marker-independent, such as the colony-forming assay for the mouse mammary tumor model or a PCR assay targeting human Alu sequences in the human breast tumor model. We did not use the colony-forming assays to assess the human breast tumor model, because the MDA-MB-231 cells have a highly variable in vitro survival rate when seeded at low numbers. 4T1.2 cells showed no difference in the overall level of cell survival when seeded at low numbers in vitro, which makes the colony-forming assay ideal for the 4T1.2 tumor model.

In our studies, suppression of tumor-produced OSM or the absence of OSM in OSM-KO mice resulted in reduced numbers of CTCs, whereas injection of recombinant OSM increased CTCs. There was no significant difference in the number of CTCs with or without TET in the MDA$^{TO/OSM}$ mouse metastasis model (data not shown). This suggests that paracrine OSM may be more important than autocrine-produced OSM for CTC development. Indeed, in our OSM-KO mouse model, where there is less paracrine OSM, total CTC numbers and lung metastatic burden were significantly reduced compared with WT mice. Although the number of CTCs appeared modest in our study, these numbers are actually higher than the low numbers of CTCs seen in previously published studies [64, 65]. It has been reported that even in advanced cancers, there can be as few as 1–5 CTCs per 7.5 ml [66]. Our higher CTC numbers may point to differences in human and mouse physiology and may explain the much more rapid progression of metastatic disease seen in mice than in patients.

To assess some of the early aspects of metastasis that could lead to generation of CTCs in vitro, tumor cell EMT, migration, and detachment were studied in the highly aggressive 4T1.2 tumor model. 4T1.2 mammary tumor cells, which are considered analogues of high-grade human TNBC, have already undergone EMT, and OSM did not cause additional EMT-like effects [67]. However, our results show that OSM does increase cell migration, detachment, and invasion in 4T1.2 cells [7], supporting the idea that OSM operates in the preintravasation steps of metastasis. Other OSM-related factors, such as IL-6 and IL-8, may promote CTCs by increasing tumor cell invasion, detachment, and EMT [68]. Furthermore, these effects may be amplified in vivo because OSM possesses a proclivity to accumulate in the acidic ECM of the tumor microenvironment [11].

On the basis of our findings, OSM may potentiate the preintravasation aspects of the metastatic cascade to increase metastasis to the lung and bone [7]. This is evidenced by the fact that intracardiac injection of 4T1.2 cells with reduced OSM (4T1.2-shOSM2) into mice, which bypasses the intravasation step of the metastatic cascade, did not result in increased survival compared with control cells (4T1.2-shLacZ). Therefore, it is highly probable that OSM functions before intravasation during cancer progression and suggests that OSM does not affect CTC survival, tumor cell extravasation, and/or secondary tumor growth.

Conclusions

The results of this study suggest that OSM increases lung metastases and CTC numbers by acting on early metastatic events (Fig. 7). Specifically, OSM increases tumor cell migration, detachment, and invasion [7], supporting the idea that OSM operates in the preintravasation steps of metastasis. Inhibition of OSM and/or OSMR has demonstrated antitumor effects and has recently been receiving increased attention as a possible cancer therapy [69, 70]. However, to our knowledge, no small-molecule inhibitors or humanized antibodies that target OSM signaling are in clinical trials for metastatic breast cancer. Taken together, the findings of this study provide a rationale for the administration of anti-OSM therapeutics before tumor resection, at the earlier stages of the disease, when the potential to improve overall survival of patients with breast cancer is greatest.

Additional files

Additional file 1: Table S1. Primer and probe sequences used for qPCR assay for the detection of CTC in blood obtained from tumor-bearing mouse. **Table S2.** Table format data for Fig. 1B show total number of patients and cores for each stage of breast tissue assessed. **Table S3.** Mean expression levels are statistically significantly different among cancerous and normal tissues for both stroma and blood vessel endothelium ($p<.001$). **Table S4.** Margin status, Her2/neu status and estrogen receptor (ER) status, were revealed by repeated measures analysis. Mean expression levels are statistically significantly different among cancerous, normal, and metastatic tissues for margin status, and ER status. For Her2 status, significant differences were found among cancerous, normal and between 0 and 1 staining intensity for metastatic tissues ($p<.001$). (DOCX 343 kb)

Additional file 2: Figure S1. qPCR standard curve derived from spiking cancer cells into mouse blood. MDA-MB-231 cells were spiked into mouse blood, and DNA was extracted and subjected to qPCR analysis. Specific cell numbers were correlated to CT values and were used to construct a standard curve for the CT values extrapolated from experimental mouse blood. (PPTX 186 kb)

Additional file 3: Figure S2. Representative OSM staining intensity in IHC. 0 = no staining (image not shown), 1 = light staining, 2 = moderate staining, 3 = heavy staining. (PPTX 27 kb)

Additional file 4: Figure S3. Deterioration of physical condition in MDA$^{TO/OSM}$ tumor-bearing mice treated with TET. **a** MDA$^{TO/OSM}$ tumor-bearing mice treated with tetracycline (+TET) lost, on average, 11.4% of their body weight during TET treatment, compared with −TET mice, which gained an average of 5.5% of their body weight over the same period. **b** Representative image of mice with MDA$^{TO/OSM}$ tumors +TET shows prominent spinal column, muscle wasting, and lack of visible adipose tissue. **c** Gross morphology of normal (left) and abnormal kidneys (right). Normal kidneys have a distinct border between the medulla and the cortex, with the cortex shown in a darker pink/red color and the medulla shown in a lighter pink color. This indicates that normal blood perfusion was taking place. Abnormal kidneys were either both pale and hypoperfused (middle) or damaged (right), with no clear distinction between the cortex and the medulla. **d** One hundred percent of mice in the +TET group have abnormal kidney morphologies, whereas only 25% of the mice in the −TET group have abnormal kidneys. **$p <$ 0.01 by Fisher's exact test. **e** Sera from mice with abnormal kidneys have a statistically significant higher level of OSM than sera from mice with normal kidneys. Data are expressed as mean ± SEM. *$p < 0.05$, **$p < 0.01$, and ***$p < 0.001$ by two-tailed Student's t test. (ZIP 135 kb)

Additional file 5: Figure S4. OSM is highly expressed in orthotopic 4T1.2 primary mammary tumors in female BALB/c mice. Histology using H&E confirmed the presence of a large primary mammary tumor (T) 32 days after 4T1.2 mouse mammary tumor cell injection into the fourth mammary fat pad of female BALB/c mice. High OSM expression is seen in the tumor, as is background expression in the normal breast connective tissue (CT). OSM expression is shown to be highest in the invasive edge of the tumor (T) closest to the normal breast connective tissue (CT). Control slides with no primary OSM antibody show low background staining. (PPTX 315 kb)

Additional file 6: Figure S5. qPCR analysis of lung metastases after intracardiac injections. 4T1.2-shLacZ cells and 4T1.2-shOSM2 cells were introduced via intracardiac injection, and qPCR analysis of the lung metastases indicated that the difference between the groups was not significant by two-tailed Student's t test. (ZIP 60 kb)

Additional file 7: Figure S6. Control colony-forming assay results derived from non-tumor-bearing mice. Blood from non-tumor-bearing mice contained no cells that formed colonies. (PPTX 53 kb)

Additional file 8: Figure S7. Test of cell line-specific variance in colony-forming assay between 4T1.2-shLacZ and 4T1.2-shOSM2 cell lines. Approximately 10 and 50 cells of 4T1.2-shLacZ or 4T1.2-shOSM2 cells were seeded onto tissue culture plates and were allowed to incubate until colony formation. No significant differences between the cells were detected with ~ 10 cells seeded; however, there was a small but significant increase in the number of colonies with 4T1.2-shOSM2 cells at 50 cells seeded. Data are expressed as mean ± SEM. *$p < 0.05$ by one-way ANOVA with Bonferroni's multiple comparisons test. (PPTX 68 kb)

Additional file 9: Figure S8. OSM inhibits proliferation of 4T1.2 cells. One hundred 4T1.2 cells were plated at day 0 and treated with 25 ng/ml of OSM. By day 7, there was a 20% reduction in total cell numbers in the OSM-treated group versus the non-OSM-treated group. Data are expressed as mean ± SEM. *$p < 0.05$, **$p < 0.01$; statistical analysis was performed for each day using a two-tailed Student's t test. (PPTX 21 kb)

Acknowledgements
The authors thank the Boise Veterans Affairs Medical Center (Boise, ID, USA), as well as the Boise State Biomedical Research Vivarium Core for use of its animal facility.

Funding
This study was partially funded by the following grants: National Institutes of Health (NIH) grants R15CA137510, P20RR016454, P20GM103408, P20GM109095, and P30CA091842, Susan G. Komen grant KG100513, and American Cancer Society grant RSG-09-276-01-CSM.

Authors' contributions
All authors contributed substantially to the concept of this study and the work presented in this paper. KT made a substantial contribution to the writing and editing of the manuscript and helped to do the experiments

presented in Figs. 2, 3, 5, and 6 as well as Additional file 3: Figure S2. KT designed and constructed Fig. 7. CB and JK made substantial contributions to the writing of the manuscript helped to generate data shown in Figs. 3 and 5 and Additional file 2: Figures S3 and Additional file 4: Figure S2. SK, JK, and LB generated the data and statistical analysis presented in Fig. 1. HC and CS generated some of the data presented in Fig. 6. CB and JRG generated the data shown in Fig. 4. CLJ provided conceptual guidance for all aspects of the project as the principal investigator. All authors read and approved the final manuscript.

Competing interests
The authors declare that they have no competing interests.

Author details
[1]Department of Biological Sciences, Biomolecular Sciences Program, Boise State University, 1910 University Drive, Boise, ID 83725, USA. [2]Mercy Medical Center, Nampa, ID, USA. [3]Mallinckrodt Institute of Radiology, Washington University, St. Louis, MO 63110, USA.

References
1. Lange C, Storkebaum E, de Almodovar CR, Dewerchin M, Carmeliet P. Vascular endothelial growth factor: a neurovascular target in neurological diseases. Nat Rev Neurol. 2016;12(8):439–54.
2. West NR, McCuaig S, Franchini F, Powrie F. Emerging cytokine networks in colorectal cancer. Nat Rev Immunol. 2015;15(10):615–29.
3. Harris HR, Willett WC, Vaidya RL, Michels KB. An adolescent and early adulthood dietary pattern associated with inflammation and the incidence of breast cancer. Cancer Res. 2017;77(5):1179–87.
4. Chang Q, Bournazou E, Sansone P, Berishaj M, Gao SP, Daly L, Wels J, Theilen T, Granitto S, Zhang X, et al. The IL-6/JAK/Stat3 feed-forward loop drives tumorigenesis and metastasis. Neoplasia. 2013;15(7):848–62.
5. West NR, Hegazy AN, Owens BMJ, Bullers SJ, Linggi B, Buonocore S, Coccia M, Görtz D, This S, Stockenhuber K, et al. Oncostatin M drives intestinal inflammation and predicts response to tumor necrosis factor-neutralizing therapy in patients with inflammatory bowel disease. Nat Med. 2017;23(5):579–89.
6. Hui W, Rowan AD, Richards CD, Cawston TE. Oncostatin M in combination with tumor necrosis factor alpha induces cartilage damage and matrix metalloproteinase expression in vitro and in vivo. Arthritis Rheum. 2003;48(12):3404–18.
7. Bolin C, Tawara K, Sutherland C, Redshaw J, Aranda P, Moselhy J, Anderson R, Jorcyk CL. Oncostatin M promotes mammary tumor metastasis to bone and osteolytic bone degradation. Genes Cancer. 2012;3(2):117–30.
8. García-Tuñón I, Ricote M, Ruiz A, Fraile B, Paniagua R, Royuela M. OSM, LIF, its receptors, and its relationship with the malignance in human breast carcinoma (in situ and in infiltrative). Cancer Investig. 2008;26(3):222–9.
9. Queen MM, Ryan RE, Holzer RG, Keller-Peck CR, Jorcyk CL. Breast cancer cells stimulate neutrophils to produce oncostatin M: potential implications for tumor progression. Cancer Res. 2005;65(19):8896–904.
10. Tripathi C, Tewari BN, Kanchan RK, Baghel KS, Nautiyal N, Shrivastava R, Kaur H, Bhatt ML, Bhadauria S. Macrophages are recruited to hypoxic tumor areas and acquire a pro-angiogenic M2-polarized phenotype via hypoxic cancer cell derived cytokines oncostatin M and eotaxin. Oncotarget. 2014;5(14):5350–68.
11. Ryan RE, Martin B, Mellor L, Jacob RB, Tawara K, McDougal OM, Oxford JT, Jorcyk CL. Oncostatin M binds to extracellular matrix in a bioactive conformation: implications for inflammation and metastasis. Cytokine. 2015;72(1):71–85.
12. Walker EC, Johnson RW, Hu Y, Brennan HJ, Poulton IJ, Zhang JG, Jenkins BJ, Smyth GK, Nicola NA, Sims NA. Murine oncostatin M acts via leukemia inhibitory factor receptor to phosphorylate signal transducer and activator of transcription 3 (STAT3) but not STAT1, an effect that protects bone mass. J Biol Chem. 2016;291(41):21703–16.
13. Smith DA, Kiba A, Zong Y, Witte ON. Interleukin-6 and oncostatin-M synergize with the PI3K/AKT pathway to promote aggressive prostate malignancy in mouse and human tissues. Mol Cancer Res. 2013;11(10):1159–65.
14. Junk DJ, Bryson BL, Smigiel JM, Parameswaran N, Bartel CA, Jackson MW. Oncostatin M promotes cancer cell plasticity through cooperative STAT3-SMAD3 signaling. Oncogene. 2017;36(28):4001–13.
15. Heinrich PC, Behrmann I, Haan S, Hermanns HM, Müller-Newen G, Schaper F. Principles of interleukin (IL)-6-type cytokine signalling and its regulation. Biochem J. 2003;374(Pt 1):1–20.
16. West NR, Murphy LC, Watson PH. Oncostatin M suppresses oestrogen receptor-α expression and is associated with poor outcome in human breast cancer. Endocr Relat Cancer. 2012;19(2):181–95.
17. Humbert L, Ghozlan M, Canaff L, Tian J, Lebrun JJ. The leukemia inhibitory factor (LIF) and p21 mediate the TGFβ tumor suppressive effects in human cutaneous melanoma. BMC Cancer. 2015;15:200.
18. Johnson RW, Finger EC, Olcina MM, Vilalta M, Aguilera T, Miao Y, Merkel AR, Johnson JR, Sterling JA, Wu JY, et al. Induction of LIFR confers a dormancy phenotype in breast cancer cells disseminated to the bone marrow. Nat Cell Biol. 2016;18(10):1078–89.
19. Kortylewski M, Heinrich PC, Mackiewicz A, Schniertshauer U, Klingmuller U, Nakajima K, Hirano T, Horn F, Behrmann I. Interleukin-6 and oncostatin M-induced growth inhibition of human A375 melanoma cells is STAT-dependent and involves upregulation of the cyclin-dependent kinase inhibitor p27/Kip1. Oncogene. 1999;18(25):3742–53.
20. West NR, Murray JI, Watson PH. Oncostatin-M promotes phenotypic changes associated with mesenchymal and stem cell-like differentiation in breast cancer. Oncogene. 2014;33(12):1485–94.
21. Jorcyk CL, Holzer RG, Ryan RE. Oncostatin M induces cell detachment and enhances the metastatic capacity of T-47D human breast carcinoma cells. Cytokine. 2006;33(6):323–36.
22. Holzer RG, Ryan RE, Tommack M, Schlekeway E, Jorcyk CL. Oncostatin M stimulates the detachment of a reservoir of invasive mammary carcinoma cells: role of cyclooxygenase-2. Clin Exp Metastasis. 2004;21(2):167–76.
23. Fossey SL, Bear MD, Kisseberth WC, Pennell M, London CA. Oncostatin M promotes STAT3 activation, VEGF production, and invasion in osteosarcoma cell lines. BMC Cancer. 2011;11:125.
24. Vollmer S, Kappler V, Kaczor J, Flügel D, Rolvering C, Kato N, Kietzmann T, Behrmann I, Haan C. Hypoxia-inducible factor 1alpha is up-regulated by oncostatin M and participates in oncostatin M signaling. Hepatology. 2009;50(1):253–60.
25. Guihard P, Boutet MA, Brounais-Le Royer B, Gamblin AL, Amiaud J, Renaud A, Berreur M, Redini F, Heymann D, Layrolle P, et al. Oncostatin M, an inflammatory cytokine produced by macrophages, supports intramembranous bone healing in a mouse model of tibia injury. Am J Pathol. 2015;185(3):765–75.
26. Lelekakis M, Moseley JM, Martin TJ, Hards D, Williams E, Ho P, Lowen D, Javni J, Miller FR, Slavin J, et al. A novel orthotopic model of breast cancer metastasis to bone. Clin Exp Metastasis. 1999;17(2):163–70.
27. Bolin C, Sutherland C, Tawara K, Moselhy J, Jorcyk CL. Novel mouse mammary cell lines for in vivo bioluminescence imaging (BLI) of bone metastasis. Biol Proced Online. 2012;14(1):6.
28. Martin-Padura I, Marighetti P, Gregato G, Agliano A, Malazzi O, Mancuso P, Pruneri G, Viale A, Bertolini F. Spontaneous cell fusion of acute leukemia cells and macrophages observed in cells with leukemic potential. Neoplasia. 2012;14(11):1057–66.
29. Eckhardt BL, Parker BS, van Laar RK, Restall CM, Natoli AL, Tavaria MD, Stanley KL, Sloan EK, Moseley JM, Anderson RL. Genomic analysis of a spontaneous model of breast cancer metastasis to bone reveals a role for the extracellular matrix. Mol Cancer Res. 2005;3(1):1–13.
30. Livak KJ, Schmittgen TD. Analysis of relative gene expression data using real-time quantitative PCR and the $2^{-\Delta\Delta C_T}$ Method. Methods. 2001;25(4):402–8.
31. Garbow JR, Dugas JP, Song S-K, Conradi MS. A simple, robust hardware device for passive or active respiratory gating in MRI and MRS experiments. Concepts Magn Reson Part B: Magn Reson Eng. 2004;21B(1):40–8.

32. Krupnick AS, Tidwell VK, Engelbach JA, Alli VV, Nehorai A, You M, Vikis HG, Gelman AE, Kreisel D, Garbow JR. Quantitative monitoring of mouse lung tumors by magnetic resonance imaging. Nat Protoc. 2012;7(1):128–42.

33. Garbow JR, Wang M, Wang Y, Lubet RA, You M. Quantitative monitoring of adenocarcinoma development in rodents by magnetic resonance imaging. Clin Cancer Res. 2008;14(5):1363–7.

34. Holliday DL, Speirs V. Choosing the right cell line for breast cancer research. Breast Cancer Res. 2011;13(4):215.

35. Jenkins DE, Hornig YS, Oei Y, Dusich J, Purchio T. Bioluminescent human breast cancer cell lines that permit rapid and sensitive in vivo detection of mammary tumors and multiple metastases in immune deficient mice. Breast Cancer Res. 2005;7(4):R444–54.

36. Mak RH, Ikizler AT, Kovesdy CP, Raj DS, Stenvinkel P, Kalantar-Zadeh K. Wasting in chronic kidney disease. J Cachexia Sarcopenia Muscle. 2011;2(1):9–25.

37. Kato Y, Ozawa S, Miyamoto C, Maehata Y, Suzuki A, Maeda T, Baba Y. Acidic extracellular microenvironment and cancer. Cancer Cell Int. 2013;13(1):89.

38. Liu J, Hadjokas N, Mosley B, Estrov Z, Spence MJ, Vestal RE. Oncostatin M-specific receptor expression and function in regulating cell proliferation of normal and malignant mammary epithelial cells. Cytokine. 1998;10(4):295–302.

39. Somlo G, Lau SK, Frankel P, Hsieh HB, Liu X, Yang L, Krivacic R, Bruce RH. Multiple biomarker expression on circulating tumor cells in comparison to tumor tissues from primary and metastatic sites in patients with locally advanced/inflammatory, and stage IV breast cancer, using a novel detection technology. Breast Cancer Res Treat. 2011;128(1):155–63.

40. Putzbach W, Gao QQ, Patel M, van Dongen S, Haluck-Kangas A, Sarshad AA, Bartom ET, Kim KA, Scholtens DM, Hafner M, et al. Many si/shRNAs can kill cancer cells by targeting multiple survival genes through an off-target mechanism. Elife. 2017;6:e29702.

41. Ramji K, Kulesza DW, Chouaib S, Kaminska B. Off-target effects of plasmid-transcribed shRNAs on NFκB signaling pathway and cell survival of human melanoma cells. Mol Biol Rep. 2013;40(12):6977–86.

42. Buehler E, Khan AA, Marine S, Rajaram M, Bahl A, Burchard J, Ferrer M. siRNA off-target effects in genome-wide screens identify signaling pathway members. Sci Rep. 2012;2:428.

43. Liu H, Zhang X, Li J, Sun B, Qian H, Yin Z. The biological and clinical importance of epithelial-mesenchymal transition in circulating tumor cells. J Cancer Res Clin Oncol. 2015;141(2):189–201.

44. Murray JI, West NR, Murphy LC, Watson PH. Intratumoural inflammation and endocrine resistance in breast cancer. Endocr Relat Cancer. 2015;22(1):R51–67.

45. Hosseini H, Obradović MM, Hoffmann M, Harper KL, Sosa MS, Werner-Klein M, Nanduri LK, Werno C, Ehrl C, Maneck M, et al. Early dissemination seeds metastasis in breast cancer. Nature. 2016;540:552–8.

46. Hazlett LD, Berk RS. Heightened resistance of athymic, nude (nu/nu) mice to experimental Pseudomonas aeruginosa ocular infection. Infect Immun. 1978; 22(3):926–33.

47. Koch J, Hau J, Pravsgaard Christensen J, Elvang Jensen H, Bagge Hansen M, Rieneck K. Immune cells from SR/CR mice induce the regression of established tumors in BALB/c and C57BL/6 mice. PLoS One. 2013;8(3): e59995.

48. Xie J, Zhu S, Dai Q, Lu J, Chen J, Li G, Wu H, Li R, Huang W, Xu B, et al. Oncostatin M was associated with thrombosis in patients with atrial fibrillation. Medicine (Baltimore). 2017;96(18):e6806.

49. Lauber S, Wong S, Cutz JC, Tanaka M, Barra N, Lhotak S, Ashkar A, Richards CD. Novel function of oncostatin M as a potent tumour-promoting agent in lung. Int J Cancer. 2015;136(4):831–43.

50. Tisdale MJ. Mechanisms of cancer cachexia. Physiol Rev. 2009;89(2):381–410.

51. Kholmukhamedov A, Czerny C, Hu J, Schwartz J, Zhong Z, Lemasters JJ. Minocycline and doxycycline, but not tetracycline, mitigate liver and kidney injury after hemorrhagic shock/resuscitation. Shock. 2014;42(3): 256–63.

52. Lokeshwar BL, Selzer MG, Zhu BQ, Block NL, Golub LM. Inhibition of cell proliferation, invasion, tumor growth and metastasis by an oral non-antimicrobial tetracycline analog (COL-3) in a metastatic prostate cancer model. Int J Cancer. 2002;98(2):297–309.

53. Miller A, McLeod L, Alhayyani S, Szczepny A, Watkins DN, Chen W, Enriori P, Ferlin W, Ruwanpura S, Jenkins BJ. Blockade of the IL-6 trans-signalling/STAT3 axis suppresses cachexia in Kras-induced lung adenocarcinoma. Oncogene. 2017;36(21):3059–66.

54. Onesti JK, Guttridge DC. Inflammation based regulation of cancer cachexia. Biomed Res Int. 2014;2014:168407.

55. Rao DD, Senzer N, Cleary MA, Nemunaitis J. Comparative assessment of siRNA and shRNA off target effects: what is slowing clinical development. Cancer Gene Ther. 2009;16(11):807–9.

56. Li C, Li J, Li Y, Lang S, Yougbare I, Zhu G, Chen P, Ni H. Crosstalk between platelets and the immune system: old systems with new discoveries. Adv Hematol. 2012;2012:384685.

57. Taucher S, Salat A, Gnant M, Kwasny W, Mlineritsch B, Menzel RC, Schmid M, Smola MG, Stierer M, Tausch C, et al. Impact of pretreatment thrombocytosis on survival in primary breast cancer. Thromb Haemost. 2003;89(6):1098–106.

58. Yuan L, Liu X. Platelets are associated with xenograft tumor growth and the clinical malignancy of ovarian cancer through an angiogenesis-dependent mechanism. Mol Med Rep. 2015;11(4):2449–58.

59. Gligorijevic B, Wyckoff J, Yamaguchi H, Wang Y, Roussos ET, Condeelis J. N-WASP-mediated invadopodium formation is involved in intravasation and lung metastasis of mammary tumors. J Cell Sci. 2012;125(Pt 3):724–34.

60. Bednarz-Knoll N, Alix-Panabieres C, Pantel K. Clinical relevance and biology of circulating tumor cells. Breast Cancer Res. 2011;13(6):228.

61. Husemann Y, Geigl JB, Schubert F, Musiani P, Meyer M, Burghart E, Forni G, Eils R, Fehm T, Riethmuller G, et al. Systemic spread is an early step in breast cancer. Cancer Cell. 2008;13(1):58–68.

62. Zhao S, Yang H, Zhang M, Zhang D, Liu Y, Liu Y, Song Y, Zhang X, Li H, Ma W, et al. Circulating tumor cells (CTCs) detected by triple-marker EpCAM, CK19, and hMAM RT-PCR and their relation to clinical outcome in metastatic breast cancer patients. Cell Biochem Biophys. 2013;65(2):263–73.

63. Gorges TM, Tinhofer I, Drosch M, Rose L, Zollner TM, Krahn T, von Ahsen O. Circulating tumour cells escape from EpCAM-based detection due to epithelial-to-mesenchymal transition. BMC Cancer. 2012;12:178.

64. Allan AL, Keeney M. Circulating tumor cell analysis: technical and statistical considerations for application to the clinic. J Oncol. 2010;2010:426218.

65. Tibbe AG, Miller MC, Terstappen LW. Statistical considerations for enumeration of circulating tumor cells. Cytometry A. 2007;71(3):154–62.

66. Tseng JY, Yang CY, Liang SC, Liu RS, Jiang JK, Lin CH. Dynamic changes in numbers and properties of circulating tumor cells and their potential applications. Cancers (Basel). 2014;6(4):2369–86.

67. Tester AM, Ruangpanit N, Anderson RL, Thompson EW. MMP-9 secretion and MMP-2 activation distinguish invasive and metastatic sublines of a mouse mammary carcinoma system showing epithelial-mesenchymal transition traits. Clin Exp Metastasis. 2000;18(7):553–60.

68. Kim MY, Oskarsson T, Acharyya S, Nguyen DX, Zhang XH, Norton L, Massagué J. Tumor self-seeding by circulating cancer cells. Cell. 2009;139(7): 1315–26.

69. Kucia-Tran JA, Tulkki V, Scarpini CG, Smith S, Wallberg M, Paez-Ribes M, Araujo AM, Botthoff J, Feeney M, Hughes K, et al. Anti-oncostatin M antibody inhibits the pro-malignant effects of oncostatin M receptor overexpression in squamous cell carcinoma. J Pathol. 2018;244(3):283–95.

70. Caffarel MM, Coleman N. Oncostatin M receptor is a novel therapeutic target in cervical squamous cell carcinoma. J Pathol. 2014;232(4):386–90.

7

Obesity promotes the expansion of metastasis-initiating cells in breast cancer

Mélanie Bousquenaud[1], Flavia Fico[2], Giovanni Solinas[3], Curzio Rüegg[1,4†] and Albert Santamaria-Martínez[2*†] (iD)

Abstract

Background: Obesity is a strong predictor of poor prognosis in breast cancer, especially in postmenopausal women. In particular, tumors in obese patients tend to seed more distant metastases, although the biology behind this observation remains poorly understood.

Methods: To elucidate the effects of the obese microenvironment on metastatic spread, we ovariectomized C57BL/6 J female mice and fed them either a regular diet (RD) or a high-fat diet (HFD) to generate a postmenopausal diet-induced obesity model. We then studied tumor progression to metastasis of Py230 and EO771 grafts. We analyzed and phenotyped the RD and HFD tumors and the surrounding adipose tissue by flow cytometry, qPCR, immunohistochemistry (IHC) and western blot. The influence of the microenvironment on tumor cells was assessed by performing cross-transplantation of RD and HFD tumor cells into other RD and HFD mice. The results were analyzed using the unpaired Student t test when comparing two variables, otherwise we used one-way or two-way analysis of variance. The relationship between two variables was calculated using correlation coefficients.

Results: Our results show that tumors in obese mice grow faster, are also less vascularized, more hypoxic, of higher grade and enriched in $CD11b^+Ly6G^+$ neutrophils. Collectively, this favors induction of the epithelial-to-mesenchymal transition and progression to claudin-low breast cancer, a subtype of triple-negative breast cancer that is enriched in cancer stem cells. Interestingly, transplanting HFD-derived tumor cells in RD mice transfers enhanced tumor growth and lung metastasis formation.

Conclusions: These data indicate that a pro-metastatic effect of obesity is acquired by the tumor cells in the primary tumor independently of the microenvironment of the secondary site.

Keywords: Obesity, Breast cancer, Metastasis-initiating cells

Background

Obesity affects more than half a billion adults worldwide and is a well-known risk factor for many cancers, including breast cancer [1], showing correlation with both increased risk and poor prognosis [2]. Of note, this association is mainly linked to postmenopausal patients, whereas in premenopausal women increased BMI correlates with decreased breast cancer risk - yet more aggressive progression and resistance to therapy [3]. However, the biology behind these links remains unclear,

in part due to the wide range of conditions associated with obesity.

Obesity-derived systemic complications, including but not restricted to inflammation, insulin resistance and hyperglycemia have been explored as potential causative effects or contributors to increased breast cancer risk and progression, albeit with mixed results [4]. Obesity is commonly characterized by macrophage-induced chronic inflammation in the adipose tissue [5, 6]. The effector cells leading to adipose tissue inflammation are M1 macrophages [7], which are initially recruited by T cells as monocytes [8]. Macrophages proliferate locally in the adipose tissue, a process that results in local and systemic subclinical inflammation leading to insulin resistance, diabetes and further increased adiposity [9]. Recent studies suggest that macrophages promote tumor progression in

* Correspondence: albert.santamaria@unifr.ch
†Curzio Rüegg and Albert Santamaria-Martínez contributed equally to this work.
[2]Tumor Ecology Laboratory, Division of Pathology, Department of Oncology, Microbiology and Immunology, Faculty of Science and Medicine, University of Fribourg, Chemin du Musée 18, PER17, CH-1700 Fribourg, Switzerland
Full list of author information is available at the end of the article

obesity through interactions with adipocytes [10], although M1 macrophages typically play protective roles in tumor formation [11]. Still, none of these studies provide experimental evidence to explain why obesity correlates with increased risk of distant metastasis, particularly in postmenopausal women [12]. Recently, two groups have found obesity to promote metastasis by two independent tumor cell extrinsic mechanisms [13, 14]. However, we and others have previously shown that metastasis relies on both tumor cell extrinsic and intrinsic factors [15]. With the aim to understand the molecular mechanisms linking obesity and poor prognosis in postmenopausal breast cancer, we generated a syngeneic orthotopic mouse model of post-menopausal breast cancer and investigated the effects of obesity on primary tumor growth and spontaneous meta-static progression. Our results reveal a novel mechanism in-volving hypoxia and neutrophil granulocytes-tumor cell interactions in the primary tumor that leads to the expan-sion of metastasis-initiating cells collectively resulting in in-creased distant metastasis formation.

Methods

Mouse work

C57BL/6 J, FVB/N, MMTV-PyMT (FVB/N) [16], and B6(Cg)-$Rag2^{tm1.1Cgn}$/J (Rag2−/−) [17] mice were housed in ventilated cages in the mouse husbandry of the Uni-versity of Fribourg. For tumor cell grafting, cells were trypsinized, resuspended in complete medium and cen-trifuged at 1300 rpm. They were washed twice in PBS, counted and resuspended in 1:3 Matrigel:PBS for injec-tion into the 4th mammary fat pad. To mimic postmeno-pausal estrogen decrease, 5–7-week-old female mice were ovariectomized and 2 weeks later they were sup-plied with either a high-fat diet (HFD) or a normal (regular) diet (RD (60% and 10% fat content, respect-ively). Mice were treated with clodronate liposomes as previously descrived [18]. All the experiments were per-formed by trained researchers holding the necessary ac-creditations and in accordance to the Swiss Animal Welfare Regulations and approved by the Cantonal Vet-erinary Service of the Canton Fribourg (2015_07_FR).

Antibodies and reagents

The following antibodies and reagents were used: TER119, CD3 (17A2), CD4 (GK1.5), CD8a (53–6.7), CD19 (6D5), CD31 (MEC13.3), CD45 (30-F11), Ly6C (HK1.4), Ly6G (RB6-8C5), CD11b (M1/70) (Biolegend), CD31, PCNA (Santa Cruz Technologies), Cytokeratin 14 (Covance), CD11b, CD31, Ki67 (Abcam), α-SMA, β-Tubulin, β-Actin (Sigma), Vimentin (Lifespan Biosci-ences), N-Cadherin, E-cadherin, p21, p53 (Cell Signal-ing), hypoxia inducible factor 1 alpha (HIF1α) (Novus Biologicals) and PIMO (Hypoxiprobes).

Cell culture

EO771 [19] and Py230 [20] cell lines were obtained from the American Type Culture Collection (ATCC) and grown as recommended. Mouse tumor tissue was disso-ciated using a mixture of Liberase TH (Roche) and DNAse at 37 °C for 45 min. Cells were filtered, washed twice in 2 mM EDTA in PBS and twice in PBS and then seeded for culture.

Fluorescence-activated cell sorting (FACS) analysis

For FACS analysis, tumor cells derived from tumor grafts (Py230 and EO771) or primary MMTV-PyMT tu-mors were obtained by disaggregating the tumors with Liberase TH (Roche) and DNAse at 37 °C for 45 min with agitation. Cells were then washed, filtered, stained with the appropriate antibodies for 30 min at 4 °C; 4',6-diamidino-2-phenylindole (DAPI) was used to stain and discard dead cells. Fluorescence was analyzed using a MACSQuant (Miltenyi) analyzer. FACS data were processed and analyzed using FlowJo.

Immunohistofluorescence

Immunostaining was performed on 4-μm-thick paraffin sections. Antigen retrieval was induced by heating the samples to 95 °C for 30 min in citrate buffer, pH 6.0. After blocking, we incubated the sections with the indi-cated antibodies overnight at 4 °C, and then used the secondary fluorescently labeled antibodies Alexa Fluor 488, 567 and 647 (Molecular Probes, Invitrogen) or HRP-conjugated secondary antibodies (Dako). Fluores-cent images were taken with a TCS-SP5 confocal micro-scope (Leica). Light images were taken with a widefield microscope (Leica).

Western blot

Protein was extracted with complete radioimmunopreci-pitation assay (RIPA) buffer, separated by electrophor-esis, transferred to polyvinylidene fluoride (PVDF) membranes, blocked with 5% BSA and incubated over-night with primary antibodies. Immunoreactive bands were visualized using HRP-conjugated secondary anti-bodies (Cell Signaling).

Real-time PCR

RNA was prepared using the mini RNeasy kit (Qiagen). Complementary DNAs (cDNAs) were generated using oligo-T priming and the M-MLV transcriptase (H-) point mutant (Promega) and quantitative PCR (qPCR) was performed in a StepOnePlus thermocycler (Applied Biosystems) using the SYBR green PCR Master Mix (Kapa). A list of the primers used is shown in Additional file 1: TableS1.

Statistics

Data were analyzed using GraphPad Prism 6. Means were compared using the unpaired Student t test. Samples were analyzed using Mann-Whitney's non-parametric test if the data were not normally distributed (with normality assessed using the D'Agostino-Pearson omnibus normality test). When comparing more than two variables, we performed one-way or two-way analysis of variance (ANOVA). To isolate differences between groups in ANOVA, we performed Fisher's least significant difference (LSD) test. We tested correlation using Pearson's correlation coefficient or Spearman's nonparametric correlation analysis depending on the data distribution. The p values are indicated for each experiment. Error bars in the figures indicate standard deviation unless stated otherwise in the figure legends. Significant differences between experimental groups are indicated with asterisks as follows: $*p < 0.05$, $**p < 0.01$, $***p < 0.001$ and $****p < 0.0001$.

Results

Mice fed with a HFD experience faster tumor growth and progression to metastasis

In order to recapitulate postmenopausal obesity and assess how it affects breast cancer progression, we first generated an experimental model following the strategy schematically depicted in Additional file 2: Figure S1A. Ovariectomizing C57BL/6 J mice and feeding them with a high-fat diet (HFD, 60% fat content) significantly increased weight gain compared to non-ovariectomized HFD-fed mice and ovariectomized or non-ovariectomized mice fed with a regular diet (RD) (Additional file 2: Figure S1B). Between 20 and 25 weeks of age, the difference between the mean of the final weight in both groups was 39.7% (Additional file 2: Figure S1C). In addition, obese mice developed the common systemic conditions frequently observed in the HFD mouse model, such as hyperinsulinemia (data not shown) [21]. Obesity is mainly associated with estrogen receptor alpha-positive (ERα^+) breast tumors [22]. To mimic human disease, we next performed syngeneic transplants in the mammary fat pad of C57BL/6 J mice with two different murine breast cancer cell lines that are hormone-sensitive in vivo, EO771 and Py230 [23, 24], and studied primary tumor growth and progression. As shown in Fig. 1a and b, E0771 and Py230 tumors in the HFD group grew significantly bigger. As with humans, in rodents the susceptibility to gain weight in response to obesogenic diets differs substantially between individuals [25, 26]. This variability is reflected within our experimental groups, since neither the RD nor the HFD body weights follow a normal distribution but are negatively and positively skewed, respectively ($p < 0.0068$; $n = 29$ and $p < 0.007$; $n = 35$, Additional file 2: Figure S1D and E). Nevertheless, our analyses revealed that body weight moderately correlated with tumor mass (Fig. 1c), which is again in agreement with observations in humans [27].

Interestingly, metastasis was also significantly increased in obese mice (Fig. 1d, e), even when there was no significant correlation between the size of the tumor and the number of metastatic foci in our control groups ($r = 0.29$, $p = 0,22$). Comparing same-sized tumors rendered similar results (Additional file 2: Figure S1F and G). To understand whether this increase in metastasis was due to tumor or host derived factors, we injected Celltracker-labeled Py230 cells into the tail vein of lean and obese mice and studied lung colonization using FACS after 2 h, as the time point for initial tumor cell trapping/seeding, and after 48 h, when most cells have extravasated. Our results show that there are no major differences in initial seeding and extravasation in lean compared to obese mice (Fig. 1f). Furthermore, we did not observe significant differences in the number of metastatic colonies formed upon tail vein injection, though there was a slight, non-significant trend toward more metastasis formation in obese mice (Fig. 1g, h). Taken together, these results demonstrated that obesity in ovariectomized mice promotes the formation of larger tumors and increased lung metastasis formation in the two models tested.

Obesity and not dietary factors is responsible for differences in tumor progression

Recent clinical data suggest that a diet rich in unsaturated fatty acids correlates with breast cancer risk independently of body mass index (BMI) [28], particularly in postmenopausal women [29]. However, it is still not clear whether the diet itself contributes to a poor prognosis in those patients with breast cancer or whether obesity is required. We then aimed at assessing whether the effects observed on tumor growth and metastasis in our model were due to obesity or to the diet. It is well-known that alternatively activated macrophages (M2) protect against obesity and insulin resistance [30]. We therefore reasoned that using M1/Th1 and M2/Th2-biased mouse strains [31] would allow us to discriminate the relevance of the diet versus obesity in our setting. Hence, we switched to the FVB/N mouse strain, an archetypical M2/Th2-biased mouse strain, in which we could use the PyMT tumor model for consistency purposes. We ovariectomized female mice, fed them with either a RD or HFD and performed syngeneic transplants with MMTV-PyMT tumor-derived cells.

Our results show that FVB/N mice did not gain weight after 12 weeks on the HFD regimen (Fig. 2a). Contrary to Py230-injected C57BL/6 mice, in which RD and HFD tumor growth rates diverge very early (Fig. 2b), we found that FVB/N mice, tumors did not differ in growth kinetics between the RD and HFD groups (Fig. 2c). Recruitment and activation of resting

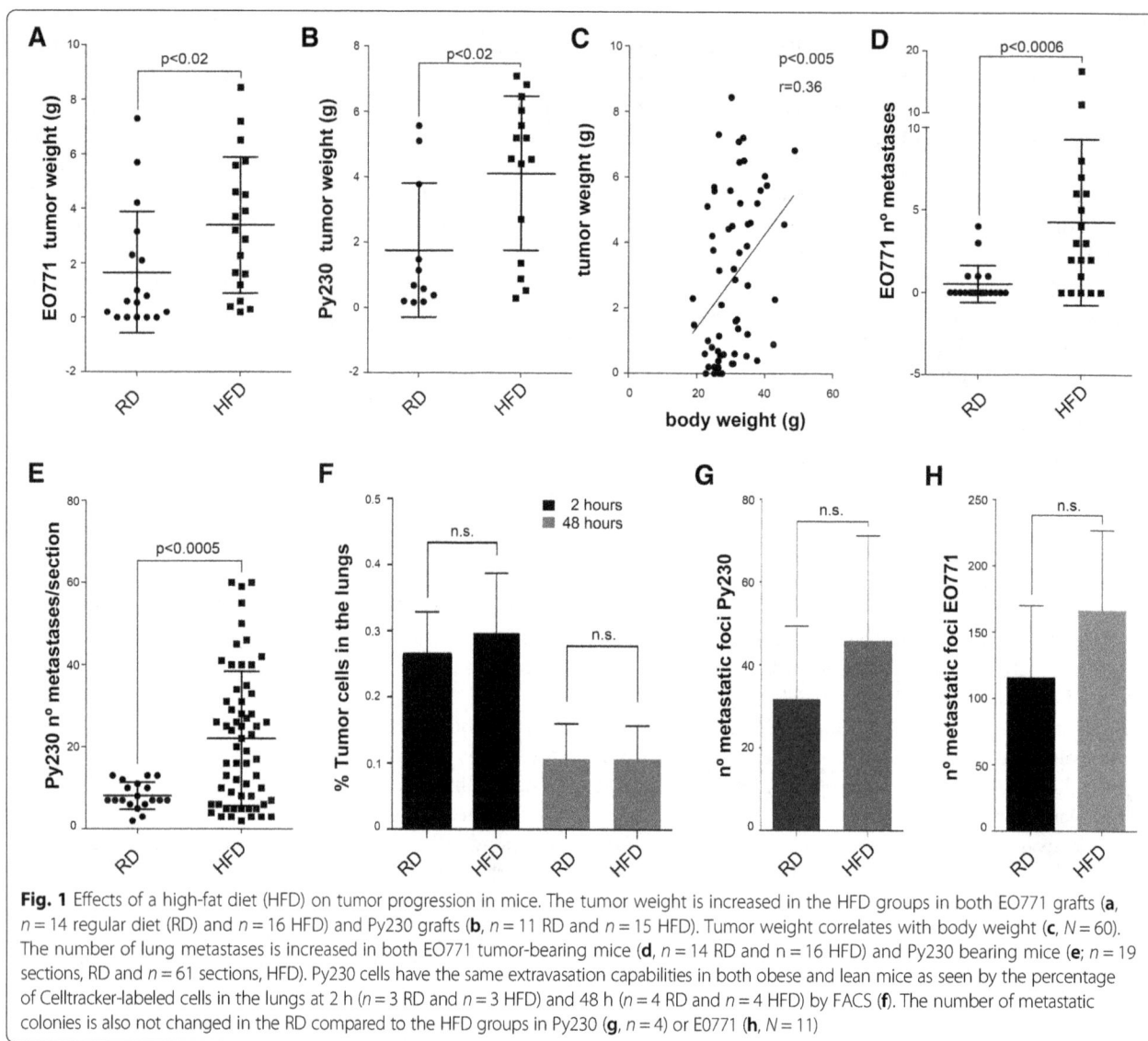

Fig. 1 Effects of a high-fat diet (HFD) on tumor progression in mice. The tumor weight is increased in the HFD groups in both EO771 grafts (**a**, $n = 14$ regular diet (RD) and $n = 16$ HFD) and Py230 grafts (**b**, $n = 11$ RD and $n = 15$ HFD). Tumor weight correlates with body weight (**c**, $N = 60$). The number of lung metastases is increased in both EO771 tumor-bearing mice (**d**, $n = 14$ RD and n = 16 HFD) and Py230 bearing mice (**e**; $n = 19$ sections, RD and $n = 61$ sections, HFD). Py230 cells have the same extravasation capabilities in both obese and lean mice as seen by the percentage of Celltracker-labeled cells in the lungs at 2 h ($n = 3$ RD and $n = 3$ HFD) and 48 h ($n = 4$ RD and $n = 4$ HFD) by FACS (**f**). The number of metastatic colonies is also not changed in the RD compared to the HFD groups in Py230 (**g**, $n = 4$) or EO771 (**h**, $N = 11$)

macrophages into proinflammatory ones in the adipose tissue requires previous infiltration by CD8$^+$ effector T cells [8]. Therefore, we argued that the absence of lymphocytes in an M1/Th1 biased strain should be sufficient to prevent obesity and rescue the obesity-mediated effects on tumor growth depicted in Fig. 1. Indeed, our results demonstrate that C57BL/6 J Rag2$^{-/-}$ mice, which lack T and B cells but not macrophages, did not become obese after 12 weeks of HFD (Fig. 2d). Consistent with the lack of T cells, overall tumor growth was faster in C57BL/6 Rag2$^{-/-}$ mice than in FVB/N mice. However, Py230 tumors did not progress faster in C57BL/6 Rag2$^{-/-}$ mice fed with HFD compared to RD controls (Fig. 2e). Moreover, in contrast to HFD-fed wild-type C57BL/6 J controls, the peritumoral adipose tissue of HFD-fed FVB/N mice had fewer crown-like structures - histologic

arrangements composed of macrophages and dead or dying adipocytes that define white adipose tissue inflammation (Fig. 2f) [32]. Likewise, the peritumoral adipose tissue of obese wild-type C57BL/6 J mice had higher expression of monocyte chemoattractants such as *Ccl2* (Fig. 2g), which is in agreement with human data [5]. Overall, these results indicate that in our experimental model, obesity promotes primary tumor growth and metastasis formation, while HFD in the absence of obesity is not sufficient to do this.

Obesity reduces angiogenesis and promotes hypoxia in the primary site

We then aimed at investigating possible reasons for faster primary tumor progression in obese mice. Not surprisingly, we observed an increase in the fraction of proliferating cancer cells in early-stage tumors in obese

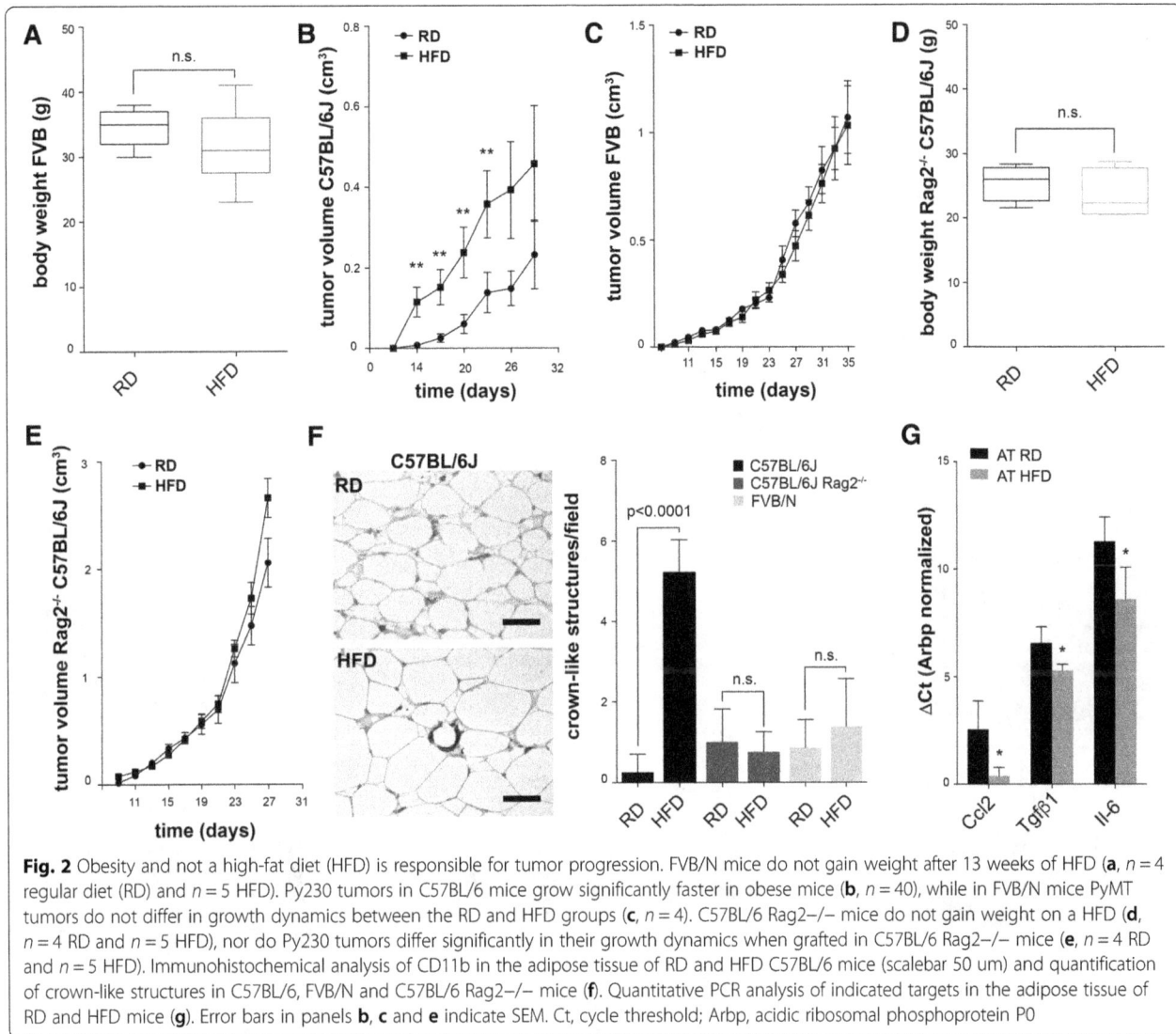

Fig. 2 Obesity and not a high-fat diet (HFD) is responsible for tumor progression. FVB/N mice do not gain weight after 13 weeks of HFD (**a**, $n = 4$ regular diet (RD) and $n = 5$ HFD). Py230 tumors in C57BL/6 mice grow significantly faster in obese mice (**b**, $n = 40$), while in FVB/N mice PyMT tumors do not differ in growth dynamics between the RD and HFD groups (**c**, $n = 4$). C57BL/6 Rag2−/− mice do not gain weight on a HFD (**d**, $n = 4$ RD and $n = 5$ HFD), nor do Py230 tumors differ significantly in their growth dynamics when grafted in C57BL/6 Rag2−/− mice (**e**, $n = 4$ RD and $n = 5$ HFD). Immunohistochemical analysis of CD11b in the adipose tissue of RD and HFD C57BL/6 mice (scalebar 50 um) and quantification of crown-like structures in C57BL/6, FVB/N and C57BL/6 Rag2−/− mice (**f**). Quantitative PCR analysis of indicated targets in the adipose tissue of RD and HFD mice (**g**). Error bars in panels **b**, **c** and **e** indicate SEM. Ct, cycle threshold; Arbp, acidic ribosomal phosphoprotein P0

mice (Fig. 3a). To study the association between obesity and faster tumor progression, we next analyzed tumor angiogenesis. A number of reports show that in obesity, angiogenesis cannot cope with adipose tissue growth [33–37]. We hypothesized that this might be mirrored in tumors, since the mammary gland is mainly composed of adipose tissue and tumors are surrounded by and in close contact with adipose tissue. In agreement with this, we found fewer vessels and lower fractions of CD31+ cells in tumors in obese mice (Fig. 3b, c and Additional file 2: Figure S2A). To understand the impact of decreased angiogenesis on oxygen levels in tumors in HFD-fed mice, we injected mice with pimonidazole and found higher hypoxic regions in tumors in obese mice (Fig. 3d). Furthermore, hypoxia in tumors from obese mice led to the accumulation of HIF1α (Additional file 3: Figure S2B), which consequently activated the transcription of specific hypoxia-target genes (Fig. 3e). Interestingly, HIF1α is known to be highly activated in triple-negative breast cancer (TNBC) [38, 39], a subset of aggressive breast cancers most of which are high-grade and present a high risk of metastasis and recurrence [40]. Indeed, histological analyses revealed that in obese mice the tumor mass was less differentiated, more often lacking glandular structures and possessing bigger nuclei (Additional file 3: Figure S2C). In addition, Py230 tumors in obese mice showed a consistent reduction in ERα, human epidermal growth factor receptor 2 (HER2), GATA3 and cytokeratin 18 and a gain in vimentin and c-Myc expression (Fig. 3f and Additional file 3: Figure S2D), suggestive of differentiation into more aggressive TNBC tumors. Overall, our results indicate that obesity causes reduced angiogenesis and triggers hypoxia in primary tumors, which promotes tumor progression.

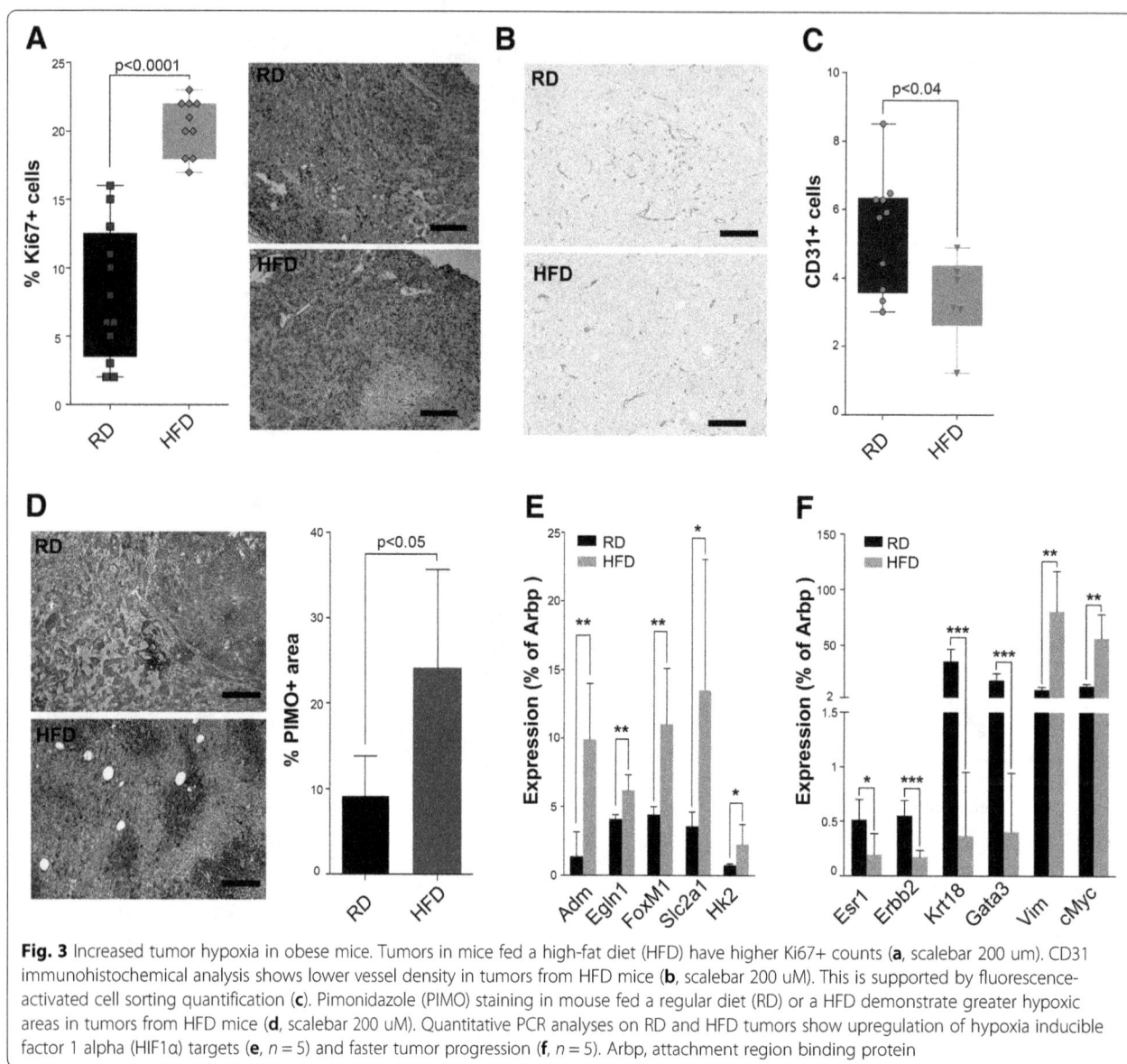

Fig. 3 Increased tumor hypoxia in obese mice. Tumors in mice fed a high-fat diet (HFD) have higher Ki67+ counts (**a**, scalebar 200 um). CD31 immunohistochemical analysis shows lower vessel density in tumors from HFD mice (**b**, scalebar 200 uM). This is supported by fluorescence-activated cell sorting quantification (**c**). Pimonidazole (PIMO) staining in mouse fed a regular diet (RD) or a HFD demonstrate greater hypoxic areas in tumors from HFD mice (**d**, scalebar 200 uM). Quantitative PCR analyses on RD and HFD tumors show upregulation of hypoxia inducible factor 1 alpha (HIF1α) targets (**e**, $n = 5$) and faster tumor progression (**f**, $n = 5$). Arbp, attachment region binding protein

The obese primary tumor microenvironment stimulates the expansion of metastasis-initiating cells

Given the essential involvement of inflammation in obesity [41], we next aimed at understanding how decreased angiogenesis and hypoxia modulate the immune compartment in the primary tumor. FACS analyses revealed that tumors from HFD mice contained 23% less CD11b$^+$F4/80$^+$ macrophages (Additional file 4: Figure S3A), which are mostly M1 macrophages in the C57BL/6 model (Additional file 4: Figure S3B). In contrast, the population of CD11b$^+$F4/80$^-$ cells showed a 31% increase in tumors from HFD mice. This population consists of CD11b$^+$Ly6C^{med}Gr1$^+$ neutrophils and CD11b$^+$Ly6C^{high} monocytes (Fig. 4a). We confirmed these results by performing western blot analyses and found increased CD11b protein in tumor tissue lysates

from HFD mice, compared to tumors from RD mice (Additional file 4: Figure S3C). Of note, this increase was not seen in tumors grown in C57BL/6 Rag2–/– or FVB/N mice fed with HFD diet (Additional file 4: Figure S3D and E), which underscores again the immunological differences between these strains. We then reasoned that if fast-growing tumors in HFD-fed mice contain fewer M1 macrophages and more tumor associated neutrophils (TANs) compared to tumors growing in RD-fed mice, macrophage may be protective against tumor growth. To test this hypothesis, we treated mice with clodronate liposomes to deplete macrophages. Indeed, clodronate liposome treatment boosted primary tumor growth in HFD-fed mice (Fig. 4b) and did not reduce metastasis (Additional file 4: Figure S3F). These results suggest that in our model, macrophages do not

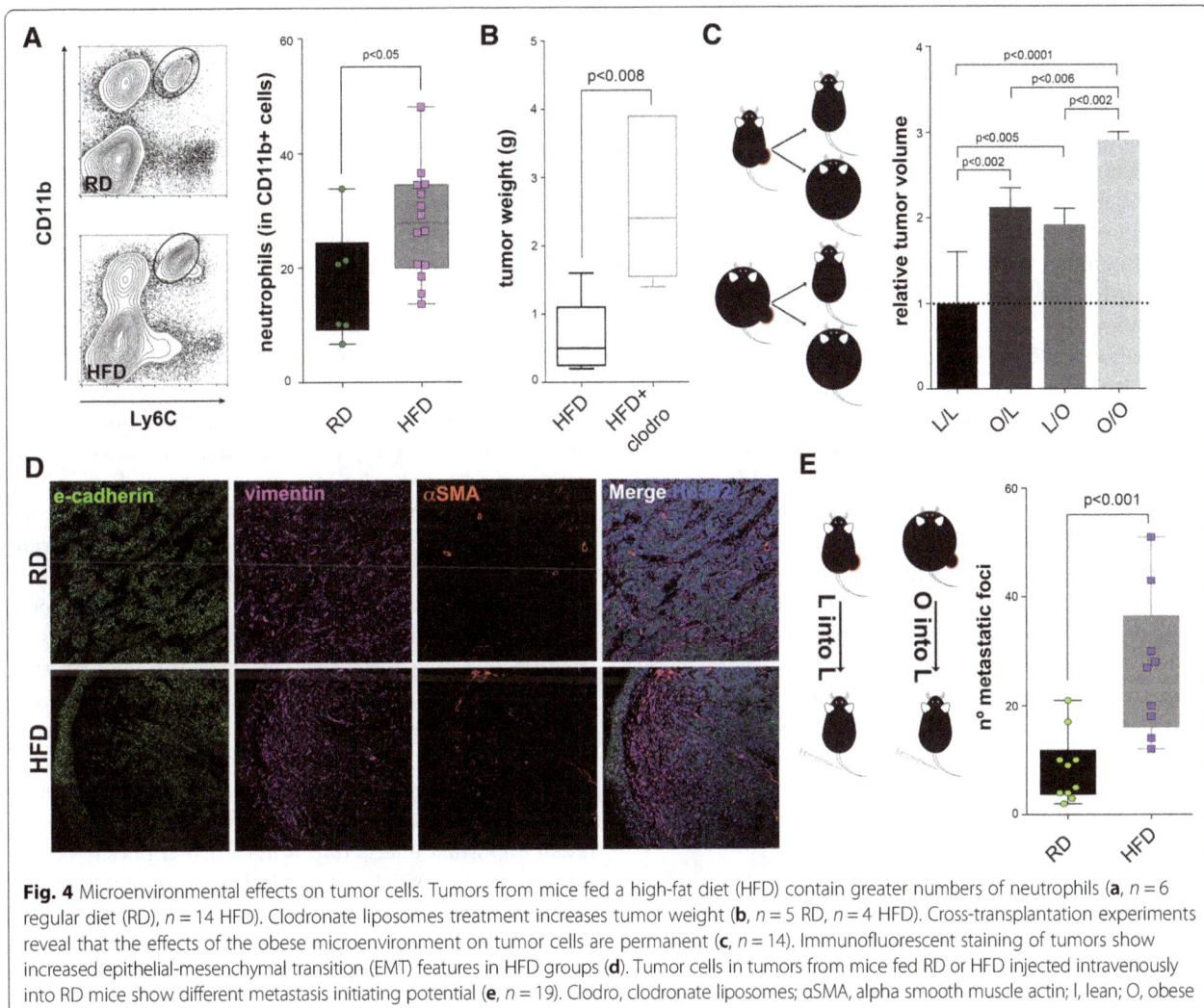

Fig. 4 Microenvironmental effects on tumor cells. Tumors from mice fed a high-fat diet (HFD) contain greater numbers of neutrophils (**a**, $n = 6$ regular diet (RD), $n = 14$ HFD). Clodronate liposomes treatment increases tumor weight (**b**, $n = 5$ RD, $n = 4$ HFD). Cross-transplantation experiments reveal that the effects of the obese microenvironment on tumor cells are permanent (**c**, $n = 14$). Immunofluorescent staining of tumors show increased epithelial-mesenchymal transition (EMT) features in HFD groups (**d**). Tumor cells in tumors from mice fed RD or HFD injected intravenously into RD mice show different metastasis initiating potential (**e**, $n = 19$). Clodro, clodronate liposomes; αSMA, alpha smooth muscle actin; l, lean; O, obese

contribute to promote tumor progression and metastatic spread, regardless of their essential involvement in obesity.

In order to evaluate the importance of the effects of the microenvironment on the tumor cells, we performed cross-transplantation of tumor cells from HFD-fed and RD-fed into RD-fed and HFD-fed mice, respectively. Interestingly, we observed that tumor cells derived from obese mice grew faster in lean recipient mice compared to cells derived from lean mice (Fig. 4c). As expected, grafting into obese mice further boosted growth of both transplanted cell populations. These results uncoupled immediate microenvironmental effects from tumor cell effects and indicate that the obese tumor microenvironment exerts contextual and sustained effects on tumor cells.

Neutrophils are known to migrate to ischemic tissues and to contribute to the epithelial-to-mesenchymal transition (EMT) [42]. EMT is a process involved in invasion and metastasis and produces cancer stem cells (CSC) [43], a subpopulation of cells that we and others have previously shown to lead metastatic colonization [15]. Indeed, tumors from HFD mice consistently lost E-cadherin and had an increase in N-cadherin and vimentin, three hallmarks of EMT (Fig. 4d and Additional file 5: Figure S4A). This effect was not observed in FVB/N tumors (Additional file 5: Figure S4B). In agreement with TANs being associated with EMT, we identified strong correlation between the expression of CD11b and N-cadherin and anti-correlation with E-cadherin in primary tumors (Additional file 5: Figure S4D).

All these assays were performed with equal-sized tumors to avoid potential confounding effects due to more rapid tumor growth in HFD-fed mice (Additional file 5: Figure S4C). EMT is a distinctive feature of claudin-low tumors, a particular subset of TNBC that is enriched in CSC-related genes [44]. Since aggressive subtypes of breast cancer such as TNBC and basal-like tumors are associated with mutations in p53 [23, 45–47], we next stained for p53, a surrogate marker for its mutational status. Our results indicate that tumors in obese mice have a higher number of p53-positive cells (Additional file 5: Figure S4E). As a consequence, they also show significantly lower levels of p21(WAF1/CIP1), an important target of p53 responsible for cell cycle arrest (Additional file 5: Figure S4A).

Claudin-low tumors are also characterized by a loss of cell-cell junction proteins. Therefore, we next performed qPCR analyses in tumors from RD and HFD mice using a number of genes from the cell-cell junction organization gene set M820 from the MSigDB database [48], as previously described [23]. The results confirmed that the obese microenvironment triggers a process that leads to the rapid expansion of claudin-low tumors (Additional file 5: Figure S4F).

Finally, to test whether the effects of obesity on the primary tumor are essential for the late steps of cancer metastasis, we digested tumors from RD and HFD mice and injected 5×10^5 tumor cells via the tail vein into tumor-free, RD mice. Our results demonstrate that tumor cells derived from obese mice metastasize more to the lungs compared to cells derived from lean mice (Fig. 4e), i.e. tumors from obese mice contain more CSC with metastasis-initiating capacity. Our data provide direct evidence that the primary tumor microenvironment of obese mice generates more tumor cells with lung metastasis-initiating capacity.

Discussion

To date, the link between obesity and worse outcomes observed in patients with breast cancer remains poorly understood, mainly due to the lack of experimental studies based on mouse models of metastasis that explore the full metastatic cascade. In this study, we used orthotopic, syngeneic models of spontaneous breast cancer metastasis and have discovered a novel experimental link between obesity and tumor progression to metastasis; collectively, our results show that the interactions between hypoxia, elements of the tumor microenvironment (likely neutrophils) and tumor cells ultimately orchestrate a shift towards TNBC/claudin-low tumors and a consequent increase in metastasis-initiating cells within primary tumors in obese mice. Overall, our data provide an experimental link with clinical observations describing higher TNBC rates in obese patients [2, 49]. Moreover, premenopausal and postmenopausal, overweight and obese patients with breast cancer are generally at higher risk of recurrence and resistance to therapy [1, 2, 12, 50–52]. Biganzoli and collaborators used data from the prospective "three-arms" trial with very long follow up to show that the patient's BMI at diagnosis is associated with specific recurrence patterns over time [53]. They observed for example that obese

patients present with at least two peaks of recurrences, one early and one late. Our results showing TNBC features and increased CSC content in tumors in obese mice might explain the higher risk of recurrence and resistance to therapy observed in overweight and obese humans, although this hypothesis requires further studies to be confirmed.

Interestingly, recent work suggests that higher neutrophil infiltration in the lungs of obese mice results in higher metastatic burden [13]. While in our setting primary tumor hypoxia could also be responsible for the generation of a neutrophilic premetastatic niche in the lungs [54], we here showed that the events in the primary tumor promote increased metastasis in obese mice without the need for preconditioning the distant metastatic site. Accordingly, in secondary transplants obese primary tumors have higher metastatic potential regardless of the host in which they are grafted. The different conclusions between this work [13] and ours are likely to be explained by experimental differences, the most significant of which is the use of orthotopic models of spontaneous lung metastasis, which is the only strategy that allows study of the whole metastatic cascade. In addition, our obese mice were ovariectomized, thereby better mimicking postmenopausal obesity in patients. In short, while our results do not exclude additional metastasis-promoting effects in the secondary site, they clearly reveal important effects of postmenopausal obesity on the primary tumor which are critical for metastatic spread and colonization. We therefore think that our model provides a more clinically relevant approach to unravel the effects of obesity on breast cancer progression.

Due to the lack of ovarian-derived estrogens, postmenopausal women are more prone to increases in their BMI. We show that in our model this is not due to dietary factors but, similarly to humans, it is linked to each individual's susceptibility to become obese [26]. Indeed, to address the importance of the diet in the progression of breast cancer, we used obesity-resistant M2/Th2 FVB/N mice and demonstrated that the diet alone, i.e. in the absence of obesity, is not sufficient to affect tumor growth.

Local estrogen production has also been linked to the increased risk of breast cancer and contributes to progression in postmenopausal women, given that after menopause the production of estrogens is thought to occur mainly in the adipose tissue [55]. However, we were not able to detect aromatase transcripts in the adipose tissue or the tumors of RD or HFD mice (data not shown), which rules out potential effects of local estrogen production on tumor growth in obese animals.

Obesity is characterized by low-grade chronic inflammation. Our results indicate correlation between the infiltration of neutrophils in the primary tumor and the acquisition of a more mesenchymal phenotype by tumor cells. In contrast, Kolb and collaborators found that the inflammasome of macrophages in primary tumors in obese mice is responsible for triggering angiogenesis through expression of vascular endothelial growth factor A (VEGFA), consequently boosting primary tumor growth [10]. Our results differ in that we did not see increased macrophage content in tumors from obese mice, and we observed a reduction in vessel density with a concomitant increase in hypoxia. We argue that this decrease in vascularization is the same as observed in the adipose tissue during obesity [56], and we suggest that higher proliferative rates may be the result of p53 dysregulation. Notwithstanding the differences between Kolb et al. and our group, it is worth noting that in our experimental setting elimination of macrophages by treatment with clodronate liposomes did not reduce tumor growth but rather the opposite. In addition, we and others have observed that clodronate treatment reduces body weight in obese mice, which is consistent with an obesity promoting effect of M1 macrophages [57]. Finally, it is known that during obesity there is an increase in neutrophil recruitment in the adipose tissue, which mediates insulin resistance [58, 59]. Overall, our results indicate that obesity-associated macrophages play a crucial role in stimulating the growth of the adipose tissue, but they have antagonistic effects on cancer progression. We here suggest that other immune cells, such as neutrophils, might be involved in primary tumor progression in obesity. Our model might prove useful in identifying further key factors relevant to breast cancer progression in obesity and to evaluate potential therapeutic strategies.

Conclusions

In summary, we have found that decreased vascularization in the primary tumors of postmenopausal obese mice triggers hypoxia, neutrophil infiltration and EMT, leading to the expansion of TNBC/claudin-low tumors and an increase in metastasis-initiating cells. These results provide an explanation for the higher incidence of metastasis and higher ratio of TNBC observed in obese patients with breast cancer and challenge the recent notion that tumor-cell extrinsic factors in the secondary site are clinically relevant to these patients.

Additional files

Additional file 1: Table S1. (DOCX 45.3 kb)

Additional file 2: Figure S1. Scheme of the experimental procedure (A). Body weight comparison between ovariectomized ($n = 12$ RD, $n = 12$ HFD) and non-ovariectomized ($n = 5$ RD, $n = 5$ HFD) mice (B). Body weight of ovariectomized RD and HFD mouse groups after 13 weeks of diet (C; $n = 29$ RD and $n = 35$ HFD). Data distribution of mouse weight in RD (D) and HFD (E) groups. Number of metastases seeded by same-sized tumors in RD and HFD mice (F and G). Error bars in panel B indicate SEM. (TIF 2261 kb)

Additional file 3: Figure S2. CD31 staining in C57BL/6 Rag2–/– mice show no differences between tumors from RD and HFD mice when they are grown in C57BL/6 Rag2–/– hosts (A, scalebar = 100uM). HIF1a staining in wild-type (wt) and C57BL/6 Rag2–/– mice show that hypoxia is increased in tumors from wt obese mice, while it is not changed in tumors in HFD-fed C57BL/6 Rag2–/– mice (B, scalebar 100 uM). HE staining of RD and HFD tumors showing enlarged nuclei and less packed chromatin in the latter (C, scalebar 50 um). IHC analyses in tumor samples show faster progression in HFD compared to RD tumors (D, $n = 5$, scalebar 50 um). (JPG 3325 kb)

Additional file 4: Figure S3. FACS analyses show lower percentages of F4/80+ macrophages in the CD11b + compartment in Py230 HFD tumors (A, $n = 18$ RD, $n = 20$ HFD). Percentages of M1 (F4/80 + CD206-) and M2 macrophages (F4/80 + CD206+) identified in the CD11b + compartment of C57BL/6 and FVB/N mice (B, n = 3 RD, $n = 7$ HFD for C57BL/6 and $n = 4$ RD, $n = 4$ HFD for FVB/N). Normalized western blot analysis for CD11b in Py230-C57BL6 tumors (C; $N = 8$), Py230-C57BL/6;Rag2–/– tumors (D; $N = 9$) and PyMT-FVB/N tumors (E; $n = 8$). Clodronate liposomes treatment increases metastasis (F, $n = 5$ RD, $n = 6$ HFD). (TIF 1676 kb)

Additional file 5: Figure S4. Western blot analysis for E-cadherin, N-cadherin, p21, and HIF1a in Py230-C57BL/6 tumor lysates of RD and HFD (A). Western blot analysis for E-cadherin in PyMT tumors grown in FVB/N mice (B). Tumor weight of groups used for qPCR and western blot analyses (C, $N = 10$). CD11b strongly correlates with N-cadherin and anti correlates with E cadherin (D, $N = 10$). IHC on RD vs HFD tumors show nuclear p53 accumulation in the latter (E, scalebar 100 uM). qPCR analyses on Py230 RD and HFD tumors show significant downregulation of claudins and other cell-cell junction genes (F, $n = 5$). (TIF 9127 kb)

Abbreviations
ANOVA: Analysis of variance; BMI: Body mass index; CSC: Cancer stem cell; EMT: Epithelial to mesenchymal transition; FACS: Fluorescence-activated cell sorting; HER2: Human epidermal growth receptor 2; HFD: High-fat diet; HIF1α: Hypoxia inducible factor 1 alpha; IHC: Immunohistochemistry; PBS: Phosphate-buffered saline; RD: Regular diet; TAN: Tumor associated neutrophil; TNBC: Triple-negative breast cancer

Acknowledgements
We thank Oriana Coquoz for excellent technical help, Dr. Elizabeth Allen for critical revision of the manuscript and Dr. Christine Desmedt and Dr. Elia Biganzoli for their invaluable scientific input.

Funding
This project was supported by a Sinergia grant to CR and GS (CRSII3_154499) and an Ambizione career award to ASM (PZ00P3_154751) from the Swiss National Science Foundation (SNSF).

Authors' contributions
Conceptualization: CR, ASM and GS; methodology: ASM and CR; experiments performed by ASM, MB and FF; formal analysis: ASM; writing: original draft, ASM; revision: ASM; funding acquisition: CR and ASM; supervision: ASM and CR. All authors read and approved the final manuscript.

Competing interests
The authors declare that they have no competing interests.

Author details

[1]Experimental and Translational Oncology Laboratory, Division of Pathology, Department of Oncology, Microbiology and Immunology, Faculty of Science and Medicine, University of Fribourg, Fribourg, Switzerland. [2]Tumor Ecology Laboratory, Division of Pathology, Department of Oncology, Microbiology and Immunology, Faculty of Science and Medicine, University of Fribourg, Chemin du Musée 18, PER17, CH-1700 Fribourg, Switzerland. [3]Department of Molecular and Clinical Medicine, The Wallenberg Laboratory, University of Gothenburg, Gothenburg, Sweden. [4]Swiss Integrative Center for Human Health, Fribourg, Switzerland.

References

1. Calle EE, Rodriguez C, Walker-Thurmond K, Thun MJ. Overweight, obesity, and mortality from cancer in a prospectively studied cohort of U.S. adults. N Engl J Med. 2003;348(17):1625–38.
2. Jiralerspong S, Goodwin PJ. Obesity and breast Cancer prognosis: evidence, challenges, and opportunities. J Clin Oncol. 2016;34(35):4203–16.
3. WCRF/AICR. Food, nutrition, physical activity, and the prevention of cancer: a global perspective. Washington DC: AICR; 2007.
4. Hernandez AV, Guarnizo M, Miranda Y, Pasupuleti V, Deshpande A, Paico S, Lenti H, Ganoza S, Montalvo L, Thota P, et al. Association between insulin resistance and breast carcinoma: a systematic review and meta-analysis. PLoS One. 2014;9(6):e99317.
5. Weisberg SP, McCann D, Desai M, Rosenbaum M, Leibel RL, Ferrante AW Jr. Obesity is associated with macrophage accumulation in adipose tissue. J Clin Invest. 2003;112(12):1796–808.
6. Solinas G, Karin M. JNK1 and IKKbeta: molecular links between obesity and metabolic dysfunction. FASEB J. 2010;24(8):2596–611.
7. Lumeng CN, Bodzin JL, Saltiel AR. Obesity induces a phenotypic switch in adipose tissue macrophage polarization. J Clin Invest. 2007;117(1):175–84.
8. Nishimura S, Manabe I, Nagasaki M, Eto K, Yamashita H, Ohsugi M, Otsu M, Hara K, Ueki K, Sugiura S, et al. CD8+ effector T cells contribute to macrophage recruitment and adipose tissue inflammation in obesity. Nat Med. 2009;15(8):914–20.
9. Amano SU, Cohen JL, Vangala P, Tencerova M, Nicoloro SM, Yawe JC, Shen Y, Czech MP, Aouadi M. Local proliferation of macrophages contributes to obesity-associated adipose tissue inflammation. Cell Metab. 2014;19(1):162–71.
10. Kolb R, Phan L, Borcherding N, Liu Y, Yuan F, Janowski AM, Xie Q, Markan KR, Li W, Potthoff MJ, et al. Obesity-associated NLRC4 inflammasome activation drives breast cancer progression. Nat Commun. 2016;7:13007.
11. Williams CB, Yeh ES, Soloff AC. Tumor-associated macrophages: unwitting accomplices in breast cancer malignancy. NPJ Breast Cancer. 2016;2
12. Ewertz M, Jensen MB, Gunnarsdottir KA, Hojris I, Jakobsen EH, Nielsen D, Stenbygaard LE, Tange UB, Cold S. Effect of obesity on prognosis after early-stage breast cancer. J Clin Oncol. 2011;29(1):25–31.
13. Quail DF, Olson OC, Bhardwaj P, Walsh LA, Akkari L, Quick ML, Chen IC, Wendel N, Ben-Chetrit N, Walker J, et al. Obesity alters the lung myeloid cell landscape to enhance breast cancer metastasis through IL5 and GM-CSF. Nat Cell Biol. 2017;19(8):974–87.
14. Baek AE, Yu YA, He S, Wardell SE, Chang CY, Kwon S, Pillai RV, McDowell HB, Thompson JW, Dubois LG, et al. The cholesterol metabolite 27 hydroxycholesterol facilitates breast cancer metastasis through its actions on immune cells. Nat Commun. 2017;8(1):864.
15. Malanchi I, Santamaria-Martinez A, Susanto E, Peng H, Lehr HA, Delaloye JF, Huelsken J. Interactions between cancer stem cells and their niche govern metastatic colonization. Nature. 2011;481(7379):85–9.
16. Guy CT, Cardiff RD, Muller WJ. Induction of mammary tumors by expression of polyomavirus middle T oncogene: a transgenic mouse model for metastatic disease. Mol Cell Biol. 1992;12(3):954–61.
17. Shinkai Y, Rathbun G, Lam KP, Oltz EM, Stewart V, Mendelsohn M, Charron J, Datta M, Young F, Stall AM, et al. RAG-2-deficient mice lack mature lymphocytes owing to inability to initiate V(D)J rearrangement. Cell. 1992; 68(5):855–67.
18. Kuonen F, Laurent J, Secondini C, Lorusso G, Stehle JC, Rausch T, Faes-Van't Hull E, Bieler G, Alghisi GC, Schwendener R, et al. Inhibition of the Kit ligand/c-Kit axis attenuates metastasis in a mouse model mimicking local breast cancer relapse after radiotherapy. Clin Cancer Res. 2012; 18(16):4365–74.
19. Sugiura K, Stock CC. Studies in a tumor spectrum. I. Comparison of the action of methylbis (2-chloroethyl)amine and 3-bis(2-chloroethyl)aminomethyl-4-methoxymethyl –5-hydroxy-6-methylpyridine on the growth of a variety of mouse and rat tumors. Cancer. 1952;5(2):382–402.
20. Biswas T, Gu X, Yang J, Ellies LG, Sun LZ. Attenuation of TGF-beta signaling supports tumor progression of a mesenchymal-like mammary tumor cell line in a syngeneic murine model. Cancer Lett. 2014;346(1):129–38.
21. Winzell MS, Ahren B. The high-fat diet-fed mouse: a model for studying mechanisms and treatment of impaired glucose tolerance and type 2 diabetes. Diabetes. 2004;53(Suppl 3):S215–9.
22. Rose DP, Komninou D, Stephenson GD. Obesity, adipocytokines, and insulin resistance in breast cancer. Obes Rev. 2004;5(3):153–65.
23. Bao L, Cardiff RD, Steinbach P, Messer KS, Ellies LG. Multipotent luminal mammary cancer stem cells model tumor heterogeneity. Breast Cancer Res. 2015;17(1):137.
24. Ewens A, Mihich E, Ehrke MJ. Distant metastasis from subcutaneously grown E0771 medullary breast adenocarcinoma. Anticancer Res. 2005;25(6B):3905–15.
25. Levin BE, Keesey RE. Defense of differing body weight set points in diet-induced obese and resistant rats. Am J Phys. 1998;274(2 Pt 2):R412–9.
26. Levine JA, Eberhardt NL, Jensen MD. Role of nonexercise activity thermogenesis in resistance to fat gain in humans. Science. 1999;283(5399): 212–4.
27. Maehle BO, Tretli S, Skjaerven R, Thorsen T. Premorbid body weight and its relations to primary tumour diameter in breast cancer patients; its dependence on estrogen and progesterone receptor status. Breast Cancer Res Treat. 2001;68(2):159–69.
28. Sieri S, Chiodini P, Agnoli C, Pala V, Berrino F, Trichopoulou A, Benetou V, Vasilopoulou E, Sanchez MJ, Chirlaque MD, et al. Dietary fat intake and development of specific breast cancer subtypes. J Natl Cancer Inst. 2014;106(5)
29. Sieri S, Krogh V, Ferrari P, Berrino F, Pala V, Thiebaut AC, Tjonneland A, Olsen A, Overvad K, Jakobsen MU, et al. Dietary fat and breast cancer risk in the European prospective investigation into cancer and nutrition. Am J Clin Nutr. 2008;88(5):1304–12.
30. Chawla A, Nguyen KD, Goh YP. Macrophage-mediated inflammation in metabolic disease. Nat Rev Immunol. 2011;11(11):738–49.
31. Mills CD, Kincaid K, Alt JM, Heilman MJ, Hill AM. M-1/M-2 macrophages and the Th1/Th2 paradigm. J Immunol. 2000;164(12):6166–73.
32. Murano I, Barbatelli G, Parisani V, Latini C, Muzzonigro G, Castellucci M, Cinti S. Dead adipocytes, detected as crown-like structures, are prevalent in visceral fat depots of genetically obese mice. J Lipid Res. 2008;49(7):1562–8.
33. Hosogai N, Fukuhara A, Oshima K, Miyata Y, Tanaka S, Segawa K, Furukawa S, Tochino Y, Komuro R, Matsuda M, et al. Adipose tissue hypoxia in obesity and its impact on adipocytokine dysregulation. Diabetes. 2007;56(4):901–11.
34. Michailidou Z, Turban S, Miller E, Zou X, Schrader J, Ratcliffe PJ, Hadoke PW, Walker BR, Iredale JP, Morton NM, et al. Increased angiogenesis protects against adipose hypoxia and fibrosis in metabolic disease-resistant 11beta-hydroxysteroid dehydrogenase type 1 (HSD1)-deficient mice. J Biol Chem. 2012;287(6):4188–97.
35. Pasarica M, Sereda OR, Redman LM, Albarado DC, Hymel DT, Roan LE, Rood JC, Burk DH, Smith SR. Reduced adipose tissue oxygenation in human obesity: evidence for rarefaction, macrophage chemotaxis, and inflammation without an angiogenic response. Diabetes. 2009;58(3):718–25.
36. Rausch ME, Weisberg S, Vardhana P, Tortoriello DV. Obesity in C57BL/6J mice is characterized by adipose tissue hypoxia and cytotoxic T-cell infiltration. Int J Obes. 2008;32(3):451–63.
37. Lee YS, Kim JW, Osborne O, Oh DY, Sasik R, Schenk S, Chen A, Chung H, Murphy A, Watkins SM, et al. Increased adipocyte O2 consumption triggers HIF-1alpha, causing inflammation and insulin resistance in obesity. Cell. 2014;157(6):1339–52.
38. Cancer Genome Atlas N. Comprehensive molecular portraits of human breast tumours. Nature. 2012;490(7418):61–70.
39. Montagner M, Enzo E, Forcato M, Zanconato F, Parenti A, Rampazzo E, Basso G, Leo G, Rosato A, Bicciato S, et al. SHARP1 suppresses breast cancer metastasis by promoting degradation of hypoxia-inducible factors. Nature. 2012;487(7407):380–4.

40. Dent R, Trudeau M, Pritchard KI, Hanna WM, Kahn HK, Sawka CA, Lickley LA, Rawlinson E, Sun P, Narod SA. Triple-negative breast cancer: clinical features and patterns of recurrence. Clin Cancer Res. 2007;13(15 Pt 1):4429–34.

41. Mraz M, Haluzik M. The role of adipose tissue immune cells in obesity and low-grade inflammation. J Endocrinol. 2014;222(3):R113–27.

42. Powell DR, Huttenlocher A. Neutrophils in the tumor microenvironment. Trends Immunol. 2016;37(1):41–52.

43. Mani SA, Guo W, Liao MJ, Eaton EN, Ayyanan A, Zhou AY, Brooks M, Reinhard F, Zhang CC, Shipitsin M, et al. The epithelial-mesenchymal transition generates cells with properties of stem cells. Cell. 2008;133(4): 704–15.

44. Prat A, Parker JS, Karginova O, Fan C, Livasy C, Herschkowitz JI, He X, Perou CM. Phenotypic and molecular characterization of the claudin-low intrinsic subtype of breast cancer. Breast Cancer Res. 2010;12(5):R68.

45. Carey LA, Perou CM, Livasy CA, Dressler LG, Cowan D, Conway K, Karaca G, Troester MA, Tse CK, Edmiston S, et al. Race, breast cancer subtypes, and survival in the Carolina breast cancer study. JAMA. 2006;295(21):2492–502.

46. Herschkowitz JI, Zhao W, Zhang M, Usary J, Murrow G, Edwards D, Knezevic J, Greene SB, Darr D, Troester MA, et al. Comparative oncogenomics identifies breast tumors enriched in functional tumor-initiating cells. Proc Natl Acad Sci U S A. 2012;109(8):2778–83.

47. Sorlie T, Perou CM, Tibshirani R, Aas T, Geisler S, Johnsen H, Hastie T, Eisen MB, van de Rijn M, Jeffrey SS, et al. Gene expression patterns of breast carcinomas distinguish tumor subclasses with clinical implications. Proc Natl Acad Sci U S A. 2001;98(19):10869–74.

48. Subramanian A, Tamayo P, Mootha VK, Mukherjee S, Ebert BL, Gillette MA, Paulovich A, Pomeroy SL, Golub TR, Lander ES, et al. Gene set enrichment analysis: a knowledge-based approach for interpreting genome-wide expression profiles. Proc Natl Acad Sci U S A. 2005;102(43):15545–50.

49. Reeves GK, Pirie K, Beral V, Green J, Spencer E, Bull D, Million Women Study Collaboration. Cancer incidence and mortality in relation to body mass index in the Million Women Study: cohort study. BMJ. 2007;335(7630):1134.

50. Lauby-Secretan B, Scoccianti C, Loomis D, Grosse Y, Bianchini F, Straif K, International Agency for Research on Cancer Handbook Working Group. Body fatness and cancer–viewpoint of the IARC working group. N Engl J Med. 2016;375(8):794–8.

51. Protani M, Coory M, Martin JH. Effect of obesity on survival of women with breast cancer: systematic review and meta-analysis. Breast Cancer Res Treat. 2010;123(3):627–35.

52. Sparano JA, Zhao F, Martino S, Ligibel JA, Perez EA, Saphner T, Wolff AC, Sledge GW Jr, Wood WC, Davidson NE. Long-term follow-up of the E1199 phase III trial evaluating the role of taxane and schedule in operable breast cancer. J Clin Oncol. 2015;33(21):2353–60.

53. Biganzoli E, Desmedt C, Fornili M, de Azambuja E, Cornez N, Ries F, Closon-Dejardin MT, Kerger J, Focan C, Di Leo A, et al. Recurrence dynamics of breast cancer according to baseline body mass index. Eur J Cancer. 2017;87:10–20.

54. Sceneay J, Chow MT, Chen A, Halse HM, Wong CS, Andrews DM, Sloan EK, Parker BS, Bowtell DD, Smyth MJ, et al. Primary tumor hypoxia recruits CD11b+/Ly6Cmed/Ly6G+ immune suppressor cells and compromises NK cell cytotoxicity in the premetastatic niche. Cancer Res. 2012;72(16):3906–11.

55. Cleary MP, Grossmann ME. Minireview: obesity and breast cancer: the estrogen connection. Endocrinology. 2009;150(6):2537–42.

56. Corvera S, Gealekman O. Adipose tissue angiogenesis: impact on obesity and type-2 diabetes. Biochim Biophys Acta. 2014;1842(3):463–72.

57. Bu L, Gao M, Qu S, Liu D. Intraperitoneal injection of clodronate liposomes eliminates visceral adipose macrophages and blocks high-fat diet-induced weight gain and development of insulin resistance. AAPS J. 2013;15(4): 1001–11.

58. Elgazar-Carmon V, Rudich A, Hadad N, Levy R. Neutrophils transiently infiltrate intra-abdominal fat early in the course of high-fat feeding. J Lipid Res. 2008;49(9):1894–903.

59. Talukdar S, Oh DY, Bandyopadhyay G, Li D, Xu J, McNelis J, Lu M, Li P, Yan Q, Zhu Y, et al. Neutrophils mediate insulin resistance in mice fed a high-fat diet through secreted elastase. Nat Med. 2012;18(9):1407–12.

8

The association of genomic lesions and PD-1/PD-L1 expression in resected triple-negative breast cancers

Michael T. Barrett[1]*(iD), Elizabeth Lenkiewicz[1], Smriti Malasi[1], Anamika Basu[1], Jennifer Holmes Yearley[2], Lakshmanan Annamalai[2], Ann E. McCullough[3], Heidi E. Kosiorek[1], Pooja Narang[4], Melissa A. Wilson Sayres[4], Meixuan Chen[5], Karen S. Anderson[5,6] and Barbara A. Pockaj[7]

Abstract

Background: Elevated PD-L1 expression on tumor cells, a context associated with an adaptive immune response, has been linked to the total burden of copy number variants (CNVs) in aneuploid tumors, to microsatellite instability (MSI), and to specific genomic driver lesions, including loss of *PTEN*, *MYC* amplification, and activating mutations in driver oncogenes such as *KRAS* and *PIK3CA*. Triple-negative breast cancers (TNBCs) typically have high levels of CNVs and diverse driver lesions in their genomes. Thus, there is significant interest in exploiting genomic data to develop predictive immunotherapy biomarkers for patients with TNBC.

Methods: Whole tissue samples from 55 resected TNBCs were screened by immunohistochemistry (IHC) for PD-1 and PD-L1 by using validated antibodies and established scoring methods for staining of tumor and non-tumor cells. In parallel, we interrogated biopsies from each resection with DNA content flow cytometry and sorted the nuclei of diploid, tetraploid, and aneuploid cell populations. CNVs were mapped with CNV oligonucleotide arrays by using purified (>95%) tumor populations. We generated whole exome data for 12 sorted tumor samples to increase the resolution within loci of interest and to incorporate somatic mutations into our genomic signatures.

Results and Conclusions: PD-L1 staining was detected on tumor cells in 29 out of 54 (54%) evaluable cases and was associated with increased overall survival ($P = 0.0024$). High levels of PD-1 and PD-L1 (IHC ≥ 4) were present in 11 out of 54 (20%) and 20 out of 54 (37%) cases with staining of PD-L1 primarily on tumor cells for 17 out of 20 (85%) cases. The latter included tumors with both high (>50) and low (<20) numbers of CNVs. Notably, homozygous deletion of *PTEN* ($n = 6$) or activating mutation in *PIK3CA* ($n = 1$) was not associated with increased expression of either immune checkpoint activator in TNBC. In contrast, two treatment-naïve cases with *EGFR* driver amplicons had high PD-L1 tumor staining. High mutational load and predicted neoepitopes were observed in MSI$^+$ and high CNV burden TNBCs but were not associated with high PD-L1 expression on tumor cells. Our results challenge current models of genomic-based immunotherapy signatures yet suggest that discrete genomic lesions may complement existing biomarkers to advance immune checkpoint therapies for patients with TNBC.

Keywords: PD-1, PD-L1, IHC, Flow sorting, Copy number, Somatic mutations, Triple-negative breast cancer

* Correspondence: barrett.michael@mayo.edu
[1]Division of Hematology and Medical Oncology, Mayo Clinic in Arizona, Scottsdale, AZ, USA
Full list of author information is available at the end of the article

Background

Multiple studies suggest that high levels of PD-L1 on tumor cell surfaces are associated with an adaptive immune resistance in the presence of active tumor-infiltrating lymphocytes (TILs) [1, 2]. Thus, this immunohistochemistry (IHC) staining pattern represents a candidate signature for those tumors that can be effectively targeted with checkpoint blockade. An emerging picture suggests that tumor-specific genomic lesions, either individually or in combination, are associated with immune checkpoint activation and the extent and duration of responses for patients to immunotherapy. These lesions include loss of tumor suppressor genes (*PTEN*), the activation of oncogenic drivers (*EGFR*, *KRAS*, and *PIK3CA*), BRCA mutant and BRCA-like homologous recombination-deficient (HRD) genomes, and high mutation burdens, including microsatellite instability (MSI), chromosomal instability (CIN), and aneuploidy [3–9]. The highly aberrant nature of triple-negative breast cancer (TNBC) genomes makes TNBC a highly favorable model to test genomic correlates of PD-1 and PD-L1 expression [10].

In this study, we interrogated a series of 55 well-annotated surgical resections from patients with TNBC with IHC for PD-1 and PD-L1 protein expression by using validated antibodies and established scoring methods that included PD-L1 staining intensities on tumor and non-tumor cells [11]. The expression patterns were correlated with clinical outcomes. We then assessed the associations of genomic lesions with expression of PD-1 and PD-L1 in each sample. We applied a systematic approach to rigorously interrogate the genomes of each TNBC sample. Tumor ploidy was initially measured with DNA content flow cytometry followed by sorting of the nuclei of distinct diploid, tetraploid, and aneuploid cell populations from each TNBC. Thus, rather than inferring ploidy on the basis of sequencing reads or single-nucleotide polymorphism (SNP) arrays, we used the direct measure of total DNA from our flow assays. The next level of analysis incorporated genome-wide copy number variant (CNV) measures with oligonucleotide arrays designed for CNV detection using purified (>95%) flow-sorted tumor populations. This enabled the discrimination and mapping of CNVs, including single copy losses and gains, focal amplifications, and homozygous deletions within each cancer genome. Finally, we generated whole exome data for flow-sorted tumor populations from a subset of samples ($n = 12$) to increase the resolution for loci of interest and to incorporate somatic mutations and predicted neoepitopes into our genomic signatures. This combined approach provides high-resolution measures of TNBC genomes from ploidy, whole chromosome and chromosome arm level CNVs, focal amplicons, breakpoints, and homozygous deletions to the level of gene-specific insertion/deletions (indels) and mutations. These data provide a unique opportunity to assess the presence of individual and different classes of genomic lesions and to determine their association with the extent of PD-1 and PD-L1 expression in TNBC.

Methods

Clinical samples

TNBC samples were obtained under a Mayo Clinic protocol 2130–00 Cancer Tissue Study (principal investigator: B. Pockaj). This study was approved by Mayo Clinic institutional review board protocol 08–006579-08 Breast Cancer Clinical Genomics Project. The samples included 23 formalin-fixed paraffin-embedded (FFPE) and 32 fresh frozen tissues available for genomic analyses. Estrogen receptor (ER) and progesterone receptor (PR) were evaluated by standard American Society of Clinical Oncology/College of American Pathologists (ASCO/CAP) guidelines, and less than 1% of the cells stained for the receptors [12]. HER2-negative was defined by ASCO/CAP guidelines as staining by IHC of 0 or 1+ [13]. HER2 IHC of 2+ was further evaluated by fluorescence *in situ* hybridization (FISH) and deemed negative by standard ASCO/CAP guidelines. All biopsies in this study were from surgically resected tissue. These include the neoadjuvant-treated patients. All patients gave informed consent for collection and use of the samples. All tumor samples were histopathologically evaluated prior to genomic analysis. All research conformed to the Helsinki Declaration (https://www.wma.net/policies-post/wma-declaration-of-helsinki-ethical-principles-for-medical-research-involving-human-subjects/).

Immunohistochemical staining

Whole tissue sections cut from FFPE tissue blocks were deparaffinized and rehydrated with serial passage through changes of xylene and graded ethanols. All slides were subjected to heat-induced epitope retrieval in Envision FLEX Target Retrieval Solution, High pH (Dako, Carpinteria, CA, USA). Endogenous peroxidase in tissues was blocked by incubation of slides in 3% hydrogen peroxide solution prior to incubation with primary antibody (anti-PD-L1, clone 22C3, Merck Research Laboratories, Palo Alto, CA, USA or anti-PD-1 clone NAT105, Cell Marque, Rocklin, CA, USA) for 60 min. Antigen-antibody binding was visualized via application of the FLEX+ polymer system (Dako) and application of 3, 3′ diaminobenzidine (DAB) chromogen (Dako). Stained slides were counterstained with hematoxylin and cover-slipped for review. For the scoring criteria, we used an established scoring system to report the PD-1 and PD-L1 expression levels in each sample [11]. Scoring of PD-1 and PD-L1 was conducted by a pathologist blinded to patient characteristics and clinical outcomes. A semi-quantitative 0–5 scoring system was applied:

negative: 0; rare: 1 = individuated positive cells or only very small focus within or directly adjacent to tumor tissue; low: 2 = infrequent small clusters of positive cells within or directly adjacent to tumor tissue; moderate: 3 = single large cluster, multiple smaller clusters, or moderately dense diffuse infiltration within or directly adjacent to tumor tissue; high: 4 = single very large dense cluster, multiple large clusters, or dense diffuse infiltration; and very high: 5 = coalescing clusters, dense infiltration throughout the tumor tissue. Evaluations were relativized to the size of the tumor sample.

Statistical analysis

Overall survival (OS) and disease-free survival (DFS) were estimated by using the Kaplan-Meier method, and differences were compared by using the log-rank test. Patients who were alive at the time of last follow-up were considered censored for OS, and patients without disease recurrence or death were considered censored for DFS. P values of less than 0.05 were considered statistically significant. Quantification of variance (Wilcoxon test) was performed for ploidy levels and CNV burden loads on tumors with high PD-1/PD-L1 expression versus tumors with low PD-1/PD-L1 expression. SAS version 9.4 (SAS Institute Inc., Cary, NC, USA) was used for analysis.

Flow cytometry

Excess paraffin was removed from each FFPE sample with a scalpel from either side of 40- to 60-μm scrolls and processed in accordance with our published methods [14, 15]. We used a single 50-μm scroll from each FFPE tissue block to obtain sufficient numbers of intact nuclei for subsequent sorting and molecular assays. Frozen tissue biopsies were minced in the presence of NST buffer and 4′,6-diamidino-2-phenylindole (DAPI) in accordance with published protocols [14, 16, 17]. Nuclei from each sample were disaggregated and filtered through a 40-μm mesh prior to flow sorting with an Influx cytometer (Becton Dickinson, San Jose, CA, USA) with ultraviolet excitation and DAPI emission collected at more than 450 nm. DNA content and cell cycle were analyzed by using the MultiCycle software program (Phoenix Flow Systems, San Diego, CA, USA).

Copy number analysis

DNAs from frozen tissue were treated with DNAse 1 prior to Klenow-based labeling. High-molecular-weight templates were digested for 30 min, whereas the smaller fragmented FFPE-derived DNA samples were digested for only 1 min. In each case, 1 μL of 10× DNase 1 reaction buffer and 2 μL of DNase 1 dilution buffer were added to 7 μL of DNA sample and incubated at room temperature and transferred to 70 °C for 30 min to deactivate DNase 1. Sample and reference templates were labeled with Cy-5 dUTP and Cy-3 dUTP, respectively, using a BioPrime labeling kit (Invitrogen, Carlsbad, CA, USA) in accordance with our published protocols [18]. All labeling reactions were assessed by using a Nanodrop assay (Nanodrop, Wilmington, DE, USA) prior to mixing and hybridization to Comparative Genomic Hybridization (CGH) arrays (Agilent Technologies, Santa Clara, CA, USA) for 40 h in a rotating 65 °C oven. All microarray slides were scanned by using an Agilent 2565C DNA scanner, and the images were analyzed with Agilent Feature Extraction version 11.0 using default settings. The array-based CGH (aCGH) data were assessed with a series of QC metrics and analyzed by using an aberration detection algorithm (ADM2) [19]. The latter identifies all aberrant intervals in a given sample with consistently high or low log ratios based on the statistical score derived from the average normalized log ratios of all probes in the genomic interval multiplied by the square root of the number of these probes. This score represents the deviation of the average of the normalized log ratios from its expected value of zero and is proportional to the height h (absolute average log ratio) of the genomic interval and to the square root of the number of probes in the interval. All aCGH data discussed in this publication have been deposited in the National Center for Biotechnology Information (NCBI) Gene Expression Omnibus (GEO) [20] and are accessible through GEO Series accession number GSE107764 (https://www.ncbi.nlm.nih.gov/geo/query/acc.cgi?acc=GSE107764).

Fluorescent in situ hybridization

Home-brew *JAK2* DNA (clones RP11-980 L14, RP11-927H16, and CTD-2506A8) labeled with SpectrumOrange dUTP (Abbott Molecular, Abbott Park, IL, USA/Vysis Products) and commercially available chromosome 9 centromere (SpectrumGreen) provided by Abbott Molecular were combined as one probe set. The enumeration probe set was applied to individual slides, hybridized, and washed in accordance with published protocols [21].

Whole exome sequencing

DNAs from each sorted tumor population and a patient-matched control sample were sequenced within the Mayo Clinic Medical Genome Facility (MGF) by using established protocols for whole exome analysis. Briefly, whole exon capture was carried out with Agilent's SureSelect Human All Exon 71 MB version 6 kit; 500 ng of the prepped library is incubated with whole exon biotinylated RNA capture baits supplied in the kit for 24 h at 65 °C. The captured DNA:RNA hybrids are recovered by using Dynabeads MyOne Streptavidin T1 (Thermo Fisher Scientific, Waltham, MA, USA). The DNA was eluted from the beads and desalted by using purified Ampure XP beads (Beckman Coulter Life Sciences, Indianapolis, IN, USA). The purified capture products were amplified by using the SureSelect Post-Capture Indexing forward and Index polymerase chain reaction (PCR) reverse primers (Agilent Technologies) for 12 cycles. Libraries were loaded onto paired-end flow cells at concentrations of 4–5 pM to generate cluster densities of 600,000–800,000/mm^2 by using the Illumina cBot and HiSeq Paired-end cluster kit version 3 (Illumina, San Diego, CA, USA). The flow cells are sequenced as 101×2 paired-end reads on an Illumina HiSeq 2500 or 4000 by using TruSeq SBS sequencing kit version 3 and HiSeq data collection version 1.4.8 software. Base-calling was performed by using Illumina's RTA version 1.12.4.2.

Variant calling and annotation

We started with aligned tumor and germline data (in bam format) for each patient. We used VarScan2 (version 2.3.9) [22] available on a high-performance cluster computing environment to call tumor-specific variants. We applied a minimum coverage of 10 reads in normal and tumor to call somatic variants, a minimum variant frequency of 0.08 to call a heterozygote, and a somatic P value of 0.05 as a threshold to call a somatic site. We further filtered the SNP calls to remove those near indel positions and also removed likely false positives associated with common sequencing- and alignment-related artifacts [23]. We used the variant effect predictor tool [24] with ensemble transcript versions for the hg19 reference genome to generate fasta sequences for a range of flanking amino acids (7, 8, 9, and 10 bp) on each side of the mutated amino acid to generate 15, 17, 19, and 21 amino acid sequences, respectively, to be used in the inference of neoepitopes (see below). We also annotated the variants functionally by using Annovar [25] with hg19 reference genome.

HLA typing

We used the POLYSOLVER (POLYmorphic loci reSOLVER) algorithm [26] to infer the HLA types present in each patient by using the germline (normal) whole exome sequencing data. The method employs a Bayesian classifier and selects and aligns putative HLA reads to an imputed library of full-length genomic library of HLA alleles. We included three major histocompatibility complex (MHC) class I (HLA-A, -B, and -C) genes for HLA typing.

Neoepitope generation and filtering

We generated all possible 8mers, 9mers, 10mers, and 11mers (neoepitopes), including the mutant amino acid, using a sliding window with the mutant amino acid at each possible position. To infer the binding of each

potential neoepitope to the patient-specific HLA alleles, we used the Immune Epitope Database (IEDB) prediction method from the IEDB [27] for all possible combinations of HLAs and neoepitopes. Our final set included only epitopes with a binding affinity (ann_ic50) of less than 500 nM for the patient-specific HLA alleles.

Results

In total, 55 TNBC cases were screened for PD-1 and PD-L1 expression by IHC (Additional file 1: Figure S1). One of these failed because of low tumor content in the tissue sample. Of the remaining 54 cases with IHC data, 39 were treatment-naïve at the time of resection. Biopsies from 48 of the 55 TNBCs were available for flow sorting. These included 32 of the 39 treatment-naïve cases. However, the biopsy for one case had only a single diploid population that was copy number–neutral. In addition, we sorted and obtained genomic data for the surgical samples of the 16 available cases that received neoadjuvant therapy. Fifteen of these 16 had corresponding IHC data. Thus, our final results include combined IHC tissue analyses and genomic data of flow-sorted tumor populations for 31 treatment-naïve and 15 treatment-positive TNBCs. In addition, we sequenced the exomes of flow-sorted tumor populations from six treatment-naïve and six treated cases and the transcriptomes of whole biopsies from three treatment-naïve and six treated cases with IHC and CNV profiles of interest.

PD-1 and PD-L1 expression patterns

There was a broad range of expression for both proteins in the 54 evaluable cases (Table 1). Eleven of 54 (20.0%) and 20 out of 54 (37%) of TNBCs had high (IHC score of 4) or very high (IHC score of 5) staining for PD-1 and PD-L1, respectively. The 11 cases with elevated expression of PD-1 had matching increases of PD-L1. Strikingly, PD-L1 expression in the 15 out of 20 (75%) cases with IHC scores of at least 4 was almost exclusively on the surfaces of tumor cells. In contrast, nine out of 54 (17%) and seven out of 54 (13%) TNBCs had negative (IHC score of 0) or rare (IHC score of 1) staining for

Table 1 PD-1 and PD-L1 expression in triple-negative cancer

IHC score	PD-1	PD-L1
Negative 0	0	3 (2)
Rare 1	9 (5)[a]	4 (2)
Low 2	17 (13)	15 (11)
Moderate 3	17 (12)	12 (9)
High 4	10 (8)	12 (7)
Very high 5	1 (1)	8 (8)

[a]Treatment-naïve cases
Abbreviation: *IHC* immunohistochemistry

PD-1 and PD-L1, respectively. The PD-L1 staining had a broader range compared with PD-1 with three negative cases in addition to the 20 cases with an IHC score of at least 4. Notably, 15 of these PD-L1 elevated expression cases, including the eight with a maximum IHC score of 5, were treatment-naïve. Despite the range of PD-L1 expression, there were no significant correlations with the level of expression on tumor or non-tumor cells and OS or PFS in our cohort. In contrast, the presence of any PD-L1 expression (IHC score of 1–5) on tumor cells was a significant correlate of OS (log-rank P value: 0.0024) and of DFS (log-rank P value: 0.0095) (Fig. 1).

Genomic lesions in resected TNBCs

Aneuploid peaks were detected and then sorted from 39 out of 48 (81%) available biopsies, providing pure tumor populations for genomic analyses (Additional file 2: Figure S2 and Additional file 3: Figure S3). In eight out of nine biopsies without an aneuploid peak, we sorted and subsequently confirmed tumor content in the $4N(G_2/M)$ fraction. The remaining sample was diploid only by flow cytometry and copy number–neutral by CNV analysis. Although the tumor ploidies varied from diploid to hypertetraploid, there was no association with high ($n = 17$) or low ($n = 6$) expression levels of PD-L1 (Wilcoxon rank-sum test, $P = 0.31$).

The DNAs from each sorted population of interest were interrogated with CGH arrays to confirm the tumor content and to provide a CNV profile of each tumor genome. We used the ADM2 step gram algorithm to distinguish aberrant copy number intervals and map their boundaries in each flow-sorted tumor population. There was extensive heterogeneity in the CNV profiles of the TNBC cases. The number of aberrant intervals varied from less than 10 to more than 80 in each TNBC genome. However, there

was no association with CNV burden and PD-L1 expression (Wilcoxon rank-sum test, $P = 0.92$). The intervals included whole chromosomes, chromosome arms, and interstitial aberrations in the TNBC genomes. Of significant interest were focal CNVs, including high-level amplicons and homozygous deletions that recurrently targeted oncogenic pathways associated with TNBCs. At least one focal amplicon defined by log_2 ratios of more than 1 and genomic boundaries of less than 10 Mb was identified in 43 out of 47 (91%) of the TNBC genomes. These included recurring focal amplicons targeting oncogenic drivers *EGFR* (5/47), *JAK2* (9/47), *AKT2* (3/47), *FGFR2* (3/47), and *MYC* (9/47) (Table 2). Amplified copies of *MYC* were present in 10 additional cases where the amplicon extended beyond 10 Mb, including six cases with whole 8q gains. The *JAK2* copy number status of our TNBC cohort, including both gains and losses of 9p24.1, was validated with a FISH assay (Additional file 4: Figure S4, Additional file 5: Figure S5, and Additional file 6: Figure S6) [28]. In addition, our use of pure flow-sorted samples revealed multiple homozygous deletions, ADM2-defined intervals with log_2 ratios of not more than −3.0, in these samples. These include deletions targeting known tumor suppressor genes (*CDKN2A*, *RB1*, *PTEN*, *ARID1B*, *JAK1*, and *BRIP1*) as well as unique targets (*EPS8*, *GRB10*, *EIF4G3*, *STK4*, and *RBM9*) in TNBC.

The combined IHC and genomic data were used to investigate associations between PD-1 and PD-L1 staining patterns and genomic aberrations of interest. These include gene and signaling pathway-specific lesions and measures of genomic instability across the genome. Of significant interest was the identification of recurring genomic lesions and profiles in those TNBCs with high levels of PD-L1 on the surface of tumor cells.

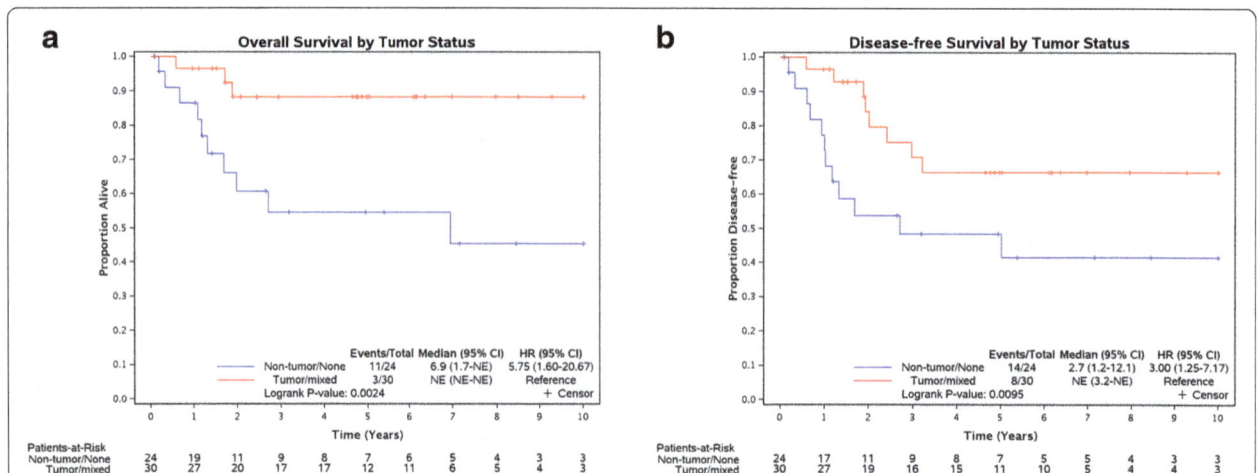

Fig. 1 Overall survival, disease-free survival, and expression of PD-L1. **a** Overall survival and (**b**) disease-free survival were estimated by using the Kaplan-Meier method and differences were compared using the log-rank test. Patients who were alive at the time of last follow-up were considered censored for overall survival. *P* values of less than 0.05 were considered statistically significant. SAS version 9.4 (SAS Institute Inc.) was used for analysis. Abbreviations: *CI* confidence interval, *HR* hazard ratio, *NE* not estimated

Table 2 Driver amplicons

Sample	MYC	EGFR	AKT2	FGFR2	JAK2
TNBC-2	+				
TNBC-4	+++++				++
TNBC-7	++			+++++	
TNBC-8	++				
TNBC-11	++				++++
TNBC-13			+++	++	
TNBC-16	++				
TNBC-17	+				
TNBC-18	++	++			+++
TNBC-19	++				
TNBC-20	++				
TNBC-23	++		++		
TNBC-27	++				
TNBC-29					+++
TNBC-30	++				
TNBC-36	++			++	
TNBC-39	+	++			
TNBC-43	++				++
TNBC-44		+++++			++
TNBC-47	+++				
TNBC-49			+++		++
TNBC-50		+++++			
TNBC-51	++				+
TNBC-53	++	++			++

+++++: log$_2$ ratio > 4
++++: log$_2$ ratio > 3
+++: log$_2$ ratio > 2
++: log$_2$ ratio > 1
+: log$_2$ ratio ≥ 1

CNVs and treatment-naïve TNBCs with increased PD-L1 expression

Whole genome CNV data were derived for 12 out of 15 treatment-naïve TNBCs with high (IHC score of 4) or very high (IHC score of 5) PD-L1 expression. The genomes of these TNBCs had a broad range of total number of CNVs, including focal amplicons targeting oncogenic drivers (Table 3). We focused on five of these treatment-naïve cases with combined IHC and CNV data to initially investigate the association of CNV burden and candidate driver amplicons with PD-L1 expression patterns (Fig. 2). One of the five cases had an aneuploid genome with a relatively simple CNV profile consisting of gain of chromosome 7, gain of chromosome 5p with an additional interstitial gain of p15.33-p15.32, a loss spanning 13q21.31-q22.2, and a homozygous deletion targeting CDKN2A (Fig. 2a). In contrast, two cases—one diploid and the other hypertetraploid by flow cytometry—had high-level (log$_2$ ratio >4.0) focal amplification of EGFR

with additional unique high-level focal amplicons targeting CDK6 and CCND1, and KIT and CCNE1, in each of the tumors (Fig. 2b). RNA-seq analysis of the latter case confirmed the high expression of EGFR, KIT, and CCNE1 with the presence of the corresponding high-level focal amplicons. The two additional treatment-naïve cases were aneuploid by flow cytometry and had extensive numbers of CNVs throughout their genomes (Fig. 2c). These included high-level amplicons targeting RUNX1 and YES1 oncogenes and a homozygous deletion of JMJD1C, a demethylase that regulates the BRCA1-mediated DNA damage response pathway [29].

CNVs and treatment-naïve TNBCs with reduced PD-L1 expression

Four of the seven TNBCs with negative (IHC score of 0) or rare (IHC score of 1) PD-L1 staining were treatment-naïve (Table 1). Two additional treatment-naïve cases with low (IHC score of 2) PD-L1 expression had a combined IHC score of only 3, suggesting low activity of the PD-1–mediated checkpoint. Genomic analysis of five of these six low-activity cases identified distinct CNVs, including focal amplicons targeting known oncogenes KRAS and JAK2 as well as homozygous deletions of variable sizes targeting tumor suppressor genes, including CDKN2A and PTEN (Fig. 3). However, there were no significant differences in the prevalence of these CNVs between TNBCs with low or high PD-L1 expression (Table 3).

DNA repair pathway lesions

There were 13 TNBCs with elevated numbers (>50) of intrachromosomal CNV aberrations often seen in BRCA mutant tumors. IHC data were obtained for 12 out of 13 of these cases. We identified DNA mutations or homozygous deletions in DNA repair pathway genes in nine out of 12 with IHC results (Table 4). Strikingly, one case had a homozygous deletion in MLH3 and another had a somatic MSH2^{F289C} mutation. Notably, the whole exome data of the MSH2 mutant case confirmed the MSI status of the tumor cells. However, both neoadjuvant-treated cases had low or moderate expression of PD-1 and PD-L1, the latter exclusive to the non-tumor cells. In seven additional high CNV burden cases with IHC data, we identified homozygous deletions of CHEK2, BRIP1, and DCLRE1C and mutations in BRCA1, FBXW7, PRKDC, and ALKBH5. Two of these—BRCA1^{mut} and PRKDC^{Q75R}—had high PD-L1 expression on the surface of tumor cells whereas the other three had rare or low expression on non-tumor cells. The genetic basis for elevated numbers of CNVs was not determined in three cases profiled by CGH only.

Table 3 Focal amplicons and PD-L1 expression

Sample	Ploidy	EGFR	JAK2	AKT2	MYC	FGFR2	PD-L1 (IHC)	Neoadjuvant
TNBC-6	4.0						5 T	–
TNBC-9	4.0						5 T	–
TNBC-14	3.1		+++		++		5 T	–
TNBC-21	2.8						5 T	–
TNBC-24	2.5						5 T	–
TNBC-33	3.6						5 T	–
TNBC-37	NB						5 T	–
TNBC-40	3.4						4 NT	–
TNBC-16	3.2				++		4 T	–
TNBC-23	3.6			++	++		4 T/NT	–
TNBC-44	4.1	+++++	++				4 T	–
TNBC-46	ND						4 T/NT	–
TNBC-50	2.0	+++++					4 T/NT	–
TNBC-55	3.0		++		++		4 NT	–
TNBC-5	3.0				++		4 T	+
TNBC-8	3.3				++		4 NT	+
TNBC-29	4.0		++				4 T	+
TNBC-36	2.0				++	++	4 T/NT	+
TNBC-43	3.2				+++		4 T/NT	+
TNBC-18	4.2	++	+++		++		1 NT	–
TNBC-30	3.1				++		1 NT	–
TNBC-4	3.2		++		+++++		1 NT	+
TNBC-7	3.8				++	+++++	1 NT	+
TNBC-51	3.5		++		++		0	+
TNBC-20	3.4				++		0	–
TNBC-56	ND						0	–

+++++: $\log_2$ ratio > 4
+++: $\log_2$ ratio > 2
++: $\log_2$ ratio > 1
Abbreviations: *IHC* immunohistochemistry, *NB* no tumor in biopsy, *ND* not done, *NT* non-tumor cells, *T* tumor cells

PTEN/PIK3CA

Homozygous deletions targeting *PTEN* were detected in six of the 46 (13%) cases profiled by CGH and IHC (Table 5, Fig. 4a). Three of these six were treatment-naïve TNBCs. We sequenced the exomes of 12 of the TNBCs, including 11 with intact *PTEN*, and detected an activating *PIK3CA*[H1047R] mutation in the aneuploid genome of another treatment-naïve tumor (Fig. 4b). Thus, in seven cases, the genomic results support an active AKT signaling context. The expression of PD-1 was rare or low in all seven cases while PD-L1 was low or moderate in six out of seven and high in one case. However, in all cases, the expression of PD-L1 was noted almost exclusively on non-tumor cells. This is in contrast to reports that loss of *PTEN* and activated AKT signaling upregulates PD-L1 and leads to its increased tumor cell surface expression in TNBC and other solid tissue tumors [30–32].

Mutation load and predicted neoepitopes

The number of non-conserved somatic mutations detected in the exomes of the 12 flow-sorted TNBCs ranged from 16 to 146 (Table 6). The number of predicted neoepitopes varied from 69 to 1368. Notably, MSI[+] TNBC-8 had an elevated number of non-conserved mutations and of predicted neoepitopes. Strikingly, TNBC-36 and TNBC-17, both microsatellite-stable (MSS) and *BRCA*[wt], had the highest mutation loads and numbers of predicted neoepitopes. We detected a 16-bp indel in DNA Cross Link Repair 1C (*DCLRE1C*) and a non-conserved *ALKBH5* mutation in these two cases. The former, also known as Artemis, plays an essential role in VDJ recombination and may mediate double-strand DNA repair, whereas *ALKBH5* is an RNA demethylase that has been implicated in direct DNA repair [33, 34]. However, PD-L1 staining was

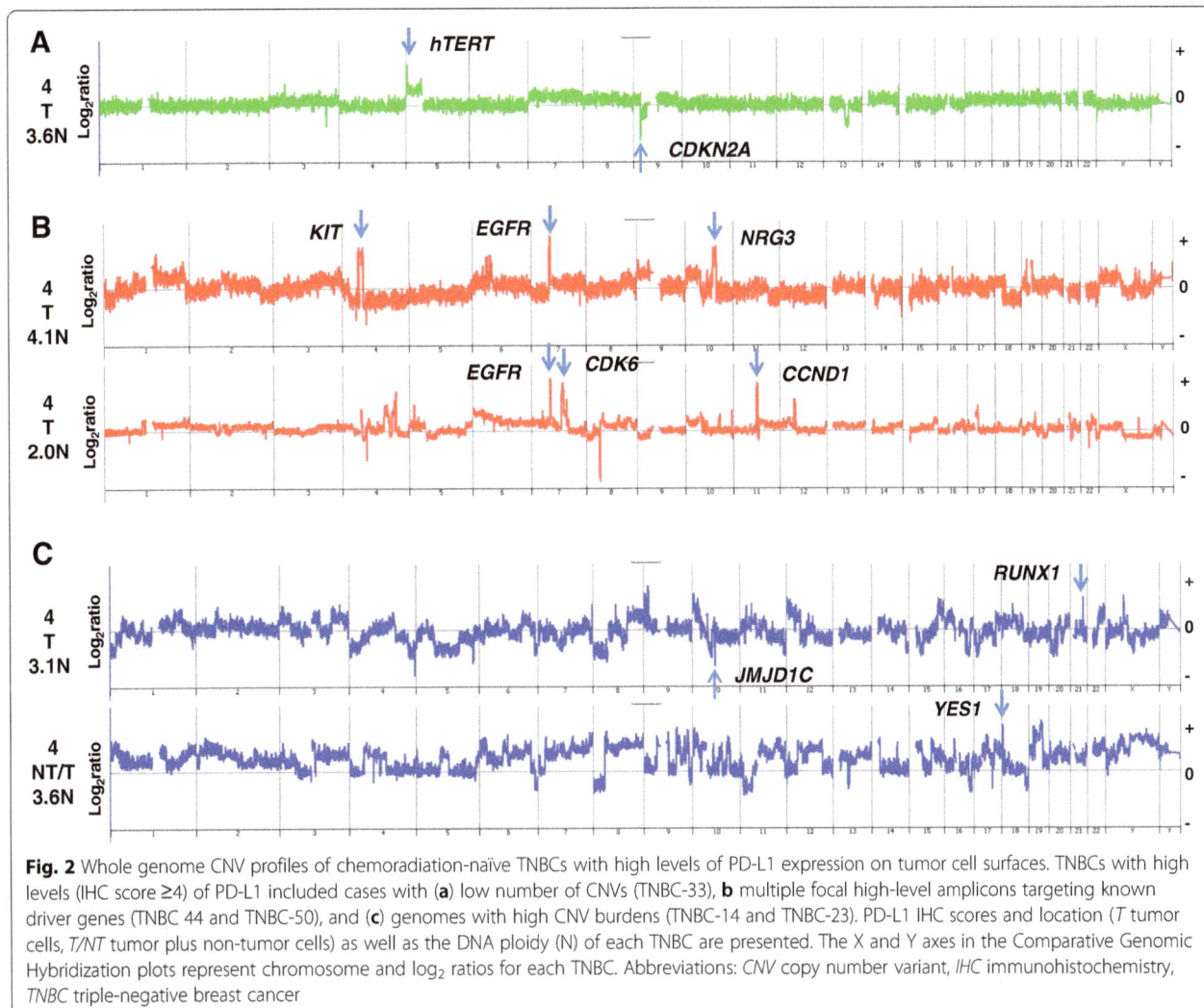

Fig. 2 Whole genome CNV profiles of chemoradiation-naïve TNBCs with high levels of PD-L1 expression on tumor cell surfaces. TNBCs with high levels (IHC score ≥4) of PD-L1 included cases with (**a**) low number of CNVs (TNBC-33), **b** multiple focal high-level amplicons targeting known driver genes (TNBC 44 and TNBC-50), and (**c**) genomes with high CNV burdens (TNBC-14 and TNBC-23). PD-L1 IHC scores and location (*T* tumor cells, *T/NT* tumor plus non-tumor cells) as well as the DNA ploidy (N) of each TNBC are presented. The X and Y axes in the Comparative Genomic Hybridization plots represent chromosome and log$_2$ ratios for each TNBC. Abbreviations: *CNV* copy number variant, *IHC* immunohistochemistry, *TNBC* triple-negative breast cancer

regionally high in TNBC-36 and low in treatment-naïve TNBC-17.

Discussion

The expression of PD-L1 on the surfaces of tumor cells has been used in clinical trials to identify and enrich for patients who will benefit from immunotherapy [35–37]. However, clinical benefit has also been seen in subsets of patients with low tumor cell PD-L1 expression [38]. The expression of PD-1 and PD-L1 can vary over time and within regions of tumors of interest. Thus, the timing of a biopsy relative to treatment and the extent of tissue and genomic heterogeneity within tumors may affect the sensitivity and specificity of IHC-based biomarkers. Furthermore, the multiple PD-1 and PD-L1 antibodies available for clinical studies and the variable scoring thresholds applied have limited the development of IHC-based prognostic assays.

Genomic-based biomarkers would provide an alternative or complementary approach to identify those patients who may benefit from or be refractory to emerging immunotherapies. Here, we used flow-sorted tumor samples from well-annotated surgically resected TNBCs for genomic analyses. We applied validated PD-1 and PD-L1 antibodies and a standardized IHC scoring system to characterize the expression patterns in these primary TNBCs, including 39 neoadjuvant treatment-naïve cases. There was a broad range of PD-1 and PD-L1 expression in our cohort with expression of PD-L1 noted exclusively on either tumor or non-tumor cells or on both within the tissue. However, our combination of IHC staining with genomic profiles of flow-sorted tumor populations in our cohort of surgically resected TNBCs represents a unique data set to test current hypotheses related to genomic lesions and signatures associated with expression of PD-1 and PD-L1.

Aneuploidy

Aneuploidy can be defined by a number of measures. DNA content flow cytometry discriminates differences

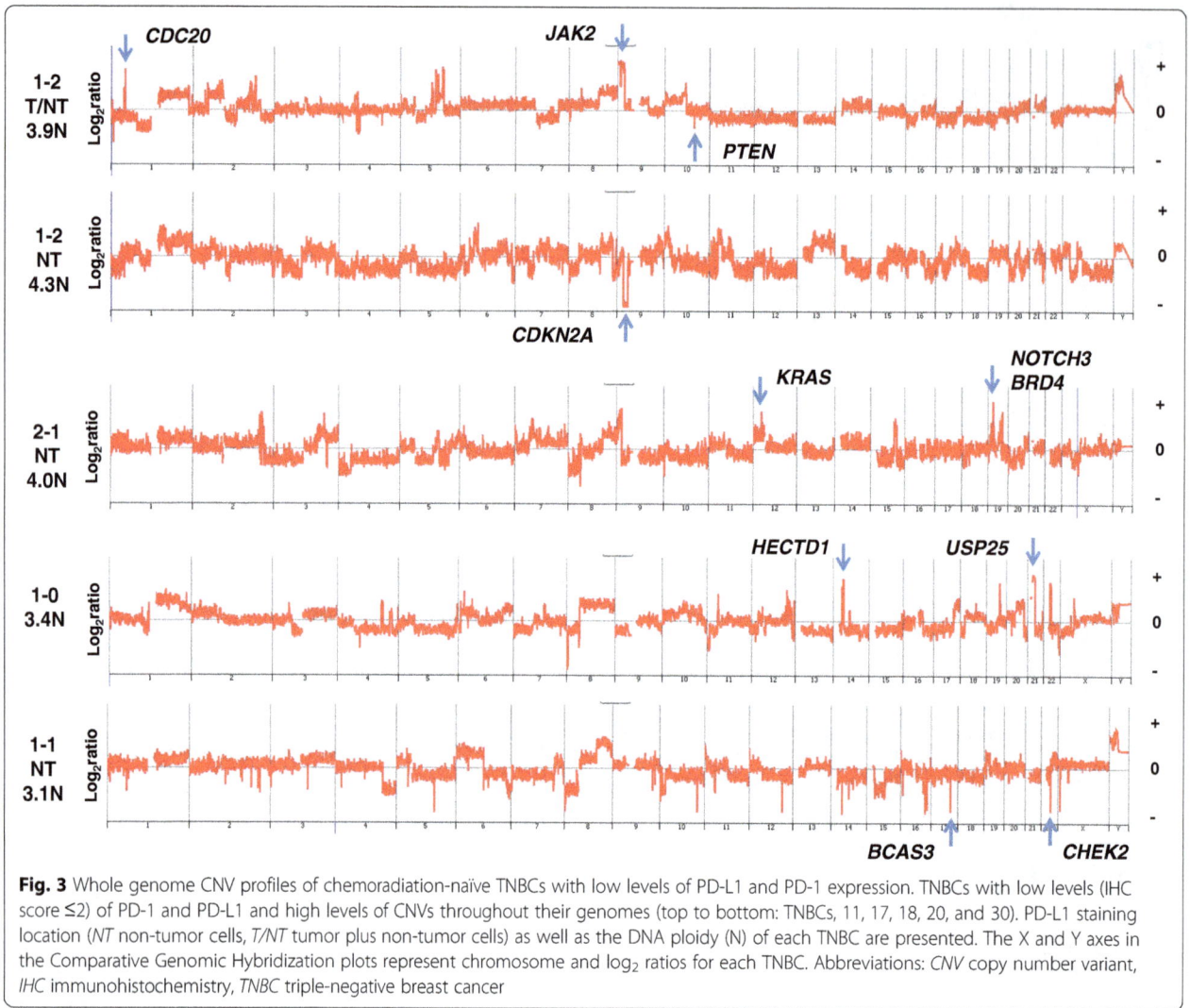

Fig. 3 Whole genome CNV profiles of chemoradiation-naïve TNBCs with low levels of PD-L1 and PD-1 expression. TNBCs with low levels (IHC score ≤2) of PD-1 and PD-L1 and high levels of CNVs throughout their genomes (top to bottom: TNBCs, 11, 17, 18, 20, and 30). PD-L1 staining location (*NT* non-tumor cells, *T/NT* tumor plus non-tumor cells) as well as the DNA ploidy (N) of each TNBC are presented. The X and Y axes in the Comparative Genomic Hybridization plots represent chromosome and log$_2$ ratios for each TNBC. Abbreviations: *CNV* copy number variant, *IHC* immunohistochemistry, *TNBC* triple-negative breast cancer

Table 4 Triple-negative breast cancers with high copy number variant burden[1]

Sample	Gene lesion	PD-1	PD-L1	Neoadjuvant
TNBC-8	MSH2^{F289C}	2	4 NT	+
TNBC-53	MLH3$^{-/-}$	3	3 NT	+
TNBC-30	CHEK2$^{-/-}$	1	1 NT	−
TNBC-31	BRIP1$^{-/-}$	3	2 NT	−
TNBC-24	BRCA^{mut}	4	5 T	−
TNBC-27	FBXW7^{S398F}	2	3 NT	+
TNBC-29	PRKDC^{Q75R}	2	4 T	+
TNBC-17	ALKBH5^{P303Q}	1	2 NT	−
TNBC-36	DCLRE1C$^{656\_671del16}$	3	4 T/NT	+
TNBC-54	TBD	2	2 T/NT	+
TNBC-51	TBD	1	0	+
TNBC-23	TBD	3	4 T/NT	−

[1]>50 intrachromosomal copy number variants
Abbreviations: *NT* non-tumor cells, *T* tumor cells, *TBD* to be determined, *TNBC* triple-negative breast cancer

in total DNA between tumor and coexisting non-tumor cells in samples of interest. Our DAPI-based flow cytometry assays have coefficients of variation (CVs) of 5–10%, allowing discrimination of nuclei with at least 2.2 N DNA content from diploid in solid tumor biopsies. The

Table 5 PD-1 and PD-L1 expression

TNBC	PD-1	PD-L1	Tumor/Non-tumor	PTEN/PIK3CA	Neoadjuvant
TNBC-1	2	2	T/NT	PTEN$^{-/-1}$	−
TNBC-8	2	3	NT	PTEN$^{-/-}$	+
TNBC-10	2	3	T/NT	PTEN$^{-/-}$	+
TNBC-11	1	2	T/NT	PTEN$^{-/-}$	−
TNBC-34	2	3	NT	PIK3CA^{H1047R}	−
TNBC-35	1	2	NT	PTEN$^{-/-}$	+
TNBC-55	2	4	NT	PTEN$^{-/-}$	−

[1]$^{-/-}$: Homozygous deletion
Abbreviations: *NT* non-tumor cells, *T* tumor cells, *TNBC* triple-negative breast cancer

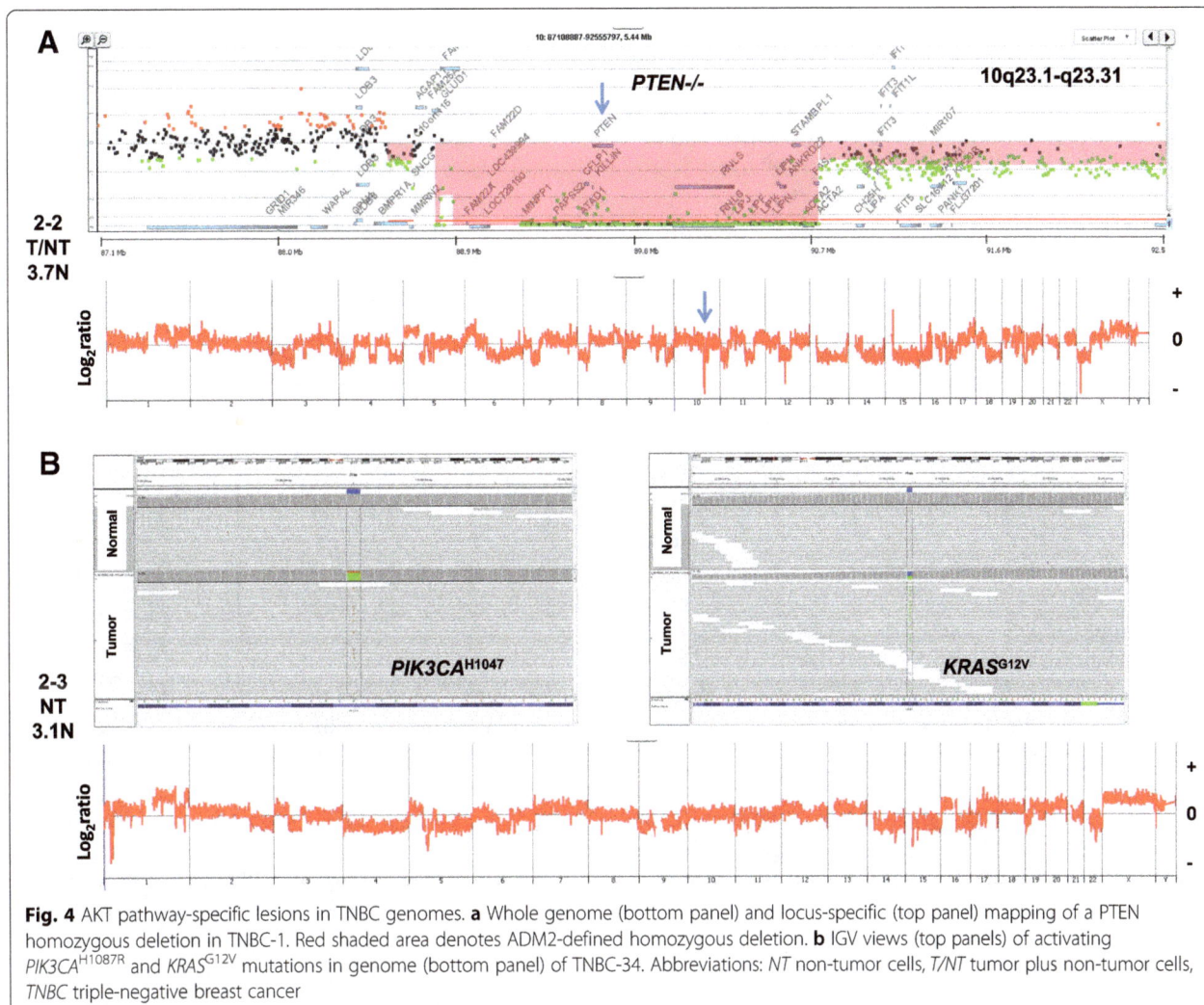

Fig. 4 AKT pathway-specific lesions in TNBC genomes. **a** Whole genome (bottom panel) and locus-specific (top panel) mapping of a PTEN homozygous deletion in TNBC-1. Red shaded area denotes ADM2-defined homozygous deletion. **b** IGV views (top panels) of activating *PIK3CA*[H1087R] and *KRAS*[G12V] mutations in genome (bottom panel) of TNBC-34. Abbreviations: *NT* non-tumor cells, *T/NT* tumor plus non-tumor cells, *TNBC* triple-negative breast cancer

Table 6 Mutation load and neoepitopes

TNBC case	Number of neoepitopes (ann < 500)	Non-synonymous mutations	Synonymous mutations	Stop gain	Stop loss
TNBC-27	129	23	19	1	0
TNBC-29	413	61	30	3	0
TNBC-44	388	50	45	5	0
TNBC-2	70	21	5	1	0
TNBC-49	69	54	54	0	0
TNBC-8	557	64	29	4	0
TNBC-25	148	16	9	0	0
TNBC-34	243	33	20	2	0
TNBC-38	187	26	25	4	0
TNBC-47	88	41	13	1	0
TNBC-36	1368	137	55	9	0
TNBC-17	1116	137	65	8	1

Abbreviation: *TNBC* triple-negative breast cancer

widths of the CVs for DNA content histograms can vary with the quality of biopsies notably with archived FFPE samples. This can affect the purity and yield of sorted tumor populations. However, careful placing of sorting gates can separate pure tumor and non-tumor populations even from suboptimal samples (Additional file 2: Figure S2 and Additional file 3: Figure S3). In contrast, cytogenetics assesses ploidy by the presence or absence of chromosomes with the resolution of a single chromosome. Thus, cells with only an extra copy of a smaller chromosome (e.g., chromosome 21), which may not be detected as a difference in total DNA in our flow cytometry assay, are classified as aneuploid by karyotype-based methods. Alternatively, tumors may contain multiple CNV regions and chromosome imbalances of gains and losses that result in an average "diploid by flow" DNA content. An additional method is to estimate DNA content from genomic data of bulk tumors [39]. Notably, recent reports of PD-1/PD-L1 checkpoint activation estimated tumor aneuploidy as the burden of whole chromosome and chromosome arm aberrations from whole exome sequencing data [6]. In total, 39 out of 48 (81%) evaluable TNBCs in our study were aneuploid by flow cytometry. The ploidies of these cases ranged from 2.3 N to 5.1 N. Eight of the remaining nine cases were sorted as diploid/tetraploid fractions and then confirmed to be aneuploid at the genome and chromosome level by CNV analysis. However, despite the range of ploidies and the variable numbers of chromosomal aberrations, we did not observe any correlation of tumor DNA content with IHC staining for either PD-1 or PD-L1.

CNVs

The use of flow-sorted tumor populations for CNV analysis enabled the identification of known driver lesions, including high-level focal amplicons targeting *EGFR*, *JAK2*, *AKT2*, *MYC*, and *FGFR2*, as well as homozygous deletions of both well-established *PTEN*, *CDKN2A*, *ARID1B*, *GRB10*, *BRIP1*, *JAK1*, and *RB1*, and unique *RBM9*, *CEBPG*, and *EIF4G3* TNBC tumor suppressor genes. The two treatment-naïve cases with the highest level ($\log_2$ ratio >4.0) focal EGFR amplicons had uniform high staining of PD-L1 on the tumor cell surfaces (Fig. 2). However, this pattern was not observed on three additional cases with moderate-level ($1.0 < \log_2$ ratio < 4.0) EGFR amplicons. Thus, the level of EGFR amplification and expression may need to exceed a threshold to elicit elevated PD-L1 levels. The two highly EGFR-amplified cases also contained high-level focal amplicons targeting other well-known oncogenic pathways (Fig. 2), suggesting that additional co-occurring genomic lesions may contribute to PD-L1 overexpression in TNBC tumor cells.

Multiple studies have interrogated clinical biopsies obtained before and after immunotherapy with the aim of identifying recurring genomic aberrations that correlate with response. Notably, loss of heterozygosity (LOH) of immune-responsive alleles has been reported to be associated with loss of clonal T cells in patients with non-small cell lung cancer who relapsed [40]. In addition, disruption of HLA alleles has been linked to loss of immunogenicity and poor outcomes [26, 41, 42]. The highly aneuploid nature of TNBCs at both the ploidy and chromosome level disrupts the ratio of alleles throughout the genome. Thus, LOH, which can be driven by ongoing genomic instability in aneuploid genomes, may have significant impact on immune signatures of TNBC. Additionally, a CRISPR screen identified a series of genes that are essential for effector function of CD8[+] T cells targeting melanoma cells [43]. We noted mutations and CNVs in multiple "hits" from this screen, including *MYO1B*, *VHL*, and *ARID2*, in our cohort. Of significant interest will be to apply our flow sorting–based genomic analyses to biopsies of relapsed TNBCs from immunotherapy trials.

PDJ amplicon

Copy number increases of the PD-L1 locus have been reported in a variety of tumors [44–47]. We and subsequently others have shown that a 9p24.1 amplicon targeting JAK2 and PD-L1 (PDJ amplicon) is enriched in TNBC [15, 48]. Notably, our study of flow-sorted tumor populations confirmed that this PDJ amplicon is present in chemoradiation-naïve resected cases and is associated with transcriptional upregulation of both genes [15]. However, the functional significance of PDJ amplification on immune regulation and response to checkpoint blockade is not known. There were three treatment-naïve TNBCs with a high-level ($\log_2$ ratio >2.0) 9p24.1 PDJ amplicon that included JAK2 and PD-L1 (Fig. 5) [15]. Only one of these three had a corresponding increase in PD-L1 on the tumor cell surface but with a striking difference in staining intensity between the undifferentiated regions of the tumor (IHC score of 5) and those that were differentiated (IHC score of 0). Expression of PD-L1 can be induced by interferon-gamma (IFN-γ) in multiple cell types, including TNBC [49, 50]. In our preliminary studies, we have observed that in TNBC cell lines with 9p24.1 copy number gain, PD-L1 expression was markedly and rapidly inducible by low-dose IFN-γ in a copy number–dependent manner, mimicking an *in situ* inflammatory response. Although RNA interference (RNAi)-mediated knockdown of JAK2 in TNBC cells did not affect constitutive PD-L1 expression, it did block IFN-γ–induced PD-L1 expression ([51] Chen et al., in press 2018). Notably, this was specific to cells with CNV gains of 9p24.1. Thus, the PDJ amplicon is associated with a dynamic IFN-inducible PD-L1 expression on tumor cells.

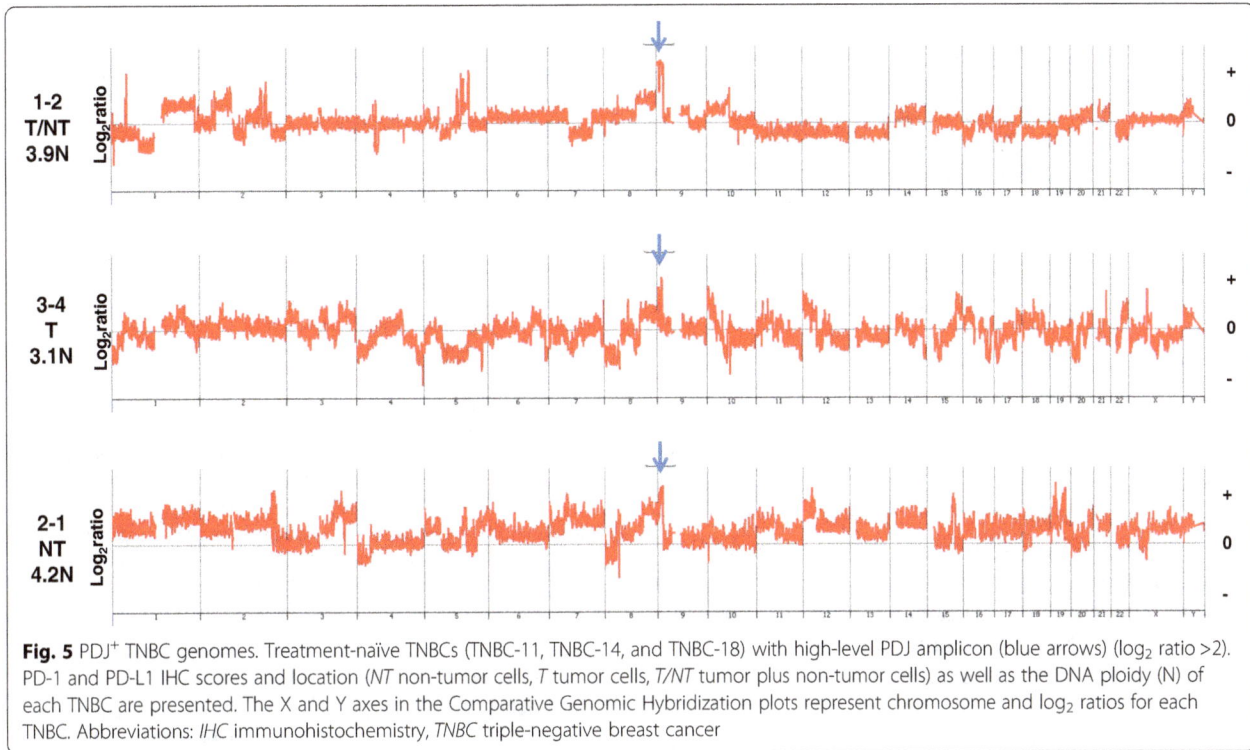

Fig. 5 PDJ⁺ TNBC genomes. Treatment-naïve TNBCs (TNBC-11, TNBC-14, and TNBC-18) with high-level PDJ amplicon (blue arrows) (log₂ ratio >2). PD-1 and PD-L1 IHC scores and location (*NT* non-tumor cells, *T* tumor cells, *T/NT* tumor plus non-tumor cells) as well as the DNA ploidy (N) of each TNBC are presented. The X and Y axes in the Comparative Genomic Hybridization plots represent chromosome and log₂ ratios for each TNBC. Abbreviations: *IHC* immunohistochemistry, *TNBC* triple-negative breast cancer

In contrast to JAK2 amplification, we also identified a 1.8-Mb homozygous deletion at 1p31.3 that included the *JAK1* locus in a post-neoadjuvant–treated case (Additional file 7: Figure S7). This TNBC had rare PD-1 expression in non-tumor cells and was negative for PD-L1 expression. Given the association of *JAK1* mutation and loss of the wild-type allele with an acquired resistance to PD-1 blockade in melanoma, this homozygous mutation may create the similar clinical context in TNBC [42, 52].

PTEN/PIK3CA
In addition to targeted amplification, homozygous deletions and somatic mutations may activate oncogenic signaling pathways. Notably, there were six cases with homozygous deletions within *PTEN* and a seventh with a common activating mutation of *PIK3CA* [53, 54]. The latter also had a $KRAS^{G12V}$ mutation (Fig. 4). Strikingly, all seven of these TNBCs lacked elevated expression of PD-L1 on tumor cell surfaces (Table 5). This is in contrast to studies of loss of *PTEN* and activation of PI3K-AKT signaling causing elevated expression of PD-L1 on the surface of most cancer cells within glioblastomas [31]. Furthermore, knockdown of *PTEN* in model systems has been reported to increase expression of PD-L1 and its appearance on the TNBC cell surface [30]. Thus, it has been hypothesized that targeting the PI3K signaling pathway in TNBC may provide additional benefit for patients treated with immunotherapy. However, our current data, which discriminate homozygous from partial *PTEN* copy number loss in flow-sorted tumors, suggest that further clinical studies applying precision genomics and well-annotated clinical samples are needed to define the role of PI3K-AKT signaling in the immune signatures and responses of TNBCs.

DNA repair lesions
Twelve of thirteen TNBC genomes with elevated numbers of interstitial CNVs, a context associated with DNA repair deficiencies, had matching IHC data (Table 1). One case had a pathogenic *BRCA1* mutation that was detected prior to surgery in a clinical laboratory. Three additional cases had homozygous deletions in genes with known roles in DNA repair pathways. We sequenced the exomes of five of the remaining seven TNBCs with this DNA repair deficiency signature to identify additional mediators of this clinical phenotype. Combined homozygous deletions and mutations accounted for 10 out of 13 TNBCs with this CNV signature. Strikingly, two cases also had lesions in mismatch repair genes, *MLH3* and *MSH2*. In the latter case, the MSI⁺ status was confirmed by whole exome next-generation sequencing. The expression of PD-L1 was exclusive to the non-tumor cells in both of these cases. Given the reports of striking responses of MSI⁺ tumors to anti-immune checkpoint therapy, additional studies are needed to determine the association of MSI status with PD-1 and PD-L1 expression in these highly aberrant TNBCs.

The mutation load varied across the 12 TNBCs whose exomes were sequenced. Strikingly, TNBC-36 and TNBC-17 had over twice as many mutations and predicted neoepitopes, 1368 and 1116, respectively, as MSI$^+$ TNBC-8 (Table 6). Both cases also had elevated CNV loads with mutations in *DCLRE1C* and *ALKBH5* (Additional file 8: Figure S8). Despite these shared genomic features, TNBC-36 had regionally high levels of PD-L1 expression on tumor cells while TNBC-17 had low PD-L1 expression on non-tumor cells.

Conclusions

PD-L1 expression on tumor cell surfaces correlated with improved OS and DFS in resected TNBCs. However, PD-L1 expression was highly variable in TNBCs even with genomic contexts such as MSI$^+$ and high CNV burden that are associated with clinical benefit from immune checkpoint inhibition. Therefore, given the complexity of TNBC genomes, simple correlations of genomic lesions with presence and levels of PD-1 and PD-L1 proteins may not provide robust predictive markers. For example, EGFR amplicons need to be well defined and placed in the context of other co-occurring aberrations. Thus, incomplete genomic and CNV profiles such as targeted panel sequences of bulk tumor samples may not provide the resolution needed to develop and validate solid tumor biomarkers for immunotherapies. Although larger studies are needed to fully develop our observations, there was a clear lack of association between pathogenic lesions targeting the PI3K-AKT pathway and increased expression of PD-L1 on tumor cell surfaces. Future studies will incorporate the location and the level of activity of tumor-infiltrating lymphocytes within TNBC tissues. In addition, T-cell receptor sequencing will prioritize tumor-specific neoepitopes identified in samples of interest. Our use of flow-sorted clinical samples will provide the resolution needed to resolve the association of genomic lesions with immune signatures and clinical responses for patients with TNBC.

Additional files

Additional file 1: Figure S1. Workflow and analyses of TNBC cohort. Fifty-five resections were screened for PD-1 and PD-L1 expression with IHC. Biopsies from 48 resections were flow-sorted and profiled for CNVs. Combined IHC and CNV data were obtained from 46 cases in this study. Abbreviations: *CNV* copy number variant, *IHC* immunohistochemistry, *TNBC* triple-negative breast cancer. (PPTX 74 kb)

Additional file 2: Figure S2. Flow-sorting formalin-fixed paraffin-embedded (FFPE) TNBC tissue samples. DNA content analysis of diploid and aneuploid populations flow-sorted from FFPE TNBC tissues. DNA content and cell cycle were analyzed by using the MultiCycle software program (Phoenix Flow Systems, San Diego, CA, USA). Abbreviation: *TNBC* triple-negative breast cancer. (PPTX 603 kb)

Additional file 3: Figure S3. Flow-sorting fresh frozen (FF) TNBC tissue samples. DNA content analysis of diploid and aneuploid populations flow-sorted from FF TNBC tissues. DNA content and cell cycle were analyzed by using the MultiCycle software program (Phoenix Flow Systems, San Diego, CA, USA). Abbreviation: *TNBC* triple-negative breast cancer. (PPTX 500 kb)

Additional file 4: Figure S4. FISH validation of high-level 9p24.1 amplicon. **A)** DNA content histogram of flow-sorted TNBC-11. **B)** Chromosome 9 Comparative Genomic Hybridization plot with high-level (log$_2$ ratio >4) gain of JAK2 locus (arrow) at 9p24.1. **C)** Multi-color FISH assay [5'JAK2[9p24](-green)/ 3'JAK2[9p24](red)/CEN 9(aqua)] image indicates more than 21 intact JAK2 signals and 1–3 CEN 9 signals. Abbreviations: *FISH* fluorescence *in situ* hybridization, *TNBC* triple-negative breast cancer. (PPTX 948 kb)

Additional file 5: Figure S5. FISH validation of 9p24.1 amplicon. **A)** DNA content histogram of flow-sorted TNBC-29. **B)** Chromosome 9 Comparative Genomic Hybridization plot with (log$_2$ ratio >1) gain of JAK2 locus (arrow) at 9p24.1. **C)** Multi-color FISH assay [5'JAK2[9p24](green)/ 3'JAK2[9p24](red)/CEN 9(aqua)] image indicates 3–5 intact JAK2 signals and 2–3 CEN 9 signals. Abbreviations: *FISH* fluorescence *in situ* hybridization, *TNBC* triple-negative breast cancer. (PPTX 776 kb)

Additional file 6: Figure S6. FISH validation of 9p24.1 copy number loss. **A)** DNA content histogram of flow-sorted TNBC-8. **B)** Chromosome 9 Comparative Genomic Hybridization plot with (log$_2$ ratio − 1) loss of JAK2 locus (arrow) at 9p24.1. **C)** Multi-color FISH assay [5'JAK2[9p24](-green)/ 3'JAK2[9p24](red)/CEN 9(aqua)] image indicates 0–2 intact JAK2 signals and 1–4 CEN 9 signals. Abbreviations: *FISH* fluorescence *in situ* hybridization, *TNBC* triple-negative breast cancer. (PPTX 700 kb)

Additional file 7: Figure S7. TNBC with JAK1 homozygous deletion. **A)** DNA content histogram of flow-sorted TNBC-51. **B)** Whole genome CNV profile of 3.5 N aneuploid TNBC-51 genome. **C)** Homozygous deletion at 1p31.3 includes the JAK1 locus. Red shaded area denotes ADM2-defined CNV interval. Abbreviations: *CNV* copy number variant, *TNBC* triple-negative breast cancer. (PPTX 226 kb)

Additional file 8: Figure S8. TNBCs with high mutation loads and predicted neoepitopes. **A, D)** DNA content histogram of flow-sorted TNBC-11 and TNBC-12. **B–E)** Whole genome CNV profiles of flow-sorted tumors. **C–F)** IGV view of DCLRE1C and ALKBH5 somatic mutations. PD-L1 staining and location (*NT* non-tumor cells, *T/NT* tumor plus non-tumor cells) are presented for each case. Abbreviations: *CNV* copy number variant, *TNBC* triple-negative breast cancer. (PPTX 196 kb)

Acknowledgments
We thank the Mayo Clinic Cancer Center for the use of the Cytogenetics Core, which provided FISH services. The Mayo Cytogenetics Core, including Sara Kloft-Nelson, Darlene Knutson and Ryan Knudson, and the director, Patricia T. Greipp, provided excellent technical support for our study of JAK2 CNVs. The Mayo Clinic Cancer Center is supported in part by an NCI Cancer Center Support Grant (5P30 CA15083-36).

Funding
This study was supported by funding from the non-profit Desert Mountain Member's CARE (Cancer Awareness through Research and Education) (Carefree, AZ, USA) and the BCRF (Breast Cancer Research Foundation) (New York, NY, USA).

Authors' contributions
EL and SM processed tissue samples for genomic analyses. AB, PN, MAWS, and MC analyzed CNV and sequencing data. JHY and LA performed and interpreted all IHC assays. HEK provided statistical analyses. AEM and BAP reviewed all TNBC samples and provided clinical annotation. MTB, KSA, and BAP wrote the manuscript. All authors read and approved the final manuscript.

Competing interests

JHY and LA are employees of Merck Research Laboratories. The other authors declare that they have no competing interests.

Author details

[1]Division of Hematology and Medical Oncology, Mayo Clinic in Arizona, Scottsdale, AZ, USA. [2]Merck Research Laboratories, Palo Alto, CA, USA. [3]Department of Pathology and Laboratory Medicine, Mayo Clinic in Arizona, Scottsdale, AZ, USA. [4]School of Life Sciences, Arizona State University, Tempe, AZ, USA. [5]Biodesign Institute, Arizona State University, Tempe, AZ, USA. [6]Division of Hematology and Medical Oncology, Mayo Clinic in Arizona, Phoenix, AZ, USA. [7]Division of General Surgery, Section of Surgical Oncology, Mayo Clinic in Arizona, Phoenix, AZ, USA.

References

1. Taube JM, Anders RA, Young GD, Xu H, Sharma R, TL MM, Chen S, Klein AP, Pardoll DM, Topalian SL, Chen L. Colocalization of inflammatory response with B7-h1 expression in human melanocytic lesions supports an adaptive resistance mechanism of immune escape. Sci Transl Med. 2012;4(127):127ra37.
2. Taube JM, Klein A, Brahmer JR, Xu H, Pan X, Kim JH, Chen L, Pardoll DM, Topalian SL, Anders RA. Association of PD-1, PD-1 ligands, and other features of the tumor immune microenvironment with response to anti-PD-1 therapy. Clin Cancer Res. 2014;20(19):5064–74.
3. Peng W, Chen JQ, Liu C, Malu S, Creasy C, Tetzlaff MT, Xu C, JA MK, Zhang C, Liang X, et al. Loss of PTEN promotes resistance to T cell-mediated immunotherapy. Cancer Discov. 2016;6(2):202–16.
4. Azuma K, Ota K, Kawahara A, Hattori S, Iwama E, Harada T, Matsumoto K, Takayama K, Takamori S, Kage M, et al. Association of PD-L1 overexpression with activating EGFR mutations in surgically resected nonsmall-cell lung cancer. Ann Oncol. 2014;25(10):1935–40.
5. Le DT UJN, Wang H, Bartlett BR, Kemberling H, Eyring AD, Skora AD, Luber BS, Azad NS, Laheru D, et al. PD-1 blockade in tumors with mismatch-repair deficiency. N Engl J Med. 2015;372(26):2509–20.
6. Davoli T, Uno H, Wooten EC, Elledge SJ. Tumor aneuploidy correlates with markers of immune evasion and with reduced response to immunotherapy. Science. 2017;355(6322):261–75.
7. Roh W, Chen PL, Reuben A, Spencer CN, Prieto PA, Miller JP, Gopalakrishnan V, Wang F, Cooper ZA, Reddy SM, et al. Integrated molecular analysis of tumor biopsies on sequential CTLA-4 and PD-1 blockade reveals markers of response and resistance. Sci Transl Med. 2017;9(379)
8. Topalian SL, Taube JM, Anders RA, Pardoll DM. Mechanism-driven biomarkers to guide immune checkpoint blockade in cancer therapy. Nat Rev Cancer. 2016;16(5):275–87.
9. Le DT DJN, Smith KN, Wang H, Bartlett BR, Aulakh LK, Lu S, Kemberling H, Wilt C, Luber BS, et al. Mismatch repair deficiency predicts response of solid tumors to PD-1 blockade. Science. 2017;357(6349):409–13.
10. Shah SP, Roth A, Goya R, Oloumi A, Ha G, Zhao Y, Turashvili G, Ding J, Tse K, Haffari G, et al. The clonal and mutational evolution spectrum of primary triple-negative breast cancers. Nature. 2012;486(7403):395–9.
11. Sabbatino F, Villani V, Yearley JH, Deshpande V, Cai L, Konstantinidis IT, Moon C, Nota S, Wang Y, Al-Sukaini A, et al. PD-L1 and HLA class I antigen expression and clinical course of the disease in intrahepatic cholangiocarcinoma. Clin Cancer Res. 2016;22(2):470–8.
12. Fitzgibbons PL, Murphy DA, Hammond ME, Allred DC, Valenstein PN. Recommendations for validating estrogen and progesterone receptor immunohistochemistry assays. Arch Pathol Lab Med. 2010;134(6):930–5.
13. Wolff AC, Hammond ME, Hicks DG, Dowsett M, LM MS, Allison KH, Allred DC, Bartlett JM, Bilous M, Fitzgibbons P, et al. Recommendations for human epidermal growth factor receptor 2 testing in breast cancer: American Society of Clinical Oncology/College of American Pathologists clinical practice guideline update. Arch Pathol Lab Med. 2014;138(2):241–56.
14. Holley T, Lenkiewicz E, Evers L, Tembe W, Ruiz C, Gsponer JR, Rentsch CA, Bubendorf L, Stapleton M, Amorese D, et al. Deep clonal profiling of formalin fixed paraffin embedded clinical samples. PLoS One. 2012;7(11):e50586.
15. Barrett MT, Anderson KS, Lenkiewicz E, Andreozzi M, Cunliffe HE, Klassen CL, Dueck AC, AE MC, Reddy SK, Ramanathan RK, et al. Genomic amplification of 9p24.1 targeting JAK2, PD-L1, and PD-L2 is enriched in high-risk triple negative breast cancer. Oncotarget. 2015;6(28):26483–93.
16. Rabinovitch PS, Longton G, Blount PL, Levine DS, Reid BJ. Predictors of progression in Barrett's esophagus III: baseline flow cytometric variables. Am J Gastroenterol. 2001;96(11):3071–83.
17. Barrett MT, Deiotte R, Lenkiewicz E, Malasi S, Holley T, Evers L, Posner RG, Jones T, Han H, Sausen M, et al. Clinical study of genomic drivers in pancreatic ductal adenocarcinoma. Br J Cancer. 2017;117(4):572–82.
18. Ruiz C, Lenkiewicz E, Evers L, Holley T, Robeson A, Kiefer J, Demeure MJ, Hollingsworth MA, Shen M, Prunkard D, et al. Advancing a clinically relevant perspective of the clonal nature of cancer. Proc Natl Acad Sci U S A. 2011;108(29):12054–9.
19. Lipson D, Aumann Y, Ben-Dor A, Linial N, Yakhini Z. Efficient calculation of interval scores for DNA copy number data analysis. J Comput Biol. 2006;13(2):215–28.
20. Edgar R, Domrachev M, Lash AE. Gene expression omnibus: NCBI gene expression and hybridization array data repository. Nucleic Acids Res. 2002;30(1):207–10.
21. Jenkins RB, Blair H, Ballman KV, Giannini C, Arusell RM, Law M, Flynn H, Passe S, Felten S, Brown PD, et al. A t(1;19)(q10;p10) mediates the combined deletions of 1p and 19q and predicts a better prognosis of patients with oligodendroglioma. Cancer Res. 2006;66(20):9852–61.
22. Koboldt DC, Zhang Q, Larson DE, Shen D, MD ML, Lin L, Miller CA, Mardis ER, Ding L, Wilson RK. VarScan 2: somatic mutation and copy number alteration discovery in cancer by exome sequencing. Genome Res. 2012;22(3):568–76.
23. Koboldt DC, Larson DE, Wilson RK. Using VarScan 2 for Germline Variant Calling and Somatic Mutation Detection. Curr Protoc Bioinformatics. 2013;44:15 4 1–17.
24. McLaren W, Gil L, Hunt SE, Riat HS, Ritchie GR, Thormann A, Flicek P, Cunningham F. The Ensembl variant effect predictor. Genome Biol. 2016;17(1):122.
25. Wang K, Li M, Hakonarson H. ANNOVAR: functional annotation of genetic variants from high-throughput sequencing data. Nucleic Acids Res. 2010;38(16):e164.
26. Shukla SA, Rooney MS, Rajasagi M, Tiao G, Dixon PM, Lawrence MS, Stevens J, Lane WJ, Dellagatta JL, Steelman S, et al. Comprehensive analysis of cancer-associated somatic mutations in class I HLA genes. Nat Biotechnol. 2015;33(11):1152–8.
27. Vita R, Zarebski L, Greenbaum JA, Emami H, Hoof I, Salimi N, Damle R, Sette A, Peters B. The immune epitope database 2.0. Nucleic Acids Res. 2010;38(Database issue):D854–62.
28. Chen M, Andreozzi M, Pockaj B, Barrett MT, Ocal IT, AE MC, Linnaus ME, Chang JM, Yearley JH, Annamalai L, et al. Development and validation of a novel clinical fluorescence in situ hybridization assay to detect JAK2 and PD-L1 amplification: a fluorescence in situ hybridization assay for JAK2 and PD-L1 amplification. Mod Pathol. 2017;30(11):1516–26.
29. Watanabe S, Watanabe K, Akimov V, Bartkova J, Blagoev B, Lukas J, Bartek J. JMJD1C demethylates MDC1 to regulate the RNF8 and BRCA1-mediated chromatin response to DNA breaks. Nat Struct Mol Biol. 2013;20(12):1425–33.
30. Mittendorf EA, Philips AV, Meric-Bernstam F, Qiao N, Wu Y, Harrington S, Su X, Wang Y, Gonzalez-Angulo AM, Akcakanat A, et al. PD-L1 expression in triple-negative breast cancer. Cancer Immunol Res. 2014;2(4):361–70.
31. Parsa AT, Waldron JS, Panner A, Crane CA, Parney IF, Barry JJ, Cachola KE, Murray JC, Tihan T, Jensen MC, et al. Loss of tumor suppressor PTEN function increases B7-H1 expression and immunoresistance in glioma. Nat Med. 2007;13(1):84–8.
32. Song M, Chen D, Lu B, Wang C, Zhang J, Huang L, Wang X, Timmons CL, Hu J, Liu B, et al. PTEN loss increases PD-L1 protein expression and affects the correlation between PD-L1 expression and clinical parameters in colorectal cancer. PLoS One. 2013;8(6):e65821.
33. Fedeles BI, Singh V, Delaney JC, Li D, Essigmann JM. The AlkB family of Fe(II)/alpha-ketoglutarate-dependent dioxygenases: repairing nucleic acid alkylation damage and beyond. J Biol Chem. 2015;290(34):20734–42.

34. Riballo E, Kühne M, Rief N, Doherty A, Smith GC, Recio MJ, Reis C, Dahm K, Fricke A, Krempler A, et al. A pathway of double-strand break rejoining dependent upon ATM, Artemis, and proteins locating to gamma-H2AX foci. Mol Cell. 2004;16(5):715–24.

35. Wolchok JD, Kluger H, Callahan MK, Postow MA, Rizvi NA, Lesokhin AM, Segal NH, Ariyan CE, Gordon RA, Reed K, et al. Nivolumab plus ipilimumab in advanced melanoma. N Engl J Med. 2013;369(2):122–33.

36. Topalian SL, Hodi FS, Brahmer JR, Gettinger SN, Smith DC, DF MD, Powderly JD, Carvajal RD, Sosman JA, Atkins MB, et al. Safety, activity, and immune correlates of anti-PD-1 antibody in cancer. N Engl J Med. 2012;366(26):2443–54.

37. Reck M, Rodríguez-Abreu D, Robinson AG, Hui R, Csőszi T, Fülöp A, Gottfried M, Peled N, Tafreshi A, Cuffe S, et al. Pembrolizumab versus chemotherapy for PD-L1-positive non-small-cell lung cancer. N Engl J Med. 2016;375(19):1823–33.

38. Antonia SJ, Villegas A, Daniel D, Vicente D, Murakami S, Hui R, Yokoi T, Chiappori A, Lee KH, de Wit M, et al. Durvalumab after Chemoradiotherapy in stage III non-small-cell lung Cancer. N Engl J Med. 2017;377(20):1919–29.

39. Andor N, Graham TA, Jansen M, Xia LC, Aktipis CA, Petritsch C, Ji HP, Maley CC. Pan-cancer analysis of the extent and consequences of intratumor heterogeneity. Nat Med. 2016;22(1):105–13.

40. Anagnostou V, Smith KN, Forde PM, Niknafs N, Bhattacharya R, White J, Zhang T, Adleff V, Phallen J, Wali N, et al. Evolution of Neoantigen landscape during immune checkpoint blockade in non-small cell lung Cancer. Cancer Discov. 2017;7(3):264–76.

41. Yeung JT, Hamilton RL, Ohnishi K, Ikeura M, Potter DM, Nikiforova MN, Ferrone S, Jakacki RI, Pollack IF, Okada H. LOH in the HLA class I region at 6p21 is associated with shorter survival in newly diagnosed adult glioblastoma. Clin Cancer Res. 2013;19(7):1816–26.

42. Zaretsky JM, Garcia-Diaz A, Shin DS, Escuin-Ordinas H, Hugo W, Hu-Lieskovan S, Torrejon DY, Abril-Rodriguez G, Sandoval S, Barthly L, et al. Mutations associated with acquired resistance to PD-1 blockade in melanoma. N Engl J Med. 2016;375(9):819–29.

43. Patel SJ, Sanjana NE, Kishton RJ, Eidizadeh A, Vodnala SK, Cam M, Gartner JJ, Jia L, Steinberg SM, Yamamoto TN, et al. Identification of essential genes for cancer immunotherapy. Nature. 2017;548(7669):537–42.

44. Comprehensive molecular characterization of gastric adenocarcinoma. Nature. 2014;513(7517):202–9. Cancer Genome Atlas Research Network.

45. Green MR, Monti S, Rodig SJ, Juszczynski P, Currie T, O'Donnell E, Chapuy B, Takeyama K, Neuberg D, Golub TR, et al. Integrative analysis reveals selective 9p24.1 amplification, increased PD-1 ligand expression, and further induction via JAK2 in nodular sclerosing Hodgkin lymphoma and primary mediastinal large B-cell lymphoma. Blood. 2010;116(17):3268–77.

46. Ikeda S, Okamoto T, Okano S, Umemoto Y, Tagawa T, Morodomi Y, Kohno M, Shimamatsu S, Kitahara H, Suzuki Y, et al. PD-L1 is upregulated by simultaneous amplification of the PD-L1 and JAK2 genes in non-small cell lung Cancer. J Thorac Oncol. 2016;11(1):62–71.

47. George J, Saito M, Tsuta K, Iwakawa R, Shiraishi K, Scheel AH, Uchida S, Watanabe SI, Nishikawa R, Noguchi M, et al. Genomic amplification of CD274 (PD-L1) in small-cell lung Cancer. Clin Cancer Res. 2017;23(5):1220–6.

48. Balko JM, Schwarz LJ, Luo N, Estrada MV, Giltnane JM, Dávila-González D, Wang K, Sánchez V, Dean PT, Combs SE, et al. Triple-negative breast cancers with amplification of JAK2 at the 9p24 locus demonstrate JAK2-specific dependence. Sci Transl Med. 2016;8(334):334ra53.

49. Soliman H, Khalil F, Antonia S. PD-L1 expression is increased in a subset of basal type breast cancer cells. PLoS One. 2014;9(2):e88557.

50. Mandai M, Hamanishi J, Abiko K, Matsumura N, Baba T, Konishi I. Dual faces of IFNgamma in Cancer progression: a role of PD-L1 induction in the determination of pro- and antitumor immunity. Clin Cancer Res. 2016;22(10):2329–34.

51. Chen M, Andreozzi M, Gonzalez-Malerva L, Eaton S, Pockaj B, Barrett MT and Anderson KS. JAK2 copy number and targeted JAK2 inhibition of TNBC cell lines. Cancer Res. 2016;76(4 Supplement):P5-04-19.

52. Shin DS, Zaretsky JM, Escuin-Ordinas H, Garcia-Diaz A, Hu-Lieskovan S, Kalbasi A, Grasso CS, Hugo W, Sandoval S, Torrejon DY, et al. Primary resistance to PD-1 blockade mediated by JAK1/2 mutations. Cancer Discov. 2017;7(2):188–201.

53. Saal LH, Holm K, Maurer M, Memeo L, Su T, Wang X, Yu JS, Malmström PO, Mansukhani M, Enoksson J, et al. PIK3CA mutations correlate with hormone receptors, node metastasis, and ERBB2, and are mutually exclusive with PTEN loss in human breast carcinoma. Cancer Res. 2005;65(7):2554–9.

54. Koren S, Reavie L, Couto JP, De Silva D, Stadler MB, Roloff T, Britschgi A, Eichlisberger T, Kohler H, Aina O, Cardiff RD, et al. PIK3CA(H1047R) induces multipotency and multi-lineage mammary tumours. Nature. 2015;525(7567):114–8.

Mucosal associated invariant T cells from human breast ducts mediate a Th17-skewed response to bacterially exposed breast carcinoma cells

Nicholas A. Zumwalde[1], Jill D. Haag[2], Michael N. Gould[2] and Jenny E. Gumperz[1]* ⓘ

Abstract

Background: Antimicrobial T cells play key roles in the disease progression of cancers arising in mucosal epithelial tissues, such as the colon. However, little is known about microbe-reactive T cells within human breast ducts and whether these impact breast carcinogenesis.

Methods: Epithelial ducts were isolated from primary human breast tissue samples, and the associated T lymphocytes were characterized using flow cytometric analysis. Functional assays were performed to determine T-cell cytokine secretion in response to bacterially treated human breast carcinoma cells.

Results: We show that human breast epithelial ducts contain mucosal associated invariant T (MAIT) cells, an innate T-cell population that recognizes specific bacterial metabolites presented by nonclassical MR1 antigen-presenting molecules. The MAIT cell population from breast ducts resembled that of peripheral blood in its innate lymphocyte phenotype (i.e., CD161, PLZF, and interleukin [IL]-18 receptor coexpression), but the breast duct MAIT cell population had a distinct T-cell receptor Vβ use profile and was markedly enriched for IL-17-producing cells compared with blood MAIT cells. Breast carcinoma cells that had been exposed to *Escherichia coli* activated MAIT cells in an MR1-dependent manner. However, whereas phorbol 12-myristate 13-acetate/ionomycin stimulation induced the production of both interferon-γ and IL-17 by breast duct MAIT cells, bacterially exposed breast carcinoma cells elicited a strongly IL-17-biased response. Breast carcinoma cells also showed upregulated expression of natural killer group 2 member D (NKG2D) ligands compared with primary breast epithelial cells, and the NKG2D receptor contributed to MAIT cell activation by the carcinoma cells.

Conclusions: These results demonstrate that MAIT cells from human breast ducts mediate a selective T-helper 17 cell response to human breast carcinoma cells that were exposed to *E. coli*. Thus, cues from the breast microbiome and the expression of stress-associated ligands by neoplastic breast duct epithelial cells may shape MAIT cell responses during breast carcinogenesis.

Keywords: Mucosal associated invariant T (MAIT) cells, Breast duct, Breast carcinoma, Microbe-reactive human T cells, NKG2D ligands, Th17 response

* Correspondence: jegumperz@wisc.edu
[1]Department of Medical Microbiology and Immunology, University of Wisconsin School of Medicine and Public Health, Madison, WI, USA
Full list of author information is available at the end of the article

Background

Most breast cancers initially arise in the epithelial ducts [1]. Although epithelial surfaces of the gastrointestinal and urogenital tracts are well known to be colonized by intricate microbial communities, it has only recently become clear that the breast ducts also contain a complex microbiota [2–8]. Because T cells that are specific for microbial antigens are now known to play key roles in the progression of tumors arising in epithelial layers of the intestine [9], the observation that the breast ducts contain microbial colonists raises the question whether antimicrobial T cells may also contribute, either positively or negatively, to the genesis of breast cancers. Consistent with this possibility, the presence of cancerous tissue has been found to be associated with alterations to the microbiome of the local breast tissue [8]. Hence, dysbiosis of the breast duct microbiome might lead to increased or altered T-cell activation. A central obstacle to assessing the role of microbe-specific T cells in breast cancer is that little is known about the T-cell compartment found within human breast ducts, and particularly, the presence of T cells that recognize microbial antigens has not yet been established.

We recently investigated the intraepithelial lymphocyte (IEL) compartment from isolated human breast epithelial duct organoids and observed that it includes T cells with $V\alpha7.2^+$ T-cell receptors (TCRs) [10]. TCR use of the $V\alpha7.2$ segment (T-cell receptor alpha variables 1 and 2 [TRAV1–2]) is one of the central characteristics of a distinctive subset called *mucosal associated invariant T cells* (MAIT cells) [11]. MAIT cells are innate T cells that recognize specific microbially synthesized precursors of riboflavin as antigens presented by the nonclassical antigen-presenting molecule MR1 [12, 13] and are thus microbially reactive T cells. They typically coexpress CD161, promyelocytic leukemia zinc finger protein (PLZF), and interleukin (IL)-18Rα and can be readily detected using MR1 tetramers loaded with 5-(2-oxopropylideneamino)-6-D-ribitylaminouracil (5RU) [12, 14–16]. MAIT cells are comparatively abundant in human peripheral blood, typically comprising 0.5–10% of the T-cell population [16]. MAIT cells have also been detected in a variety of other tissues, including liver, lung, kidney, intestine, female genital tract, prostate, and ovary [14, 17–22]. MAIT cells from blood mainly produce interferon (IFN)-γ and tumor necrosis factor (TNF)-α upon activation, and they efficiently mediate cytolytic responses [23]. In contrast, compared with those from the blood, MAIT cells from the female genital tract expressed higher levels of T-helper 17 cell (Th17) cytokines (IL-17A and IL-22) and lower levels of Th1 cytokines (IFN-γ and TNF-α) in response to *Escherichia coli* [20]. Thus, MAIT cells from distinct anatomical locations may have important functional differences.

Intriguingly, recent studies suggest that MAIT cells may play a role in the etiology of colon adenocarcinomas. MAIT cells were found to accumulate at tumor sites in patients with colon cancer, and the tumor-associated MAIT cells produced lower levels of IFN-γ than those obtained from healthy intestinal tissue from the same donor [24]. In another study, circulating MAIT cells from patients with colorectal cancer were found to have reduced expression of IFN-γ and TNF-α and elevated levels of IL-17A compared with MAIT cells from the blood of healthy control subjects [25]. It is not yet clear whether the apparent Th17 bias of tumor-associated and blood MAIT cells observed in patients with colon cancer is due to a functional skewing that occurs in the context of malignancy or whether it is a result of the expansion of a MAIT cell subset that is normally present only within select mucosal epithelial sites. Similarly, the role of microbial stimulation and/or dysbiosis in the MAIT cell response during colon cancer is as yet unknown. Nevertheless, the observation that Th17-biased MAIT cells are recruited to the sites of colon adenocarcinomas raises the possibility that these T cells also play a role in breast carcinomas. Therefore, in this analysis, we sought to investigate the phenotypes and functional characteristics of breast epithelium-derived MAIT cells, as well as to determine the ability of microbially exposed breast carcinoma cells to elicit responses from human MAIT cells.

Methods

Breast tissue acquisition and preparation

Noncancerous breast tissue from reduction mammoplasties or prophylactic mastectomies was obtained from the Cooperative Human Tissue Network (a National Cancer Institute-supported resource) or from the UW Translational Science BioCore-BioBank, in accordance with an institutional review board (IRB)-approved protocol. Human breast epithelial organoids were isolated as previously described [10]. Briefly, breast tissue was minced and digested overnight in a 37 °C shaker with 1× collagenase/hyaluronidase in Complete EpiCult B Human Media (STEMCELL Technologies, Vancouver, BC, Canada) supplemented with 5% FBS (HyClone; GE Healthcare Bio-Sciences, Pittsburgh, PA, USA). After incubation, digested tissue was spun for ≤ 1 minute at 80–100 × g to produce a pellet enriched for epithelial ductal organoids. The pellet was washed, and organoids were collected on a 40-μm filter. Organoids were cryopreserved in 50% FBS/6% dimethyl sulfoxide and stored in liquid nitrogen. Single-cell suspensions from organoids were prepared for all experiments by trypsinizing the organoids using 2-3 ml of 0.1% ethylenediaminetetraacetic acid (EDTA)/trypsin solution (diluted in PBS from 0.5%; Life Technologies, Carlsbad, CA, USA) for ≥ 3 - minutes. EDTA/trypsin reaction was quenched using serum-containing media and spun. Pellets were resuspended and filtered using 40–70-μm filters. Cells were spun, supernatants discarded, and breast organoid-derived cells resuspended for experimentation.

Peripheral blood mononuclear cell isolation

Peripheral blood mononuclear cells (PBMCs) were isolated from healthy donors according to an IRB-approved protocol. Written informed consent was obtained from all donors. PBMCs were isolated from blood using Ficoll-Paque PLUS (GE Healthcare Bio-Sciences) as previously described [10].

Flow cytometric analyses

For surface stains, cells were washed with PBS, blocked with 20% human AB serum (Atlanta Biologicals, Flowery Branch, GA, USA) for 15 minutes, stained with fluorochrome-conjugated antibodies for 30 minutes at 4 °C, washed, resuspended in PBS, and analyzed by flow cytometry (BD LSR II cytometer; BD Biosciences, San Jose, CA, USA) with FlowJo analysis software (version 9.3.1; FlowJo, Ashland, OR, USA). MR1 tetramers (5RU and 6FP provided by National Institutes of Health, Bethesda, MD, USA) were used at a 1:100 final dilution. In general, optimal staining was seen when tetramers were stained for 40 minutes in the dark at room temperature prior to surface staining. Intracellular cytokine staining was performed according to the manufacturer's recommendations using the BD Cytofix/Cytoperm kit in the presence of BD GolgiStop or BD GolgiPlug protein transport inhibitors (BD Biosciences). PLZF staining was performed with the BD Cytofix/Cytoperm kit.

The following fluorochrome-conjugated flow cytometry antibodies were used for analysis: CD45 (clone HI30), CD3 (OKT3), Vα7.2 (3C10), CD161 (HP-3G10), IL-18Rα (H44), TNF-α (Mab11), IFN-γ (4S.B3), IL-17A (BL168), natural killer group 2 member D (NKG2D) (1D11), CD31 (WM59), epithelial cell adhesion molecule (9C4), CD49f (GoH3), major histocompatibility complex class I-related chains A and B (MICA/B) (6D4), CD56 (HCD56), MR1 (26.5), and NKp46 (9E2) (all from BioLegend, San Diego, CA, USA); Vβ2 (MPB2D5), Vβ8 (56C5.2), Vβ13.1 (IMMU 222), Vβ13.2 (H132), and Vβ13.6 (JU74.3) (all from Beckman Coulter Life Sciences, Indianapolis, IN, USA); UL16-binding protein 1 (ULBP1) (170818), ULBP2/5/6 (165903), ULBP3 (166510), ULBP4 (709116), immunoglobulin G2A (IgG2A) (20102), and IgG2B (133303) (R&D Systems, Minneapolis, MN, USA); and PLZF (R17-809; BD Pharmingen, San Diego, CA, USA).

Short-term in vitro expansion of MAIT cells

Single-cell suspensions prepared from breast duct organoids or freshly isolated PBMCs were stained using 5RU-loaded MR1 tetramer and antibodies against CD45,

CD3, Vα7.2 TCR, and CD161. MAIT cells (1–1000 cells/well) were sorted into 96-well round-bottomed plates. Irradiated PBMCs were added at a density of 1×10^5 cells/well in T-cell medium (RPMI 1640, 15% heat-inactivated bovine calf serum, 3% human AB serum, 1% penicillin/streptomycin [P/S], 200 U/ml recombinant human IL-2) containing 5 μg/ml phytohemagglutinin (PHA; Sigma-Aldrich, St. Louis, MO, USA), and the cultures were maintained at 37 °C in a humidified incubator with 5% CO_2. If necessary, the cells were restimulated after 4–6 weeks to induce another round of proliferation by adding irradiated PBMCs in T-cell medium containing 5 μg/ml PHA. The MAIT cell composition of the expanded cells was assessed by flow cytometry after ~ 8 weeks of in vitro expansion using 5RU-loaded MR1 tetramer staining, and lines that were comprised of ≥ 95% MAIT cells were used for functional analyses.

Phorbol 12-myristate 13-acetate and ionomycin stimulation

Cells were washed and resuspended in culture medium (RPMI 1640, 15% HI-BCS, 3% human AB serum, 1% P/S) containing a final concentration of 50 ng/ml phorbol 12-myristate 13-acetate (PMA) (Sigma-Aldrich) and 500 ng/ml ionomycin (Sigma-Aldrich) in the presence of monensin or brefeldin A (BD Biosciences). The cells were stimulated for ~ 6 hours at 37 °C. Unstimulated control cells were incubated in parallel in culture medium alone. Because we observed that effector cytokine production decreased as cell density increased (data not shown), we used a maximum density of 2.5×10^5 cells/well for stimulation. After stimulation, cells were harvested and prepared for flow cytometry.

Breast carcinoma cells and bacterial exposure

The breast carcinoma cell line MDA-MB-231 was obtained from the American Type Culture Collection (Manassas, VA, USA) as an authenticated cell line and maintained in DMEM/F-12 medium (Corning, Corning, NY, USA) supplemented with 10% HI-BCS or 10% FBS and 1% P/S; Mediatech, Manassas, VA, USA). To prepare carcinoma cells for functional assays, the carcinoma cells were plated at a subconfluent density in flat-bottomed tissue culture plates and allowed to adhere for ~ 3 hours at 37 °C. E. coli strain K12 was cultured in Luria-Bertani (LB) broth in a 37 °C shaker overnight and then stored frozen in 40% glycerol/LB broth. Aliquots were thawed prior to use, and E. coli was washed in PBS three times. Bacteria were fixed in 1% formalin for 3 minutes, then washed three times with PBS and resuspended in the DMEM/F-12 medium used to culture the tumor cells. Carcinoma cells were exposed to E. coli overnight at a multiplicity of infection of 400–500 or incubated in medium alone (mock). The wells were then washed with PBS, and fresh DMEM culture medium containing 10% serum and 1% P/S was added.

Enrichment of primary MAIT cells from PBMCs
We performed a magnetic sorting step to remove potential MR1$^+$ antigen-presenting cell (APC) types (e.g., monocytes, B cells, dendritic cells) from PBMC samples prior to using them to test the responses of primary MAIT cells to MDA-MB-231 cells as APCs. CD161$^+$ cells were positively selected using indirect magnetic bead separation (Miltenyi Biotec, Bergisch Gladbach, Germany). The PBMCs were incubated first with an anti-CD161-phycoerythrin (PE) antibody and then with anti-PE microbeads, followed by passage over a Miltenyi Biotec LS column. Purity of the resulting cell preparations was assessed by flow cytometric analysis, as shown in Additional file 1: Figure S4.

Functional assays
Cell preparations containing primary MAIT cells (CD161$^+$ PBMCs or breast epithelial organoid cells) or in vitro-expanded MAIT cultures were added to wells containing *E. coli*-exposed or mock-treated MDA-MB-231 breast carcinoma cells. CD161$^+$ PBMCs and in vitro-expanded MAIT cells were added at a 1:1 ratio to breast carcinoma cells, whereas the breast epithelial organoid cells (which are composed of both IELs and epithelial cells) were added at a 3:1 ratio. Where indicated, the following blocking antibodies were added to the cocultures: 20 μg/ml anti-MR1 (clone 26.5; BioLegend) or 5 μg/ml anti-NKG2D (1D11; BioLegend). The carcinoma and effector cells were coincubated at 37 °C for ~ 18 hours, then monensin (GolgiStop) or brefeldin A (GolgiPlug) was added to all cultures, and the cells were coincubated for an additional 6 hours. After ~ 24 hours of coincubation, the effector cells were resuspended using cold EDTA (500 mM) in PBS, washed, and analyzed by flow cytometry.

Statistical analysis
To assess statistical significance, samples from different tissues (e.g., PBMC vs. breast duct organoids) were analyzed using a Mann-Whitney U test. Different populations of cells within the same sample (e.g., MAIT cells vs. non-MAIT cells from breast duct organoid preparations) were evaluated using a Wilcoxon matched pairs analysis. Where indicated, a two-tailed, one-sample t test was used to assess whether individual treatment groups showed a significant difference compared with a hypothetical value of 100%.

Results
Identification of MAIT cells in human breast epithelium
Breast tissue was obtained from human subjects who had undergone reduction mammoplasty or prophylactic mastectomy, and these tissues were subjected to a purification protocol that was optimized to isolate tissue fragments representing ductal organoids [10]. Purified ductal organoids were trypsinized to yield single-cell suspensions, and flow cytometric analysis was performed to identify T cells expressing Vα7.2 (Fig. 1a, left panel). Analysis of breast tissue samples from 16 unrelated donors revealed that the percentage of Vα7.2$^+$ T cells varied over more than a 10-fold range, but the mean was nearly identical to that for Vα7.2$^+$ T cells from blood of control donors (Fig. 1a, right panel). We next investigated staining by MR1 tetramers loaded with the 5RU antigen. For both PBMC and breast tissue samples, nearly 100% of the events stained by the MR1-5RU tetramer were positive for Vα7.2 (Fig. 1b, left panel). Neither PBMC nor breast duct organoid samples showed more than a marginal amount of staining using an MR1 tetramer loaded with a compound (6FP) that has been shown to have little or no antigenicity for MAIT cells (Additional file 2: Figure S1) [12, 26]. Surprisingly, whereas MR1-5RU tetramer-positive cells typically comprised at least half of the Vα7.2$^+$ T cells in PBMCs, only a minority of the Vα7.2$^+$ T cells from breast organoids were positively stained by the MR1-5RU tetramer (Fig. 1b, right panel). Nearly all of the Vα7.2$^+$ MR1-5RU tetramer-positive cells from the breast duct were positive for CD161, and they also coexpressed IL-18Rα and PLZF (Fig. 1c). Together, these results establish that a population of Vα7.2$^+$ T cells is present in human breast ducts that can be classified as MAIT cells, in that they bind MR1 molecules loaded with the 5RU antigen and coexpress CD161, IL-18Rα, and PLZF.

In contrast, the Vα7.2$^+$ but MR1-5RU tetramer-negative population did not coexpress CD161, IL-18Rα, or PLZF (Additional file 3: Figure S2A), suggesting that they are not innate T lymphocytes. It remains unclear whether these Vα7.2$^+$ T cells that are not stained by the MR1-5RU tetramer are simply not MR1-restricted T cells or whether they are MR1-restricted but fail to bind the 5RU-loaded tetramer because they recognize structurally distinct antigens. Notably, however, whereas most peripheral blood T cells are negative for CD69 and CD103 (αE integrin), nearly all of the T cells from breast duct (including both the MR1-5RU tetramer-positive and tetramer-negative populations) showed uniformly positive expression of CD69, and a large fraction coexpressed CD103 (Additional file 3: Figure S2B). Thus, the T cells associated with our breast duct organoid preparations had a phenotype similar to

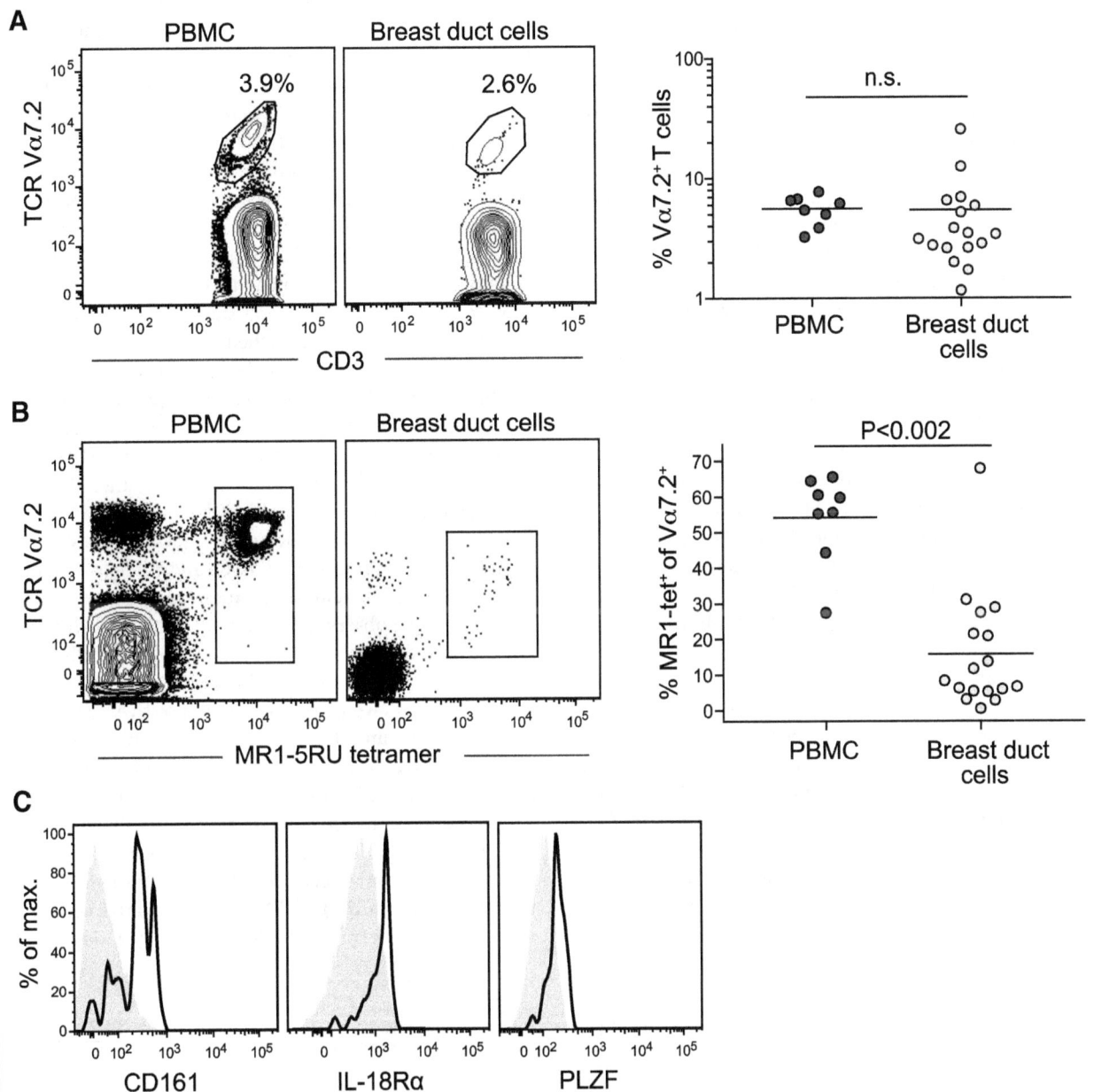

Fig. 1 Detection of mucosal associated invariant T cells from human breast ducts. **a** Left plots: Staining for Vα7.2 T-cell receptor TCR expression by T cells from peripheral blood (peripheral blood mononuclear cells [PBMCs]) or human breast ducts. Right plot: Quantification of Vα7.2⁺ T-cell frequencies in PBMCs vs. breast duct tissue. PBMCs and breast tissue samples were not obtained from the same donors. **b** Left plots: Costaining of CD3⁺ cells from blood vs. breast ducts by anti-Vα7.2 antibody and 5-(2-oxopropylideneamino)-6-ᴅ-ribitylaminouracil (5RU)-loaded MR1 tetramer. Right plot: Quantification of the fraction of the Vα7.2⁺ T cells costained by the MR1-5RU tetramer for PBMCs vs. breast duct cells. **c** Flow cytometric analysis of CD161, interleukin (IL)-18Rα, and promyelocytic leukemia zinc finger protein (PLZF) staining for the subset of breast duct T cells that costain for Vα7.2 and MR1-5RU tetramer (*black line histogram*) compared with Vα7.2-negative T cells from the breast (*gray filled histogram*). *n.s.* Not significant

tissue-resident memory T-cell populations that have recently been described [27].

TCR Vβ use

Although the TCR α-chain sequences of MAIT cells are highly constrained (Vα7.2 paired with a limited set of Jα segments), their TCR β-chains are much more diverse and use a variety of different Vβ segments [22, 28, 29]. It has recently been shown that the specific TCR Vβ segments used by MAIT cells can influence their responsiveness to different bacterial species [30]. Because the microbial species encountered by breast duct MAIT cells likely differ at least in part from those encountered by MAIT cells circulating in blood, we investigated TCR Vβ use. Prior studies have established that the majority of MAIT cells in human blood express either Vβ2 or Vβ13.2, and MAIT cells with these Vβ chains are highly responsive to *E. coli* [30]. We found that, on average, less than 20% of the breast duct MR1-5RU tetramer-positive T cells expressed either of these two Vβ chains (Fig. 2a and b), and the frequency of breast duct MAIT cells expressing Vβ2 or Vβ13.2 appeared significantly lower than that for blood MAIT cells from a group of sex-matched control donors (Fig. 2b).

Conversely, MAIT cells using Vβ8, Vβ13.1, or Vβ13.6, which together made up only a minor fraction of the MAIT cells in blood, were previously found to have lower levels of responsiveness to *E. coli* [30]. There was little or no detectable expression of these Vβ segments by MAIT cells from most of the breast tissue samples we tested, although they appeared to be expanded in a few of the samples (Fig. 2b). Based on the low representation in the breast duct MAIT population of Vβ2 or Vβ13.2 TCRs, which are typically highly represented in the blood MAIT population, these results suggest that the breast duct MAIT cell population may have antigen specificity differences compared with those from blood.

Cytokine production

We next compared the cytokine production profile of breast duct MAIT cells with those in PBMC samples. Total breast duct cells or PBMCs were stimulated with PMA and ionomycin, then stained them with MR1-5RU tetramer and anti-CD3 to detect MAIT cells and fixed, permeabilized, and stained them for expression of TNF-α, IFN-γ, and IL-17A. As also previously observed by others [20], blood MAIT cells produced almost exclusively IFN-γ and TNF-α (Fig. 3a, left panels). In contrast, the breast

duct MAIT cells included cells producing TNF-α, IFN-γ, and IL-17A (Fig. 3a, right panels). Although the production of TNF-α and IFN-γ was not statistically different between MAIT cells from breast duct or blood, IL-17-producing MAIT cells were significantly enriched in breast duct compared with blood (Fig. 3b). Moreover, comparison of cytokine production by breast duct MAIT cells vs. the non-MAIT cells present in the breast duct organoid samples demonstrated significantly higher IL-17 production by the MAIT cell subset (Fig. 3c). These results demonstrate that, similar to what has recently been reported for the female genital tract [20], the breast duct MAIT cell population is enriched for IL-17 producers.

Costaining for IL-17A and IFN-γ indicated that most of the breast duct MAIT cells were single producers of these cytokines (data not shown). To further investigate, we generated short-term in vitro expansions of MAIT cells derived from breast ducts or blood. Five lines that each contained at least 95% MAIT cells as assessed by MR1 tetramer staining were selected for further analysis (two MAIT lines from breast duct tissue and three from blood). Using PMA/ionomycin stimulation to activate cytokine production, we observed that one of the breast duct lines (B11) showed mainly IL-17A single-positive cells (59%), along with 7.4% that were double-positive for IL-17/IFN-γ and 12% that were IFN-γ single-positive. The other breast-derived line (C12) showed mainly IL-17/IFN-γ double-positive cells (82%), along with 9% IL-17A single-positive cells and only very few (2.6%) IFN-γ single-positive cells. In contrast, two of the PBMC-derived MAIT lines (B12 and C4) contained nearly exclusively IFN-γ single-positive cells, whereas the third (F12) contained a majority (57%) of IFN-γ single-positive cells along with 39% that coexpressed IFN-γ and IL-17A (Fig. 3d and

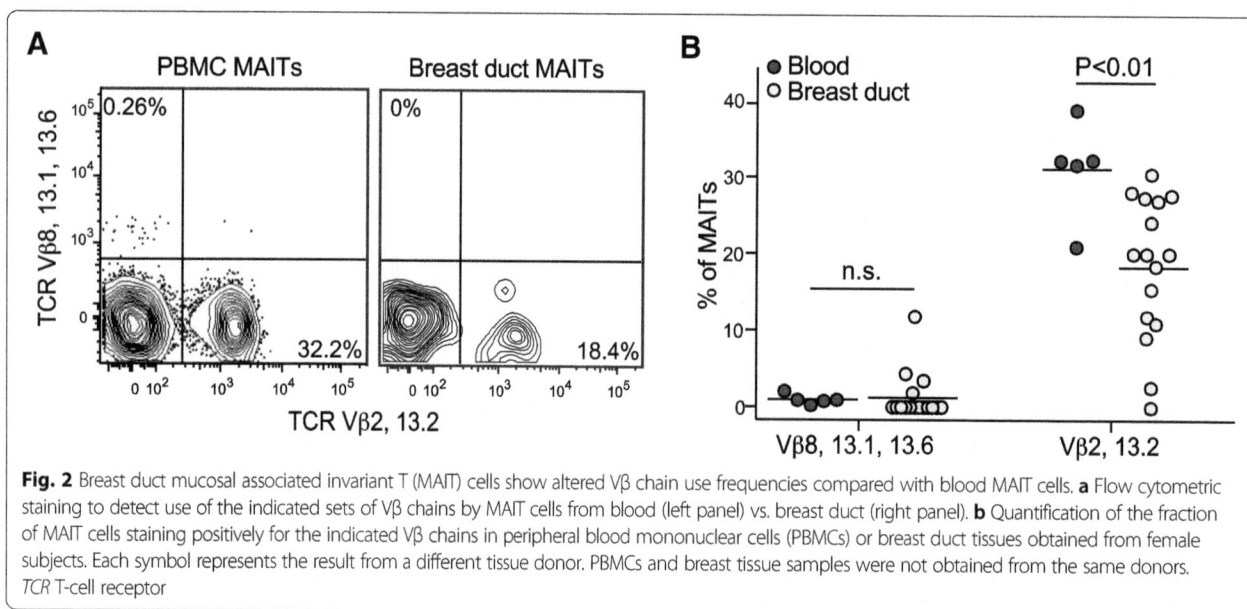

Fig. 2 Breast duct mucosal associated invariant T (MAIT) cells show altered Vβ chain use frequencies compared with blood MAIT cells. **a** Flow cytometric staining to detect use of the indicated sets of Vβ chains by MAIT cells from blood (left panel) vs. breast duct (right panel). **b** Quantification of the fraction of MAIT cells staining positively for the indicated Vβ chains in peripheral blood mononuclear cells (PBMCs) or breast duct tissues obtained from female subjects. Each symbol represents the result from a different tissue donor. PBMCs and breast tissue samples were not obtained from the same donors. *TCR* T-cell receptor

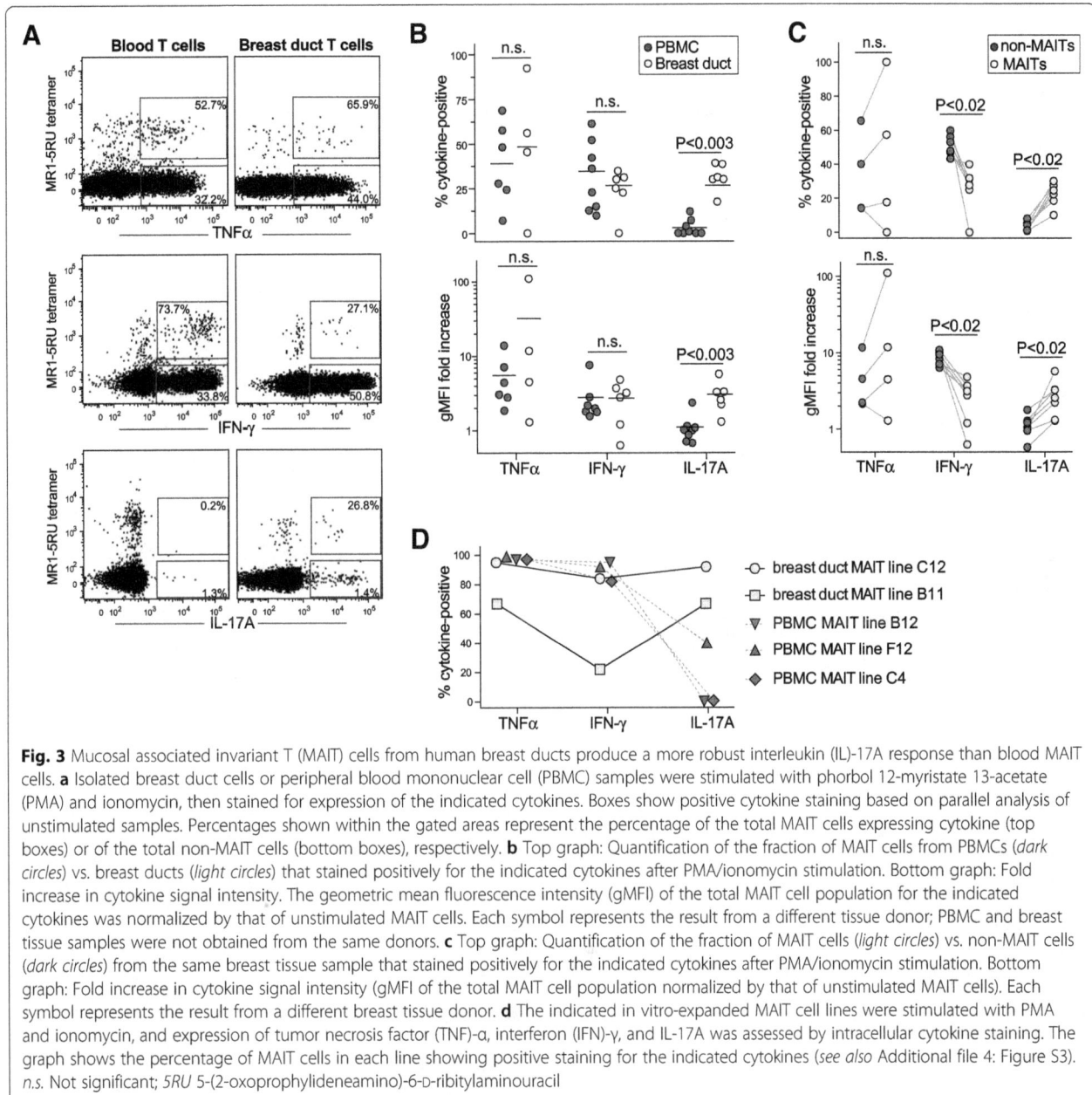

Fig. 3 Mucosal associated invariant T (MAIT) cells from human breast ducts produce a more robust interleukin (IL)-17A response than blood MAIT cells. **a** Isolated breast duct cells or peripheral blood mononuclear cell (PBMC) samples were stimulated with phorbol 12-myristate 13-acetate (PMA) and ionomycin, then stained for expression of the indicated cytokines. Boxes show positive cytokine staining based on parallel analysis of unstimulated samples. Percentages shown within the gated areas represent the percentage of the total MAIT cells expressing cytokine (top boxes) or of the total non-MAIT cells (bottom boxes), respectively. **b** Top graph: Quantification of the fraction of MAIT cells from PBMCs (*dark circles*) vs. breast ducts (*light circles*) that stained positively for the indicated cytokines after PMA/ionomycin stimulation. Bottom graph: Fold increase in cytokine signal intensity. The geometric mean fluorescence intensity (gMFI) of the total MAIT cell population for the indicated cytokines was normalized by that of unstimulated MAIT cells. Each symbol represents the result from a different tissue donor; PBMC and breast tissue samples were not obtained from the same donors. **c** Top graph: Quantification of the fraction of MAIT cells (*light circles*) vs. non-MAIT cells (*dark circles*) from the same breast tissue sample that stained positively for the indicated cytokines after PMA/ionomycin stimulation. Bottom graph: Fold increase in cytokine signal intensity (gMFI of the total MAIT cell population normalized by that of unstimulated MAIT cells). Each symbol represents the result from a different breast tissue donor. **d** The indicated in vitro-expanded MAIT cell lines were stimulated with PMA and ionomycin, and expression of tumor necrosis factor (TNF)-α, interferon (IFN)-γ, and IL-17A was assessed by intracellular cytokine staining. The graph shows the percentage of MAIT cells in each line showing positive staining for the indicated cytokines (*see also* Additional file 4: Figure S3). *n.s.* Not significant; *5RU* 5-(2-oxoprophylideneamino)-6-ᴅ-ribitylaminouracil

Additional file 4: Figure S3). These results suggest that MAIT cells which are stably polarized toward a Th17 phenotype are present in the breast duct compartment. Additionally, some of the breast duct MAIT cells may be Th1-polarized, and some may maintain plasticity in the ability to produce IFN-γ and IL-17.

Activation of MAIT cells by breast carcinoma cells

We next investigated the ability of human breast carcinoma cells to activate MAIT cells in an MR1-dependent manner. Prior researchers have observed MR1 gene expression by a variety of different cell types, including neoplastic cells of epithelial origin, such as HeLa cells (cervical carcinoma) and A549 (lung carcinoma) [31, 32]. However, it has typically been difficult to detect cell surface expression of endogenous MR1 molecules by flow cytometry, likely because antigen binding is strictly required for export of MR1 molecules to the cell surface and because MR1 expression at the cell surface is highly transient [33, 34]. We therefore used intracellular flow cytometric staining to confirm that the human breast carcinoma cell line MDA-MB-231 endogenously expresses the MR1 antigen-presenting molecule (Fig. 4a).

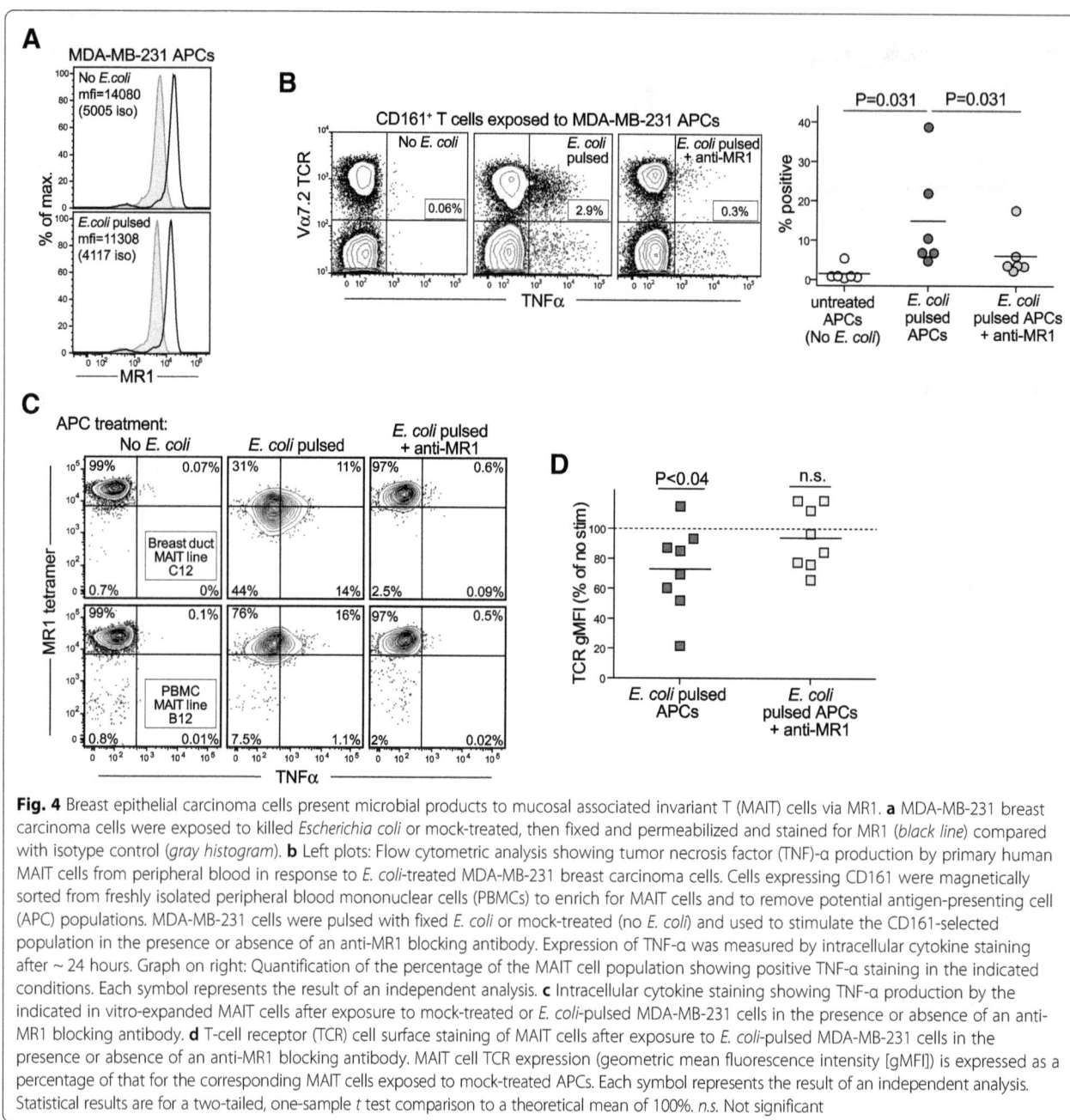

Fig. 4 Breast epithelial carcinoma cells present microbial products to mucosal associated invariant T (MAIT) cells via MR1. **a** MDA-MB-231 breast carcinoma cells were exposed to killed *Escherichia coli* or mock-treated, then fixed and permeabilized and stained for MR1 (*black line*) compared with isotype control (*gray histogram*). **b** Left plots: Flow cytometric analysis showing tumor necrosis factor (TNF)-α production by primary human MAIT cells from peripheral blood in response to *E. coli*-treated MDA-MB-231 breast carcinoma cells. Cells expressing CD161 were magnetically sorted from freshly isolated peripheral blood mononuclear cells (PBMCs) to enrich for MAIT cells and to remove potential antigen-presenting cell (APC) populations. MDA-MB-231 cells were pulsed with fixed *E. coli* or mock-treated (no *E. coli*) and used to stimulate the CD161-selected population in the presence or absence of an anti-MR1 blocking antibody. Expression of TNF-α was measured by intracellular cytokine staining after ∼ 24 hours. Graph on right: Quantification of the percentage of the MAIT cell population showing positive TNF-α staining in the indicated conditions. Each symbol represents the result of an independent analysis. **c** Intracellular cytokine staining showing TNF-α production by the indicated in vitro-expanded MAIT cells after exposure to mock-treated or *E. coli*-pulsed MDA-MB-231 cells in the presence or absence of an anti-MR1 blocking antibody. **d** T-cell receptor (TCR) cell surface staining of MAIT cells after exposure to *E. coli*-pulsed MDA-MB-231 cells in the presence or absence of an anti-MR1 blocking antibody. MAIT cell TCR expression (geometric mean fluorescence intensity [gMFI]) is expressed as a percentage of that for the corresponding MAIT cells exposed to mock-treated APCs. Each symbol represents the result of an independent analysis. Statistical results are for a two-tailed, one-sample *t* test comparison to a theoretical mean of 100%. *n.s.* Not significant

Although MAIT cells can produce IFN-γ in a TCR-independent manner in response to IL-18 exposure [35, 36], it has recently been shown that they produce TNF-α selectively as a result of TCR-mediated activation [30]. Therefore, we investigated the ability of primary human MAIT cells to produce TNF-α in response to MDA-MB-231 breast carcinoma cells. Freshly isolated PBMCs were enriched for CD161+ cells by magnetic sorting, yielding a preparation that contained almost exclusively CD161+ T cells and natural killer (NK) cells (Additional file 1: Figure S4). MDA-MB-231 breast carcinoma cells were exposed to killed *E. coli* bacteria or mock-treated, then washed and coincubated with the isolated CD161+ cells in the presence or absence of an anti-MR1 blocking antibody. There was little evidence of TNF-α production by MAIT cells in response to the mock-treated breast carcinoma lines, whereas the *E. coli*-treated cells elicited a robust TNF-α response (Fig. 4b). MAIT cell cytokine production was markedly reduced in the presence of the anti-MR1 blocking antibody (Fig. 4b), indicating that the *E. coli*-dependent response was due to recognition of MR1. We also observed similar MR1-dependent TNF-α production in response to *E. coli*-pulsed MDA-MB-231 cells by our in vitro expanded MAIT lines (Fig. 4c). These results suggested that the MDA-MB-231 cells are able to take up bacterially derived extracellular antigens and present them to MAIT cells via MR1.

Further supporting a role for TCR recognition in MAIT cell responses to the MDA-MB-231 cells, we noted that the responding MAIT cells showed somewhat reduced staining by reagents specific for MAIT TCRs (i.e., either Vα7.2 monoclonal antibody or MR1 tetramer; *see* flow cytometric analyses shown in Fig. 4b and c). It is now well established that antigenic activation of T cells results in increased internalization of TCR-CD3 complexes and thus leads to reduced cell surface expression levels of these molecules [37]. MAIT cells that were exposed to *E. coli*-pulsed MDA-MB-231 cells reproducibly showed reduced TCR cell surface expression compared with MAIT cells that were exposed to mock-treated MDA-MB-231 cells (Fig. 4d). Moreover, the TCR downregulation was prevented in the presence of an anti-MR1 blocking antibody (Fig. 4d). Together, these results demonstrate that MAIT cells are activated in a TCR-, MR1-, and microbe-dependent manner by MDA-MB-231 breast carcinoma cells.

Breast carcinoma cells elicit an IL-17-skewed response by breast duct MAIT cells

On the basis of our analyses of MAIT cell responses to PMA/ionomycin stimulation (Fig. 3a–c), it was clear that the breast duct MAIT population includes both IFN-γ and IL-17A producers. We were therefore surprised to observe that primary breast duct MAIT cells showed production of IL-17A but no detectable IFN-γ in response to *E. coli*-pulsed MDA-MB-231 cells (Fig. 5a). To further investigate, we tested the responses of two in vitro expanded MAIT lines to *E. coli*-pulsed MDA-MB-231 cells. Whereas most MAIT cells within the C12 breast duct-derived MAIT line produced both IFN-γ and IL-17A in response to PMA/ionomycin stimulation, their response to the breast carcinoma cells was nearly exclusively limited to IL-17A production (Fig. 5b, top panels). The PBMC-derived MAIT line B12, which produced IFN-γ but not IL-17A in response to PMA/ionomycin, showed only modest IFN-γ secretion in response to *E. coli*-pulsed MDA-MB-231 cells and no detectable IL-17A (Fig. 5b, bottom panels). Addition of an anti-MR1 blocking antibody nearly completely prevented these cytokine responses to the *E. coli*-pulsed APCs, and neither MAIT cell line showed detectable responses to mock-treated MDA-MB-231 cells (data not shown). Thus, these results reveal a surprising

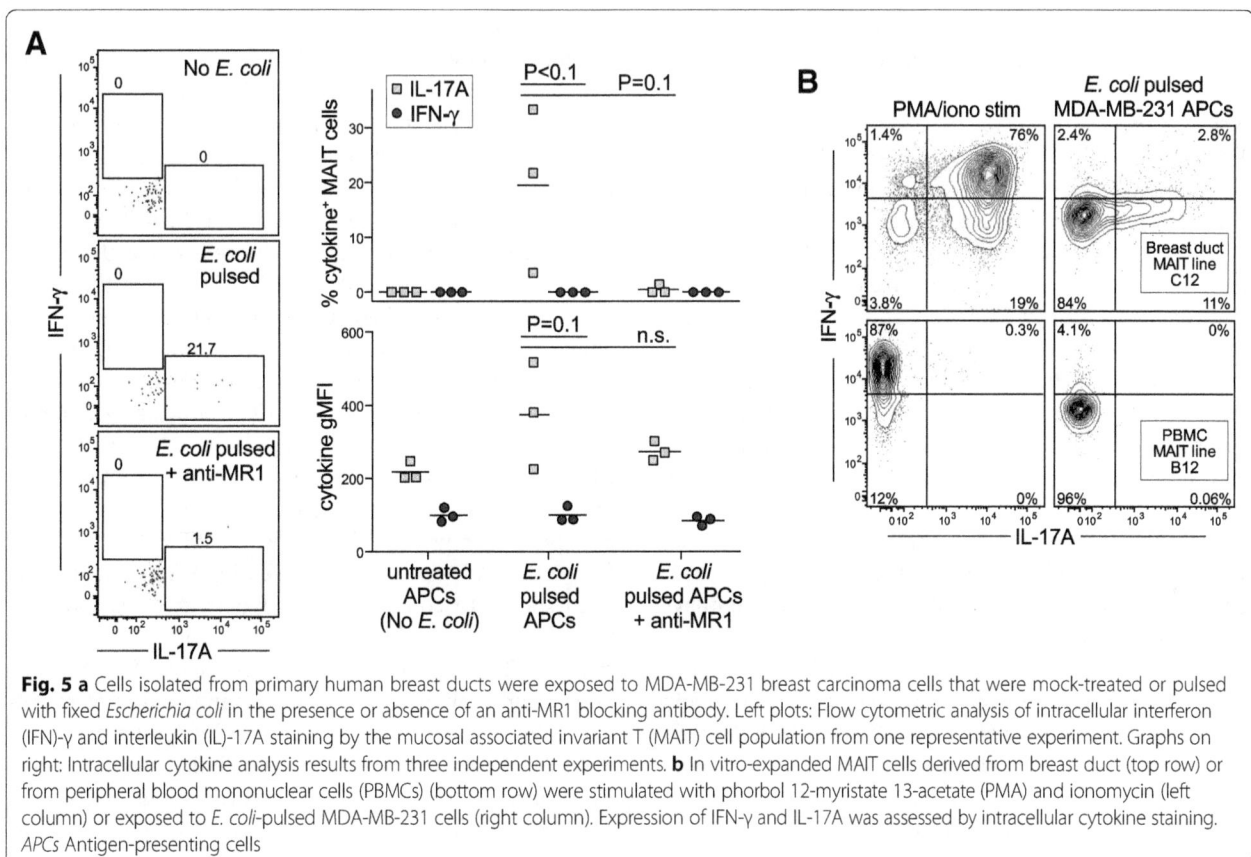

Fig. 5 a Cells isolated from primary human breast ducts were exposed to MDA-MB-231 breast carcinoma cells that were mock-treated or pulsed with fixed *Escherichia coli* in the presence or absence of an anti-MR1 blocking antibody. Left plots: Flow cytometric analysis of intracellular interferon (IFN)-γ and interleukin (IL)-17A staining by the mucosal associated invariant T (MAIT) cell population from one representative experiment. Graphs on right: Intracellular cytokine analysis results from three independent experiments. **b** In vitro-expanded MAIT cells derived from breast duct (top row) or from peripheral blood mononuclear cells (PBMCs) (bottom row) were stimulated with phorbol 12-myristate 13-acetate (PMA) and ionomycin (left column) or exposed to *E. coli*-pulsed MDA-MB-231 cells (right column). Expression of IFN-γ and IL-17A was assessed by intracellular cytokine staining. *APCs* Antigen-presenting cells

bias toward IL-17A production by breast duct MAIT cells in response to bacterially treated breast carcinoma cells.

Role of NKG2D in MAIT cell responses to breast carcinoma cells

Prior analyses have revealed that peripheral blood MAIT cells are positive for NKG2D, a receptor that recognizes a series of ligands that become upregulated on stressed and neoplastic cells [14]. We found that most MAIT cells from breast ducts show intermediate to high levels of NKG2D expression, although most non-MAIT cells from breast ducts also expressed NKG2D (Fig. 6a). Comparing NKG2D counterligand expression by primary breast duct epithelial cells with that of MDA-MB-231 carcinoma cells, we found that primary epithelial cells of either a luminal or basal phenotype lacked detectable expression of MICA/B or ULBP isoform 1, 2, 3, 5, or 6 (Fig. 6b). However, there was detectable expression of ULBP4 on both luminal and basal epithelial cells (Fig. 6b). In contrast, MDA-MB-231 cells showed positive staining for MICA/B and also for some of the ULBP isoforms (Fig. 6b). MAIT cells that were exposed to *E. coli*-pulsed MDA-MB-231 cells in the presence of an anti-NKG2D blocking antibody consistently showed a partial reduction in TNF-α production (Fig. 6c). These results suggest that, though not the dominant pathway of activation, NKG2D-mediated stimulation may costimulate the TCR-mediated activation of MAIT cells by *E. coli*-pulsed breast carcinoma cells.

Discussion

We show in the present study that MAIT cells are present in the epithelial ducts of human breast tissue and that MAIT cells mediate effector responses to breast carcinoma cells that have been exposed to microbial compounds. The role that the breast duct microbiome plays in breast cancer initiation and progression is currently completely uncharted, because the composition and dynamics of the breast duct microbiota are just beginning to be explored. However, intriguing hints are starting to emerge that dysbiosis of the normal breast duct microbiota may be associated with breast cancer, because recent studies have documented differences in the composition of the microbial taxa associated with breast cancer tissue compared with healthy breast tissue [2–4, 6–8]. Given that MAIT cells specifically recognize riboflavin metabolites as antigens presented by MR1 molecules, it is of particular interest that riboflavin-producing bacterial species have been found to be present at higher relative abundance in women with breast cancer, including *Enterobacteriaceae* (the family that includes *E. coli*), *Bacillus*, and *Staphylococcus* species [5, 6]. Thus, understanding the phenotypic and functional properties of the MAIT cells found within breast ducts is an important step in determining whether these cells play a role during the carcinogenesis of breast duct epithelial cells.

In contrast to MAIT cells from peripheral blood, which show almost exclusively a Th1 phenotype, we observed that about one-third of the breast duct MAIT cell population produced IL-17A. Similarly, MAIT cells from the female genital tract were recently shown to be enriched for IL-17A and IL-22 production [20]. Hence, Th17 polarization may be a common feature of MAIT cells from ductal and skin epithelial tissues. Because IL-17A enhances epithelial barrier integrity, MAIT cells with Th17 polarization might contribute to the maintenance of a healthy epithelial surface. It is not clear whether secretion of IL-17A promotes or hinders the initial stages of epithelial carcinogenesis. However, there is a growing body of evidence that after tumors are established, IL-17A has protumorigenic functions, because IL-17A has been shown to be produced by breast cancer tumor-infiltrating lymphocytes and thereby to promote chemoresistance, proliferation, and migration of breast cancer cells [38]. Thus, it will be of great interest to determine whether IL-17A-producing MAIT cells are selectively expanded within breast carcinoma tissue, as has been observed recently for colon carcinomas [24].

In contrast, the IFN-γ-producing subset of breast duct MAIT cells might be expected to have antitumor functions. However, we found that breast MAIT cells that were exposed to *E. coli*-pulsed breast carcinoma cells produced only IL-17A and TNF-α. It is not clear whether the breast carcinoma cells somehow selectively suppress MAIT cell IFN-γ production. Alternatively, it is possible that cancerous cells that have taken up enterobacterial antigens selectively activate only the Th17-polarized subset of breast duct MAIT cells. One mechanism that might explain the selective activation of a particular functional subset of MAIT cells is the observation that the Vβ chain use of the TCR influences the ability of MAIT cells to respond to microbial species, presumably as a result of structural or quantitative variations in the antigenic compounds produced by different types of bacteria [30]. We found that the breast duct MAIT cell population appeared to have a comparatively low frequency of TCRs that use the two Vβ chains that are most common in the blood MAIT cell population (i.e., Vβ2 and Vβ13.2). Because these Vβ chains have been shown to confer stronger reactivity to *E. coli* [30], this observation would be consistent with the possibility that the TCR repertoire of the breast duct MAIT cell population is shaped by a distinct composition of microbial colonists. If this is the case, an intriguing extension of this hypothesis is the possibility that specific functional subsets of MAIT cells (e.g., Th1- vs. Th17-polarized) bear distinct TCR Vβ uses and thus differ in their microbial reactivity.

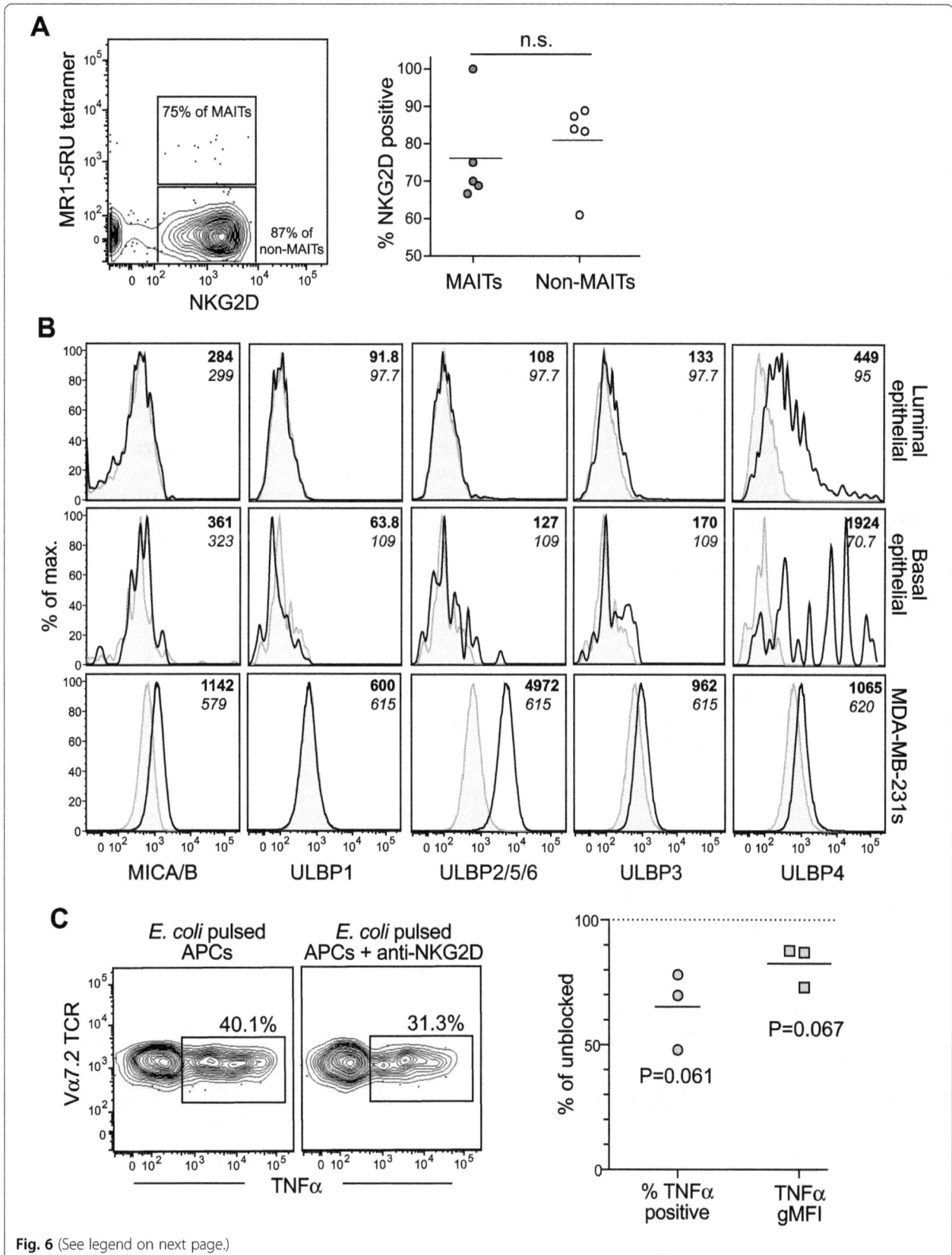

Fig. 6 (See legend on next page.)

(See figure on previous page.)

Fig. 6 Natural killer group 2 member D (NKG2D) plays a role in mucosal associated invariant T (MAIT) cell activation by breast carcinoma cells. **a** Left plot: Flow cytometric analysis showing NKG2D receptor expression by primary MAIT cells in a breast duct tissue sample. Right graph: Aggregated results from five different breast tissue samples showing the percentage of MAIT cells or non-MAIT cells staining positively for NKG2D. **b** Flow cytometric analysis of the expression of known NKG2D ligands (major histocompatibility complex class I-related chain A and B [MICA/B], UL16-binding proteins 1–6 [ULBP1–6]) by primary nontransformed breast duct epithelial cells (top row, luminal subset; middle row, basal subset) compared with MDA-MB-231 breast carcinoma cells (bottom row). Staining with specific antibodies is shown as an *open histogram* with a *heavy black line* with geometric mean fluorescence intensity (gMFI) indicated in bold; *gray filled histograms* show isotype-matched negative control antibody staining with gMFI indicated in italic font. **c** Left plots: Tumor necrosis factor (TNF)-α expression by primary MAIT cells in CD161-selected peripheral blood mononuclear cell samples in response to *Escherichia coli*-pulsed MDA-MB-231 breast carcinoma cells in the presence or absence of an anti-NKG2D blocking antibody. Right graph: Quantification of anti-NKG2D blocking effect. The percentage of MAIT cells showing positive cytokine expression in the NKG2D blockade condition was normalized by the percentage positive in the unblocked condition. Symbols represent the results of independent experiments. *P* values are derived from two-tailed, one-sample *t* tests. *APCs* Antigen-presenting cells, *n.s.* Not significant, *5RU* 5-(2-oxoprophylideneamino)-6-D-ribitylaminouracil

It is also interesting that in contrast to the blood, where more than half of the Vα7.2$^+$ T cells typically are stained by the MR1-5RU tetramer, only about one-third of the breast duct Vα7.2$^+$ T cells were tetramer-positive. One potential explanation for this is that the tetramer-negative Vα7.2$^+$ T cells recognize completely distinct antigens presented by MR1 and therefore are not bound by MR1 tetramers loaded with the 5RU compound. Alternatively, these cells may simply not be MR1-restricted. If this is the case, it is intriguing to speculate that they may belong to another conserved Vα7.2$^+$ T-cell population that is now known as germline-encoded mycolyl-reactive T cells. This subset of T cells also uses Vα7.2 and has been shown to be restricted by CD1b and to recognize mycolate antigens produced by mycobacterial species [39].

A further question of interest relates to the features of breast duct epithelial cells that are required to activate the responses of breast duct MAIT cells. We found that MAIT cells are readily activated by breast carcinoma cells and that this activation is dependent on prior bacterial exposure of the carcinoma cells and can be blocked by an anti-MR1 antibody. It is not yet clear whether normal (i.e., nontransformed) breast duct epithelial cells are also able to activate MAIT cells via MR1-mediated antigen presentation or whether their activation is normally mediated by other immune cell types present in the local tissues (e.g., monocytes, macrophages, or dendritic cells). However, because neoplastic cells often upregulate ligands for NKG2D, and because the addition of an NKG2D blocking antibody resulted in a partial reduction of MAIT cell effector responses, it is possible that the NKG2D pathway promotes the ability of MAIT cells to detect and respond to breast carcinomas.

Conclusions

Together, these findings underscore the likelihood that there exists a tripartite interaction among MAIT cells, breast duct epithelial cells, and the breast microbiome that may play a role in breast carcinogenesis or during the progression of established tumors. Because breast duct MAIT cells appear to use distinct TCR sequences and include multiple functional subsets (e.g., Th1- or Th17-polarized), the breast-resident MAIT cell population likely mediates divergent responses to different types of challenge. Our data suggest that microbially exposed breast carcinoma cells may selectively activate only Th17-polarized MAIT cells from breast ducts and not the Th1-polarized subset. Therefore, a critical question for future analysis is to investigate whether Th17-polarized MAIT cells are enriched in breast carcinomas and how this impacts prognosis.

Additional files

Additional file 1: Figure S4. Magnetic sorting of CD161$^+$ cells from PBMCs yields enrichment of MAIT cells and depletion of nonlymphocytic antigen-presenting cells. Flow cytometric analysis of the CD161-enriched fraction, showing the MAIT cell population (far right plot) and demonstrating that the CD3$^-$ population is almost entirely comprised of NK cells as assessed by NKp46 and CD56 expression. (PDF 235 kb)

Additional file 2: Figure S1. Validation of MR1 tetramer staining. MR1-5RU tetramer staining (1:100 dilution) and MR1-6FP tetramer (1:100 dilution) in combination with Vα7.2 on CD3$^+$ cells from (**a**) PBMCs and (**b**) breast ducts. (PDF 401 kb)

Additional file 3: Figure S2. Phenotypic analyses of breast duct lymphocytes. **a** CD161, IL-18Rα, and PLZF expression on Vα7.2$^+$ T cells that do *not* costain with MR1-5RU tetramer (*black line*) compared with Vα7.2$^-$CD3$^+$ T cells (*filled gray histogram*). **b** In contrast to most T cells from PBMCs, T lymphocytes from breast ducts show a tissue-resident memory phenotype (CD69$^+$ and CD103$^+$). (PDF 270 kb)

Additional file 4: Figure S3. IFN-γ vs. IL-17A production by in vitro-expanded MAIT lines after PMA/ionomycin stimulation. In vitro-expanded MAIT cells derived from breast duct (left column) or from PBMCs (right column) were stimulated with PMA and ionomycin, and expression of IFN-γ and IL-17A was assessed by intracellular cytokine staining. (PDF 252 kb)

Funding
NAZ is supported by a postdoctoral fellowship (PF-17-002-01-CCE) from the American Cancer Society. Funding for this project was provided by the Wisconsin Partnership Program at the UW School of Medicine and Public

Health and by an award to JEG from the Graduate School of the University of Wisconsin-Madison. None of the funding bodies played any role in the design of the study; in the collection, analysis, or interpretation of data; or in the writing of the manuscript.

Authors' contributions

NAZ designed and performed experiments; collected, analyzed, and interpreted data; prepared figures; and wrote the manuscript. JDH performed experiments. MNG designed experiments and interpreted data. JEG designed experiments, analyzed and interpreted data, prepared figures, and wrote the manuscript. All authors read and approved the final manuscript.

Competing interests

The authors declare that they have no competing interests.

Author details

[1]Department of Medical Microbiology and Immunology, University of Wisconsin School of Medicine and Public Health, Madison, WI, USA. [2]McArdle Laboratory for Cancer Research, Department of Oncology, University of Wisconsin School of Medicine and Public Health, Madison, WI, USA.

References

1. Visvader JE. Keeping abreast of the mammary epithelial hierarchy and breast tumorigenesis. Genes Dev. 2009;23(22):2563–77.
2. Chan AA, Bashir M, Rivas MN, Duvall K, Sieling PA, Pieber TR, Vaishampayan PA, Love SM, Lee DJ. Characterization of the microbiome of nipple aspirate fluid of breast cancer survivors. Sci Rep. 2016;6:28061.
3. Hieken TJ, Chen J, Hoskin TL, Walther-Antonio M, Johnson S, Ramaker S, Xiao J, Radisky DC, Knutson KL, Kalari KR, et al. The microbiome of aseptically collected human breast tissue in benign and malignant disease. Sci Rep. 2016;6:30751.
4. Thompson KJ, Ingle JN, Tang X, Chia N, Jeraldo PR, Walther-Antonio MR, Kandimalla KK, Johnson S, Yao JZ, Harrington SC, et al. A comprehensive analysis of breast cancer microbiota and host gene expression. PLoS One. 2017;12(11):e0188873.
5. Urbaniak C, Cummins J, Brackstone M, Macklaim JM, Gloor GB, Baban CK, Scott L, O'Hanlon DM, Burton JP, Francis KP, et al. Microbiota of human breast tissue. Appl Environ Microbiol. 2014;80(10):3007–14.
6. Urbaniak C, Gloor GB, Brackstone M, Scott L, Tangney M, Reid G. The microbiota of breast tissue and its association with breast cancer. Appl Environ Microbiol. 2016;82(16):5039–48.
7. Wang H, Altemus J, Niazi F, Green H, Calhoun BC, Sturgis C, Grobmyer SR, Eng C. Breast tissue, oral and urinary microbiomes in breast cancer. Oncotarget. 2017;8(50):88122–38.
8. Xuan C, Shamonki JM, Chung A, Dinome ML, Chung M, Sieling PA, Lee DJ. Microbial dysbiosis is associated with human breast cancer. PLoS One. 2014; 9(1):e83744.
9. Russo E, Taddei A, Ringressi MN, Ricci F, Amedei A. The interplay between the microbiome and the adaptive immune response in cancer development. Therap Adv Gastroenterol. 2016;9(4):594–605.
10. Zumwalde NA, Haag JD, Sharma D, Mirrielees JA, Wilke LG, Gould MN, Gumperz JE. Analysis of immune cells from human mammary ductal epithelial organoids reveals Vδ2⁺ T cells that efficiently target breast carcinoma cells in the presence of bisphosphonate. Cancer Prev Res (Phila). 2016;9(4):305–16.
11. Treiner E, Duban L, Bahram S, Radosavljevic M, Wanner V, Tilloy F, Affaticati P, Gilfillan S, Lantz O. Selection of evolutionarily conserved mucosal-associated invariant T cells by MR1. Nature. 2003;422(6928):164–9.
12. Kjer-Nielsen L, Patel O, Corbett AJ, Le Nours J, Meehan B, Liu L, Bhati M, Chen Z, Kostenko L, Reantragoon R, et al. MR1 presents microbial vitamin B metabolites to MAIT cells. Nature. 2012;491(7426):717–23.
13. Reantragoon R, Kjer-Nielsen L, Patel O, Chen Z, Illing PT, Bhati M, Kostenko L, Bharadwaj M, Meehan B, Hansen TH, et al. Structural insight into MR1-mediated recognition of the mucosal associated invariant T cell receptor. J Exp Med. 2012;209(4):761–74.
14. Dusseaux M, Martin E, Serriari N, Peguillet I, Premel V, Louis D, Milder M, Le Bourhis L, Soudais C, Treiner E, et al. Human MAIT cells are xenobiotic-resistant, tissue-targeted, CD161hi IL-17-secreting T cells. Blood. 2011;117(4):1250–9.
15. Savage AK, Constantinides MG, Han J, Picard D, Martin E, Li B, Lantz O, Bendelac A. The transcription factor PLZF directs the effector program of the NKT cell lineage. Immunity. 2008;29(3):391–403.
16. Reantragoon R, Corbett AJ, Sakala IG, Gherardin NA, Furness JB, Chen Z, Eckle SB, Uldrich AP, Birkinshaw RW, Patel O, et al. Antigen-loaded MR1 tetramers define T cell receptor heterogeneity in mucosal-associated invariant T cells. J Exp Med. 2013;210(11):2305–20.
17. Gold MC, Cerri S, Smyk-Pearson S, Cansler ME, Vogt TM, Delepine J, Winata E, Swarbrick GM, Chua WJ, Yu YY, et al. Human mucosal associated invariant T cells detect bacterially infected cells. PLoS Biol. 2010;8(6):e1000407.
18. Peterfalvi A, Gomori E, Magyarlaki T, Pal J, Banati M, Javorhazy A, Szekeres-Bartho J, Szereday L, Illes Z. Invariant Vα7.2-Jα33 TCR is expressed in human kidney and brain tumors indicating infiltration by mucosal-associated invariant T (MAIT) cells. Int Immunol. 2008;20(12):1517–25.
19. Serriari NE, Eoche M, Lamotte L, Lion J, Fumery M, Marcelo P, Chatelain D, Barre A, Nguyen-Khac E, Lantz O, et al. Innate mucosal-associated invariant T (MAIT) cells are activated in inflammatory bowel diseases. Clin Exp Immunol. 2014;176(2):266–74.
20. Gibbs A, Leeansyah E, Introini A, Paquin-Proulx D, Hasselrot K, Andersson E, Broliden K, Sandberg JK, Tjernlund A. MAIT cells reside in the female genital mucosa and are biased towards IL-17 and IL-22 production in response to bacterial stimulation. Mucosal Immunol. 2017;10(1):35–45.
21. Leeansyah E, Loh L, Nixon DF, Sandberg JK. Acquisition of innate-like microbial reactivity in mucosal tissues during human fetal MAIT-cell development. Nat Commun. 2014;5:3143.
22. Lepore M, Kalinichenko A, Colone A, Paleja B, Singhal A, Tschumi A, Lee B, Poidinger M, Zolezzi F, Quagliata L, et al. Parallel T-cell cloning and deep sequencing of human MAIT cells reveal stable oligoclonal TCRβ repertoire. Nat Commun. 2014;5:3866.
23. Dias J, Sobkowiak MJ, Sandberg JK, Leeansyah E. Human MAIT-cell responses to Escherichia coli: activation, cytokine production, proliferation, and cytotoxicity. J Leukoc Biol. 2016;100(1):233–40.
24. Sundstrom P, Ahlmanner F, Akeus P, Sundquist M, Alsen S, Yrlid U, Borjesson L, Sjoling A, Gustavsson B, Wong SB, et al. Human mucosa-associated invariant T cells accumulate in colon adenocarcinomas but produce reduced amounts of IFN-γ. J Immunol. 2015;195(7):3472–81.
25. Ling L, Lin Y, Zheng W, Hong S, Tang X, Zhao P, Li M, Ni J, Li C, Wang L, et al. Circulating and tumor-infiltrating mucosal associated invariant T (MAIT) cells in colorectal cancer patients. Sci Rep. 2016;6:20358.
26. Patel O, Kjer-Nielsen L, Le Nours J, Eckle SB, Birkinshaw R, Beddoe T, Corbett AJ, Liu L, Miles JJ, Meehan B, et al. Recognition of vitamin B metabolites by mucosal-associated invariant T cells. Nat Commun. 2013;4:2142.
27. Kumar BV, Ma W, Miron M, Granot T, Guyer RS, Carpenter DJ, Senda T, Sun X, Ho SH, Lerner H, et al. Human tissue-resident memory T cells are defined by Core transcriptional and functional signatures in lymphoid and mucosal sites. Cell Rep. 2017;20(12):2921–34.
28. Gold MC, McLaren JE, Reistetter JA, Smyk-Pearson S, Ladell K, Swarbrick GM, Yu YY, Hansen TH, Lund O, Nielsen M, et al. MR1-restricted MAIT cells display ligand discrimination and pathogen selectivity through distinct T cell receptor usage. J Exp Med. 2014;211(8):1601–10.
29. Eckle SB, Birkinshaw RW, Kostenko L, Corbett AJ, McWilliam HE, Reantragoon R, Chen Z, Gherardin NA, Beddoe T, Liu L, et al. A molecular basis underpinning the T cell receptor heterogeneity of mucosal-associated invariant T cells. J Exp Med. 2014;211(8):1585–600.
30. Dias J, Leeansyah E, Sandberg JK. Multiple layers of heterogeneity and subset diversity in human MAIT cell responses to distinct microorganisms and to innate cytokines. Proc Natl Acad Sci U S A. 2017;114(27):E5434–43.
31. Laugel B, Lloyd A, Meermeier EW, Crowther MD, Connor TR, Dolton G, Miles JJ, Burrows SR, Gold MC, Lewinsohn DM, et al. Engineering of isogenic cells deficient for MR1 with a CRISPR/Cas9 lentiviral system: tools to study

microbial antigen processing and presentation to human MR1-restricted T cells. J Immunol. 2016;197(3):971–82.

32. Riegert P, Wanner V, Bahram S. Genomics, isoforms, expression, and phylogeny of the MHC class I-related MR1 gene. J Immunol. 1998;161(8): 4066–77.

33. Chua WJ, Kim S, Myers N, Huang S, Yu L, Fremont DH, Diamond MS, Hansen TH. Endogenous MHC-related protein 1 is transiently expressed on the plasma membrane in a conformation that activates mucosal-associated invariant T cells. J Immunol. 2011;186(8):4744–50.

34. McWilliam HE, Eckle SB, Theodossis A, Liu L, Chen Z, Wubben JM, Fairlie DP, Strugnell RA, Mintern JD, McCluskey J, et al. The intracellular pathway for the presentation of vitamin B-related antigens by the antigen-presenting molecule MR1. Nat Immunol. 2016;17(5):531–7.

35. Loh L, Wang Z, Sant S, Koutsakos M, Jegaskanda S, Corbett AJ, Liu L, Fairlie DP, Crowe J, Rossjohn J, et al. Human mucosal-associated invariant T cells contribute to antiviral influenza immunity via IL-18-dependent activation. Proc Natl Acad Sci U S A. 2016;113(36):10133–8.

36. Ussher JE, Bilton M, Attwod E, Shadwell J, Richardson R, de Lara C, Mettke E, Kurioka A, Hansen TH, Klenerman P, et al. CD161++CD8+T cells, including the MAIT cell subset, are specifically activated by IL-12+IL-18 in a TCR-independent manner. Eur J Immunol. 2014;44(1):195–203.

37. Alcover A, Alarcon B. Internalization and intracellular fate of TCR-CD3 complexes. Crit Rev Immunol. 2000;20(4):325–46.

38. Cochaud S, Giustiniani J, Thomas C, Laprevotte E, Garbar C, Savoye AM, Cure H, Mascaux C, Alberici G, Bonnefoy N, et al. IL-17A is produced by breast cancer TILs and promotes chemoresistance and proliferation through ERK1/2. Sci Rep. 2013;3:3456.

39. Van Rhijn I, Kasmar A, de Jong A, Gras S, Bhati M, Doorenspleet ME, de Vries N, Godfrey DI, Altman JD, de Jager W, et al. A conserved human T cell population targets mycobacterial antigens presented by CD1b. Nat Immunol. 2013;14(7):706–13.

Simultaneous blockade of IL-6 and CCL5 signaling for synergistic inhibition of triple-negative breast cancer growth and metastasis

Kideok Jin[1]*(iD), Niranjan B. Pandey[2] and Aleksander S. Popel[2,3]

Abstract

Background: Metastatic triple-negative breast cancer (TNBC) is a heterogeneous and incurable disease. Numerous studies have been conducted to seek molecular targets to treat TNBC effectively, but chemotherapy is still the main choice for patients with TNBC. We have previously presented evidence of the important roles of interleukin-6 (IL-6) and chemokine (C-C motif) ligand 5 (CCL5) in TNBC tumor growth and metastasis. These experiments highlighted the importance of the crosstalk between cancer cells and stromal lymphatic endothelial cells (LECs) in tumor growth and metastasis.

Methods: We examined the viability and migration of MDA-MB-231-LN, SUM149, and SUM159 cells co-cultured with LECs when treated with maraviroc (CCR5 inhibitor) and tocilizumab (anti-IL-6 receptor antibody). To assess the anti-tumor effects of the combination of these two drugs in an athymic nude mouse model, MDA-MB-231-LN cells were implanted in the mammary fat pad and maraviroc (8 mg/kg, orally daily) and cMR16-1 (murine surrogate of the anti-IL-6R antibody, 10 mg/kg, IP, 3 days a week) were administrated for 5 weeks and effects on tumor growth and thoracic metastasis were measured.

Results: In this study, we used maraviroc and tocilizumab to confirm that IL-6 and CCL5 signaling are key pathways promoting TNBC cell proliferation and migration. Further, in a xenograft mouse model, we showed that tumor growth was dramatically inhibited by cMR16-1, the mouse version of the anti-IL6R antibody. The combination of maraviroc and cMR16-1 caused significant reduction of TNBC tumor growth compared to the single agents. Significantly, the combination of maraviroc and cMR16-1 abrogated thoracic metastasis.

Conclusion: Taken together, these findings show that IL-6 and CCL5 signaling, which promote crosstalk between TNBC and lymphatic vessels, are key enhancers of TNBC tumor growth and metastasis. Furthermore, these results demonstrate that a drug combination inhibiting these pathways may be a promising therapy for TNBC patients.

Keywords: Triple negative breast cancer, Tumor microenvironment, Secretome, Drug repurposing, Maraviroc, Tocilizumab

* Correspondence: kideok.jin@acphs.edu
[1]Department of Pharmaceutical Sciences, Albany College of Pharmacy and Health Sciences, Albany, NY 12208, USA
Full list of author information is available at the end of the article

Background

Lymphangiogenesis plays a critical role in tumor invasion, distal metastasis, and immune unresponsiveness. Crosstalk between tumor-associated lymphatic endothelial cells (LEC) and cancer cells enhances the recruitment of cancer cells to the lymphatic system from primary tumors. This recruitment is increased by various secreted factors such as CCL21, CXCL12, CCL27, IL6 and KAI1 [1], which also induce lymphangiogenesis in tumor-draining lymph nodes (LNs). Lymphangiogenesis, which promotes tumor metastasis, is induced in the pre-metastatic niche by lymphangiogenic growth factors such as vascular endothelial growth factor (VEGF)-C, VEGF-D, angiopoietins, platelet-derived growth factor (PDGF)-BB/AA and basic fibroblast growth factor (bFGF) [2–6]. The recruitment of immune cells such as myeloid-derived suppressor cells (MDSCs), tumor-associated macrophages (TAMs), and immature dendritic cells (DCs) contribute to tumor-induced immunosuppression in the lymph nodes [7]. Due to a paucity of lymphatic markers the role of lymphangiogenesis in tumor growth and metastasis has not been studied as well as the role of blood endothelial cells (BEC). We have previously demonstrated that the crosstalk between LEC secreting CCL5 and triple-negative breast cancer (TNBC) cells expressing CCR5, the CCL5 receptor, promotes the recruitment of TNBC cells towards the lymphatic vessels, induces lymphangiogenesis, and facilitates subsequent lung metastasis. Consistent with these finding, we showed that maraviroc, a CCR5 inhibitor with anti-retroviral activity, inhibited TNBC lymphangiogenesis and lung metastasis. Furthermore, we discovered that IL-6, which is secreted by TNBC cells, is a key factor in upregulating CCL5 expression in LECs by activating the IL6 receptor and subsequently STAT3, which enhances transcription of the CCL5 gene. In our earlier study, we showed that inhibiting the IL-6 signaling pathway by depleting IL-6 levels using an anti-IL-6 antibody or a STAT3 inhibitor decreased CCL5 expression and consequently lymphogenous metastasis [8]. Here, we present more evidence that both IL-6 and CCL5 are key factors in TNBC lymphangiogenesis, tumor growth, and thoracic metastasis. Furthermore, by using maraviroc (CCR5 inhibitor) and cMR16-1 Ab (murine surrogate of the anti-IL-6 receptor antibody) we showed that simultaneous blockade of CCR5 and IL-6 receptor signaling strongly inhibits TNBC tumor growth and profoundly inhibits TNBC tumor metastasis.

Methods
Cell lines

MDA-MB-231-luc-D3H2LN (MDA-MB-231-LN) cells were purchased from Caliper and propagated in RPMI-1640 medium supplemented with 10% FBS and 1% penicillin/streptomycin (Sigma). SUM149 and SUM159 breast cancer cells were cultured in F-12 medium supplemented with 5% FBS, 1 ng/ml hydrocortisone, 5 μg/ml insulin (Sigma, St. Louis, MO, USA), and 0.1 mM HEPES (ThermoFisher Scientific, Waltham, MA, USA). LECs were purchased from Lonza, and grown in EGM-2MV. Cells were maintained under standard conditions of 37 °C and 5% CO^2. Cells were cultured for a maximum of 4 weeks after thawing fresh, early passage cells and confirmed to be Mycoplasma negative (Hoechst stain).

Conditioned medium

When TNBC cells had grown to confluence in T175 tissue culture flasks, the normal cancer cell growth medium was replaced with 8 ml serum-free medium (SFM) after extensive washing. After 24 h incubation in a tissue culture incubator, the supernatant was centrifuged and filtered through 0.2-μm syringe filters (Corning). The resulting tumor-conditioned medium (TCM) was stored in aliquots at – 80 °C. When LECs reached 30–40% confluence in T75 tissue culture flasks, the growth medium (GM) was replaced with 30% TCM in GM (TCM:GM = 3:7) to allow the TCM to activate the LECs. For education of LECs by TCM, the cells were allowed to grow in the medium for 3–4 days at which point the medium was replaced with 3 ml SFM containing 2% FBS. After 48 h, the supernatant was centrifuged and filtered. The resulting tumor-educated LEC conditioned medium, (TCM-LEC)CM, was stored in aliquots at – 80 °C to avoid multiple freeze thaws.

Cell migration and proliferation assays

Cancer cell migration was assessed using the Oris™ cell migration kit (Platypus), as previously described [8]. The (TCM-LEC)CM (100 μl) with or without 20 μM maraviroc (R&D Systems) or 200 μg/ml tocilizumab (Genentech) was added once the cancer cells had attached. Migration and proliferation assays using CIM (cell invasion and migration) plates and the RTCA system (ACEA Bioscience) were performed as previously described [9].

Mouse xenograft studies

Before tumor inoculation, athymic nude mice (female, 5–6 weeks, 18–20 g) were pre-treated by injecting 50 μl TCM or SFM subcutaneously for 2 weeks daily as described previously [8]. MDA-MB-231-LN cells were grown to 90% confluence, trypsinized, resuspended in serum-free medium, and mixed 1:1 with Matrigel (BD Biosciences) and 2×10^6 cells were injected into the upper inguinal mammary fat pad of the animals induced for 2 weeks with TCM as described above. Tumor sizes were measured using calipers, and the volume was calculated, using the formula: $V = 0.52 \times (length) \times (width)^2$. Animals were imaged every week to track anterior tumor metastases, using the IVIS Xenogen 200 optical imager

(Xenogen) after intraperitoneal (i.p.) injection of D-luciferin (Caliper, 150 mg/kg body weight). After 5 weeks, organs were harvested and bathed in D-luciferin solution for 5–10 min and placed in the IVIS imager to detect metastases ex vivo. Luciferase-mediated photon flux was quantified using Living Image® 3D Analysis (Xenogen). Maraviroc (8 mg/kg body weight, R&D systems) was administered orally daily; cMR16-1 (10 mg/kg, Genentech) was administered intraperitoneally 3 days per week for 5 weeks.

Immunofluorescence and immunohistochemical analysis

Immunofluorescence and immunohistochemical analysis (IHC) were performed using monoclonal antibodies against CD31 and pan-cytokeratin (Sigma). For immunofluorescence, after blocking with 5% normal goat or normal chicken serum (Jackson Immunoresearch) in PBS/Tween (PBST) (0.3% Triton) for 1 h at room temperature (RT), the sections were treated with anti-CD31 primary antibodies overnight at 4 °C. After three rinses with PBST, the sections were incubated for 1 h at RT with FITC-conjugated goat anti-rabbit secondary antibodies (1:500). After three rinses with PBST, the samples were counterstained with 4′,6-diamidino-2-phenylindole (DAPI) (1:10,000, Roche) (5 min at RT). The samples were washed with PBST once and mounted with the ProLong Gold anti-fade reagent (Invitrogen) in the dark. Fluorescent signals were visualized and digital images were obtained using the Zeiss LSM-700 confocal microscope (Carl Zeiss). For IHC, after blocking with 5% goat serum in PBST for 1 h at room temperature, the sections were treated with the pan-cytokeratin antibody overnight at 4 °C, then the peroxidase conjugated streptavidin complex method was performed, followed by the 3, 3′ diaminobenzidine (DAB) procedure according to the manufacturers' protocols (VECTASTAIN Elite ABC Kit, Vector Lab).

Statistical analysis

Error bars represent the SEM. All statistical tests were two sided, and differences were considered statistically significant at $P < 0.05$. The synergy calculation was performed using the Chou-Talalay method as previously described [10–12].

Results

Maraviroc and tocilizumab block TNBC cell proliferation

We have previously shown that lymphatic endothelial cells (LECs) promote TNBC tumor growth [13]. Furthermore, we have discovered that IL-6 secreted by TNBC cells binds to the IL-6 receptor on LECs and activates the STAT3 signaling pathway. The phosphorylated ternary complex of STAT3, c-Jun, and ATF-2 binds to a CRE site on the CCL5 promoter to enhance CCL5

transcriptional activity in LECs. The CCL5 secreted by LECs recruits CCR5-positive TNBC cells and guides them towards the lymphatic system [8]. This finding motivated the hypothesis that inhibition of both CCL5 and IL-6 signaling would attenuate TNBC tumor growth and thoracic metastasis. In our earlier work we elucidated the role of IL-6 in TNBC growth and metastasis by depleting its levels in the TCM administered to the animals prior to tumor inoculation. To facilitate translation of our work to patients, here we tested the effect of an antibody against the IL-6 receptor on the growth and metastasis of TNBC tumors. We examined the viability of MDA-MB-231-LN cells co-cultured with LECs in the presence of maraviroc (CCR5 inhibitor, Pfizer) and tocilizumab (anti-IL-6 receptor antibody, Genentech) (Fig. 1a). The proliferation of MDA-MB-231-LN cells was increased when co-cultured with LECs (Fig. 1b). We observed that maraviroc had no significant effect, whereas tocilizumab decreased MDA-MB-231-LN cellular viability in a concentration-dependent manner (Fig. 1c and d). Using transwell plates, real-time co-culture E-plates (RTCA system ACEA Biosciences Inc.) and crystal violet staining, we confirmed that tocilizumab inhibited the cell viability of three different TNBC cells including MDA-MB-231-LN, SUM149, and SUM159 compared to control and maraviroc. The viability of TNBC cells was decreased further in the combination of maraviroc and tocilizumab compared to the single agents as seen above. Furthermore, we analyzed tocilizumab with maraviroc in the TNBC cellular viability according to the Chou-Talalay method for drug synergy analysis. We found that the combination of maraviroc and tocilizumab is highly synergistic with CI < 1 (Fig. 1e, f, and Additional file 1: Figure S1). These results suggest that the crosstalk between TNBC cells and LECs enhances TNBC cell proliferation, and that the IL-6 signaling plays a critical role in TNBC cellular viability.

Decrease of TNBC cell migration by inhibition of IL-6 and CCL5 signaling

In previous studies, we showed that the TCM from TNBC cells induced LECs, and the conditioned medium from LECs induced by TCM, (TCM-LEC)CM, facilitated TNBC cell migration. We found that IL-6 in TCM plays an important role in upregulating CCL5 expression in LECs. The CCL5 in (TCM-LEC)CM plays a key role in TNBC cell motility and maraviroc efficiently inhibited this migratory effect [8]. Here we investigated the effect of the combination of maraviroc and tocilizumab on TNBC cell migration in conditioned medium from LECs induced by TCM of TNBC cells, (TCM-LEC)CM, using a CIM-plate from ACEA Biosciences. We cultured TNBC cells (top chamber) with (TCM-LEC)CM (bottom chamber) in treatment with maraviroc, tocilizumab, and the

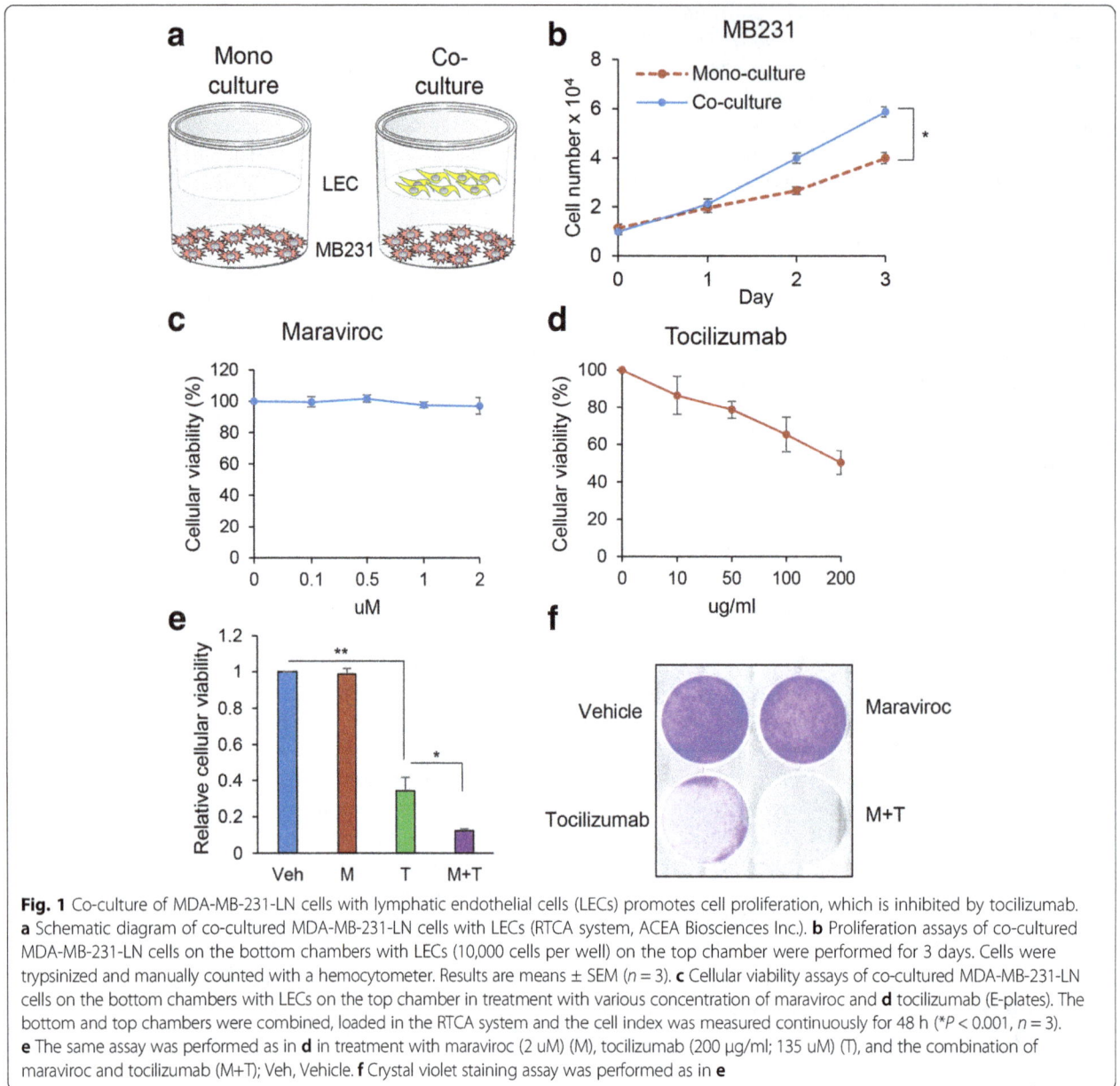

Fig. 1 Co-culture of MDA-MB-231-LN cells with lymphatic endothelial cells (LECs) promotes cell proliferation, which is inhibited by tocilizumab. **a** Schematic diagram of co-cultured MDA-MB-231-LN cells with LECs (RTCA system, ACEA Biosciences Inc.). **b** Proliferation assays of co-cultured MDA-MB-231-LN cells on the bottom chambers with LECs (10,000 cells per well) on the top chamber were performed for 3 days. Cells were trypsinized and manually counted with a hemocytometer. Results are means ± SEM ($n = 3$). **c** Cellular viability assays of co-cultured MDA-MB-231-LN cells on the bottom chambers with LECs on the top chamber in treatment with various concentration of maraviroc and **d** tocilizumab (E-plates). The bottom and top chambers were combined, loaded in the RTCA system and the cell index was measured continuously for 48 h (*$P < 0.001$, $n = 3$). **e** The same assay was performed as in **d** in treatment with maraviroc (2 uM) (M), tocilizumab (200 µg/ml; 135 uM) (T), and the combination of maraviroc and tocilizumab (M+T); Veh, Vehicle. **f** Crystal violet staining assay was performed as in **e**

combination of maraviroc and tocilizumab, and measured the migration of TNBC cells in the RTCA system. Maraviroc significantly inhibited TNBC cell migration by inhibiting CCR5 of TNBC cells in response to (TCM-LEC)CM including CCL5 compared to control. Compared to maraviroc, tocilizumab had less effect on the migration of TNBC cells by blocking IL-6 receptor in TNBC cells. Significantly, TNBC cell migration was decreased by the combination of maraviroc and tocilizumab, about three fold compared to treatment with maraviroc alone. It implied that both CCR5 and IL-6 receptor signaling in TNBC cells play an important role in TNBC cell migration (Fig. 2a and Additional file 1: Figure S2A and B). We wanted to confirm that TNBC cell migration

depended on the crosstalk between TNBC cells and LECs through IL-6 and CCL5 signaling so LECs were cultured in TCM of TNBC cells pre-treated with tocilizumab (scheme shown in Fig. 2b). Inhibition of the IL-6 signaling pathway by tocilizumab should result in reduced levels of CCL5. We found that TNBC cell migration was enhanced in (TCM-LEC)CM compared to (SFM-LEC)CM as expected. However, we found that TNBC cell migration was significantly inhibited in tocilizumab-pre-treated (TCM-LEC)CM compared to control (TCM-LEC)CM (Fig. 2c and Additional file 1: Figure S2C). As expected, the secretion of CCL5 was decreased in tocilizumab-pre-treated (TCM-LEC)CM compared to control (TCM-LEC)CM (Fig. 2d and

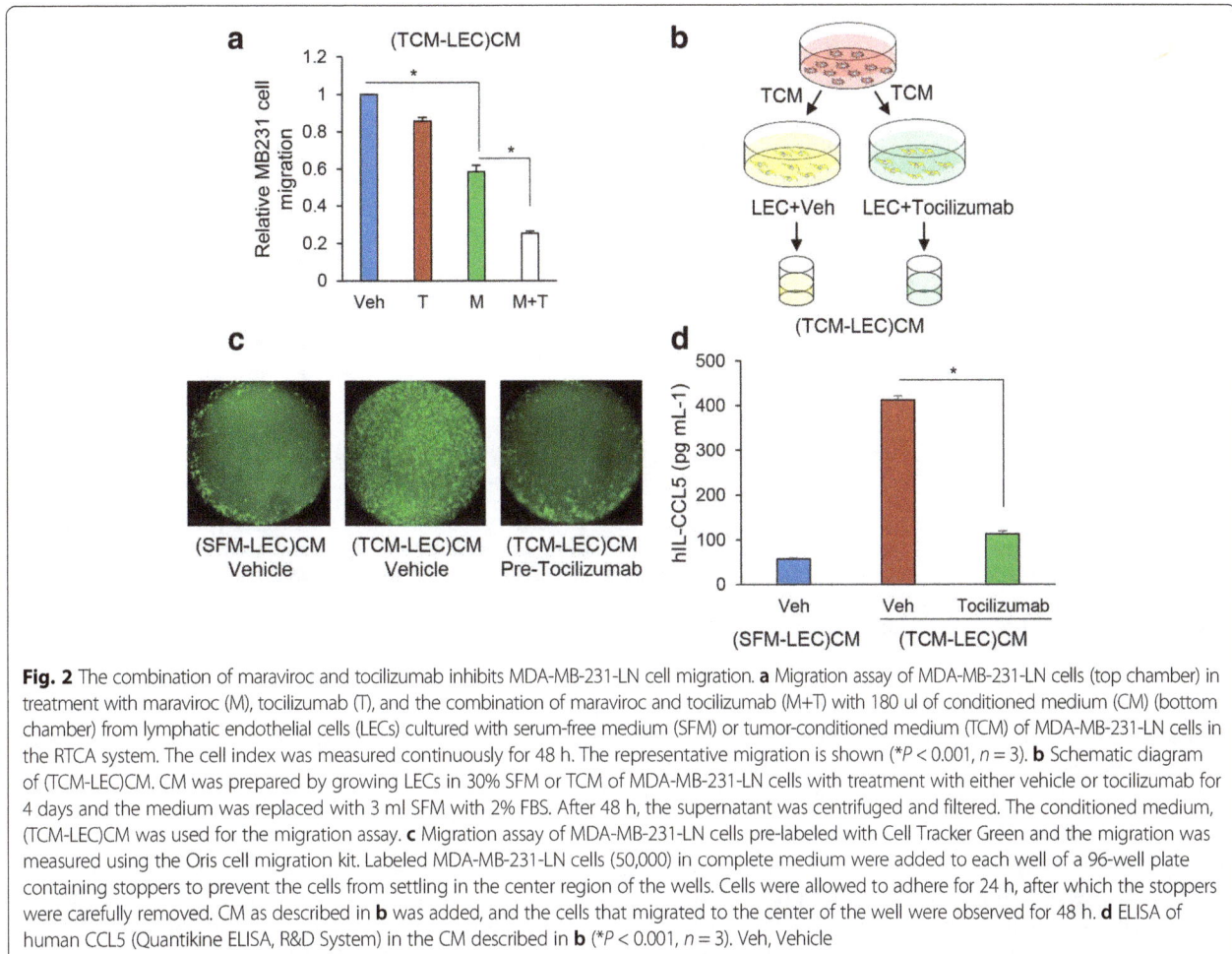

Fig. 2 The combination of maraviroc and tocilizumab inhibits MDA-MB-231-LN cell migration. **a** Migration assay of MDA-MB-231-LN cells (top chamber) in treatment with maraviroc (M), tocilizumab (T), and the combination of maraviroc and tocilizumab (M+T) with 180 ul of conditioned medium (CM) (bottom chamber) from lymphatic endothelial cells (LECs) cultured with serum-free medium (SFM) or tumor-conditioned medium (TCM) of MDA-MB-231-LN cells in the RTCA system. The cell index was measured continuously for 48 h. The representative migration is shown (*$P < 0.001$, $n = 3$). **b** Schematic diagram of (TCM-LEC)CM. CM was prepared by growing LECs in 30% SFM or TCM of MDA-MB-231-LN cells with treatment with either vehicle or tocilizumab for 4 days and the medium was replaced with 3 ml SFM with 2% FBS. After 48 h, the supernatant was centrifuged and filtered. The conditioned medium, (TCM-LEC)CM was used for the migration assay. **c** Migration assay of MDA-MB-231-LN cells pre-labeled with Cell Tracker Green and the migration was measured using the Oris cell migration kit. Labeled MDA-MB-231-LN cells (50,000) in complete medium were added to each well of a 96-well plate containing stoppers to prevent the cells from settling in the center region of the wells. Cells were allowed to adhere for 24 h, after which the stoppers were carefully removed. CM as described in **b** was added, and the cells that migrated to the center of the well were observed for 48 h. **d** ELISA of human CCL5 (Quantikine ELISA, R&D System) in the CM described in **b** (*$P < 0.001$, $n = 3$). Veh, Vehicle

Additional file 1: Figure S2D and E). These results show that crosstalk between TNBC cells and LECs mediated by IL-6 and CCL5 signaling is important for TNBC cell migration.

The combination of maraviroc and cMR16-1, an anti-mouse anti-IL6 receptor antibody, inhibits growth of MDA-MB-231-LN tumors

Next we investigated the inhibitory effect of maraviroc and tocilizumab on the growth of orthotopic MDA-MB-231-LN tumors in athymic mice. We administered maraviroc (8 mg/kg body weight, orally daily) and cMR16-1 (murine surrogate of the anti-IL-6R antibody, 10 mg/kg body weight, i.p., 3 days a week), and monitored tumor growth for 5 weeks (Fig. 3a). We used the cMR16-1 in these experiments because the LEC cells on lymphatic vessels, which are from the mouse host, carry the mouse IL6 receptor. The growth of MDA-MB-231-LN tumors treated with cMR16-1 was significantly inhibited compared to control while maraviroc had no significant effect on tumor growth. The combination of maraviroc and cMR16-1 enhanced the inhibition of MDA-MB-231-LN

cell tumor growth significantly (Fig. 3b and c) compared to cMR16-1 alone. These results demonstrate that the IL-6 receptor is an attractive target in TNBC and that the combination of maraviroc and an anti-IL6 receptor antibody could be beneficial in the treatment of TNBC.

Inhibition of IL-6 and CCL5 signaling prevents TNBC metastasis

In previous work, we developed a metastatic mouse model in which TCM of MDA-MB-231-LN cells was administered to mice for 2 weeks subcutaneously prior to tumor inoculation. MDA-MB-231-LN cells were then injected into the mammary fat pad to establish orthotopic tumor xenografts [14]. The primary tumors robustly gave rise to thoracic metastases including to the lymph nodes (LNs) and lungs within 4–5 weeks [8]. Utilizing this mouse model, we monitored the effect of maraviroc and cMR16-1 on thoracic metastasis of MDA-MB-231-LN tumors by weekly IVIS imaging over a period of 5 weeks. We observed that MDA-MB-231-LN cell tumors metastasized to the LNs and thoracic region in all the mice of the control group (10/10) within 5 weeks as shown by the

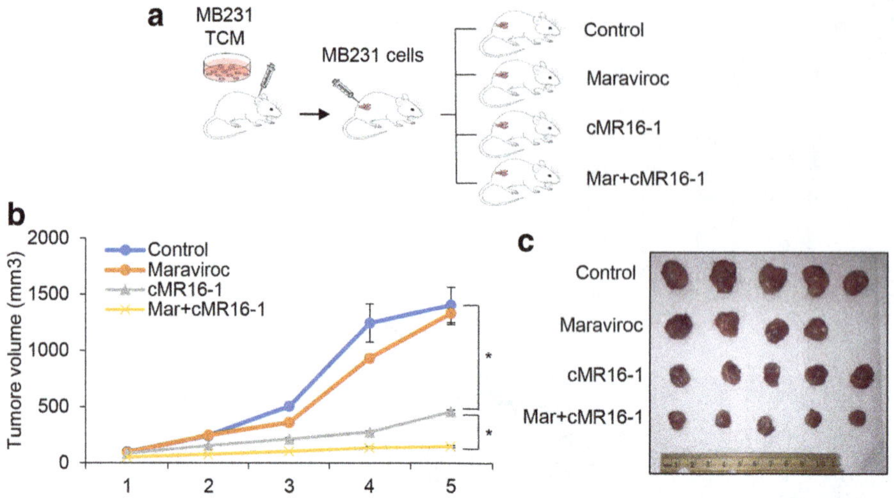

Fig. 3 MDA-MB-231-LN cell tumor growth was inhibited by the combination of maraviroc and tocilizumab. **a** Generation of MDA-MB-231-LN cell xenografts administered maraviroc, tocilizumab, and the combination of maraviroc and tocilizumab. **b** Tumor growth curves of MDA-MB-231-LN cells implanted mammary fat pad in athymic mice treated with maraviroc (8 mg/kg body weight, R&D systems) orally daily; cMR16-1 (10 mg/kg, Genentech) intraperitoneally 3 days per week for 5 weeks (mean ± SEM, **P < 0.005, n = 10). **c** Size of MDA-MB-231-LN cells xenografts in athymic nude mice after 5 weeks of treatment with maraviroc and cMR16-1. TCM, tumor-conditioned medium

increase in photon flux in these tissues. However, thoracic metastases were found in only 20% of the mice (2/10) in the maraviroc treated group and in 30% of the mice (3/10) in the cMR16-1 treated group. Remarkably, we observed no metastasis in LNs and in thoracic tissues in the group of mice treated with the combination of maraviroc and cMR16-1 (Fig. 4a-c). We assayed for the presence of the lung metastasis by IHC with cytokeratin in the lung (Fig. 4d and e) and the lymphangiogenesis in LNs by immunostaining with CD31 (Fig. 4f and g). The results demonstrate that IL-6 and CCL5 signaling in the crosstalk of TNBC cells with LECs plays a key role in metastasis and drugs targeting them could be used to minimize metastasis in patients with TNBC.

Discussion

Tumor cells are commonly spread to tumor-draining lymph nodes in many types of cancer. There is ample evidence that lymphangiogenesis is actively induced by tumor cells and lymphangiogenic growth factors play an important role in lymphangiogenesis and distal organ metastasis [15–17]. For example, the proteolytic matured VEGF-C and VEGF-D interact with VEGFR-3 and upregulate lymphangiogenic activity [18, 19]; the VEGF-A-VEGFR-2 axis also induces tumor lymphangiogenesis by inducing LEC proliferation [20, 21]. Angiogenin 1 (Ang1) and Ang2 were also shown to be important for stimulating lymphangiogenesis and lymphatic metastasis in a tumor xenograft model [22, 23]. Hepatocyte growth factor receptor (HGF c-MET) is also known to be an inducer of lymphangiogenesis in vivo [24–26]. Studies by our laboratory and others showed that fibroblast growth factor (FGF), epidermal growth factor (EGF), PDGF, and insulin-like growth factor (IGF) play critical roles in lymphangiogenesis [13, 27–30]. In our previous studies, we have shown that crosstalk between MDA-MB-231-LN cells and LECs induce upregulation of EGF to promote MDA-MB-231-LN cell proliferation and LECs co-injected with MDA-MB-231-LN cells into nude mice enhanced tumor growth. In addition, we demonstrated that an interaction of MDA-MB-231-LN and LEC stimulated PDGF-BB expression and recruited pericytes to the neovasculature in a xenograft mouse model; SU16f, a PDGFRβ inhibitor, inhibited the recruitment of pericytes in this model [13]. It has been reported that the CCL5-CCR5 axis enhanced metastasis of basal breast cancer cells [31–33], but detailed mechanisms of how this happens are not yet clear. We have tried to clarify these mechanisms in this and earlier studies. In a previous study, we discovered that IL-6 secreted by TNBC cells upregulates CCL5 and VEGF in LECs through the IL-6-STAT3 signaling pathway. Additionally, we showed that the secreted CCL5 recruited CCR5-positive TNBC breast cancer to LNs resulting in LN angiogenesis and lung metastasis. In addition, the increased levels of VEGF induced LN angiogenesis and supported tumor cell extravasation into the lung. In agreement with these results, we have also found a significant inhibitory effect on TNBC metastasis by the following manipulations: depleting IL-6 in the tumor-conditioned medium injected into mice prior to tumor inoculation using an anti-IL-6 antibody, inhibiting CCL5 by maraviroc, inhibiting VEGF by an anti-VEGF antibody, and inhibiting STAT3 by S3I-201 [8]. Maraviroc exerts its anti-retroviral activity by inhibiting the CCR5 receptor and it is commonly utilized as a treatment for HIV

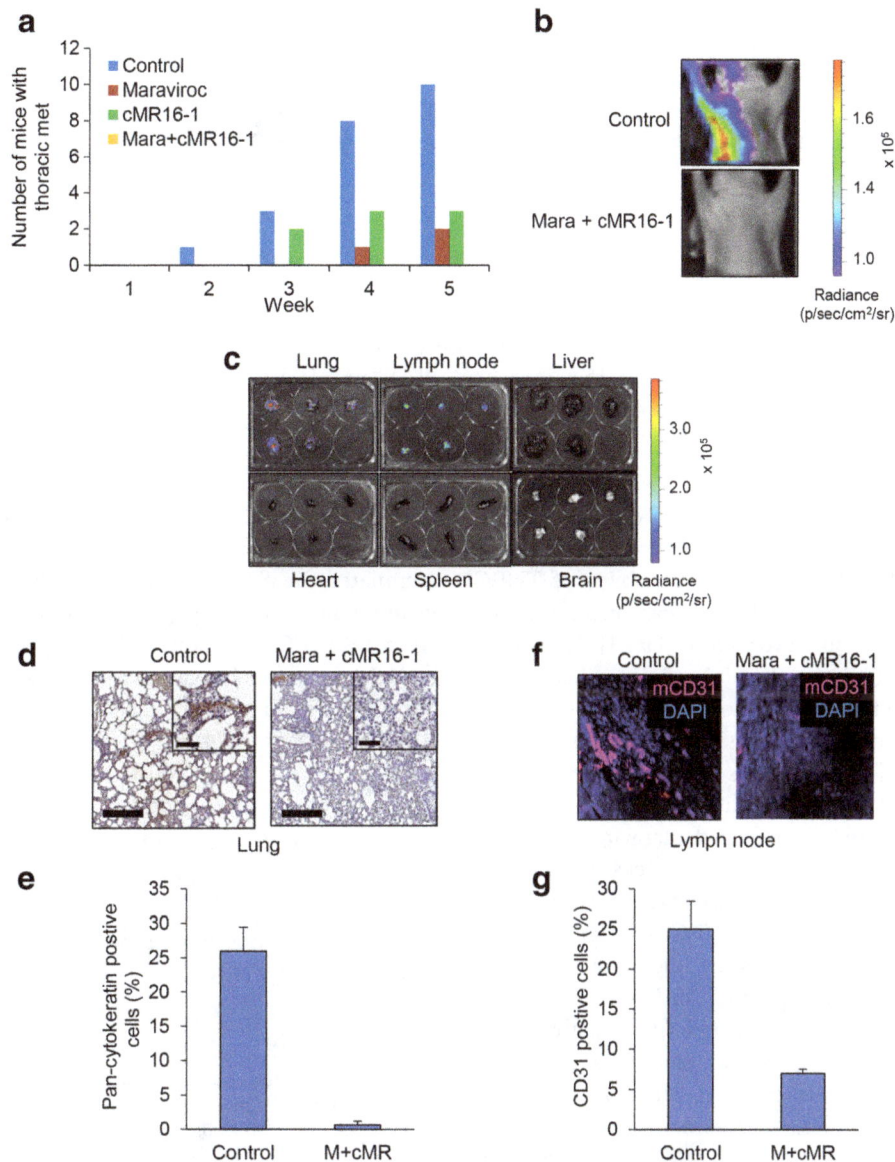

Fig. 4 The thoracic metastasis of MDA-MB-231-LN cell tumor was inhibited by the combination of maraviroc and tocilizumab. **a** Athymic nude mice (4–5 weeks, female, from Charles river) were pretreated with tumor-conditioned medium (50 ul) of MDA-MB-231-LN cells for 2 weeks before inoculation with MDA-MB-231-LN cells. After maraviroc and tocilizumab were administered for 5 weeks, the number of mice with thoracic metastasis was counted using the IVIS imager. The incidence of thoracic metastasis was significantly effective in the combination treatment compared to both single agents (P < 0.0325, Fisher's exact test). **b** Representative thoracic metastasis in the control group and the group treated with a combination of maraviroc and tocilizumab as demonstrated by the IVIS imager. **c** Representative organ images of luciferase-mediated photon flux from lung, lymph node, liver, heart, spleen and brain. **d** Formalin-fixed paraffin embedded tissues from the tumor in the control and the combination of maraviroc (Mara) and cMR16-1 groups were used for immunohistochemistry (IHC) with anti-cytokeratin antibodies on the lungs to indicate metastatic colonies. Low-power microscopes are at × 10 magnification (scale bar 200 um). High-power insets are × 40 magnification (50 um). **e** The IHC results were examined and quantified by ImageJ. **f** Representative immunofluorescence images of mouse CD31 in the lymph node and **g** quantification of results

infection. Our results show that maraviroc inhibits TNBC metastasis so we propose repurposing this drug to treat patients with TNBC. In order to produce even more effective treatments for TNBC using repurposed drugs, we tested tocilizumab, a Food and Drug Administration (FDA)-approved anti-inflammatory IL-6 receptor inhibitor drug for the treatment of rheumatoid arthritis. Application of these two drugs allowed us to directly test the hypothesis that drugs against both IL-6 and CCL5 could be used to treat TNBC. We discovered that co-cultures of MDA-MB-231-LN cells with LECs enhanced proliferation of MDA-MB-231-LN cells. It has been reported that

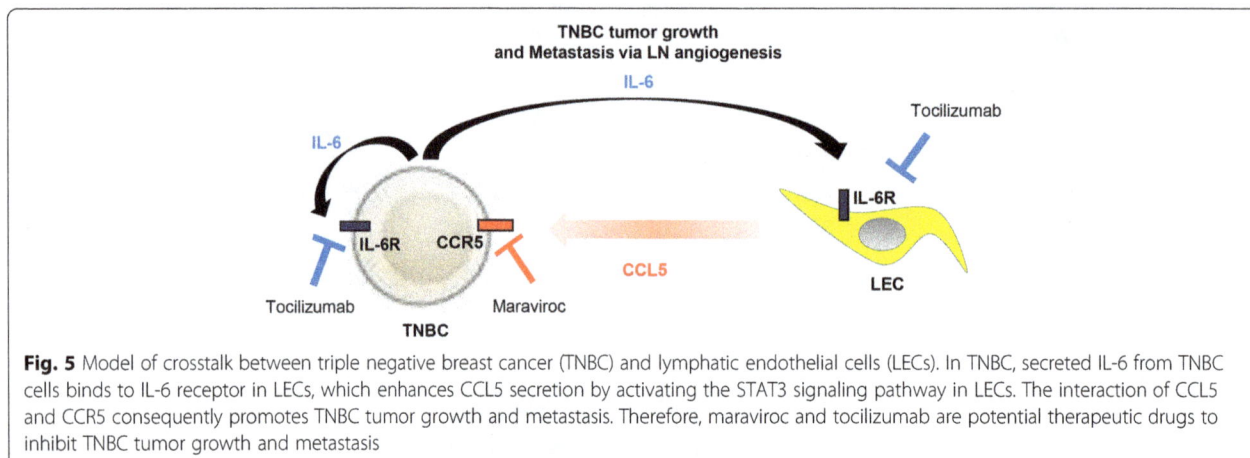

Fig. 5 Model of crosstalk between triple negative breast cancer (TNBC) and lymphatic endothelial cells (LECs). In TNBC, secreted IL-6 from TNBC cells binds to IL-6 receptor in LECs, which enhances CCL5 secretion by activating the STAT3 signaling pathway in LECs. The interaction of CCL5 and CCR5 consequently promotes TNBC tumor growth and metastasis. Therefore, maraviroc and tocilizumab are potential therapeutic drugs to inhibit TNBC tumor growth and metastasis

autocrine IL-6 is a key promoter of TNBC cell proliferation [34, 35]. In support of our hypothesis, in our experiments, tocilizumab significantly decreased the viability of TNBC cells and the combination of tocilizumab and maraviroc decreased cellular viability even more (Fig. 1). Consistent with this result, we observed no significant difference in the viability of TNBC cells in the presence of maraviroc. Our data demonstrate that IL-6 signaling in the crosstalk between TNBC cells and LECs is a major determinant of TNBC cell proliferation and viability.

We next investigated the effect of maraviroc and tocilizumab on the migration of TNBC cells induced by (TCM-LEC)CM. The results indicate that the migration of TNBC cells is dependent on CCL5-CCR5 signaling and that IL-6 indirectly contributes to migration of TNBC cells by regulating CCL5 expression in LECs (Fig. 2). We tested agents targeting the IL-6 and CCR5 pathways in athymic mice with TNBC tumor xenografts to extend these findings. The growth of MDA-MB-231-LN tumors was inhibited by cMR16-1, whereas maraviroc had no effect on tumor growth, consistent with our observation that maraviroc had no effect on the proliferation of MDA-MB-231-LN cells. The combination of maraviroc and cMR16-1 resulted in greater inhibition of tumor growth compared to the single agents (Fig. 3). Next, we were interested in determining whether maraviroc and cMR16-1 could inhibit TNBC tumor metastasis. Thoracic metastasis was detected in all control group mice while mice treated with either maraviroc or cMR16-1 had low incidences of metastasis. Strikingly, we observed no metastasis in any of the mice treated with a combination of maraviroc and cMR16-1 (Fig. 4). These observations demonstrate that CCL5-CCR5 and IL-6-IL-6R signaling between TNBC cells and LECs plays a critical role in TNBC tumor growth and metastasis.

Evidence from our previous studies suggests that TNBC cells secrete IL-6, which interacts with the IL-6 receptor on tumor-associated lymphatic vessels in the tumor microenvironment or on lymphatic vessels in distant organs and that the activated IL-6 receptor stimulates the STAT3 signaling pathway, which results in upregulated CCL5 expression and secretion by LECs. As a result, CCL5 induces LN angiogenesis, and lung and thoracic metastasis. We propose using maraviroc and tocilizumab to block TNBC metastasis through the lymphatic system (Fig. 5).

Conclusions

Taken together, these studies confirmed that IL-6 and CCL5 function as critical molecules in TNBC growth and metastasis. Furthermore, maraviroc and tocilizumab could be repurposed and provide a new clinical approach to treat TNBC.

Additional file

Additional file 1: Figure S1. Cellular viability assays of co-cultured SUM149 (**A**) and SUM159 (**B**) cells on the bottom chambers with LECs on the top chamber in treatment with various concentration of maraviroc and d tocilizumab (transwell plates). The cellular viability was measured for 72 h by MTT assay (*$P < 0.001$, $n = 3$). **C** Crystal violet staining assay was performed in treatment with maraviroc (2 uM), tocilizumab (200 μg/ml), and the combination of maraviroc and tocilizumab. **Figure S2.** Migration assay of SUM149 (**A**) and SUM159 (**B**) cells (top chamber) in CM (bottom chamber) from LECs co-cultured with two TNBC cells with treatment with maraviroc, tocilizumab, and the combination of both. The migrated cells were counted for 24 h by the crystal violet staining. The representative migration is shown. (**$P < 0.001$, $n = 3$). **C** Migration assay of TNBC cells in CM from LECs co-cultured with TNBC cells with tocilizumab pre-treatment. The cells were pre-labeled with Cell Tracker Green and the migration was measured using the Oris cell migration kit. ELISA of human CCL5 (Quantikine ELISA, R&D System) in the CM of LECs co-cultured with SUM149 (**D**) and SUM159 (**E**) cells pre-treated tocilizumab (*$P < 0.001$, $n = 3$). (PDF 271 kb)

Abbreviations

Ang: Angiogenin; BEC: Blood endothelial cell; CCL5: Chemokine (C-C motif) ligand 5; CCR5: CCL receptor 5; CIM: Cell invasion and migration; CM: Conditioned medium; c-MET: Hepatocyte growth factor receptor; DCs: Immature dendritic cells; EGF: Epidermal growth factor; ELISA: Enzyme-linked immunosorbent assay; FBS: Fetal bovine serum; FGF: Fibroblast growth factor; GM: Growth medium; HGF: Hepatocyte growth factor; IGF: Insulin-like growth factor; IL-6: Interleukin-6; i.p.: Intraperitoneal/intraperitoneally; LECs: Lymphatic endothelial cells; LNs: Lymph nodes; PBS: Phosphate-buffered saline; PDGF: Platelet-derived growth factor; RT: Room temperature; SFM: Serum-free medium; STAT3: Signal transducer and activator of transcription 3; TAMs: Tumor-associated macrophages; TCM: Tumor-conditioned medium; TNBC: Triple-negative breast cancer; VEGF: Vascular endothelial growth factor; VEGFR: Vascular endothelial growth factor receptor

Acknowledgments
We thank Pfizer for providing maraviroc, Genentech for providing tocilizumab and cMR16-1, and ACEA Biosciences and Dr. Yama Abassi for technical advice in using the RTCA system.

Funding
This work was supported by the National Institutes of Health grant R01 CA138264.

Authors' contributions
Conception and design: KJ, NBP, and ASP. Development of methodology: KJ and NBP. Laboratory experiments: KJ. Analysis and interpretation of data: KJ, NBP, and ASP. Writing and review of the manuscript: KJ, NBP, and ASP. Administrative, technical, or material support: KJ, NBP, and ASP. All authors read and approved the final manuscript.

Competing interests
The authors declare that they have no competing interests.

Author details
[1]Department of Pharmaceutical Sciences, Albany College of Pharmacy and Health Sciences, Albany, NY 12208, USA. [2]Department of Biomedical Engineering, Johns Hopkins University School of Medicine, Baltimore, MD 21205, USA. [3]Department of Oncology and Sidney Kimmel Comprehensive Cancer Center, Johns Hopkins University School of Medicine, Baltimore, MD, USA.

References
1. Lee E, Pandey NB, Popel AS. Crosstalk between cancer cells and blood endothelial and lymphatic endothelial cells in tumour and organ microenvironment. Expert Rev Mol Med. 2015;17:e3.
2. Karnezis T, Shayan R, Caesar C, Roufail S, Harris NC, Ardipradja K, Zhang YF, Williams SP, Farnsworth RH, Chai MG, et al. VEGF-D promotes tumor metastasis by regulating prostaglandins produced by the collecting lymphatic endothelium. Cancer Cell. 2012;21(2):181–95.
3. Wakisaka N, Hasegawa Y, Yoshimoto S, Miura K, Shiotani A, Yokoyama J, Sugasawa M, Moriyama-Kita M, Endo K, Yoshizaki T. Primary tumor-secreted lymphangiogenic factors induce pre-metastatic lymphvascular niche formation at sentinel lymph nodes in oral squamous cell carcinoma. PLoS One. 2015;10(12):e0144056.
4. Cao Y. Opinion: emerging mechanisms of tumour lymphangiogenesis and lymphatic metastasis. Nat Rev Cancer. 2005;5(9):735–43.
5. Von Marschall Z, Scholz A, Stacker SA, Achen MG, Jackson DG, Alves F, Schirner M, Haberey M, Thierauch KH, Wiedenmann B, et al. Vascular endothelial growth factor-D induces lymphangiogenesis and lymphatic metastasis in models of ductal pancreatic cancer. Int J Oncol. 2005;27(3):669–79.
6. Kesler CT, Liao S, Munn LL, Padera TP. Lymphatic vessels in health and disease. Wiley Interdiscip Rev Syst Biol Med. 2013;5(1):111–24.
7. Sleeman JP. The lymph node pre-metastatic niche. J Mol Med (Berl). 2015;93(11):1173–84.
8. Lee E, Fertig EJ, Jin K, Sukumar S, Pandey NB, Popel AS. Breast cancer cells condition lymphatic endothelial cells within pre-metastatic niches to promote metastasis. Nat Commun. 2014;5:4715.
9. Lee E, Rosca EV, Pandey NB, Popel AS. Small peptides derived from somatotropin domain-containing proteins inhibit blood and lymphatic endothelial cell proliferation, migration, adhesion and tube formation. Int J Biochem Cell Biol. 2011;43(12):1812–21.
10. Chou TC, Talalay P. Quantitative analysis of dose-effect relationships: the combined effects of multiple drugs or enzyme inhibitors. Adv Enzym Regul. 1984;22:27–55.
11. Chou TC. Drug combination studies and their synergy quantification using the Chou-Talalay method. Cancer Res. 2010;70(2):440–6.
12. Koskimaki JE, Lee E, Chen W, Rivera CG, Rosca EV, Pandey NB, Popel AS. Synergy between a collagen IV mimetic peptide and a somatotropin-domain derived peptide as angiogenesis and lymphangiogenesis inhibitors. Angiogenesis. 2013;16(1):159–70.
13. Lee E, Pandey NB, Popel AS. Lymphatic endothelial cells support tumor growth in breast cancer. Sci Rep. 2014;4:5853.
14. Lee E, Pandey NB, Popel AS. Pre-treatment of mice with tumor-conditioned media accelerates metastasis to lymph nodes and lungs: a new spontaneous breast cancer metastasis model. Clin Exp Metastasis. 2014;31(1):67–79.
15. Achen MG, Stacker SA. Tumor lymphangiogenesis and metastatic spread-new players begin to emerge. Int J Cancer. 2006;119(8):1755–60.
16. Dieterich LC, Detmar M. Tumor lymphangiogenesis and new drug development. Adv Drug Deliv Rev. 2016;99(Pt B):148–60.
17. Steinskog ES, Sagstad SJ, Wagner M, Karlsen TV, Yang N, Markhus CE, Yndestad S, Wiig H, Eikesdal HP. Impaired lymphatic function accelerates cancer growth. Oncotarget. 2016;7(29):45789–802.
18. Joukov V, Sorsa T, Kumar V, Jeltsch M, Claesson-Welsh L, Cao Y, Saksela O, Kalkkinen N, Alitalo K. Proteolytic processing regulates receptor specificity and activity of VEGF-C. EMBO J. 1997;16(13):3898–911.
19. Stacker SA, Stenvers K, Caesar C, Vitali A, Domagala T, Nice E, Roufail S, Simpson RJ, Moritz R, Karpanen T, et al. Biosynthesis of vascular endothelial growth factor-D involves proteolytic processing which generates non-covalent homodimers. J Biol Chem. 1999;274(45):32127–36.
20. Hirakawa S, Kodama S, Kunstfeld R, Kajiya K, Brown LF, Detmar M. VEGF-A induces tumor and sentinel lymph node lymphangiogenesis and promotes lymphatic metastasis. J Exp Med. 2005;201(7):1089–99.
21. Bjorndahl MA, Cao R, Burton JB, Brakenhielm E, Religa P, Galter D, Wu L, Cao Y. Vascular endothelial growth factor-a promotes peritumoral lymphangiogenesis and lymphatic metastasis. Cancer Res. 2005;65(20):9261–8.
22. Schulz P, Fischer C, Detjen KM, Rieke S, Hilfenhaus G, von Marschall Z, Bohmig M, Koch I, Kehrberger J, Hauff P, et al. Angiopoietin-2 drives lymphatic metastasis of pancreatic cancer. FASEB J. 2011;25(10):3325–35.
23. Fagiani E, Lorentz P, Kopfstein L, Christofori G. Angiopoietin-1 and -2 exert antagonistic functions in tumor angiogenesis, yet both induce lymphangiogenesis. Cancer Res. 2011;71(17):5717–27.
24. Kajiya K, Hirakawa S, Ma B, Drinnenberg I, Detmar M. Hepatocyte growth factor promotes lymphatic vessel formation and function. EMBO J. 2005;24(16):2885–95.
25. Jiang WG, Davies G, Martin TA, Parr C, Watkins G, Mansel RE, Mason MD. The potential lymphangiogenic effects of hepatocyte growth factor/scatter factor in vitro and in vivo. Int J Mol Med. 2005;16(4):723–8.
26. Cao R, Bjorndahl MA, Gallego MI, Chen S, Religa P, Hansen AJ, Cao Y. Hepatocyte growth factor is a lymphangiogenic factor with an indirect mechanism of action. Blood. 2006;107(9):3531–6.
27. Platonova N, Miquel G, Regenfuss B, Taouji S, Cursiefen C, Chevet E, Bikfalvi A. Evidence for the interaction of fibroblast growth factor-2 with the lymphatic endothelial cell marker LYVE-1. Blood. 2013;121(7):1229–37.
28. Marino D, Angehrn Y, Klein S, Riccardi S, Baenziger-Tobler N, Otto VI, Pittelkow M, Detmar M. Activation of the epidermal growth factor receptor promotes lymphangiogenesis in the skin. J Dermatol Sci. 2013;71(3):184–94.
29. Cao R, Bjorndahl MA, Religa P, Clasper S, Garvin S, Galter D, Meister B, Ikomi F, Tritsaris K, Dissing S, et al. PDGF-BB induces intratumoral lymphangiogenesis and promotes lymphatic metastasis. Cancer Cell. 2004;6(4):333–45.
30. Li ZJ, Ying XJ, Chen HL, Ye PJ, Chen ZL, Li G, Jiang HF, Liu J, Zhou SZ. Insulin-like growth factor-1 induces lymphangiogenesis and facilitates lymphatic metastasis in colorectal cancer. World J Gastroenterol. 2013;19(43):7788–94.

31. Velasco-Velazquez M, Jiao X, De La Fuente M, Pestell TG, Ertel A, Lisanti MP,
      Pestell RG. CCR5 antagonist blocks metastasis of basal breast cancer cells.
      Cancer Res. 2012;72(15):3839–50.
32. Velasco-Velazquez M, Xolalpa W, Pestell RG. The potential to target CCL5/CCR5
      in breast cancer. Expert Opin Ther Targets. 2014;18(11):1265–75.
33. Velasco-Velazquez M, Pestell RG. The CCL5/CCR5 axis promotes metastasis
      in basal breast cancer. Oncoimmunology. 2013;2(4):e23660.
34. Hartman ZC, Poage GM, den Hollander P, Tsimelzon A, Hill J, Panupinthu N,
      Zhang Y, Mazumdar A, Hilsenbeck SG, Mills GB, et al. Growth of triple-negative
      breast cancer cells relies upon coordinate autocrine expression of the
      proinflammatory cytokines IL-6 and IL-8. Cancer Res. 2013;73(11):3470–80.
35. Lin C, Liao W, Jian Y, Peng Y, Zhang X, Ye L, Cui Y, Wang B, Wu X, Xiong Z,
      et al. CGI-99 promotes breast cancer metastasis via autocrine interleukin-6
      signaling. Oncogene. 2017;36(26):3695-705.

Hyperprolactinemia-inducing antipsychotics increase breast cancer risk by activating JAK-STAT5 in precancerous lesions

A. N. Johnston[1,2,3], W. Bu[2,3,4], S. Hein[2,3,4], S. Garcia[5], L. Camacho[2,3], L. Xue[2,3], L. Qin[2,3], C. Nagi[3], S. G. Hilsenbeck[2,3], J. Kapali[2], K. Podsypanina[6,7], J. Nangia[3] and Y. Li[1,2,3,4,8]* (iD)

Abstract

Background: Psychiatric medications are widely prescribed in the USA. Many antipsychotics cause serum hyperprolactinemia as an adverse side effect; prolactin-Janus kinase 2 (JAK2)-signal transducer and activator of transcription 5 (STAT5) signaling both induces cell differentiation and suppresses apoptosis. It is controversial whether these antipsychotics increase breast cancer risk.

Methods: We investigated the impact of several antipsychotics on mammary tumorigenesis initiated by retrovirus-mediated delivery of either *ErbB2* or *HRas* or by transgenic expression of *Wnt-1*.

Results: We found that the two hyperprolactinemia-inducing antipsychotics, risperidone and pimozide, prompted precancerous lesions to progress to cancer while aripiprazole, which did not cause hyperprolactinemia, did not. We observed that risperidone and pimozide (but not aripiprazole) caused precancerous cells to activate STAT5 and suppress apoptosis while exerting no impact on proliferation. Importantly, we demonstrated that these effects of antipsychotics on early lesions required the *STAT5* gene function. Furthermore, we showed that only two-week treatment of mice with ruxolitinib, a JAK1/2 inhibitor, blocked STAT5 activation, restored apoptosis, and prevented early lesion progression.

Conclusions: Hyperprolactinemia-inducing antipsychotics instigate precancerous cells to progress to cancer via JAK/STAT5 to suppress the apoptosis anticancer barrier, and these cancer-promoting effects can be prevented by prophylactic anti-JAK/STAT5 treatment. This preclinical work exposes a potential breast cancer risk from hyperprolactinemia-inducing antipsychotics in certain patients and suggests a chemoprevention regime that is relatively easy to implement compared to the standard 5-year anti-estrogenic treatment in women who have or likely have already developed precancerous lesions while also requiring hyperprolactinemia-inducing antipsychotics.

Keywords: Cancer, Breast cancer, Antipsychotics, Neuroleptics, Prolactin, STAT5, JAK, Ruxolitinib, Mammary gland

Background

Psychiatric medications are among the top five drugs in sales in the USA [1]. Both typical (class 1) and atypical (class 2) antipsychotics (also known as neuroleptics) act by antagonizing dopamine and thus blocking post-synaptic dopamine D2 receptors in the pituitary gland; atypical antipsychotics additionally suppress serotonin

receptors [2]. Dopaminergic receptors typically suppress prolactin (PRL) production and secretion; thus, a multitude of antipsychotics are associated with elevated serum PRL [2]. A retrospective study of 422 psychiatric patients found that antipsychotic therapy was strongly associated with hyperprolactinemia [3], and that serum PRL levels were affected in a dose-dependent manner [4–6].

PRL binds to its receptor PRLR to activate Janus kinase 2 (JAK2). JAK2 then phosphorylates and activates the signal transducer and activator of transcription 5 (STAT5). Once phosphorylated, STAT5 forms homodimers or heterodimerizes with another STAT family

* Correspondence: liyi@bcm.edu
[1]Translational Biology and Molecular Medicine, Baylor College of Medicine, Houston, TX 77030, USA
[2]Lester and Sue Smith Breast Center, Baylor College of Medicine, Baylor College of Medicine, Houston, TX 77030, USA
Full list of author information is available at the end of the article

member, translocates to the nucleus, and transactivates its targets, which regulate alveolar differentiation and milk production and proliferation and apoptosis [7]. PRL-JAK2-STAT5 signaling is highly activated during late pregnancy and lactation, and is required for alveolar expansion and milk production [7]. Transgenic or retrovirus-mediated expression of constitutively activated STAT5 in normal mammary epithelia in nulliparous mice causes alveolar differentiation and milk production [8, 9]. Hyperprolactinemia associated with the use of antipsychotics of both classes often causes mammary swelling and lactation that are not associated with pregnancy [10]. Mammary cell differentiation caused by PRL-PRLR-JAK2-STAT5 signaling is a mechanism by which an early-age pregnancy reduces breast cancer risk [11]. However, we have also reported that STAT5 activation in preexistent precancerous lesions in mice instigates accelerated progression to cancer via suppression of the apoptosis anticancer barrier [11]. This finding provides an explanation for increased breast cancer risk associated with a late-age pregnancy when early lesions may have already formed. Activated forms of JAK2 and STAT5 have been reported in human early breast lesions and cancer [7, 12–16] and in other human cancers [7, 17].

While it explains the dichotomous effects of early versus late-age pregnancy on breast cancer risk, the dual-role of PRL-JAK2-STAT5 in both promoting normal cell differentiation and suppressing the anticancer barrier in precancerous cells also predicts that hyperprolactinemia-inducing antipsychotics may have a similar dichotomous impact on breast tumorigenesis – reducing breast cancer risk when taken at a young age but increasing breast cancer risk if started at an older age or when early lesions have already been diagnosed. However, when started at an early age, this type of medication is usually taken for decades or for lifetime [18], likely leading to protection against breast cancer earlier on but increased risk later in life. Therefore, epidemiological studies of breast cancer risk in patients on antipsychotics must consider hyperprolactinemia, starting age and length of treatment, precancerous lesion status, and multiple other confounding factors such as obesity and poor health status [2, 19–23]. The limited work in this area has not stratified patients to consider all of these variables. Not surprisingly, these studies have resulted in inconclusive or contradictory reports [19, 24–31], although a few studies have detected a significant increase in breast cancer in women who were prescribed dopamine antagonists compared to age-matched controls who were not prescribed antipsychotics [32, 33]. Data from well-controlled laboratory studies may provide the experimental foundation for sophisticated epidemiological studies that will involve multiple patient registries and are stringently controlled. Importantly, laboratory studies may especially expose potential cancer risk of administering hyperprolactinemia-inducing antipsychotics in patients who may have already developed precancerous lesions. However, there have been no significant laboratory studies to investigate the influence of antipsychotics on breast cancer risk. Here, we report that in mouse models that closely mimic human breast cancer initiation, hyperprolactinemia-inducing antipsychotics accelerate early lesion progression to cancer via activation of JAK-STAT5 signaling to suppress the apoptosis anticancer barrier. These findings highlight the potential risk associated with the use of hyperprolactinemia-inducing antipsychotics in women at risk of breast cancer and urgently calls for epidemiological studies specifically designed to examine breast cancer risk in women who have already developed precancerous lesions while also requiring hyperprolactinemia-inducing antipsychotics.

Methods

Experimental animals

The mouse mammary tumour virus promoter (MMTV-tva) (MA line) and STAT5a$^{-/-}$ mice used in this study are on a Friend virus B (FVB) genetic background and have been previously reported [34, 35]. Briefly, lesion initiation is achieved by intraductal injection of a Rous sarcoma virus-based vector - replication-competent avian sarcoma (RCAS) - to deliver an oncogene into a minute subset of mammary epithelial cells in an otherwise normally developed mammary gland [34]. This allows cancer to initiate in a "field" of normal mammary cells in a normal mammary gland as human breast cancer usually initiates and evolves [34]. This subset of mammary epithelial cells was made susceptible to RCAS infection by transgenic expression of the gene encoding the RCAS receptor TVA from the MMTV promoter (MMTV-tva) [34]. STAT5a$^{-/-}$ mice have been previously described [35]; the STAT5a knockout mice on the FVB background have normal mammary development unlike those on the 129 background [11, 35]. All animals were handled according to the animal protocol approved by Baylor College of Medicine (BCM) Institutional Animal Care and Use Committee (IACUC).

Early lesion and tumor studies

RCAS virus was prepared as previously described [34, 36] and was intraductally injected into MMTV-tva mice at 10 weeks of age. Five days later they were randomized and treated with either a drug or diluent for 2 weeks (early lesion studies) or until euthanasia (tumor study). Mice in the tumor latency study were palpated thrice weekly and tumor size was recorded. When tumors reached 2.0 cm in diameter, cumulatively, the mice were euthanized. Tumor-free mice were euthanized 12 months post injection.

Drug treatments

Pimozide (cat. no. P1793; Sigma-Aldrich) was intraperitoneally (IP) administered daily at 5 mg/kg. Risperidone (cat. no. 1604654; Sigma-Aldrich) was delivered IP daily (3 mg/kg) for 2 weeks (early lesion study) or in drinking water (1.56 mg/l) until euthanasia (tumor latency study), resulting in the same daily dose based on the calculation previously reported [37]. Aripiprazole (cat. no. SML0935; Sigma-Aldrich) was delivered via IP injection in a daily dose of 3 mg/kg for 2 weeks, and clomipramine (cat. no. 1140247; Sigma-Aldrich) was delivered in drinking water (190 mg/l), resulting in a daily dose of 28 mg/kg. All drugs were diluted in dimethyl sulfoxide (DMSO) to the appropriate concentrations. Both ruxolitinib and control chow was provided by Incyte Corp. Ruxolitinib chow was packaged in a pre-determined measurement of 2000 mg/kg chow; mice were allowed to free-feed for the duration of the study.

Serum PRL

Serum PRL was determined using the Sigma-Aldrich Mouse Prolactin ELISA kit (RAB0408) using the manufacturer's protocol.

Immunostaining and microscopy

Immunohistochemistry analysis (IHC) and immunofluorescence (IF) were performed as previously described [9, 11, 34]. MOM and vectastain Elite ABC rabbit kits (cat.no. PK-2200 and PK-6101; Vector Laboratories) were used according to the manufacturer's protocols. Primary antibodies used included mouse monoclonal antibodies against HA (1:250; cat.no.901503; Covance) and BCL-xL (1:50; cat.no. K1308; Santa Cruz) and rabbit antibodies against pSTAT5 1:300; cat.no. 9359 L; Cell Signaling), cleaved caspase 3 (1:300; cat.no. Asp175; Cell Signaling), and Ki67 (1:300; cat.no. MIB-1; Lycra). Secondary antibodies for IF were Alexa Fluor 568 goat-anti-rabbit, and Alexa 488 goat-anti-mouse. Nuclei were counterstained with 4′-6-diamidino-2-phenylindole (DAPI)-containing mounting medium and hematoxylin, respectively, for IF and IHC. TUNEL assay was performed using the ApopTag Red in situ TUNEL detection Kit (Chemicon, S7165). Bright-field images were captured using a Leica DMLB microscope. IF images were captured using the Zeiss Axiskop2 plus microscope.

Quantification of stained sections

For quantification of cells stained for a marker, 10 random fields of early lesions in each mammary gland were captured, and both positively stained cells and the total number of cells in the lesion as identified by DAPI or hematoxylin staining were counted to determine the percentage of positivity. ImageJ software was used for counting cells and determining lesion size. The total

numbers of cells in IF images were counted using a semi-automotive program that has been previously described [38]. Fixed thresholds were set to analyze both experimental and control mammary glands.

Lung metastasis study

Lung metastases were detected by the quantitative-PCR (qPCR) method using a set of primers specific for the RCAS provirus (CTTCCCTGCCGCTTCC; FWD: AGCCGCCTCAAGTCATGATG; GCTCTTTCCAATG-TACCGATAACCT). DNA was extracted from the largest, left-most lobe of the lung. A mammary tumor induced by RCAS-caErbB2 was used as positive control, and a lung from a FVB mouse without virus injection was used as negative control. The relative amounts of the RCAS provirus with respect to the endogenous gene β-actin were determined using the 7500 Fast System software provided by Applied Biosystems.

Statistical analysis

All numbers in this study are reported as medians and interquartile ranges in the format median (IQR). Statistical analyses of quantification of stained sections were performed using analysis of variance (ANOVA) or the Mann-Whitney test. In cases where data were distributed normally, Student's t test for independent samples with Holm's correction for multiple comparisons was used. Tumor-free survival analysis was performed using the generalized Gehan-Wilcoxon test with Rho = 1, and Kaplan-Meier survival curves. All tumor-free survival analyses were performed in R with the survival package using R commander interface. All other graphs were generated using Prism software. Each dot in the dot plots generated for this study represents one mouse.

Results

Treatment with hyperprolactinemia-inducing antipsychotics accelerates tumorigenesis from breast cancer cells with an oncogenic mutation

We have reported a mouse model that closely mimics human breast cancer initiation and is ideally suited for studying hormones and other factors that may impact breast cancer risk [9, 11, 34, 38–42]. Tumor initiation is achieved by intraductal injection of a Rous sarcoma virus-based vector, RCAS, to deliver an oncogene into a small subset of mammary epithelial cells (< 0.3% of the mammary gland) in a normally developed mammary gland so that cancer initiates in a "field" of normal mammary cells in a normal mammary gland as most human breast cancers initiate and evolve [34]. This subset of mammary epithelial cells was made susceptible to RCAS infection by transgenic expression of the gene encoding the RCAS receptor TVA from the MMTV promoter (MMTV-tva) [34]. The transgenic avian tva is only required for the initial virus infection; the virus does not replicate in mammalian cells. Additionally, the oncogene is transcriptionally controlled by the proviral RCAS long terminal repeat (LTR); it is constitutively active and is not influenced by the presence of reproductive hormones such as prolactin [39, 43]. Using this method, we explored the effect of several antipsychotics on mammary cancer development from preexisting early lesions. We injected 10 week-old MMTV-*tva* mice intraductally with RCAS-caErbB2 to infect approximately 0.3% of the luminal epithelial cells [34, 44]. RCAS-caErbB2 expresses a constitutively active form of rat *ErbB2* (*HER2/ Neu*); *ErbB2* is amplified/mutated in 20–25% of human breast cancers [45]. Five days following injection, mice were randomized for treatment with risperidone (3 mg/ kg daily), a commonly prescribed class 2, "atypical" antipsychotic that is known to cause hyperprolactinemia [2], or with vehicle. Introduction of the oncogene took place before drug treatment so as to specifically investigate antipsychotic effects on preexisting precancerous early

lesions rather than the overall risk that antipsychotics may pose on the normal mammary epithelia. Mice were continually treated with either risperidone or the diluent control in drinking water for the duration of the study. While vehicle-treated mice developed tumors with a median latency of 112 days, the risperidone cohort developed tumors with a median latency of only 59 days (*p* = 0.000138; Fig. 1a). Additionally, the risperidone-treated cohort had a greater tumor multiplicity than the control (*p* = 0.002; Fig. 1b). When the tumor size reached 2.0 cm in diameter, mice were euthanized. As expected, serum PRL levels were significantly increased in the risperidone cohort (*p* = 0.004; Fig. 1c). Tumors from both cohorts were high-grade, poorly differentiated, and highly mitotic with areas of necrosis. Many of the tumor cells were highly pleomorphic with large nuclei, often with metaplastic features. These tumors extensively invaded the surrounding fibroadipose tissue, skeletal muscle, and nerves (Additional file 1: Figure S1A). Likewise, incidence of pulmonary metastasis was

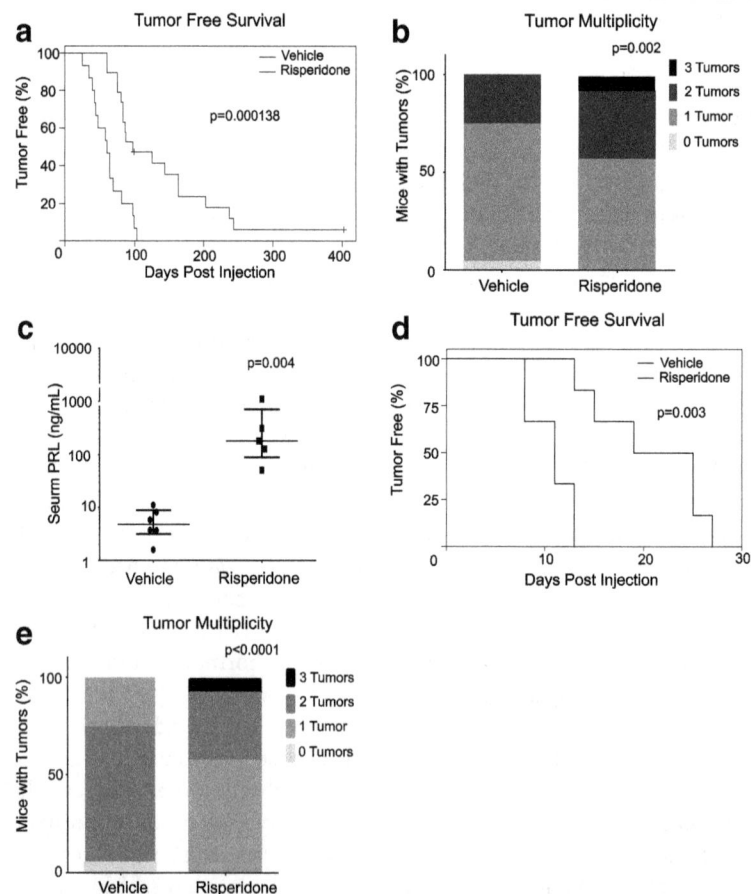

Fig. 1 Risperidone promotes carcinogenesis initiated by ca*ErbB2* and *HrasQ61L*. **a** Kaplan-Meier tumor-free survival curve of mice infected by replication-competent avian sarcoma (RCAS)-caErbB2. The *p* value was determined by the generalized Gehan-Wilcoxon test with Rho = 1. **b** Tumor multiplicity. The chi square test was for used comparison. **c** Serum prolactin (PRL) levels. The Mann-Whitney test was used to determine the *p* values. Each dot in this plot represents one mouse. **d** Kaplan-Meier tumor-free survival curve of mice infected by RCAS-HRasQ61L. The *p* value was determined by the generalized Gehan-Wilcoxon test with Rho = 1. **e** Tumor multiplicity. The chi square test was for used comparison

similar in the two cohorts of mice based on qPCR analysis of the RCAS-proviral load ($p = 0.753$; Additional file 1: Figure S1B). Therefore, we conclude that treatment with risperidone accelerates tumorigenesis and increases tumor multiplicity in mice with preexisting precancerous mammary lesions, while not influencing the grade, aggressiveness, or metastatic potential of the resulting tumors.

To investigate whether risperidone also accelerated tumorigenesis initiated by other oncogenic events, we injected MMTV-*tva* mice (n = 25), at 10 weeks of age, with RCAS carrying an activated form of *HRas*, *HRasQ61L* (RCAS-HRasQ61L). *RAS* genes are known to be amplified/overexpressed/mutated in a subset of human breast cancer, and their protein products often activated [46–49]. Five days following injection, mice were continually treated with risperidone or vehicle in their drinking water. While vehicle-treated mice developed tumors with a median latency of 25 days, the

risperidone cohort developed tumors with a median latency of only 11 days ($p = 0.003$; Fig. 1d). Additionally, the risperidone-treated cohort had a higher tumor multiplicity than the control ($p < 0.0001$; Fig. 1e). Taken together, these data suggest that risperidone stimulates tumorigenesis initiated by multiple oncogenic events.

We next determined if this tumorigenic acceleration was due to antipsychotic effects on early lesion development. Here we used RCAS-caErbB2-infected mice and treated them with risperidone or vehicle for only 2 weeks. Early lesions were defined as any hyperplastic ductal foci comprised of three or more layers of epithelial cells stained positively for the provirus-encoded oncogene product HA tag. Risperidone-treated mice had more early lesions and higher early lesion burden than the vehicle control cohort (Fig. 2a). Therefore, we conclude that risperidone promotes early lesion progression.

To test whether the above-observed risperidone effect on mammary early lesions is broadly applicable across

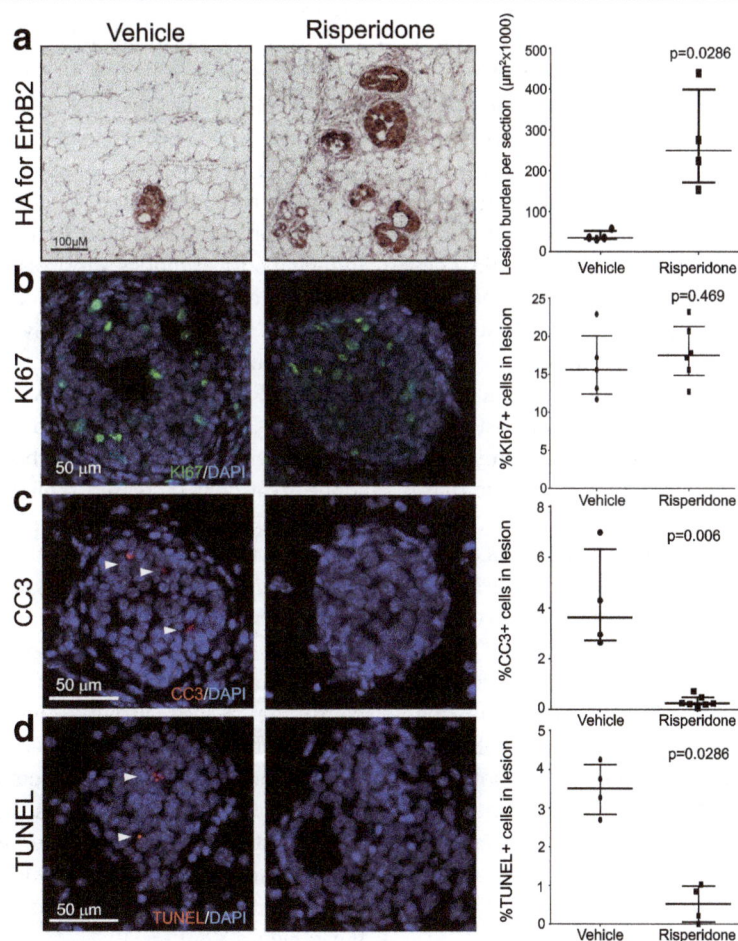

Fig. 2 Risperidone increases early lesion burden and lowers the level of apoptosis. **a** Immunohistochemistry analysis and the accompanying dot plot for the HA tag on replication-competent avian sarcoma (RCAS)-caErbB2 provirus. **b** Immunofluorescence for Ki67 and the accompanying dot plot. **c** and **d** Immunofluorescence staining for cleaved caspase 3 (**c**) and TUNEL assay (**d**) with the accompanying dot plots. The *p* values were determined by the Mann-Whitney test. Each dot in these plots represents one mouse

different subtypes of breast cancer, we administered risperidone or vehicle to mice transgenic for MMTV-*Wnt1* [50], which develops basal-like tumors and some estrogen receptor (ER)-positive tumors [51–53]. Mice treated with risperidone for 2 weeks developed extensive ductal branching and many more and larger early lesions compared to vehicle-treated mice (Additional file 2: Figure S2A-2B). Taken together, these data suggest that risperidone stimulates the progression of early lesions that are the precursor to multiple breast cancer subtypes.

To determine the underlying mechanisms by which risperidone spurred early lesion expansion, we first compared the precancerous cell proliferation in these two cohorts of mice injected with RCAS-caErbB2. Ki67 staining detected approximately 20% of positive cells in both sets of early lesions ($p = 0.469$; Fig. 2b), suggesting that proliferation did not play a significant role in risperidone acceleration of early lesion development. Besides cell proliferation, evasion of apoptosis serves a key role in the progression of precancerous early lesions to cancer [54, 55]. We have reported that apoptosis was rapidly activated in mammary cells following *ErbB2* activation to provide a barrier to cancer [11, 42, 44]. Both cleaved caspase 3 (CC3) and TUNEL detected robust apoptosis (3.6% (2.7–6.3%) and 3.5% (2.8–4.1%), respectively) in early lesions in vehicle-treated mice, as expected; however, these apoptosis levels were diminished in the risperidone cohort (0.2% (0.07–0.5%), $p = 0.006$ and 0.5% (0.05–0.9%), $p = 0.0286$, respectively) (Fig. 2c-d). These results demonstrate that treatment with risperidone allows precancerous cells to suppress the apoptotic anticancer barrier to increase early lesion burden.

To test whether other hyperprolactinemia-inducing antipsychotics also instigate early lesion progression, we treated a separate cohort of early lesion-bearing mice with pimozide, which is a "typical", class 1 antipsychotic that is also known to induce hyperprolactinemia [10]. As expected, this antipsychotic also led to hyperprolactinemia in these mice ($p = 0.007$; Additional file 3: Figure S3A). Like risperidone, pimozide (5 mg/kg daily) for 2 weeks increased early lesion numbers (from 22 (12.8–31) to 64 (42.5–98), $p = 0.004$) and led to a greater early lesion burden (Additional file 4: Figure S4A). While not affecting cell proliferation (Additional file 4: Figure S4B), pimozide suppressed apoptosis in early lesions based on both CC3 and TUNEL ($p = 0.0002$ and $p = 0.0007$, respectively; Additional file 4: Figure S4C-3D). Taken together, these data indicate that hyperprolactinemia-inducing antipsychotics dismantle the apoptosis anticancer barrier in early lesions and instigate their progression to cancer.

To investigate whether antipsychotics that do not cause hyperprolactinemia have the potential to accelerate early lesion progression, we tested aripiprazole, a widely prescribed class 2, "atypical" antipsychotic that

does not elevate prolactin levels but is otherwise mechanistically similar to risperidone [2]. Two weeks of aripiprazole (28 mg/kg daily) did not elevate serum prolactin levels (Additional file 5: Figure S5A), and failed to increase the load of RCAS-caErbB2-initiated early lesions (Additional file 5: Figure S5B). Likewise, this drug did not affect cell proliferation (Additional file 5: Figure S5C) or apoptosis as tested by TUNEL (Additional file 5: Figure S5D). In addition, clomipramine, a commonly prescribed antidepressant that did not cause hyperprolactinemia in our mouse model ($p = 0.151$; Additional file 5: Figure S5E) also failed to increase early lesion burden ($p = 0.687$; Additional file 5: Figure S5F). Together, we conclude that hyperprolactinemia-inducing antipsychotics cause preexisting early lesion to suppress the apoptosis anticancer barrier and to accelerate progression to cancer; these cancer-promoting effects are associated with hyperprolactinemia.

Hyperprolactinemia-inducing antipsychotics activate STAT5

PRL is a key hormone released during pregnancy and lactation, and activates STAT5 via its receptor PRLR and the receptor-associated JAK2 [7]. Forced or pregnancy-associated JAK2/STAT5 activation lowers the apoptosis anticancer barrier in preexisting early lesions and advances the progression to cancer [11]. To understand the underlying mechanism by which hyperprolactinemia-inducing antipsychotics suppress the apoptosis anticancer barrier and increase breast cancer risk, we asked whether treatment with risperidone activates the STAT5 signaling pathway. In vehicle-treated mice bearing early lesions initiated by RCAS-caErbB2, pSTAT5+ cells were detected in 11% (5.7–30.3%) of precancerous cells, a level similar to those previously reported [11]; however, 2 weeks of risperidone treatment increased their population size to 86.4% (84.2–94.3%) ($p = 0.0079$; Fig. 3a). Induction of STAT5 activity was also detected in normal ducts that did not gain ca*ErbB2* (Fig. 3a). We confirmed that serum PRL levels were significantly increased in the risperidone cohort ($p = 0.029$; Fig. 3c). *Bcl-xL* and *β-casein* are genes that are transactivated by STAT5, and their gene products contribute to cell survival and alveolar differentiation, respectively [56, 57]. As expected, β-casein was induced in early lesions and in normal ducts (Fig. 3b). Likewise, Bcl-xL was induced in early lesions (Fig. 3d). Additionally, we found that pSTAT5 levels were elevated in lesions of the risperidone-treated MMTV-Wnt1 transgenic mice compared to the vehicle-treated control cohort (Additional file 2: Figure S2C).

Next, we tested whether pSTAT5 and its transcriptional target β-casein were also upregulated by pimozide. While 7.3% (3.4–14.6%) of cells in the early lesions of vehicle-treated mice were pSTAT5+, 58% (50–89%) of

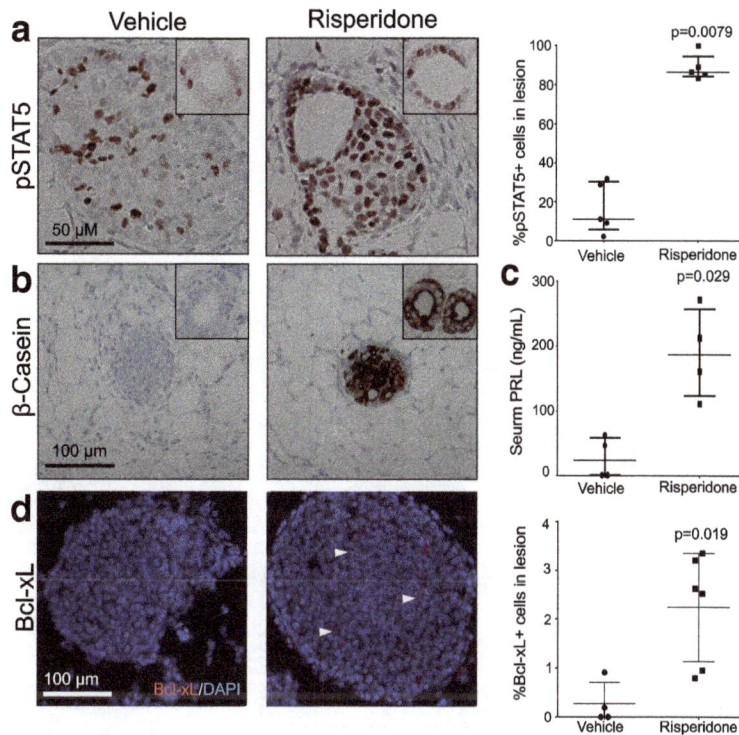

Fig. 3 Risperidone treatment increases signal transducer and activator of transcription 5 (STAT5) activity. **a** Immunohistochemistry staining for pSTAT5 in early precancerous lesions and in normal ducts (inset) and the accompany dot plot. **b** Immunohistochemistry analysis of the downstream effector of STAT5, β-casein, in early lesions and normal ducts (inset). **c** Serum prolactin (PRL) levels. **d** Immunofluorescence and the accompanying dot plot for Bcl-xL. The p values were determined by the Mann-Whitney test. Each dot in these plots represents one mouse

cells in the early lesions of pimozide-treated mice were pSTAT5+ ($p = 0.0007$; Additional file 3: Figure S3B). β-casein was also induced following pimozide administration (Additional file 3: Figure S3C). Of note, pimozide has been reported to block STAT5 activation in cultured cells [58, 59], but this potential direct effect on STAT5 was overridden in vivo by hyperprolactinemia-induced PRL signaling. To further test the association between hyperprolactinemia and activation of STAT5, we also stained for pSTAT5 in early lesions in mice treated with aripiprazole, which did not increase PRL. No evidence of STAT5 activation was detected (Additional file 3: Figure S3D). Together, these data suggest that hyperprolactinemia-inducing antipsychotics activate STAT5 and its transcriptional targets to suppress the apoptosis-anticancer barrier in preexisting precancerous cells, while simultaneously inducing alveolar differentiation in both early lesions and normal ducts.

STAT5a is required for antipsychotic promotion of mammary tumorigenesis

PRL-PRLR signaling activates STAT5 and possibly several other pathways including extracellular

signal-related kinase (Erk) and protein kinase B (Akt) [60]. We tested whether the gene encoding STAT5a, the predominant form of STAT5 in the mammary gland and tumorigenesis [35, 61], is required for the above-observed effects of risperidone on early lesion progression, to investigate whether STAT5 activation is the crucial factor mediating antipsychotic stimulation of carcinogenesis. We utilized $STAT5a^{-/-}$ mice on the FVB background as $STAT5a$ ablation on this background does not significantly impair normal mammary development and lactogenesis [11]. These $STAT5a$ knockout mice were bred to MMTV-tva mice, infected with RCAS-caErBb2, and 5 days later, continually treated with either risperidone or vehicle control for 2 weeks. $STAT5a^{+/+}$/MMTV-tva mice infected with RCAS-caErbB2 were also treated with risperidone for 2 weeks for comparison. Risperidone treatment failed to activate STAT5 in $STAT5a^{-/-}$ mice – the percentage of pSTAT5+ cells was comparable to that in the vehicle-treated mice ($p = 0.908$) and much lower than that in $STAT5a$ wild-type mice treated with risperidone ($p = 0.004$; Fig. 4a). The residual levels of pSTAT5 in $STAT5a^{-/-}$ mice were likely due to the minor player pSTAT5b. Additionally, β-casein, a transcriptional target of STAT5,

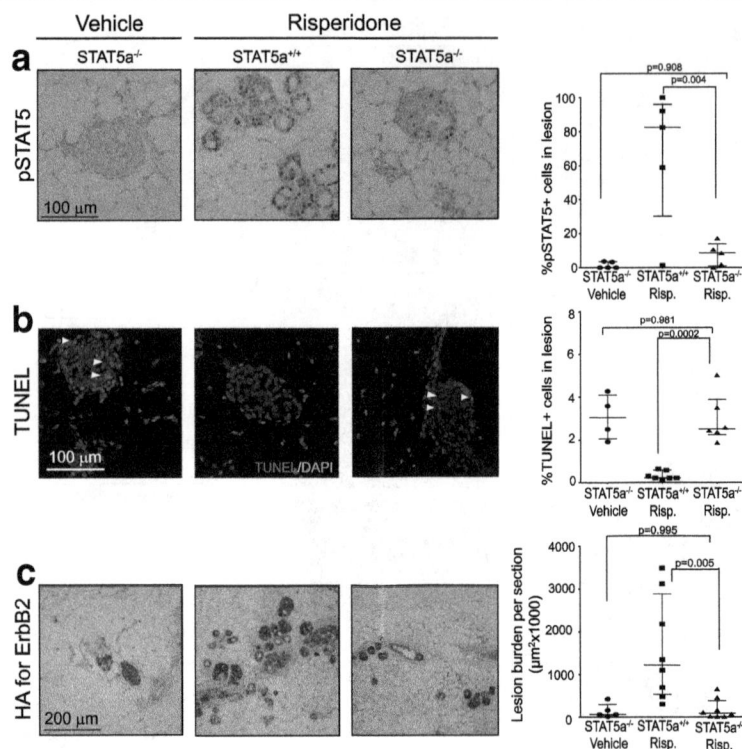

Fig. 4 Genetic ablation of signal transducer and activator of transcription 5 (*STAT5*)*a* dismantles the effects of risperidone on early lesions. **a** pSTAT5 immunohistochemistry analysis and the accompanying dot plot. **b** TUNEL assay and the accompanying dot plot. **c** Immunohistochemistry analysis and the accompanying dot plot for the HA tag on replication-competent avian sarcoma (RCAS)-*caErbB2* provirus. The *p* values were determined by analysis of variance. Each dot in these plots represents one mouse

was elevated in the risperidone-treated *STAT5a* wild-type mice, but severely diminished in the *STAT5a* knockout risperidone-treated group (Additional file 6: Figure S6). Next, we asked if *STAT5a*-knockout-induced diminishment of STAT5 activity restored apoptosis in early lesions in the risperidone cohort. In comparison to the wild-type mice treated with risperidone, the $STAT5a^{-/-}$ mice treated with risperidone had significantly elevated levels of apoptosis as measured by TUNEL ($p = 0.0002$; Fig. 4b), which were comparable to those in the vehicle-treated $STAT5a^{-/-}$ mice ($p = 0.981$; Fig. 4b). This finding indicates that *STAT5a* plays a pivotal role in the effects of risperidone on evading the apoptotic anticancer barrier. Next, we examined whether STAT5 activity reduction also led to a lower early lesion burden in risperidone-treated mice. Indeed, $STAT5a^{-/-}$ mice treated with risperidone had significantly lower levels of the early lesion burden than the $STAT5a^{+/+}$ mice treated with risperidone ($p = 0.005$; Fig. 4c), and further, these low levels were comparable to the levels in the vehicle control $STAT5a^{-/-}$ mice ($p = 0.995$; Fig. 4c). Taken together, these results demonstrate that STAT5 activity is responsible for evading the apoptosis anticancer barrier in early lesions and for instigating early lesion progression.

Prophylactic treatment with an inhibitor of the JAK/STAT signaling pathway restores the apoptosis anticancer barrier in early lesions and decelerates their progression
Many older women on hyperprolactinemia-inducing antipsychotics may have already accumulated early lesions and subsequently may be at increased risk of breast cancer due to family history, older age, or other reasons. Our aforementioned findings suggest that these antipsychotics likely also stimulate the progression of the early lesions in these high-risk women. For these women, it may be advisable to switch to another antipsychotic that does not cause hyperprolactinemia; however, switching to another drug is often difficult for fear of relapse and/or withdrawal effects. Consequently, it is important to identify effective breast cancer preventive strategies in high-risk women who need to take these types of antipsychotics. There are currently only a few US Food and Drug Administrtion (FDA)-approved drugs for breast cancer chemoprevention, all of which antagonize estrogen signaling [62]. As these drugs require 5 years of continuous treatment to lower breast cancer risk by 50%, do not prevent estrogen receptor (ER)-negative cancer, and can have significant side effects, they are not widely used for prevention [62].

However, we have previously reported that short-term suppression of either pSTAT5 or JAK1/2 activity can restore the apoptosis anticancer barrier and reduce mammary tumor risk in mouse models [11]. Ruxolitinib is an FDA-approved small molecule inhibitor of JAK1/2 for the treatment of myelofibrosis and polycythemia vera; it has minimal significant side effects following short-term use in healthy individuals [63–66]. Therefore, we asked whether short-term ruxolitinib treatment could prevent mammary tumors in early lesion-bearing mice on risperidone. Here, ruxolitinib-supplemented or control chow was fed to risperidone-treated mice bearing early lesions initiated by RCAS-caErbB2. After 2 weeks of treatment, serum PRL levels in both cohorts remained elevated, as expected ($p = 0.98$; Additional file 7: Figure S7A); however, ruxolitinib significantly lowered the percentages of pSTAT5+ cells in early lesions ($p < 0.0001$; Additional file 7: Figure S7B), indicating that risperidone-induced activation of STAT5

depends on JAK1/2 activity. Ruxolitinib did not affect precancerous cell proliferation based on Ki67 ($p = 0.629$; Fig. 5a), as expected from non-detectable impact on precancerous cell proliferation by risperidone; however, mice fed with ruxolitinib chow had restored apoptosis in early lesions as measured by CC3 and TUNEL ($p = 0.006$ and 0.0357, respectively; Fig. 5b-c), reaching/surpassing the levels detected in early lesions in mice not treated with any antipsychotic (Fig. 2c-d). Importantly, these mice had a much lower early lesion burden than the mice on the control chow ($p = 0.024$; Fig. 5d). Furthermore, we investigated whether ruxolitinib could prevent/delay tumor appearance. Here, we injected MMTV-*tva* mice ($n = 14$), 10 weeks of age, with RCAS-HrasQ61L virus. Five days later, we randomized the mice into two groups for risperidone water plus ruxolitinib-supplemented chow or for risperidone water plus control chow. While the control-chow-

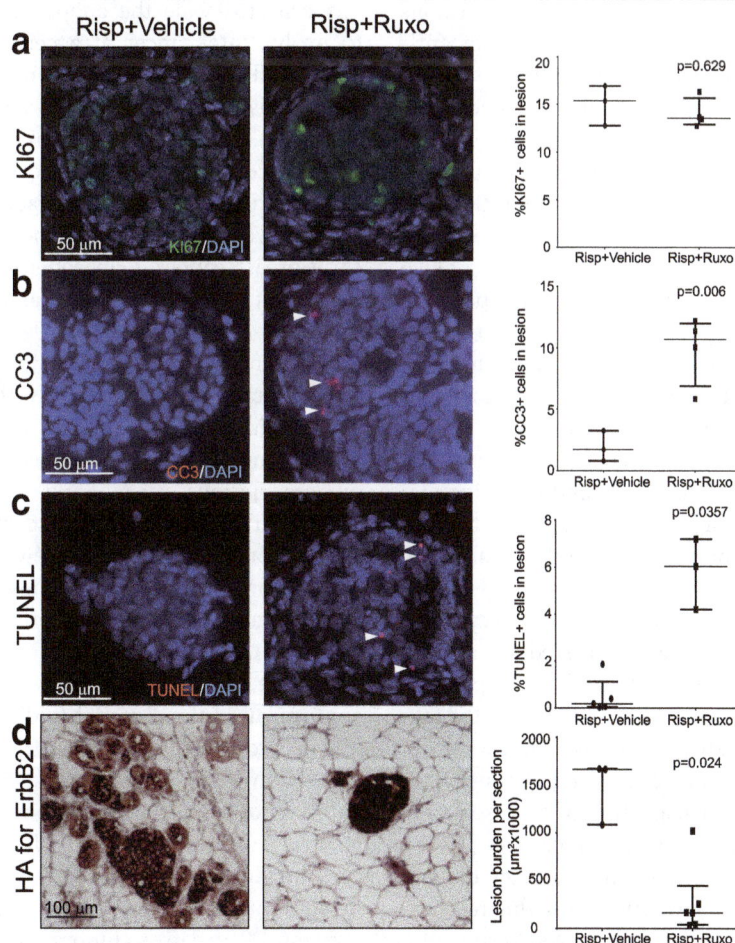

Fig. 5 Ruxolitinib (Ruxo) treatment restore the apoptosis anticancer barrier and blocks early lesion expansion. **a** Immunofluorescence staining for Ki67 and the resulting dot plot. **b** and **c** Immunofluorescence staining for cleaved caspase 3 (**b**) and TUNEL assay (**c**) with the accompanying dot plots. **d** Immunohistochemistry analysis and the accompanying dot plot for the HA tag on RCAS-ca*ErbB2* provirus. The *p* values were determined by the Mann-Whitney test. Each dot in these plots represents one mouse. Risp, risperidone

treated mice on risperidone developed tumors with a median latency of 9 days, the ruxolitinib-chow cohort on risperidone developed tumors with an extended median latency of 13 days ($p = 0.008$; Additional file 7: Figure S7C). These data further confirmed the importance of PRL-stimulated JAK-STAT5 signaling in lowering the apoptosis anticancer barrier and in increasing early lesion burden and progression in mice on risperidone. Taken together, short-term treatment with ruxolitinib restores apoptosis in early lesions, reduces early lesion burden, and lowers mammary tumor risk in mice on hyperprolactinemia-inducing antipsychotics; therefore, these data suggest that prophylactic treatment with ruxolitinib may lower breast cancer risk in high-risk women who are on these antipsychotics.

Discussion

Using three different mouse models of breast cancer, we demonstrated that hyperprolactinemia-inducing antipsychotics cause preexisting premalignant lesions in the mammary gland to lower the apoptosis anticancer barrier and to accelerate the progression to cancer. We further demonstrated that this cancer-instigating effect is via upregulation of the STAT5 signaling pathway, which is known to transactivate anti-apoptosis genes including *Bcl-xL*. Antipsychotics and other pharmaceuticals of similar classes that do not induce hyperprolactinemia do not activate the STAT5 signaling pathway, nor do they lower the apoptosis barrier; consequently, they do not confer a tumorigenic advantage to precancerous cells. These preclinical findings have important clinical implications. For women who already have preexisting early lesions such as atypical ductal hyperplasia (ADH) or ductal carcinoma in situ (DCIS), taking hyperprolactinemia-inducing antipsychotics for a long term may increase breast cancer risk and should be carefully considered for psychiatric benefits versus breast cancer risk. Unless necessary, perhaps non-hyperprolactinemia-inducing alternatives could be considered as a first-line therapy and should be suggested as a possible substitute in high-risk women who are currently taking hyperprolactinemia-inducing antipsychotics.

Our data also offer an explanation for the contradictory findings in epidemiological studies of association between antipsychotic use and breast cancer risk [19, 24, 27, 28, 30, 31, 67]. First, many of these studies did not differentiate between hyperprolactinemia-inducing antipsychotics and other drugs that do not raise serum PRL levels significantly. Second, and perhaps as equally important, PRL-mediated JAK2-STAT5 signaling has a dichotomous effect on mammary cells. Elevated JAK2-STAT5 signaling can weaken the apoptosis anticancer

barrier in precancerous lesions that have already formed in the otherwise normal breast epithelia and thus may potentially increase breast cancer risk [11]. The same signaling pathway can cause the mammary cells to undergo differentiation potentially leading to lower cell proliferation rates and thus may reduce the chance of gaining mutations and consequently breast cancer risk [68]. This dichotomous function of JAK2-STAT5 has been reported by us as a major mechanism to explain the dichotomous effects of pregnancy on breast cancer risk - while an early-age pregnancy protects against breast cancer, a late-age pregnancy increases breast cancer risk [11]. At a young age, the breast epithelia are unlikely to have accumulated mutated cells. Pregnancy at this time induces these normal cells to differentiate. As a result, they become less proliferative and less likely to suffer mutations, and cancer risk is reduced. In contrast, at an older age, mutated cells are more likely to have accumulated. Pregnancy at this time with elevated JAK2-STAT5 activity can cause these precancerous cells to evade the apoptosis anticancer barrier and to evolve into cancer at accelerated speeds. The same may hold true in patients on antipsychotics. While hyperprolactinemia-inducing antipsychotics may increase breast cancer in women who have already gained precancerous cells, they may even lower the cancer risk in women who have not yet accumulated early lesions, such as younger women without any family history of early breast cancer. Consequently, it may not be a surprise that these more general epidemiological studies have generated inconclusive data on antipsychotics and breast cancer risk. Our findings suggest that it is now important to specifically study the association between hyperprolactinemia-inducing antipsychotics and the breast cancer risk in women with preexisting precancerous early lesions.

In order to avoid relapse and withdrawal effects, most patients on antipsychotics receive the same antipsychotic medication for extended periods of time and are sometimes unable to switch to other types of medication, such as those that do not cause hyperprolactinemia. Therefore, if carefully designed epidemiological studies confirm our animal model findings in the human population, prophylactic treatment will then be needed to alleviate the increased breast cancer risk caused by antipsychotics so that patients can still receive the psychiatric care that they need without elevated breast cancer incidence. Currently available chemoprevention drugs require 5 years of continuous treatment, cannot prevent ER-negative tumors that are more difficult to treat, and can have significant side effects [69]. These drawbacks discourage women who are as yet cancer-free from using them. The FDA-approved JAK1/2 inhibitor ruxolitinib has few adverse side effects when used short-term [66, 70, 71]. Even used for only 2 weeks, ruxolitinib was previously found to restore apoptosis in early lesions and to decelerate early lesion progression [11]. In the current study, prophylactic treatment with ruxolitinib induced apoptosis in early lesions and reduced early lesion burden in risperidone-treated mice. This finding predicts that in women with risk factors suggesting the presence of early lesions (ADH and DCIS), short-term or intermittent treatment with ruxolitinib may also reduce precancerous lesion burden and thus negate the elevated breast cancer risk induced by hyperprolactinemia-inducing antipsychotics. Since JAK2-STAT5 signaling plays a crucial role in stimulating early lesion progression even in the absence of antipsychotics [7], such prophylactic treatment may reduce breast cancer risk both associated with and independent of antipsychotic use. An additional benefit of our chemoprevention modality is that it also has the potential to prevent both ER+ and ER- breast cancers, in contrast to current cancer prevention therapies that antagonize estrogen signaling and prevent ER+ breast cancer only [62]. Therefore, this chemoprevention strategy may be highly valuable for women with high breast cancer risk whether they are on antipsychotics or not.

Conclusions

In conclusion, this mouse model study demonstrates that hyperprolactinemia-inducing antipsychotics activate JAK-STAT5 signaling to lower the apoptosis anticancer barrier in preexisting precancerous early lesions and to incite their progression to cancer. To our knowledge, this is the first study that decisively links antipsychotic use to increased breast cancer risk while also providing a mechanistic insight. Our work also suggests short-term or intermittent ruxolitinib treatment as a potentially effective and more acceptable approach for preventing breast cancer risk in women on these antipsychotics.

Additional files

Additional file 1: Figure S1. Risperidone treatment does not affect tumor histopathology or lung metastatic potential. **(A)** H&E staining of tumor sections. **(B)** qPCR analysis of lung metastasis and the resulting dot plot analyzed using the Mann-Whitney test. Each dot in this plot represents one mouse. (AI 4884 kb)

Additional file 2: Figure S2. Risperidone treatment accelerates early lesion development of MMTV-Wnt1 transgenic mice. **(A)** Carmine whole mount staining of mammary glands from MMTV-Wnt1 transgenic mice. **(B)** H&E staining of mammary gland sections of MMTV-Wnt1 mice. **(C)** pSTAT5 immunohistochemical staining of mammary gland sections of MMTV-Wnt1 mice. (AI 22593 kb)

Additional file 3: Figure S3. Pimozide increases serum prolactin levels, pSTAT5 in early lesions, and β-casein, while aripiprazole does not impact pSTAT5. **(A)** Serum prolactin levels. **(B)** pSTAT5+ cells determined by immunohistochemistry analysis. **(C)** Immunohistochemistry analysis of β-casein. **(D)** pSTAT5+ cells determined by immunohistochemistry analysis. The p values were determined using the Mann-Whitney test. Each dot in these plots represents one mouse. (AI 6764 kb)

Additional file 4: Figure S4. Pimozide accelerates the development of early lesions initiated by RCAS-caErbB2 while lowering the anticancer barrier of apoptosis. **(A)** Immunohistochemical staining for the HA tag on the RCAS-ErbB2 provirus with the corresponding dot plot. **(B)** Immunofluorescence staining for Ki67 with the accompanying dot plot. **(C and D)** Immunofluorescence staining for cleaved caspase 3 **(C)** and TUNEL assay **(D)** with the accompanying dot plots. The Mann-Whitney test was used to determine the p values. Each dot in these plots represents one mouse. (AI 15221 kb)

Additional file 5: Figure S5. Effects of aripiprazole and clomipramine on biomarkers and lesion burden. **(A)** Serum prolactin levels of mice in the aripiprazole study. **(B)** Lesion burden determined by immunohistochemical staining for the HA tag on RCAS-caErbB2. **(C)** Ki67 + cells determined by immunofluorescence staining. **(D)** TUNEL+ cells. **(E)** Serum prolactin levels of mice in the clomipramine study. **(F)** Lesion burden determined by immunohistochemical staining for the HA tag on RCAS-caErbB2. The p values were determined using the Mann-Whitney test. Each dot in these plots represents one mouse. (AI 713 kb)

Additional file 6: Figure S6. Effects of genetic ablation of STAT5a on downstream factors of STAT5. Immunohistochemistry analysis of β-casein in caErbB2 early lesions. (AI 4570 kb)

Additional file 7: Figure S7. Effects of ruxolitinib on pSTAT5 and tumor latency. **(A)** Serum prolactin levels of mice. **(B)** Immunohistochemistry analysis and the accompanying dot plot for pSTAT5+ cells. The p values were determined using the Mann-Whitney test. Each dot in this plot represents one mouse. **(C)** Kaplan-Meier tumor-free survival curve of mice infected by RCAS-HRasQ61L. The p value was determined by generalized Gehan-Wilcoxon test with Rho = 1. (AI 6247 kb)

Acknowledgements
We thank Weiyu Jiang and Ashaki Nehisi for technical assistance and Suzanne Fuqua, Phung Thuy, Mothaffar Rimawi, Xiang Zhang, Daniel Medina, Jeffrey Rosen, Michael Lewis, and Gary Chamness for stimulating discussions and/or critical review of this manuscript.

Funding
This work was supported in part by funds from NIH R01CA205594 (to YL) and P50CA186784 (YL); from DOD CDMRP BC123368 (to YL); and from Susan G. Komen for the Cure PDF15330612 (YL); and by the resources from the Dan L. Duncan Cancer Center (P30CA125123). AJ was supported by T32GM088129. SMH was supported by the CPRIT Training Program (RP101499) and by NIH training award T32AG000183.

Authors' contributions
AJ performed the majority of the experiments and statistical analyses. WB oversaw much of the experimental planning, ideas, and data analyses. SH participated in the IHC/IF staining for the risperidone early lesion section. SG participated in IHC/IF for the ruxolitinib studies. LC performed the lung metastasis analysis. LX participated in tumor procurement and IHC. LQ performed the initial experiments in this study. CN determined tumor histopathology. HS confirmed all statistical analyses. KP constructed RCAS-HRasQ61L. JK performed β-casein immunostaining and participated in STAT5 knockout and ruxolitinib tumor studies. JN provided clinical input. YL is the principal investigator for this project. All authors read and approved the final manuscript.

Competing interests
Dr. Li receives the ruxolitinib and research support from Incyte Corp. The authors declare that they have no other competing interests

Author details

[1]Translational Biology and Molecular Medicine, Baylor College of Medicine, Houston, TX 77030, USA. [2]Lester and Sue Smith Breast Center, Baylor College of Medicine, Baylor College of Medicine, Houston, TX 77030, USA. [3]Dan L. Duncan Cancer Center, Baylor College of Medicine, Houston, TX 77030, USA. [4]Molecular and Cellular Biology, Baylor College of Medicine, Houston, TX 77030, USA. [5]SMART PREP Program, Baylor College of Medicine, One Baylor Plaza, Houston, TX 77030, USA. [6]Institut Curie, PSL Research University, CNRS, UMR3664, Equipe Labellisée Ligue contre le Cancer, F-75005 Paris, France. [7]Sorbonne Universités, UPMC Université Paris 06, CNRS, UMR3664, F-75005 Paris, France. [8]Molecular Virology and Microbiology, Baylor College of Medicine, One Baylor Plaza, Houston, TX 77030, USA.

References

1. Lindsley CW. The top prescription drugs of 2011 in the United States: antipsychotics and antidepressants once again lead CNS therapeutics. ACS Chem Neurosci. 2012;3(8):630–1.
2. Peuskens J, Pani L, Detraux J, De Hert M. The effects of novel and newly approved antipsychotics on serum prolactin levels: a comprehensive review. CNS drugs. 2014;28(5):421–53.
3. Montgomery J, Winterbottom E, Jessani M, Kohegyi E, Fulmer J, Seamonds B, Josiassen RC. Prevalence of hyperprolactinemia in schizophrenia: association with typical and atypical antipsychotic treatment. J Clin Psychiatry. 2004;65(11):1491–8.
4. Suliman AM, Smith TP, Gibney J, McKenna TJ. Frequent misdiagnosis and mismanagement of hyperprolactinemic patients before the introduction of macroprolactin screening: application of a new strict laboratory definition of macroprolactinemia. Clin Chem. 2003;49(9):1504–9.
5. Meltzer HY, Fang VS. The effect of neuroleptics on serum prolactin in schizophrenic patients. Arch Gen Psychiatry. 1976;33(3):279–86.
6. Haddad PM, Wieck A. Antipsychotic-induced hyperprolactinaemia: mechanisms, clinical features and management. Drugs. 2004;64(20):2291–314.
7. Haricharan S, Li Y. STAT signaling in mammary gland differentiation, cell survival and tumorigenesis. Mol Cell Endocrinol. 2014;382(1):560–9.
8. Iavnilovitch E, Groner B, Barash I. Overexpression and forced activation of stat5 in mammary gland of transgenic mice promotes cellular proliferation, enhances differentiation, and delays postlactational apoptosis. Mol Cancer Res. 2002;1(1):32–47.
9. Dong J, Tong T, Reynado AM, Rosen JM, Huang S, Li Y. Genetic manipulation of individual somatic mammary cells in vivo reveals a master role of STAT5a in inducing alveolar fate commitment and lactogenesis even in the absence of ovarian hormones. Dev Biol. 2010;346(2):196–203.
10. Torre DL, Falorni A. Pharmacological causes of hyperprolactinemia. Ther Clin Risk Manag. 2007;3(5):929–51.
11. Haricharan S, Dong J, Hein S, Reddy JP, Du Z, Toneff M, Holloway K, Hilsenbeck SG, Huang S, Atkinson R, et al. Mechanism and preclinical prevention of increased breast cancer risk caused by pregnancy. elife. 2013;2(0):e00996.
12. Peck AR, Witkiewicz AK, Liu C, Stringer GA, Klimowicz AC, Pequignot E, Freydin B, Tran TH, Yang N, Rosenberg AL, et al. Loss of nuclear localized and tyrosine phosphorylated Stat5 in breast cancer predicts poor clinical outcome and increased risk of antiestrogen therapy failure. J Clin Oncol. 2011;29(18):2448–58.
13. Nevalainen MT, Xie J, Bubendorf L, Wagner KU, Rui H. Basal activation of transcription factor signal transducer and activator of transcription (Stat5) in nonpregnant mouse and human breast epithelium. Mol Endocrinol. 2002; 16(5):1108–24.
14. Cotarla I, Ren S, Zhang Y, Gehan E, Singh B, Furth PA. Stat5a is tyrosine phosphorylated and nuclear localized in a high proportion of human breast cancers. Int J Cancer. 2004;108(5):665–71.
15. Walker SR, Xiang M, Frank DA. Distinct roles of STAT3 and STAT5 in the pathogenesis and targeted therapy of breast cancer. Mol Cell Endocrinol. 2014;382(1):616–21.
16. Shi A, Dong J, Hilsenbeck S, Bi L, Zhang H, Li Y. The status of STAT3 and STAT5 in human breast atypical ductal hyperplasia. PLoS One. 2015;10(7):e0132214.
17. Thomas SJ, Snowden JA, Zeidler MP, Danson SJ. The role of JAK/STAT signalling in the pathogenesis, prognosis and treatment of solid tumours. Br J Cancer. 2015;113(3):365–71.
18. Gilbert PL, Harris MJ, McAdams LA, Jeste DV. Neuroleptic withdrawal in schizophrenic patients. A review of the literature. Arch Gen Psychiatry. 1995;52(3):173–88.
19. De Hert M, Peuskens J, Sabbe T, Mitchell AJ, Stubbs B, Neven P, Wildiers H, Detraux J. Relationship between prolactin, breast cancer risk, and antipsychotics in patients with schizophrenia: a critical review. Acta Psychiatr Scand. 2016;133(1):5–22.
20. Mitchell AJ, Pereira IE, Yadegarfar M, Pepereke S, Mugadza V, Stubbs B. Breast cancer screening in women with mental illness: comparative meta-analysis of mammography uptake. Br J Psychiatry. 2014;205(6):428–35.
21. Kisely S, Crowe E, Lawrence D. Cancer-related mortality in people with mental illness. JAMA Psychiat. 2013;70(2):209–17.
22. Smith DJ, Langan J, McLean G, Guthrie B, Mercer SW. Schizophrenia is associated with excess multiple physical-health comorbidities but low levels of recorded cardiovascular disease in primary care: cross-sectional study. BMJ Open. 2013;3(4):e002808.
23. Carney CP, Jones L, Woolson RF. Medical comorbidity in women and men with schizophrenia: a population-based controlled study. J Gen Intern Med. 2006;21(11):1133–7.
24. Goode DJ, Corbett WT, Schey HM, Suh SH, Woodie B, Morris DL, Morrisey L. Breast cancer in hospitalized psychiatric patients. Am J Psychiatry. 1981; 138(6):804–6.
25. Kanhouwa S, Gowdy JM, Solomon JD. Phenothiazines and breast cancer. J Natl Med Assoc. 1984;76(8):785–8.
26. Overall JE. Prior psychiatric treatment and the development of breast cancer. Arch Gen Psychiatry. 1978;35(7):898–9.
27. Ettigi P, Lal S, Friesen HG. Prolactin, phenothiazines, admission to mental hospital, and carcinoma of the breast. Lancet. 1973;2(7823):266–7.
28. Wagner S, Mantel N. Breast cancer at a psychiatric hospital before and after the introduction of neuroleptic agents. Cancer Res. 1978;38(9):2703–8.
29. Seeman MV. Secondary effects of antipsychotics: women at greater risk than men. Schizophr Bull. 2009;35(5):937–48.
30. Rahman T, Clevenger CV, Kaklamani V, Lauriello J, Campbell A, Malwitz K, Kirkland RS. Antipsychotic treatment in breast cancer patients. Am J Psychiatry. 2014;171(6):616–21.
31. Froes Brandao D, Strasser-Weippl K, Goss PE. Prolactin and breast cancer: the need to avoid undertreatment of serious psychiatric illnesses in breast cancer patients: a review. Cancer. 2016;122(2):184–8.
32. Halbreich U, Shen J, Panaro V. Are chronic psychiatric patients at increased risk for developing breast cancer? Am J Psychiatry. 1996;153(4):559–60.
33. Wang PS, Walker AM, Tsuang MT, Orav EJ, Glynn RJ, Levin R, Avorn J. Dopamine antagonists and the development of breast cancer. Arch Gen Psychiatry. 2002;59(12):1147–54.
34. Du Z, Podsypanina K, Huang S, McGrath A, Toneff MJ, Bogoslovskaia E, Zhang X, Moraes RC, Fluck M, Allred DC, et al. Introduction of oncogenes into mammary glands in vivo with an avian retroviral vector initiates and promotes carcinogenesis in mouse models. Proc Natl Acad Sci U S A. 2006; 103(46):17396–401.
35. Liu X, Robinson GW, Wagner KU, Garrett L, Wynshaw-Boris A, Hennighausen L. Stat5a is mandatory for adult mammary gland development and lactogenesis. Genes Dev. 1997;11(2):179–86.
36. Reddy JP, Li Y. The RCAS-TVA system for introduction of oncogenes into selected somatic mammary epithelial cells in vivo. J Mammary Gland Biol Neoplasia. 2009;14(4):405–9.
37. Bachmanov AA, Reed DR, Beauchamp GK, Tordoff MG. Food intake, water intake, and drinking spout side preference of 28 mouse strains. Behav Genet. 2002;32(6):435–43.
38. Hein SM, Haricharan S, Johnston AN, Toneff MJ, Reddy JP, Dong J, Bu W, Li Y. Luminal epithelial cells within the mammary gland can produce basal cells upon oncogenic stress. Oncogene. 2016;35(11):1461–7.
39. Toneff MJ, Du Z, Dong J, Huang J, Sinai P, Forman J, Hilsenbeck S, Schiff R, Huang S, Li Y. Somatic expression of PyMT or activated ErbB2 induces estrogen-independent mammary tumorigenesis. Neoplasia. 2010;12(9):718–26.
40. Holloway KR, Sinha VC, Bu W, Toneff M, Dong J, Peng Y, Li Y. Targeting oncogenes into a defined subset of mammary cells demonstrates that the

initiating oncogenic mutation defines the resulting tumor phenotype. Int J Biol Sci. 2016;12(4):381–8.

41. Holloway KR, Sinha VC, Toneff MJ, Bu W, Hilsenbeck SG, Li Y. Krt6a-positive mammary epithelial progenitors are not at increased vulnerability to tumorigenesis initiated by ErbB2. PLoS One. 2015;10(1):e0117239.

42. Sinha VC, Qin L, Li Y. A p53/ARF-dependent anticancer barrier activates senescence and blocks tumorigenesis without impacting apoptosis. Mol Cancer Res. 2015;13(2):231–8.

43. Li Y, Ferris A, Lewis BC, Orsulic S, Williams BO, Holland EC, Hughes SH. The RCAS/TVA somatic gene transfer method in modeling human cancer. In: Green JE, Ried T, editors. Genetically-engineered mice for cancer research: design, analysis, pathways, validation and pre-clinical testing: Springer; 2011. p. 83–111.

44. Reddy JP, Peddibhotla S, Bu W, Zhao J, Haricharan S, Du YC, Podsypanina K, Rosen JM, Donehower LA, Li Y. Defining the ATM-mediated barrier to tumorigenesis in somatic mammary cells following ErbB2 activation. Proc Natl Acad Sci U S A. 2010;107(8):3728–33.

45. Slamon DJ, Godolphin W, Jones LA, Holt JA, Wong SG, Keith DE, Levin WJ, Stuart SG, Udove J, Ullrich A, et al. Studies of the HER-2/neu proto-oncogene in human breast and ovarian cancer. Science. 1989;244(4905):707–12.

46. Zheng ZY, Tian L, Bu W, Fan C, Gao X, Wang H, Liao YH, Li Y, Lewis MT, Edwards D, et al. Wild-type N-Ras, overexpressed in basal-like breast cancer, promotes tumor formation by inducing IL-8 secretion via JAK2 activation. Cell Rep. 2015;12(3):511–24.

47. Hoadley KA, Weigman VJ, Fan C, Sawyer LR, He X, Troester MA, Sartor CI, Rieger-House T, Bernard PS, Carey LA, et al. EGFR associated expression profiles vary with breast tumor subtype. BMC Genomics. 2007;8:258.

48. Cancer Genome Atlas Network. Comprehensive molecular portraits of human breast tumours. Nature. 2012;490(7418):61–70.

49. Cerami E, Gao J, Dogrusoz U, Gross BE, Sumer SO, Aksoy BA, Jacobsen A, Byrne CJ, Heuer ML, Larsson E, et al. The cBio cancer genomics portal: an open platform for exploring multidimensional cancer genomics data. Cancer Dis. 2012;2(5):401–4.

50. Tsukamoto AS, Grosschedl R, Guzman RC, Parslow T, Varmus HE. Expression of the int-1 gene in transgenic mice is associated with mammary gland hyperplasia and adenocarcinomas in male and female mice. Cell. 1988;55(4):619–25.

51. Herschkowitz JI, Simin K, Weigman VJ, Mikaelian I, Usary J, Hu Z, Rasmussen KE, Jones LP, Assefnia S, Chandrasekharan S, et al. Identification of conserved gene expression features between murine mammary carcinoma models and human breast tumors. Genome Biol. 2007;8(5):R76.

52. Zhang X, Podsypanina K, Huang S, Mohsin SK, Chamness GC, Hatsell S, Cowin P, Schiff R, Li Y. Estrogen receptor positivity in mammary tumors of Wnt-1 transgenic mice is influenced by collaborating oncogenic mutations. Oncogene. 2005;24(26):4220–31.

53. Li Y, Welm B, Podsypanina K, Huang S, Chamorro M, Zhang X, Rowlands T, Egeblad M, Cowin P, Werb Z, et al. Evidence that transgenes encoding components of the Wnt signaling pathway preferentially induce mammary cancers from progenitor cells. Proc Natl Acad Sci U S A. 2003;100(26):15853–8.

54. Hanahan D, Weinberg RA. Hallmarks of cancer: the next generation. Cell. 2011;144(5):646–74.

55. Tomlinson IP, Bodmer WF. Failure of programmed cell death and differentiation as causes of tumors: some simple mathematical models. Proc Natl Acad Sci U S A. 1995;92(24):11130–4.

56. Walton KD, Wagner KU, Rucker EB 3rd, Shillingford JM, Miyoshi K, Hennighausen L. Conditional deletion of the bcl-x gene from mouse mammary epithelium results in accelerated apoptosis during involution but does not compromise cell function during lactation. Mech Dev. 2001;109(2):281–93.

57. Rosen JM, Wyszomierski SL, Hadsell D. Regulation of milk protein gene expression. Annu Rev Nutr. 1999;19(1):407–36.

58. Nelson EA, Walker SR, Weisberg E, Bar-Natan M, Barrett R, Gashin LB, Terrell S, Klitgaard JL, Santo L, Addorio MR, et al. The STAT5 inhibitor pimozide decreases survival of chronic myelogenous leukemia cells resistant to kinase inhibitors. Blood. 2011;117(12):3421–9.

59. Nelson EA, Walker SR, Xiang M, Weisberg E, Bar-Natan M, Barrett R, Liu S, Kharbanda S, Christie AL, Nicolais M, et al. The STAT5 inhibitor pimozide displays efficacy in models of acute myelogenous leukemia driven by FLT3 mutations. Genes Cancer. 2012;3(7–8):503–11.

60. Neilson LM, Zhu J, Xie J, Malabarba MG, Sakamoto K, Wagner KU, Kirken RA, Rui H. Coactivation of janus tyrosine kinase (Jak)1 positively modulates prolactin-Jak2 signaling in breast cancer: recruitment of ERK and signal transducer and activator of transcription (Stat)3 and enhancement of Akt and Stat5a/b pathways. Mol Endocrinol. 2007;21(9):2218–32.

61. Liu X, Robinson GW, Gouilleux F, Groner B, Hennighausen L. Cloning and expression of Stat5 and an additional homologue (Stat5b) involved in prolactin signal transduction in mouse mammary tissue. Proc Natl Acad Sci U S A. 1995;92(19):8831–5.

62. Brown P. Prevention: targeted therapy-anastrozole prevents breast cancer. Nat Rev Clin Oncol. 2014;11(3):127–8.

63. Ogama Y, Mineyama T, Yamamoto A, Woo M, Shimada N, Amagasaki T, Natsume K. A randomized dose-escalation study to assess the safety, tolerability, and pharmacokinetics of ruxolitinib (INC424) in healthy Japanese volunteers. Int J Hematol. 2013;97(3):351–9.

64. Shi JG, Chen X, Emm T, Scherle PA, McGee RF, Lo Y, Landman RR, McKeever EG Jr, Punwani NG, Williams WV, et al. The effect of CYP3A4 inhibition or induction on the pharmacokinetics and pharmacodynamics of orally administered ruxolitinib (INCB018424 phosphate) in healthy volunteers. J Clin Pharmacol. 2012;52(6):809–18.

65. Sonbol MB, Firwana B, Zarzour A, Morad M, Rana V, Tiu RV. Comprehensive review of JAK inhibitors in myeloproliferative neoplasms. Ther Adv Hematol. 2013;4(1):15–35.

66. Quintas-Cardama A, Vaddi K, Liu P, Manshouri T, Li J, Scherle PA, Caulder E, Wen X, Li Y, Waeltz P, et al. Preclinical characterization of the selective JAK1/2 inhibitor INCB018424: therapeutic implications for the treatment of myeloproliferative neoplasms. Blood. 2010;115(15):3109–17.

67. Reutfors J, Wingard L, Brandt L, Wang Y, Qiu H, Kieler H, Bahmanyar S. Risk of breast cancer in risperidone users: a nationwide cohort study. Schizophr Res. 2017;182:98–103.

68. Medina D. Breast cancer: the protective effect of pregnancy. Clin Cancer Res. 2004;10(1 Pt 2):380S–4S.

69. Hutchinson L. Prevention: Mapping out breast cancer chemoprevention. Nat Rev Clin Oncol. 2011;8(8):445.

70. Mesa RA. Ruxolitinib, a selective JAK1 and JAK2 inhibitor for the treatment of myeloproliferative neoplasms and psoriasis. IDrug. 2010;13(6):394–403.

71. Swaim SJ. Ruxolitinib for the treatment of primary myelofibrosis. AJHP. 2014;71(6):453–62.

12

Evaluation of anti-PD-1-based therapy against triple-negative breast cancer patient-derived xenograft tumors engrafted in humanized mouse models

Roberto R. Rosato[*†], Daniel Dávila-González[†], Dong Soon Choi, Wei Qian, Wen Chen, Anthony J. Kozielski, Helen Wong, Bhuvanesh Dave and Jenny C. Chang

Abstract

Background: Breast cancer has been considered not highly immunogenic, and few patients benefit from current immunotherapies. However, new strategies are aimed at changing this paradigm. In the present study, we examined the in vivo activity of a humanized anti-programmed cell death protein 1 (anti-PD-1) antibody against triple-negative breast cancer (TNBC) patient-derived xenograft (PDX) tumor models.

Methods: To circumvent some of the limitations posed by the lack of appropriate animal models in preclinical studies of immunotherapies, partially human leukocyte antigen-matched TNBC PDX tumor lines from our collection, as well as human melanoma cell lines, were engrafted in humanized nonobese diabetic/severe combined immunodeficiency $IL2R\gamma^{null}$ (hNSG) mice obtained by intravenous injection of CD34$^+$ hematopoietic stem cells into nonlethally irradiated 3–4-week-old mice. After both PDXs and melanoma cell xenografts reached ~ 150–200 mm^3, animals were treated with humanized anti-PD-1 antibody or anti-CTLA-4 and evaluated for tumor growth, survival, and potential mechanism of action.

Results: Human CD45$^+$, CD20$^+$, CD3$^+$, CD8$^+$, CD56$^+$, CD68$^+$, and CD33$^+$ cells were readily identified in blood, spleen, and bone marrow collected from hNSG, as well as human cytokines in blood and engrafted tumors. Engraftment of TNBC PDXs in hNSG was high (~ 85%), although they grew at a slightly slower pace and conserved their ability to generate lung metastasis. Human CD45$^+$ cells were detectable in hNSG-harbored PDXs, and consistent with clinical observations, anti-PD-1 antibody therapy resulted in both a significant reduction in tumor growth and increased survival in some of the hNSG PDX tumor lines, whereas no such effects were observed in the corresponding non-hNSG models.

Conclusions: This study provides evidence associated with anti-PD-1 immunotherapy against TNBC tumors supporting the use of TNBC PDXs in humanized mice as a model to overcome some of the technical difficulties associated with the preclinical investigation of immune-based therapies.

Keywords: Triple-negative breast cancer, TNBC, Immunotherapy, Anti-PD-1, PD-L1, Humanized mouse model

* Correspondence: rrrosato@houstonmethodist.org
[†]Roberto R. Rosato and Daniel Dávila-González contributed equally to this work.
Houston Methodist Cancer Center, Houston Methodist Hospital, Houston, TX 77030, USA

Background

Immunotherapy has revolutionized the treatment regimens for various cancer types, leading to improved clinical responses in otherwise untreatable advanced cancers [1]. Observations showing accumulation of tumor-infiltrating lymphocytes (TILs) within the tumor microenvironment (TME), as well as work highlighting the efficacy of immune checkpoint inhibitors (CPIs), have sparked interest in the further development of these approaches. Studies have focused on the development of CPIs, including cytotoxic T-lymphocyte-associated protein 4 (CTLA-4) [2, 3] as well as programmed cell death 1 (PD-1) receptor and its ligands programmed death ligand 1 (PD-L1) and PD-L2 [4–6]. PD-1 is found on cytotoxic T cells and T-regulatory cells and is expressed when T cells become activated in response to inflammation or infection in peripheral tissues [7, 8]. Binding of the PD-1 ligand to its receptor inactivates the T cell, limiting the immune response to the stimuli, thereby causing immune suppression [7, 8]. Cancer cells, however, induce PD-1 L expression, enhancing the immunosuppressive action of this pathway, ultimately allowing them to "hide" from natural immune attack [7, 8]. Anti-PD-1/PD-L1 therapies disrupt this pathway by preventing these interactions, leaving activated cytotoxic T cells available to attack the cancer cells [7, 8]. In triple-negative breast cancer (TNBC), a minority of patients benefit from these approaches, and further studies are urgently needed, especially those designed to evaluate combinatorial therapies.

The recent evolution of these therapeutic strategies (i.e., allowing the immune system to identify neoplastic growth in order to prevent carcinogenesis and eliminate cancer cells) has led to the urgent need for having available a range of appropriate small-animal models that may serve in testing these interactions [9, 10]. To this end, mouse models injected with human CD34$^+$ hematopoietic stem cells (HSCs; "humanized" mice) are currently commercially available for studies in cancer, infectious diseases, and gene therapy, among others. However, these models remain relatively expensive, beyond the means of most academic laboratories, especially when used in large-scale studies.

Important advances have been made in the recent years in establishing mouse models to be used in cancer-related studies, including patient-derived xenografts (PDXs). PDXs, by conserving the characteristic of the human primary tumor, are useful for addressing critical questions regarding tumor biology and response to newly developed therapeutic concepts [11, 12]. In contrast to cell lines used for in vivo studies, PDXs retain morphology, cellular heterogeneity, and molecular profiles of the original patient tumors [12–18], representing an effective model for screening potential chemotherapeutics and translating them to enhanced efficacy in clinical trials [19–22]. New experimental designs have recently been used as valid approaches to perform large-scale PDX-based preclinical trials to evaluate and predict the clinical efficacy and drug response of new therapeutics following the so-called 1 × 1 × 1 design [15, 23, 24]. By using this design (i.e., one animal per model per treatment), PDX models provide the ability to place the same "patient" on all arms of a trial in a given preclinical study.

We have developed an extensive cohort of breast cancer PDXs that retain the morphology, cellular heterogeneity, and molecular profiles of the original patient tumors, serving as a renewable, quality-controlled tissue resource for preclinical evaluation of novel treatment regimens for what are in some cases extremely aggressive cancer types that currently lack adequate targeted therapeutic options [12]. These PDXs have been characterized and classified according to Perou PAM50 and Pietenpol subtypes [11, 25, 26] and their *TP53* mutational status [11, 12, 27]. However, new therapies involving, among others, immune CPIs emphasize the need for the appropriate small-animal models to examine xenograft growth and response to therapy in the context of a "human" immune system and TME.

In the present study, we investigated the in vivo activity of anti-immune CPI-based therapies against TNBC PDX tumor models established in models of "humanized" nonobese diabetic/severe combined immunodeficiency *IL2Rγ^{null}* (hNSG) mice by the engraftment of human CD34$^+$ HSCs, as previously described [28, 29]. We show that, in terms of the animal model, engrafted human HSCs displayed self-renewal and multilineage differentiation capacities and that anti-PD-1 antibody therapy may result, as observed in clinical studies, in varying effects, with some PDXs responding positively to the treatment (i.e., significant reduction in tumor growth and increased survival), whereas others show no signs of improvement. Importantly, in those models that responded to the anti-PD-1 therapy, the effects were differentially displayed and observed only in the hNSG mice, indicating that despite potential limitations of the model, it may still represent an important tool for the preclinical evaluation of immunotherapies in breast cancer.

Methods

Mice

All the present study protocols involving mice followed the standard regulations and were approved by the Houston Methodist Research Institute Institutional Animal Care and Use Committee. "Humanized" mouse models refer to immunodeficient mice engrafted with human hematopoietic and lymphoid cells or tissues. NOD.Cg-*Prkdc^{scid} Il2rg^{tm1Wjl}*/SzJ (NOD scid γ [NSG];

The Jackson Laboratory, Bar Harbor, ME, USA) mice were used as the recipient strain to intravenously (i.v.) engraft human CD34+ HSCs (STEMCELL Technologies, Vancouver, BC, Canada) as previously described [28, 29]. Briefly, 21-day-old NSG mice were irradiated with 240 cGy (sublethal) whole-body γ-irradiation. After 4–6 hours, mice were inoculated via the lateral tail vein with 3×10^4 CD34+ HSCs. HSCs were allowed to engraft, and peripheral blood of recipient mice was collected from the retro-orbital sinus and analyzed by flow cytometry as indicated in the corresponding figure legends herein. "hNSG" is used to denote that the mice have HSC cells engrafted.

PDXs were originally derived by transplanting a fresh patient breast tumor biopsy into the cleared mammary gland fat pad of immunocompromised mice. Tumor samples (2×2 mm) were serially passaged in NSG mice by fat pad transplant under general anesthesia [12]. Low-passage TNBC MC1 [30], BCM-2147, BCM-4913, BCM-4664, and BCM-5471 [12] samples were transferred into hNSG mice for engraftment approximately 6–8 weeks after initial human CD34+ HSC cells tail vein injection. The weight of the mice was recorded and tumor volumes were measured and calculated $[0.5 \times (\text{long dimension}) \times (\text{short dimension})^2]$ twice weekly. When tumors reached an average size of 150–200 mm^3, mice were randomized ($n \geq 5$ per group) and used to determine the response to the treatment.

As validation of the humanized model, immunogenic A375 melanoma cell lines (American Type Culture Collection, Manassas, VA, USA) were maintained in DMEM (Life Technologies, Carlsbad, CA, USA), 10% FBS (HyClone; Life Technologies), and 1% antibiotic-antimycotic in a humidified 5% CO_2 incubator at 37 °C. Cells (5×10^5) were injected orthotopically into the skin of NSG and hNSG mice and after 7–10 days (palpable tumors), and mice were randomly sorted into treatment groups.

Reagents

Humanized antibodies were obtained from Merck Oncology (Kenilworth, NJ, USA; pembrolizumab [Keytruda™], anti-PD-1) and Bristol-Myers Squibb (New York, NY, USA; nivolumab [Opdivo™], anti-PD-1; and ipilimumab, anti-CTL-4). Serum and tumor contents of human cytokine and chemokine biomarkers were determined by using the MILLIPLEX MAP Human High Sensitivity T Cell Panel Premixed 13-plex, Immunology Multiplex Assay (EMD Millipore, Billerica, MA, USA). Lymphoprep (STEMCELL Technologies) was used to isolate human peripheral blood mononuclear cells from tumor.

IHC

IHC assays were performed following established protocols [31]. After antigen retrieval (Tris-Cl, pH 9.0), paraffin-embedded sections of PDX tumors were incubated for 1 hour at room temperature with the following antibodies: antihuman CD45 (leukocyte common antigen, clones 2B11 + PD7/26); antihuman CD68, clone KP1; antihuman CD8 (clone C8/144B); antihuman CD4, clone 4B12; antihuman Ki-67, clone MIB-1 (Dako, Glostrup, Denmark); antihuman CD3, clone UCHT1 (STEMCELL Technologies); antihuman CD20, clone EP459Y; antihuman CD56, clone EPR2566 (Abcam, Cambridge, MA, USA); antihuman cytokeratin 19 (CK19), clone A53-B/A2.26, also known as Ks19.1 (Thermo Scientific, Waltham, MA, USA).

Western blot analysis

Protein analysis was performed by Western blotting [31]. Briefly, whole-cell lysates were made in 1× lysis buffer (Cell Signaling Technology, Danvers, MA, USA) with protease/phosphatase inhibitor cocktail (Thermo Scientific). Samples (30 μg) were boiled in sample buffer (Thermo Scientific) containing β-mercaptoethanol (Sigma-Aldrich, St. Louis, MO, USA) and subjected to SDS-PAGE electrophoresis in 4–20% polyacrylamide gels (Bio-Rad Laboratories, Hercules, CA, USA), transferred onto nitrocellulose membranes (Bio-Rad Laboratories), and incubated overnight at 4 °C with primary antibodies (1:1000; anti-PD-L1, catalogue no. 13684; anti-β-actin, catalogue no. 4970; Cell Signaling Technology), followed after washes by the appropriate secondary antibodies for 1 hour (1:2000). Protein bands were developed in autoradiography films (Denville Scientific Inc., South Plainfield, NJ, USA).

Fluorescence-activated cell sorting analysis

Analysis of mouse and human blood, spleen, and bone marrow mononuclear cells was performed by fluorescence-activated cell sorting analysis [29, 32]. The antibodies used were as follows: antimouse CD45-fluorescein isothiocyanate (FITC), clone 30-F11; antihuman CD45-allophycocyanin (APC), clone HI30; antihuman CD3-phycoerythrin (PE), clone UCHT1; antihuman CD20-FITC, clone 2H7; PE-cyanine 7 mouse antihuman CD68, clone Y1/82A; Alexa Fluor 700 mouse antihuman CD56, clone B159; antimouse CD45-PE, clone 30-F11; antimouse CD45-peridinin chlorophyll protein complex, clone 30-F11; mouse immunoglobulin G2b (IgG2b), κ isotype-FITC, clones 27–35; mouse IgG1, κ isotype-PE, clone MOPC-21; and mouse IgG2b κ isotype-APC (BD Biosciences, San Jose, CA, USA); Pacific Blue antihuman CD33 eFluor® 450, clone P67; and Pacific Blue Mouse IgG1 K Isotype Control eFluor® 450 (eBioscience, San Diego, CA, USA). Briefly, erythrocytes were lysed, after which lymphoid cells were incubated with the corresponding antibodies and fixed following standard procedures [29, 32]. Flow cytometric analysis was performed at the Houston Methodist Research Institute Flow

Cytometry Core using a BD LSRFortessa flow cytometer for acquisition of data and FACSDiva software (both from BD Biosciences) for analysis.

Tumor-infiltrating lymphocyte cytotoxic activity assay

Following a four-cycle treatment with anti-PD-1 antibody (nivoluzumab 10 mg/kg), MC1-engrafted tumors growing in hNSG mice were collected and mechanically disaggregated into single cells, and TILs were isolated by using Ficoll gradient (Lymphoprep; STEMCELL Technologies). These TILs were cocultured with MC1 tumor cells extracted from nonhumanized NSG mice for 6 hours (250:7 ratio of target cells to effector cells), and TIL cytotoxic activity was measured with the CytoTox 96® Non-Radioactive Cytotoxicity Assay (Promega, Madison, WI, USA) as per the manufacturer's instructions. Granzyme B tumor levels were measured by incubating tumor protein lysates with antibody-immobilized magnetic beads (HGRNZMB-MAG; EMD Millipore, Billerica, MA) and evaluated using a Luminex LX-200 multiplexing assay system (Luminex Corp., Austin, TX, USA).

Statistical analysis

All data were analyzed using Prism software (GraphPad Software, La Jolla, CA, USA). Data are presented as mean ± SEM. Statistical significance between two groups was analyzed by two-tailed Student's t test. Experiments with more than three groups were analyzed with one-way analysis of variance (ANOVA) and Bonferroni's post hoc test. Statistical analysis of tumor volume was assessed by two-way ANOVA and Bonferroni's post hoc test. Survival proportions were assessed by using the Kaplan-Meier method and further analyzed with either Wilcoxon or log-rank test. A P value less than 0.05 was considered significant.

Results

Establishment of hNSG models

As mentioned above, one of the major limitations of preclinical studies with immunotherapies in breast cancer is the lack of availability of appropriate experimental models. Although human CD34+ HSC-engrafted NSG (hNSG) mice harboring different types of PDXs are commercially available, the high costs of these animal models limit, to some extent, their use by academic research groups. We have developed in-house established humanized mouse models that were generated by i.v. injection of hCD34+ HSCs as per protocols previously described [28, 29]. Briefly, 3–4-week-old NSG mice received a low, sublethal dose of irradiation, followed after 4 hours by tail vein injection of CD34+ HSCs. The presence of human cells was evaluated in blood collected from these animals at different time intervals starting at 6 weeks after the i.v. administration of

hCD34+ HSC cells. The percentage of HSC engraftment was ~ 90% (on average) per group of mice injected (~ 80–100 mice/group). In agreement with multiple previous reports [29, 33, 34], the presence in blood of human CD45+ cells was readily detectable by week 6 (mean, 13 ± 2.26%), reaching percentages ~ 25% by weeks 8–16 (26.01 ± 1.76% and 25.24 ± 4.26%, respectively) and up to ~ 30% at week 22 (30.3 ± 4.98%) (Fig. 1a and Additional file 1: Figure S1). Analysis of hCD45+ subpopulations of cells, evaluated at week 22, showed the following distribution (expressed as percentage of hCD45+): hCD20+ (B cells), 10.76 ± 2.15%; hCD3+ (T cells), 78.5 ± 4.09%; hCD33+ (myeloid cells), 5.84 ± 5.26%; hCD56+ (natural killer [NK] cells), 3.2 ± 2.36%; and hCD68+ (macrophages), 0.48 ± 0.17% (Fig. 1b). The composition of human cell populations was also analyzed in cells collected from bone marrow and spleen, where levels of hCD45+ represented 50.98 ± 9.27% and 54.94 ± 10.53%, respectively. Additional details showing cell lineage distribution are depicted in Fig. 1b. IHC analysis was performed in samples from spleens of both humanized and nonhumanized NSG mice using an anti-hCD45 antibody, showing a robust presence of these cells only in hNSG mice (Fig. 1c, upper panels). Additional characterization of human cells showed expression of markers corresponding to B cells (hCD20+), macrophages/myeloid lineage (hCD68+), and NK cells (hCD56+). Importantly, none of the human markers were detected in samples from non-hNSG, confirming the specificity and level of humanization achieved in hNSG mice (Fig. 1c, bottom panels).

Breast cancer tumor transplant and development in hNSG mice

In order to develop and establish the appropriate mouse models to test immunotherapies against TNBC, we next directed our efforts toward obtaining PDX models harbored in the hNSG mice. To this end, we used patient-derived breast cancer tumor lines from our existing collection, previously established in immune-compromised SCID/beige mice [12]. Low-passage fresh xenograft tumor fragments of the breast cancer line MC1 [30] were transplanted into the cleared mammary gland fat pad of recipient nonhumanized and humanized NSG mice. Tumor volume was then evaluated over time. Approximately 80–85% positive tumor engraftment was observed, slightly lower than what is normally achieved in nonhumanized mice (i.e., ~ 95–100% under the same experimental conditions). As depicted in Fig. 2, after the tumors were palpable (~ 100–150 mm³; day 0), fast and aggressive tumor growth was observed in non-hNSG mice, reaching the maximum humane size before killing by day 10. In the case of hNSG mice, the growth of MC1 tumors was slower, achieving a similar volume only after day 18. To further characterize the hNSG model,

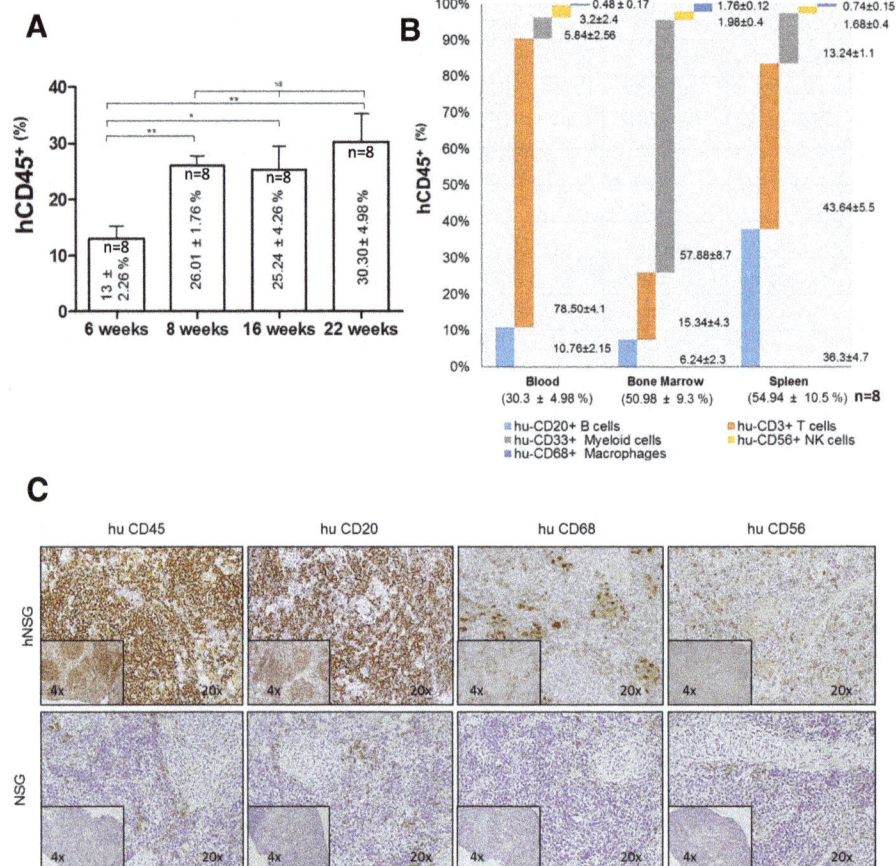

Fig. 1 Analysis of human immune cell engraftment. **a** Evolution of the percentage of human CD45$^+$ cells after intravenous (i.v.) injection of hCD34$^+$ hematopoietic stem cells. Cells were identified by flow cytometry in circulating blood collected from humanized mice at the indicated time intervals ($n = 8$). **b** Analysis of hCD45$^+$ and corresponding subpopulations, including hCD20$^+$ (B cells), hCD3$^+$ (T cells), hCD33$^+$ (myeloid lineage), hCD56$^+$ (natural killer [NK] cells), and hCD68$^+$ (macrophages) cells, was determined by flow cytometry in blood, bone marrow, and spleen samples collected from humanized nonobese diabetic/severe combined immunodeficiency *IL2Rγ*^{null} (hNSG) mice after 22 weeks of i.v. injection of human hematopoietic stem cells ($n = 8$). **c** Representative IHC analysis of human CD45$^+$, CD20$^+$, CD68$^+$, and CD56$^+$ cells performed in preparations of spleen from humanized (upper row) and nonhumanized (lower row) NSG mice. Counterstain, hematoxylin; magnifications, 20× and 4× (inset)

A375 melanoma cell xenografts were grown in both non-humanized and humanized NSG mice. As was the case with TNBC PDXs, melanoma cell xenograft growth also appeared to be delayed in hNSG animals when compared with nonhumanized NSG mice (Fig. 2b), highlighting the potential role of humanization and acquisition of a competent immunological status in affecting the growth of a tumor [35], as previously shown in similar models [36, 37]. To further investigate these observations, human leukocyte antigen (HLA) subtyping was performed in both the original hCD34$^+$ HSCs and two of the PDXs used in this study by using standard protocols used at the Department of Pathology & Genomic Medicine, Immunobiology & Transplant Science Center, Houston Methodist Hospital (Houston, TX, USA). Both PDX tumor models displayed different HLA subtypes (Additional file 2: Table S1), whereas the analysis of hCD34$^+$ HSCs resulted in the possibility of multiple patterns consistent with a mix of HLA types, which did not allow for a specific identification. These results are consistent with the fact that the hCD34$^+$ HSCs (STEMCELL Technologies) used in this study are basically formed by a pool of cells from different donors. This situation of partially matched HLA typing between hNSG mice and the PDXs may have contributed to lower tumor immunogenic rejection while simultaneously resulting in reduced percentages of engraftment and slower growing tumors (Fig. 2), as previously observed in similar studies showing that human PDX tumors can grow in hNSG with

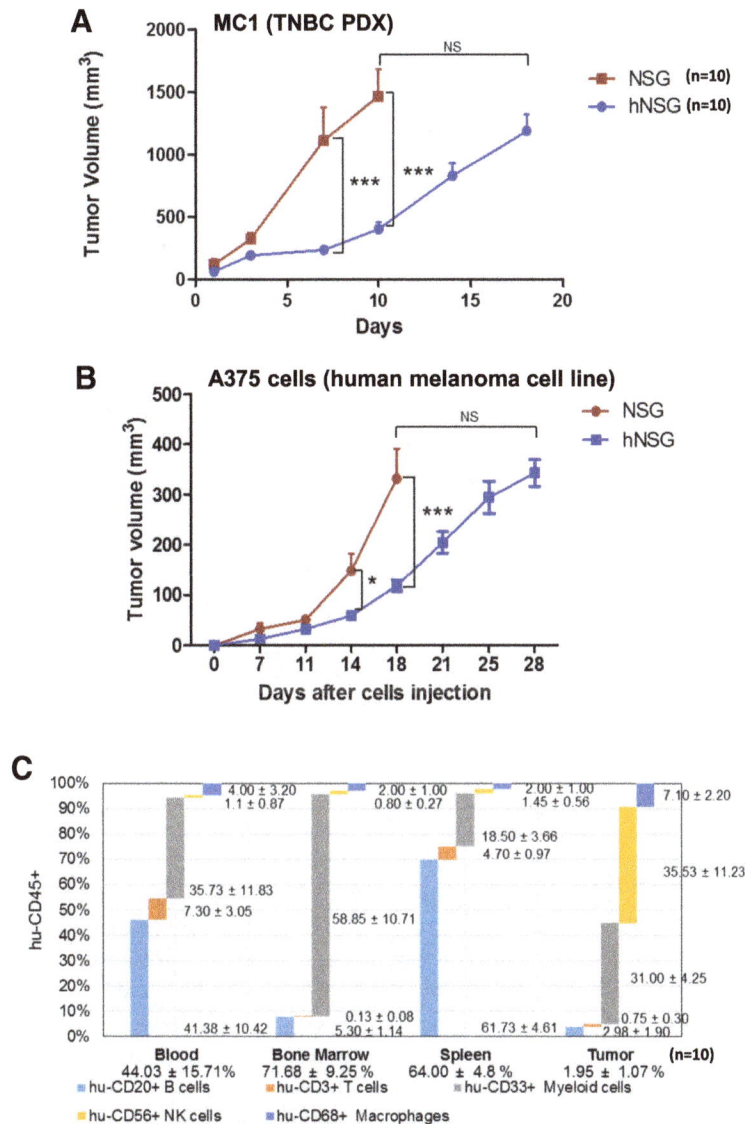

Fig. 2 In vivo effects of humanization of nonobese diabetic/severe combined immunodeficiency *IL2Rγ^null* (NSG) mice in the growth and engraftment of triple-negative breast cancer (TNBC) patient-derived xenograft (PDX) tumor line MC1 (**a**) and human melanoma A375 cell line (**b**). Both humanized and nonhumanized female NSG mice (*n* = 10 in each group) were transplanted orthotopically with pieces of either the PDX tumor line MC1 (into the cleared mammary fat pad) or A375 cells (into the skin) and allowed to grow. Tumor volume was determined twice weekly. *NS* Nonsignificant; *P < 0.05, *** P < 0.001. **c** Flow cytometric analysis of human CD45+ cells and hCD20+ (B cells), hCD3+ (T cells), hCD33+ (myeloid lineage), hCD56+ (natural killer [NK] cells) and hCD68+ (macrophages) cell subpopulations determined in blood, spleen, bone marrow, and MC1 PDX tumors of the corresponding samples shown in (**a**) (*n* = 10)

partially HLA-matched allogeneic human immune systems [36, 37].

Analysis of hCD45+ cells in blood, spleen, and bone marrow, performed at the moment the tumors reached their maximum size, showed profiles similar to those observed in animals not harboring tumors (i.e., hCD45+, 44.03 ± 15.71, 71.68 ± 9.25, and 64.00 ± 4.8 for blood, bone marrow, and spleen, respectively). A detailed distribution of the different CD45+ subpopulations is displayed in Fig. 2c, including the corresponding TILs isolated from the tumors (hCD45+, 1.95 ± 1.07).

To further characterize the humanized PDX model, levels of human cytokines known to be involved in the response to immunomodulatory therapies were determined in samples of serum and tumor lysates collected from nonhumanized NSG and hNSG mice harboring PDXs (Table 1) [38, 39]. As expected, significant increases were found in both circulating and tumor contents in the humanized mice. Importantly, taking into account the species specificity of the antibodies included in the assay, the presence of some circulating human cytokines detected in the nonhumanized NSG mice

Table 1 Levels of specific human cytokines

Human cytokines				
	Serum		Tumor	
	Non-hNSG	hNSG	Non-hNSG	hNSG
IL-1B	0	0	5.3 ± 1.0	10.9 ± 0.8*
TNF-α	0	1.3 ± 0.5	25.4 ± 2.1	250.2 ± 35.4**
IL-5	0	1.5 ± 0.4	0	0
IL-2	0	1.8 ± 0.3	0	0
IL-7	0	2.1 ± 0.6	10.4 ± 0.2	28.4 ± 0.6**
IL-12	0	3.6 ± 0.3	0	0
IFN-γ	0	19.8 ± 5.4	0	11.75 ± 0.6**
IL-13	0	0	7.8 ± 0.5	16.60 ± 0.6**
IL-4	0	0	8.3 ± 0.4	21.40 ± 1.0**
GM-CSF	93.7 ± 5.6	94.8 ± 9.7	841.8 ± 93.9	3296.3 ± 235.2**
IL-6	45.1 ± 2.5	73.3 ± 2.6*	217.8 ± 12.5	1039.2 ± 100.4**
IL-8	2989.5 ± 527.8	2798.3 ± 503.9	1208.1 ± 114.9	1310 ± 61.7

Abbreviations: GM-CSF Granulocyte-macrophage colony-stimulating factor, *hNSG* Humanized nonobese diabetic/severe combined immunodeficiency *IL2Rγ^null^*, *IFN-γ* Interferon-γ, *IL* Interleukin, *TNF-α* Tumor necrosis factor-α
Cytokines were measured in samples of serum and tumor lysates of non-hNSG and hNSG mice harboring triple-negative breast cancer MC1 patient-derived xenografts. Values are expressed in picograms per milliliter (± SEM) ($n = 4$ NSG; $n = 6$ hNSG).*$P < 0.05$, **$P < 0.01$

(e.g., granulocyte-macrophage colony-stimulating factor [GM-CSF], interleukin [IL]-6, and IL-8) were considered to have originated from the PDX because their levels, which were among the highest of the panel, were also clearly detected in the tumor collected from nonhumanized NSG mice. One of the recognized limitations of the hNSG mouse model resides in the absence of key cytokines that may support the stable engraftment of myeloid lineages, notably GM-CSF [40]. Interestingly, as the present results show, PDX-mediated production of GM-CSF may have contributed to this situation, as clearly evidenced by the fact that, despite the total levels of hCD45+ cells being similar between hNSG mice with/without PDXs, the percentage of the myeloid lineage subpopulation, represented by hCD33+ cells, was significantly increased in those mice harboring the tumors (Fig. 2c). Consequently, this may have resulted in a better reconstitution of the human immune system in the blood and thereby improved the accuracy of the studies that were performed with them.

IHC analysis was then performed on the tumors after they were collected. As shown in Fig. 3, the presence of hCD45+ cells was detectable in all the tumors screened (samples from different individual animals are shown), localizing both toward the periphery of the tumors as well as inside them. Analysis of hCD45+ cell subpopulations also showed hCD20+ cells (B cells), hCD68+ (macrophages), hCD56+ (NK cells), hCD4+ (T-helper cells), and hCD8+ T-cytotoxic cells.

Importantly, the expression of human cell markers remained negative in MC1 tumors developed in non-humanized NSG mice, indicating the specificity of the cells detected in the corresponding humanized MC1 tumor engraftments.

Breast cancer metastasis to the lung in hNSG mice

One of the most relevant characteristics of PDX models is their ability to retain the morphology, cellular heterogeneity, and molecular profiles of the original patient tumors [11]. To determine whether the immunological condition of the host (i.e., non-hNSG vs. hNSG) may have altered the genetic profile of the tumors, gene expression analysis of MC1, BCM-2147, and BCM-4913 PDXs growing in either non-hNSG or hNSG mice was performed by RNA sequencing (RNA-seq). Importantly, only minimal differences in the number of genes differentially expressed were found, demonstrating that the immunological status of the host played no significant role in the genetic stability of the tumors during the time course of the study (Additional file 2: Table S2).

Orthotopic breast cancer transplant models have been shown to recapitulate the same metastatic lesions and sites [11]. To determine whether the metastatic characteristics were maintained in the hNSG mouse model, PDXs corresponding to TNBC MC1, BCM-2147, and BCM-4913 tumor lines, all of which are known to produce metastatic lesions to the lung, were analyzed [12]. PDXs were transplanted into the cleared mammary gland fat pad of hNSG mice as described in the Methods section. At the moment of tumor removal, mice were checked for the appearance of metastasis in the lungs. As shown in Fig. 4 (representative results of each tumor line are shown; not all the animals analyzed displayed lung metastasis), IHC performed in the primary breast tumor showed expression of the human proliferation marker Ki-67 and the breast cancer marker CK19, confirming the human nature of the primary PDX. Importantly, as previously described in models using the MC1 tumor (Fig. 3), the presence of hCD45+ cells was detectable in all three primary tumor lines (Fig. 4). IHC assays using Ki-67 and CK19 identified the lung metastatic microscopic regions corresponding to the tumor localization (Fig. 4). As in the primary breast tumor, the presence of hCD45+ cells was also observed in both the lung and the proximities of the metastatic tumor (Fig. 4). Analyses of hCD45+ subpopulations in lung and lung metastasis, including hCD4, hCD3, hCD8, hCD20, hCD68, and hCD56, were also performed by IHC (Additional file 3: Figure S2). Together, these results demonstrate that one of the main characteristics of the TNBC PDXs (i.e., their capability to metastasize to the lungs) remains conserved in humanized mouse models.

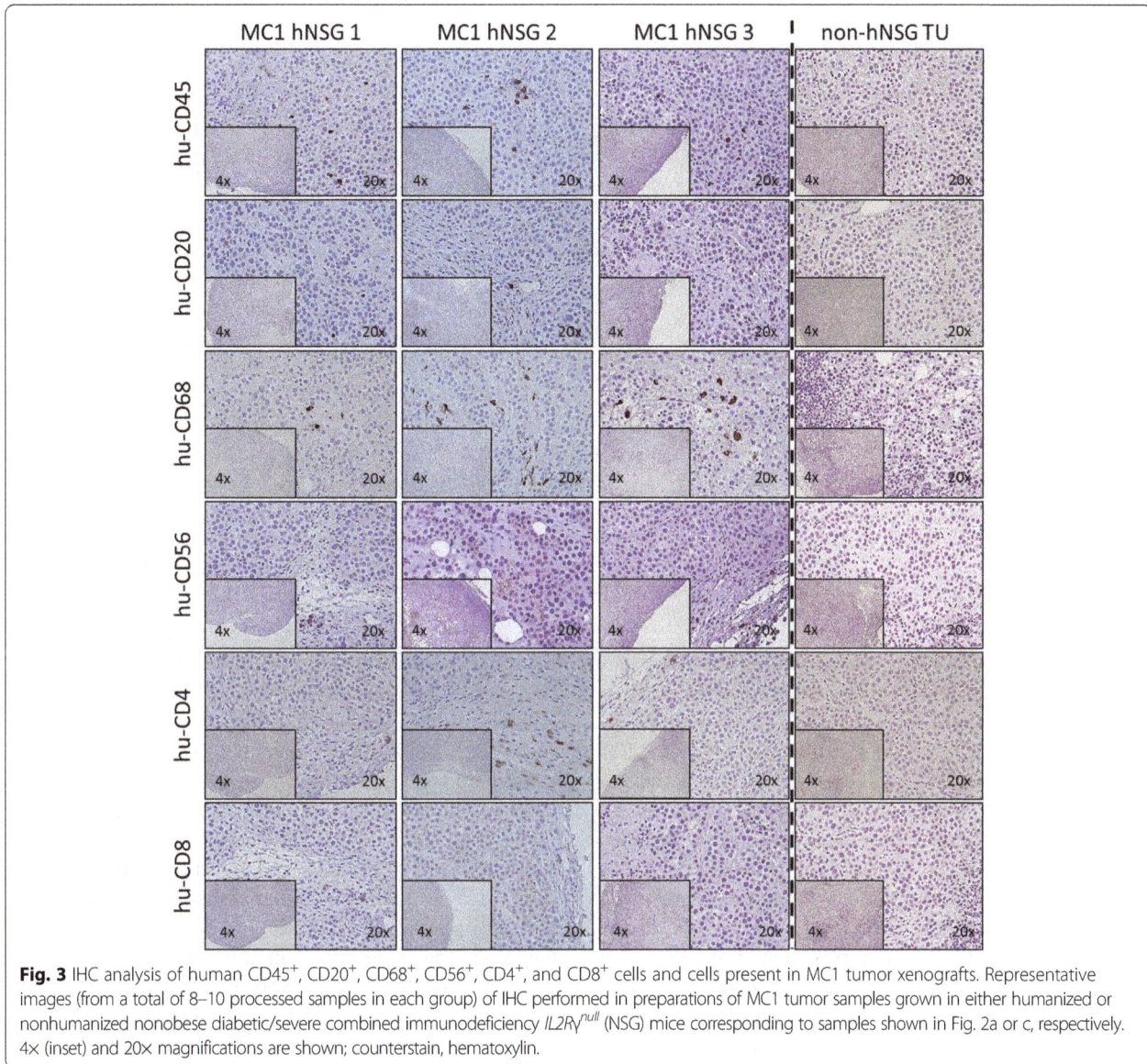

Fig. 3 IHC analysis of human CD45$^+$, CD20$^+$, CD68$^+$, CD56$^+$, CD4$^+$, and CD8$^+$ cells and cells present in MC1 tumor xenografts. Representative images (from a total of 8–10 processed samples in each group) of IHC performed in preparations of MC1 tumor samples grown in either humanized or nonhumanized nonobese diabetic/severe combined immunodeficiency $IL2R\gamma^{null}$ (NSG) mice corresponding to samples shown in Fig. 2a or c, respectively. 4× (inset) and 20× magnifications are shown; counterstain, hematoxylin.

Expression of PD-L1 in TNBC PDXs

Although still under continuous evaluation, both the expression of PD-L1 and a high mutational load have been associated with response to immune CPIs in clinical trials evaluating the efficacy of anti-PD-1-based therapies in melanoma, lung cancer, and TNBC [41–45]. The expression of PD-L1 was then determined in cell lysates of several PDX tumor lines by both Western blotting and IHC. As shown in Fig. 5a, a robust expression of PD-L1 was observed in MC1 PDXs collected from both non-hNSG and hNSG mice. Furthermore, this expression was not affected by the immunological status (i.e., humanized or nonhumanized) of the mice. Similarly, strong expression was also observed in PDX BCM-4913, as determined by both Western blotting and IHC (Fig. 5b and c). However, individual samples from two additional PDX tumor lines,

BCM-4664 and BCM-5471, displayed significantly lower expression of PD-L1 (Fig. 5c and d, Western blot and IHC, respectively). Together, these results provide evidence showing the variability of PD-L1 expression over different TNBC PDXs, recapitulating the situation often found in the clinical field [46].

Effects of anti-PD-1 therapy in the treatment of TNBC PDXs

Next, the efficacy of an anti-PD-1-based therapy was evaluated in our established hNSG PDX models. First, both non-hNSG and hNSG mice were implanted with MC1 PDXs and treated following a weekly schedule of humanized anti-PD-1 (10 mg/kg i.v.). As depicted in Fig. 6a (left graph), administration of anti-PD-1 antibody (nivolumab) to non-hNSG mice had no effect on the tumor size and growth, because tumors in both vehicle-

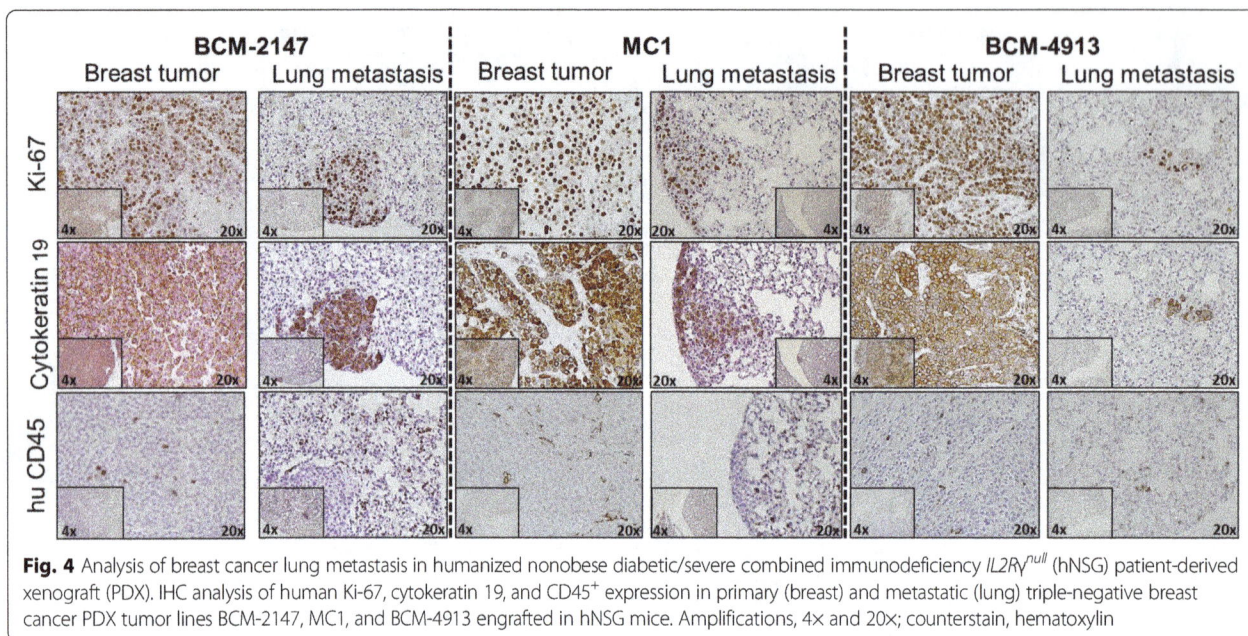

Fig. 4 Analysis of breast cancer lung metastasis in humanized nonobese diabetic/severe combined immunodeficiency *IL2Rγ^{null}* (hNSG) patient-derived xenograft (PDX). IHC analysis of human Ki-67, cytokeratin 19, and CD45$^+$ expression in primary (breast) and metastatic (lung) triple-negative breast cancer PDX tumor lines BCM-2147, MC1, and BCM-4913 engrafted in hNSG mice. Amplifications, 4× and 20×; counterstain, hematoxylin

and anti-PD-1-treated animals reached similar volume after days 10–12 of therapy (corresponding to two cycles of i.v. administered anti-PD-1 antibody). However, when the same schedule was applied to MC1-harboring hNSG animals, a significant reduction in the rate of MC1 tumor growth/volume was observed in the group of anti-PD-1-treated animals (Fig. 6a, right graph). In agreement with these results, analysis of survival rates, with endpoint based on the time that animals needed to be killed because of the tumor size, showed improved survival in the anti-PD-1-treated group vs. the corresponding vehicle-treated controls (Fig. 6b). The anti PD-1 monotherapy was then tested in additional TNBC PDX tumor lines. hNSG mice harboring the BCM-4913 PDXs were treated with pembrolizumab (10 mg/kg), following the same schedule used with the MC1 PDXs (i.e., weekly i.v. injections), resulting also in a significant reduction in tumor growth (Fig. 6c). Importantly, and consistent with the results observed in clinical settings showing despair activity of anti-PD-1/PD-L1 therapies in TNBC tumors [47–49], anti-PD-1 treatment resulted ineffective in two additional PDX models, BCM-4664 and BCM-5471 (Fig. 6d).

In addition, the effects of ipilimumab, a U.S. Food and Drug Administration-approved immune CPI directed against CTLA-4, were also evaluated for efficacy against MC1 PDXs. Once tumors reached ∼ 150 mm^3, animals were treated weekly with 10 mg/kg i.v. injections for up to 3 weeks. In contrast to the anti-PD-1-based therapies and in line with previous reports on breast cancer [50, 51], anti-CTLA-4 monotherapy did not result in a therapeutic benefit in MC1 PDXs (Additional file 4: Figure S3).

To identify potential mechanisms of action involved in the anti-PD-1-mediated TNBC tumor growth inhibition, the amount of TILs present in MC1 PDX tumors collected from both vehicle- and anti-PD-1-treated animals was determined by flow cytometry. Interestingly, no significant differences were observed in the percentage of human immunological cells infiltrating the tumor tissue (Additional file 5: Figure S4A). We then evaluated the cytotoxic activity of TILs by measuring the levels of lactate dehydrogenase, a stable cytosolic enzyme that is released upon TIL-induced tumor cell lysis. The experimental setting is described in the Methods section and in Additional file 5: Figure S4B. Briefly, TILs from MC1 PDX tumors engrafted in hNSG mice treated with either vehicle or anti-PD-1 antibody were isolated and then cocultured with disaggregated MC1 tumor cells obtained from the corresponding PDX grown in nonhumanized NSG mice. As shown in Fig. 6e, TILs corresponding to mice treated with the anti-PD-1 antibody displayed significantly higher cytotoxic activity than those corresponding to mice treated with vehicle control. Consistently, levels of granzyme B, a serine protease found in and released by TILs, were also significantly higher in lysates from tumors treated with anti-PD-1 than in those from vehicle-treated control lysates (Fig. 6f). In line with these findings, it is noteworthy that levels of IFN-γ, a cytokine secreted by activated T cells [52], was detected only in both serum and tumor lysates of PDX-harboring hNSG mice, indicating that it may have originated from human cytotoxic lymphocytes in response to the presence of PDXs. Together, these observations suggest that treatment with the anti-PD-1 resulted in increased cytotoxic activity of TILs present in the TNBC PDX tumors

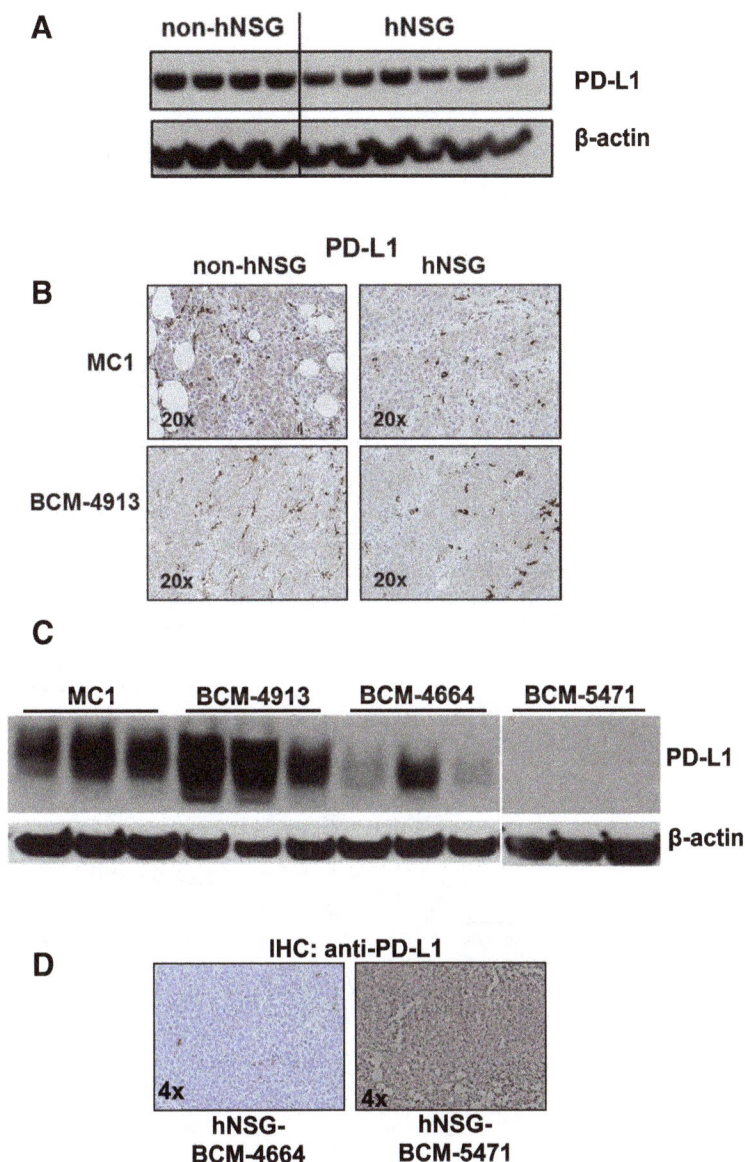

Fig. 5 Analysis of programmed death ligand 1 (PD-L1) protein expression in patient-derived xenograft (PDX) tumor samples engrafted in both nonhumanized and humanized nonobese diabetic/severe combined immunodeficiency *IL2Rγ^null* (hNSG) mice performed by Western blotting (**a**, MC1) or IHC (**b**, upper panels, MC1; lower panels, BCM-4913). In Western blotting experiments, samples were blotted with an anti-β-actin antibody as a loading control. The blots were processed in parallel, and they were all sourced from the same experiment. **c** Comparative analysis of PD-L1 levels was performed using four different PDX tumor lines (MC1, BCM-4913, BCM-4664, BCM-5471) engrafted in hNSG mice. Three independent tumors (animals) of each PDX line were evaluated by Western blot analysis. Samples were blotted with an anti-β-actin antibody as a loading control. **d** PD-L1 analysis performed by IHC of BCM-4664 and BCM-5471 PDXs engrafted in hNSG mice. 4× magnifications are shown; counterstain, hematoxylin

rather than in a higher number of TILs locating in the tumor tissue.

To further characterize and validate our humanized mouse models and their use in immunotherapy-targeted preclinical studies, similar studies were performed by generating xenografts with the immunogenic A375 melanoma cell line implanted orthotopically into the skin of both non-hNSG and hNSG mice (Fig. 7). As previously shown with MC1 TNBC PDXs (Fig. 6a), treatment with

either anti-CTLA-4 or anti-PD-1 antibodies had no effect on the progression of melanoma tumors implanted in non-hNSG mice (Fig. 7a). However, consistent with previous clinical studies [3, 53, 54] and its highly immunogenic profile, both anti-CTLA-4 and anti-PD-1 antibodies were highly effective in suppressing the growth of the melanoma cell xenografts (Fig. 7b and c), including a significant dose-dependent response with anti-CTLA-4 therapy (Fig. 7b). These results provide

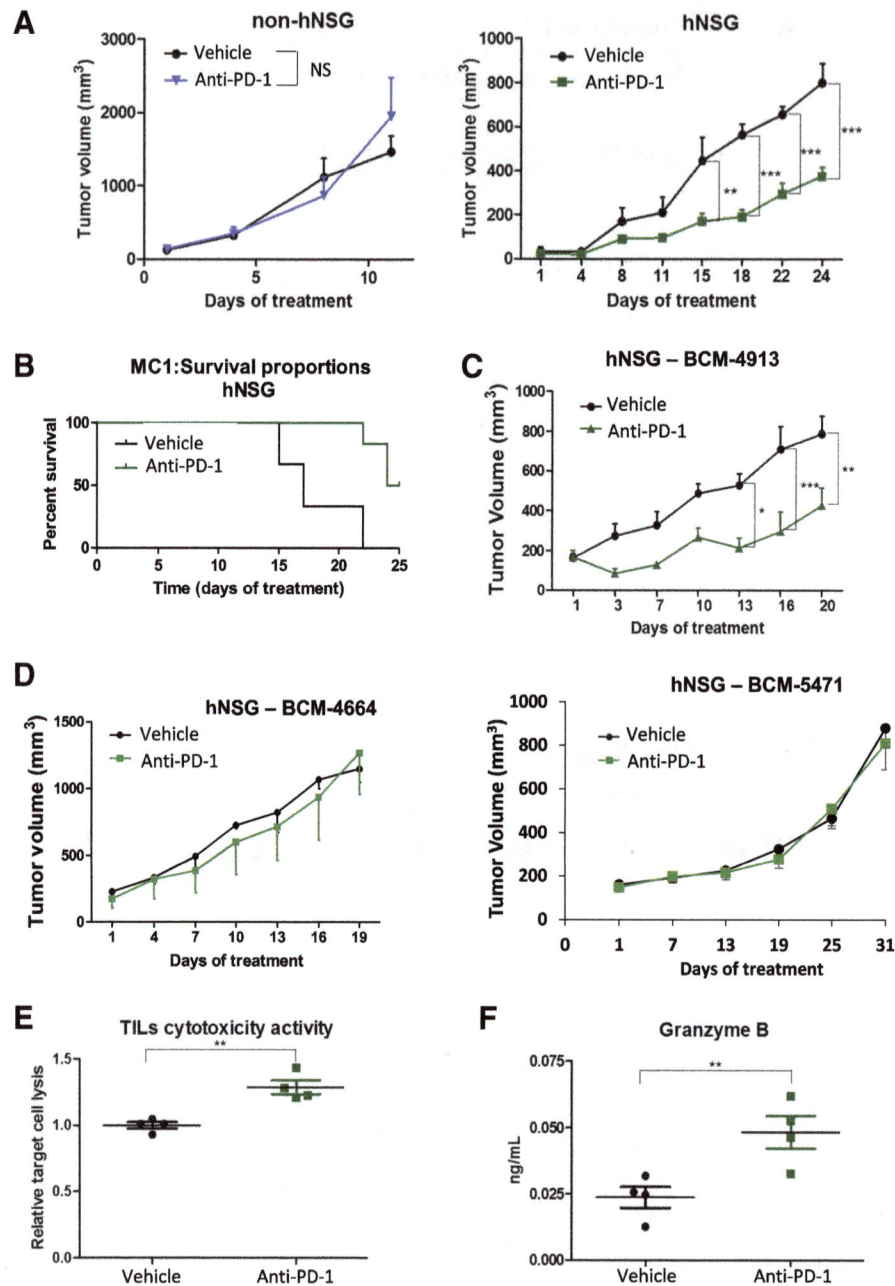

Fig. 6 Response of triple-negative breast cancer (TNBC) patient-derived xenografts (PDXs) to the anti-programmed cell death protein 1 (anti-PD-1) therapy. **a** In vivo treatment with anti-PD-1 antibody (10 mg/kg intravenous [i.v.] once weekly) of either TNBC MC1 PDX-engrafted nonhumanized (left graph, $n = 5$) or humanized (right graph, $n = 5$) nonobese diabetic/severe combined immunodeficiency $IL2R\gamma^{null}$ (hNSG) mice. Tumor volume was measured twice weekly. **b** Kaplan-Meier analysis of median survival of mice treated with vehicle ($n = 6$) vs. anti-PD-1 antibody ($n = 6$). **c** hNSG mice engrafted with an additional TNBC BCM-4913 PDX tumor line were treated with either vehicle control or anti-PD-1 antibody (10 mg/kg i.v. once weekly). Tumor volumes were measured twice weekly. **d** In vivo treatment with anti-PD-1 antibody (10 mg/kg i.v. once weekly) of TNBC BCM-4664 ($n = 5$) and HM-3818 ($n = 5$) PDXs engrafted in hNSG mice. Tumor volume was measured twice weekly. **e** Analysis of tumor-infiltrating lymphocyte (TIL) cytotoxic activity. TILs isolated by Ficoll gradient from vehicle- or anti-PD-1 antibody-treated MC1 PDX tumors engrafted in hNSG mice were cocultured with disaggregated MC1 tumor cells obtained from the corresponding PDX grown in nonhumanized NSG mice. Cytotoxic activity was measured using the CytoTox 96® Non-Radioactive Cytotoxicity Assay as per the manufacturer's instructions. **f** Levels of granzyme B tumor were measured by incubating tumor protein lysates with antibody-immobilized magnetic beads and evaluated using a Luminex LX200 Multiplexing Assay System. **$P < 0.01$, ***$P < 0.001$. *NS* Nonsignificant

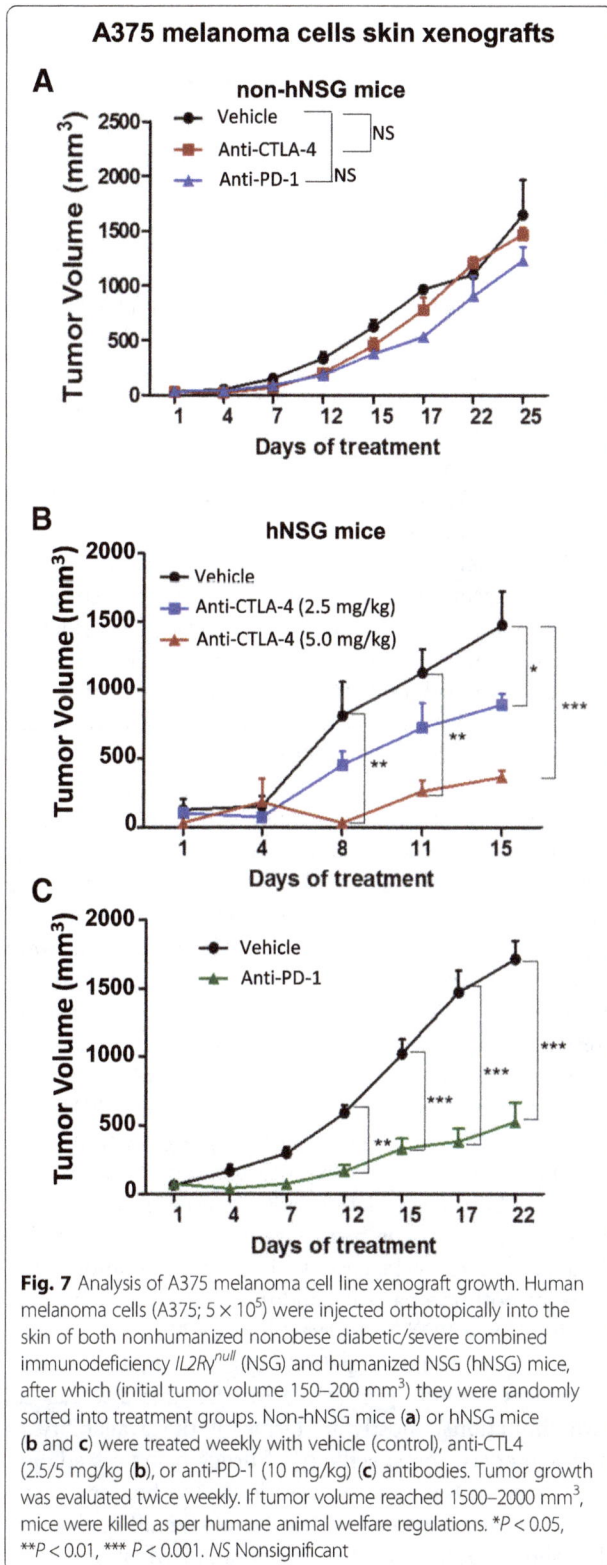

Fig. 7 Analysis of A375 melanoma cell line xenograft growth. Human melanoma cells (A375; 5×10^5) were injected orthotopically into the skin of both nonhumanized nonobese diabetic/severe combined immunodeficiency $IL2R\gamma^{null}$ (NSG) and humanized NSG (hNSG) mice, after which (initial tumor volume 150–200 mm³) they were randomly sorted into treatment groups. Non-hNSG mice (**a**) or hNSG mice (**b** and **c**) were treated weekly with vehicle (control), anti-CTL4 (2.5/5 mg/kg) (**b**), or anti-PD-1 (10 mg/kg) (**c**) antibodies. Tumor growth was evaluated twice weekly. If tumor volume reached 1500–2000 mm³, mice were killed as per humane animal welfare regulations. *$P < 0.05$, **$P < 0.01$, *** $P < 0.001$. *NS* Nonsignificant

additional evidence of both the humanization of the NSG model used and the relevance that such a model may have for testing immunotherapy-based regimens.

Discussion

The use of immunotherapies in breast cancer has been limited by breast cancer's relatively low immunogenicity [55]. However, newly developed strategies and/or approaches are rapidly changing the field, and novel immune CPIs are already approved or under different phases of clinical evaluation. Examples of these studies include clinical evaluation of anti-PD-1 and anti-PD-L1 therapies, administered either as single drugs or as part of multiple combinations [56, 57]. Enrichment strategies to select for patients more likely to respond have identified the expression and testing of PD-L1 to be a potentially useful predictive marker in guiding this process [58–60]. Following these criteria, in the present study, we investigated the expression of PD-L1 and its correlation with the anti-PD-1 activity. Although we did not evaluate a number of PDX tumor lines large enough to have the power required to achieve a statistically supported conclusion, our results showed a trend: Those PDXs that expressed high levels of PD-L1 appeared to respond to the anti-PD-1 therapy. Several clinical studies have evaluated the expression of PD-L1 and tried to identify possible associations with the therapeutic response. For example, positive expression of PD-L1 in TNBC stromal tissue or in $\geq 1\%$ of tumor cells has been used as a potential predictive biomarker in the phase Ib KEYNOTE-012 clinical trial [47]. Here, an 18.5% overall response rate was observed in the PD-L1-positive group, which represented ~60% of the total number of heavily pretreated patients with advanced TNBC under evaluation [47]. Other studies included a retrospective analysis (between 2004 and 2013) of 136 TNBC cases without neoadjuvant therapy, showing that stromal PD-L1 expression was significantly associated with better disease-free survival (DFS), whereas no association was found between PD-1 expression and DFS, overall survival, or metastasis [61]. Additional observations made by Botti et al. also showed a strong association between PD-L1 expression and better DFS [62]. Similar outcomes have resulted from a phase Ia study of the anti-PD-L1 antibody atezolizumab in previously treated patients with TNBC [63], altogether adding supporting evidence to the notion that PD-L1 expression may represent an important biomarker for prognostic stratification and CPI-based therapies. Nonetheless, the current consensus is that in addition to the expression of PD-L1 and mutation burden, multiple biomarkers may be needed to determine which patients will likely benefit from immunotherapies, including, notably in TNBC and HER2-positive patients, the presence of CD8$^+$ TILs, immune-related gene signatures, and multiplex IHC assays that may take into account the pharmacodynamic and spatial interactions of the TME [55, 56, 64–66]. As we demonstrated in the present study, our hNSG PDX model displayed clear evidence of several of these parameters (i.e., a humanized immune system with detectable presence of hCD45[+] TILs and cytokine levels) and robust expression of PD-L1 in some of the tumor lines. These results are in line with the clinical studies previously mentioned where the therapeutic benefits of regimens containing immunomodulatory CPI were observed mainly in patients where both TILs and PD-L1 were present, which provides additional support for the use of the humanized TNBC PDX mouse model used in this work. Similarly, also in agreement with observations in clinical trials [51, 67], the present model showed limited or no activity when TNBC tumor line MC1 was treated with an anti-CTLA-4 antibody, further validating the humanized mouse model because it reproduces some of the most relevant results observed during the clinical evaluation of immune CPIs. In fact, anti-CTLA-4 monotherapies have shown no or very limited therapeutic advantage against breast cancer when administered alone [67], although their efficacy has been improved by combination with other agents [50, 51, 68], which opens the field to new investigations. The mechanisms leading to the apparent lack of anti-CTLA-4 activity when administered as a monotherapy in certain solid tumors, including breast cancer, are still not well understood. However, it is thought to be associated with tumors' low antigenicity and microenvironment conditions that may not favor immune recognition [65, 69, 70].

From a potential mechanistic point of view, our studies indicate that the effects of blocking PD-1/PD-L1 interactions, thereby improving the immunological response [7, 8], may have resulted from increased activation of TILs rather than changes in the number of cells infiltrating the tumor. These observations are consistent with the established mode of action of these compounds (i.e., interfering the immune-inhibitory effects of the PD-1/PD-L1 interactions) [71]. In addition, our results may also suggest that amelioration of the therapeutic efficacy of immune CPIs could be achieved by modifying the TME as a way to enhance their activity, and in fact, multiple ongoing studies at both our and other laboratories are currently addressing this hypothesis. In addition, further studies are being designed to determine the long-term effects of CPIs in terms of tumor growth inhibition and mechanisms of resistance, notably in comparison to established chemotherapies, because the present report spanned a relatively short time frame.

In terms of the animal model that we used in the present study, it is clear that although these animals represent a very useful tool, humanization of NSG mice may still pose some technical challenges and/or limitations. Notably, one of those well-recognized limiting factors is the lack of GM-CSF, important for the differentiation and maturation of the myeloid lineage [72]. To address this point, several newer, genetically modified NSG-based (The Jackson Laboratory) or NOG (NOD/Shi-*scid*/IL-2Rγ[null])-based (Taconic Biosciences, Rensselaer, NY, USA) models are being developed, which, by expressing the human cytokines GM-CSF and IL-3 and human stem cell factor gene (*SCF*; also known as KIT ligand, *KITLG*), allow for better engraftment of HSCs and cell lineage differentiation [73]. In our case, it is important to note that some of these limitations appeared to be compensated by the presence of the TNBC PDX. Indeed, as our results show, PDXs were associated with the presence of several cytokines, including GM-CSF, which consequently may have played an important role in improving the levels of the myeloid lineage (hCD33[+] cells) when compared with the hNSG mice not harboring tumors. These results suggest, as previously mentioned, that the simultaneous presence of the PDX during hHSC engraftment may have compensated for the lack of this and other factors, contributing to a better reconstitution of the immune system.

Another important factor that was considered in our study was the potential role of matching HLA typing between the hNSG host and the PDXs. Our observations showed some differences in the PDX growth rate based on whether the mice were humanized or not, most likely owing to the incipient presence of an active immune system. However, as also shown by others, including the case of commercially available humanized PDX models [36, 37], no signs of graft-versus-host reaction were found. Furthermore, on the basis of the fact that the HLA typing of HSCs did not conclusively demonstrate compatibility with more than one pattern, it is plausible to postulate that the slower growth of PDXs may have resulted from partially HLA-matched hNSG/PDX engraftment, which allowed a seemingly regular tumor engraftment. This is an important observation because the ideal situation (i.e., isolating HSCs from the same cancer patient whose PDX is being used) may prove extremely difficult to achieve in large-scale preclinical studies, because of both the patient condition and the time usually required for a PDX to be established [73]. Alternatively, the use of immunocompetent syngeneic mouse models represents a valid approach. However, this also has its own limitations, mostly in terms of the availability of tumor models, the specificity of drugs being tested, and the extrapolation of observations to human cases. Together, despite some of the factors mentioned above that should be taken into consideration whenever using humanized PDX mouse models, these models still represent very helpful and sophisticated tools for preclinical evaluation of immune-based therapies, notably as they become more available and improved animal versions are generated.

Conclusions

In the present work, we evaluated the preclinical efficacy of anti-PD-1 therapies developed in humanized mouse models of TNBC PDXs. Our results in this study (1) indicate that breast cancer PDX models engrafted in hNSG mice represent a valuable tool to test for immune-based therapies, as demonstrated by the differential effects of the anti-PD-1 therapy in either nonhumanized or humanized NSG mice; and (2) highlight the validity of our methodology developed "in-house."

Additional files

Additional file 1: Representative figure showing the results of flow cytometric analysis of human cells collected from blood of nonhumanized and humanized NSG mice after 8, 16, and 22 weeks of intravenous injection of human CD34+ hematopoietic stem cells (HSCs). Procedures and antibodies used in these studies are described in the Methods section. (PPTX 722 kb)

Additional file 2: Table S1 Analysis of HLA type in PDX BCM-2147/-4913 and CD34+ HSCs. HLA typing was performed by using PCR-SSO DNA-based procedures. The serological phenotype is an interpretation based on molecular typing data. *ND* Not determined. **Table S2** Gene expression analysis (RNA-Seq) comparing MC1, BCM-2147, and BCM-4913 PDXs growing in nonhumanized vs. humanized NSG mice. Differentially expressed genes (DEGs) were selected by edge R-based *p* value and fold change (FC). Supplemental Methods. (DOCX 22 kb)

Additional file 3: IHC analysis of human CD4-, CD3-, CD8-, CD20-, CD68-, CD4-, and CD8-positive cells present in BCM-2147, MC1, and BCM-4913 tumor xenograft lung micrometastases. Representative IHC images of obtained using preparations of tumor samples grown in humanized NSG mice; 4× and 20× magnifications are shown counterstained with hematoxylin. (PPTX 3007 kb)

Additional file 4: Effects of the anti-CTLA-4 immune checkpoint inhibitor antibody ipilimumab against MC1 PDXs implanted in hNSG mice. Once tumors reached ~ 150 mm^3, animals were treated weekly with 10 mg/kg intravenous injections for up to 3 weeks; tumor volumes were evaluated twice weekly. The values represent the mean ± SEM ($n = 8$). (PPTX 50 kb)

Additional file 5: a Evaluation of the percentages of human CD45+ TILs present in MC1 PDX tumors engrafted in hNSG mice and collected from animals treated with either vehicle control or anti-PD-1 antibody. The values represent the mean ± SEM ($n = 8$). **b** Schematic representation of the method used to determine the cytotoxic activity of TILs by measuring the levels of the lactate dehydrogenase (LDH), a stable cytosolic enzyme that is released upon TIL-induced tumor cell lysis. TILs were isolated from MC1 PDX tumors engrafted in hNSG mice and treated with either vehicle or anti-PD1 antibody that were cocultured with disaggregated MC1 tumor cells obtained from the corresponding PDX grown in nonhumanized NSG mice. (PPTX 131 kb)

Abbreviations
ANOVA: Analysis of variance; APC: Allophycocyanin; CK19: Cytokeratin 19; CPI: Checkpoint inhibitor; CTLA-4: Cytotoxic T-lymphocyte-associated protein 4; DFS: Disease-free survival; FITC: Fluorescein isothiocyanate; GM-CSF: Granulocyte-macrophage colony-stimulating factor; HLA: Human leukocyte antigen; hNSG: Humanized nonobese diabetic/severe combined immunodeficiency *IL2Rγ^null*; HSC: Hematopoietic stem cell; IgG: Immunoglobulin G; IL: Interleukin; i.v.: Intravenous(ly); NK: Natural killer cells; PD-1: Programmed cell death protein 1; PD-L1: Programmed death ligand 1; PDX: Patient-derived xenograft; PE: Phycoerythrin; RNA-seq: RNA sequencing; TIL: Tumor-infiltrating lymphocyte; TME: Tumor microenvironment; TNBC: Triple-negative breast cancer

Acknowledgements
The RNA-seq data were generated and analyzed by the Genome Sequencing Facility of Greehey Children's Cancer Research Institute at the University of Texas Health San Antonio. We thank Dr. Zhao Lai for RNA-seq assistance and Hung-I Chen and Dr. Yidong Chen for RNA-seq data analysis. Low-resolution HLA typing was performed by the transplant immunology laboratory at Houston Methodist Hospital, Houston, TX, USA. DDG is grateful for support from the Instituto Tecnológico y de Estudios Superiores de Monterrey, Monterrey, Mexico, and Consejo Nacional de Ciencia y Tecnología, Mexico (CONACyT 490148/278957). The authors acknowledge the help provided by the Flow Cytometry and Comparative Medicine core facilities at the Houston Methodist Research Institute. DDG is a current graduate student at the Instituto Tecnológico y de Estudios Superiores de Monterrey, Monterrey, Mexico.

Funding
This research was supported by National Cancer Institute grants R01 CA138197 and U54 CA149196 from the National Institutes of Health, Golfers Against Cancer, the Breast Cancer Research Foundation, Causes for a Cure, Team Tiara, the Emily W. Herrman Cancer Research Laboratory, Department of Defense Innovator Expansion Award BC104158, and Komen for Cure grant KG 081694 (to JCC). None of the funding sources had any role in the design of the study, the analysis or interpretation of data, or the writing of the present manuscript.

Authors' contributions
JCC and RRR conceived of and designed the study in collaboration with DDG, DSC, and BD. DDG, WQ, WC, AJK, and HW performed experiments, including animal studies, IHC, flow cytometry, and Western blotting. JCC, RRR, and DDG performed statistical analysis, interpreted the results, and drafted the manuscript. All authors contributed with critical revision, editing of the final version of the manuscript, and approval of the final version for publication, and all authors agree to be accountable for the accuracy and integrity of the work.

Competing interests
The authors declare that they have no competing interests.

References
1. Wolchok JD, Kluger H, Callahan MK, Postow MA, Rizvi NA, Lesokhin AM, et al. Nivolumab plus ipilimumab in advanced melanoma. N Engl J Med. 2013; 369:122–33.
2. Linsley PS, Brady W, Grosmaire L, Aruffo A, Damle NK, Ledbetter JA. Binding of the B cell activation antigen B7 to CD28 costimulates T cell proliferation and interleukin 2 mRNA accumulation. J Exp Med. 1991;173:721–30.
3. Robert C, Thomas L, Bondarenko I, O'Day S, Weber J, Garbe C, et al. Ipilimumab plus dacarbazine for previously untreated metastatic melanoma. N Engl J Med. 2011;364:2517–26.
4. Butte MJ, Keir ME, Phamduy TB, Sharpe AH, Freeman GJ. Programmed death-1 ligand 1 interacts specifically with the B7-1 costimulatory molecule to inhibit T cell responses. Immunity. 2007;27:111–22.
5. Freeman GJ, Long AJ, Iwai Y, Bourque K, Chernova T, Nishimura H, et al. Engagement of the PD-1 immunoinhibitory receptor by a novel B7 family member leads to negative regulation of lymphocyte activation. J Exp Med. 2000;192:1027–34.

6.   Okazaki T, Honjo T. PD-1 and PD-1 ligands: from discovery to clinical application. Int Immunol. 2007;19:813–24.

7.   Pardoll DM. The blockade of immune checkpoints in cancer immunotherapy. Nat Rev Cancer. 2012;12:252–64.

8.   Tumeh PC, Harview CL, Yearley JH, Shintaku IP, Taylor EJ, Robert L, et al. PD-1 blockade induces responses by inhibiting adaptive immune resistance. Nature. 2014;515:568–71.

9.   Morton JJ, Bird G, Keysar SB, Astling DP, Lyons TR, Anderson RT, et al. XactMice: humanizing mouse bone marrow enables microenvironment reconstitution in a patient-derived xenograft model of head and neck cancer. Oncogene. 2016;35:290–300.

10. Morton JJ, Bird G, Refaeli Y, Jimeno A. Humanized mouse xenograft models: narrowing the tumor-microenvironment gap. Cancer Res. 2016;76(21):6153–8.

11. Landis MD, Lehmann BD, Pietenpol JA, Chang JC. Patient-derived breast tumor xenografts facilitating personalized cancer therapy. Breast Cancer Res. 2013;15:201.

12. Zhang X, Claerhout S, Prat A, Dobrolecki LE, Petrovic I, Lai Q, et al. A renewable tissue resource of phenotypically stable, biologically and ethnically diverse, patient-derived human breast cancer xenograft models. Cancer Res. 2013;73:4885–97.

13. DeRose YS, Wang G, Lin YC, Bernard PS, Buys SS, Ebbert MT, et al. Tumor grafts derived from women with breast cancer authentically reflect tumor pathology, growth, metastasis and disease outcomes. Nat Med. 2011;17:1514–20.

14. Ding L, Ellis MJ, Li S, Larson DE, Chen K, Wallis JW, et al. Genome remodelling in a basal-like breast cancer metastasis and xenograft. Nature. 2010;464:999–1005.

15. Gao H, Korn JM, Ferretti S, Monahan JE, Wang Y, Singh M, et al. High-throughput screening using patient-derived tumor xenografts to predict clinical trial drug response. Nat Med. 2015;21:1318–25.

16. Marangoni E, Vincent-Salomon A, Auger N, Degeorges A, Assayag F, de Cremoux P, et al. A new model of patient tumor-derived breast cancer xenografts for preclinical assays. Clin Cancer Res. 2007;13:3989–98.

17. Townsend EC, Murakami MA, Christodoulou A, Christie AL, Koster J, DeSouza TA, et al. The public repository of xenografts enables discovery and randomized phase II-like trials in mice. Cancer Cell. 2016;29:574–86.

18. Visonneau S, Cesano A, Torosian MH, Miller EJ, Santoli D. Growth characteristics and metastatic properties of human breast cancer xenografts in immunodeficient mice. Am J Pathol. 1998;152:1299–311.

19. Fiebig HH, Maier A, Burger AM. Clonogenic assay with established human tumour xenografts: correlation of in vitro to in vivo activity as a basis for anticancer drug discovery. Eur J Cancer. 2004;40:802–20.

20. Hidalgo M, Amant F, Biankin AV, Budinská E, Byrne AT, Caldas C, et al. Patient-derived xenograft models: an emerging platform for translational cancer research. Cancer Discov. 2014;4(9):998–1013.

21. Voskoglou-Nomikos T, Pater JL, Seymour L. Clinical predictive value of the in vitro cell line, human xenograft, and mouse allograft preclinical cancer models. Clin Cancer Res. 2003;9:4227–39.

22. Krepler C, Sproesser K, Brafford P, Beqiri M, Garman B, Xiao M, et al. A comprehensive patient-derived xenograft collection representing the heterogeneity of melanoma. Cell Rep. 2017;21:1953–67.

23. Bertotti A, Migliardi G, Galimi F, Sassi F, Torti D, Isella C, et al. A molecularly annotated platform of patient-derived xenografts ("xenopatients") identifies HER2 as an effective therapeutic target in cetuximab-resistant colorectal cancer. Cancer Discov. 2011;1:508–23.

24. Migliardi G, Sassi F, Torti D, Galimi F, Zanella ER, Buscarino M, et al. Inhibition of MEK and PI3K/mTOR suppresses tumor growth but does not cause tumor regression in patient-derived xenografts of RAS-mutant colorectal carcinomas. Clin Cancer Res. 2012;18:2515–25.

25. Lehmann S, Walther T, Kempfert J, Leontyev S, Bakhtiary F, Rastan A, et al. Ten-year follow up after prospectively randomized evaluation of stentless versus conventional xenograft aortic valve replacement. J Heart Valve Dis. 2011;20:681–7.

26. Nielsen TO, Parker JS, Leung S, Voduc D, Ebbert M, Vickery T, et al. A comparison of PAM50 intrinsic subtyping with immunohistochemistry and clinical prognostic factors in tamoxifen-treated estrogen receptor-positive breast cancer. Clin Cancer Res. 2010;16:5222–32.

27. Schott AF, Landis MD, Dontu G, Griffith KA, Layman RM, Krop I, et al. Preclinical and clinical studies of γ secretase inhibitors with docetaxel on human breast tumors. Clin Cancer Res. 2013;19:1512–24.

28. Hasgur S, Aryee KE, Shultz LD, Greiner DL, Brehm MA. Generation of immunodeficient mice bearing human immune systems by the engraftment of hematopoietic stem cells. Methods Mol Biol. 2016;1438:67–78.

29. Pearson T, Greiner DL, Shultz LD. Creation of "humanized" mice to study human immunity. Curr Protoc Immunol. 2008;Chapter 15:Unit 15.21.

30. Ginestier C, Hur MH, Charafe-Jauffret E, Monville F, Dutcher J, Brown M, et al. ALDH1 is a marker of normal and malignant human mammary stem cells and a predictor of poor clinical outcome. Cell Stem Cell. 2007;1:555–67.

31. Granados-Principal S, Liu Y, Guevara ML, Blanco E, Choi DS, Qian W, et al. Inhibition of iNOS as a novel effective targeted therapy against triple-negative breast cancer. Breast Cancer Res. 2015;17:25.

32. Choi DS, Blanco E, Kim YS, Rodriguez AA, Zhao H, Huang TH, et al. Chloroquine eliminates cancer stem cells through deregulation of Jak2 and DNMT1. Stem Cells. 2014;32:2309–23.

33. Wang Q, Li N, Wang X, Kim MM, Evers BM. Augmentation of sodium butyrate-induced apoptosis by phosphatidylinositol 3′-kinase inhibition in the KM20 human colon cancer cell line. Clin Cancer Res. 2002;8:1940–7.

34. Wege AK, Schmidt M, Ueberham E, Ponnath M, Ortmann O, Brockhoff G, et al. Co-transplantation of human hematopoietic stem cells and human breast cancer cells in NSG mice: a novel approach to generate tumor cell specific human antibodies. MAbs. 2014;6:968–77.

35. Dunn GP, Bruce AT, Ikeda H, Old LJ, Schreiber RD. Cancer immunoediting: from immunosurveillance to tumor escape. Nat Immunol. 2002;3:991–8.

36. Wang M, Keck JG, Cheng M, Cai D, Shultz L, Palucka K, et al. Abstract LB-050: Patient-derived tumor xenografts in humanized NSG mice: a model to study immune responses in cancer therapy [abstract]. Cancer Res. 2015; 75(15 Suppl):LB-050.

37. Wang M, Yao LC, Cheng M, Cai D, Martinek J, Pan CX, et al. Humanized mice in studying efficacy and mechanisms of PD-1-targeted cancer immunotherapy. FASEB J. 2018;32(3):1537–49.

38. Mischinger J, Comperat E, Schwentner C, Stenzl A, Gakis G. Inflammation and cancer: what can we therapeutically expect from checkpoint inhibitors? Curr Urol Rep. 2015;16(9):59.

39. Ribas A. Adaptive immune resistance: how cancer protects from immune attack. Cancer Discov. 2015;5:915–9.

40. Yao L-C, Riess J, Cheng M, Wang M, Banchereau J, Shultz L, et al. Patient-derived tumor xenografts in humanized NSG-SGM3 mice: a new immuno-oncology platform [abstract]. J Clin Oncol. 2016;34(15 Suppl):3074.

41. Carbone DP, Reck M, Paz-Ares L, Creelan B, Horn L, Steins M, et al. First-line Nivolumab in stage IV or recurrent non–small-cell lung cancer. N Engl J Med. 2017;376:2415–26.

42. Festino L, Botti G, Lorigan P, Masucci GV, Hipp JD, Horak CE, et al. Cancer treatment with anti-PD-1/PD-L1 agents: is PD-L1 expression a biomarker for patient selection? Drugs. 2016;76:925–45.

43. Mori H, Kubo M, Yamaguchi R, Nishimura R, Osako T, Arima N, et al. The combination of PD-L1 expression and decreased tumor-infiltrating lymphocytes is associated with a poor prognosis in triple-negative breast cancer. Oncotarget. 2017;8:15584–92.

44. Rizvi NA, Mazieres J, Planchard D, Stinchcombe TE, Dy GK, Antonia SJ, et al. Activity and safety of nivolumab, an anti-PD-1 immune checkpoint inhibitor, for patients with advanced, refractory squamous non-small-cell lung cancer (CheckMate 063): a phase 2, single-arm trial. Lancet Oncol. 2015;16:257–65.

45. Snyder A, Makarov V, Merghoub T, Yuan J, Zaretsky JM, Desrichard A, et al. Genetic basis for clinical response to CTLA-4 blockade in melanoma. N Engl J Med. 2014;371:2189–99.

46. Mittendorf EA, Philips AV, Meric-Bernstam F, Qiao N, Wu Y, Harrington S, et al. PD-L1 expression in triple-negative breast cancer. Cancer Immunol Res. 2014;2:361–70.

47. Nanda R, Chow LQM, Dees EC, Berger R, Gupta S, Geva R, et al. Pembrolizumab in patients with advanced triple-negative breast cancer: phase Ib KEYNOTE-012 study. J Clin Oncol. 2016;34:2460–7.

48. Nanda R, Liu MC, Yau C, Asare S, Hylton N, van 't Veer L, et al. Pembrolizumab plus standard neoadjuvant therapy for high-risk breast cancer (BC): results from I-SPY 2 [abstract]. J Clin Oncol. 2017;35(15 Suppl):506.

49. Schmid P, Park YH, Muñoz-Couselo E, Kim S-B, Sohn J, Im SA, et al. Pembrolizumab (pembro) + chemotherapy (chemo) as neoadjuvant treatment for triple negative breast cancer (TNBC): preliminary results from KEYNOTE-173 [abstract]. J Clin Oncol. 2017;35(15 Suppl):556.

50. Calabro L, Danielli R, Sigalotti L, Maio M. Clinical studies with anti-CTLA-4 antibodies in non-melanoma indications. Semin Oncol. 2010;37:460–7.

51. McArthur HL, Diab A, Page DB, Yuan J, Solomon SB, Sacchini V, et al. A pilot study of preoperative single-dose ipilimumab and/or cryoablation in women with early-stage breast cancer with comprehensive immune profiling. Clin Cancer Res. 2016;22:5729–37.

52. Schoenborn JR, Wilson CB. Regulation of interferon-γ during innate and adaptive immune responses. Adv Immunol. 2007;96:41–101.

53. Robert C, Long GV, Brady B, Dutriaux C, Maio M, Mortier L, et al. Nivolumab in previously untreated melanoma without BRAF mutation. N Engl J Med. 2015;372:320–30.

54. Robert C, Schachter J, Long GV, Arance A, Grob JJ, Mortier L, et al. Pembrolizumab versus Ipilimumab in Advanced Melanoma. N Engl J Med. 2015;372:2521–32.

55. Luen SJ, Savas P, Fox SB, Salgado R, Loi S. Tumour-infiltrating lymphocytes and the emerging role of immunotherapy in breast cancer. Pathology. 2017;49: 141–55.

56. Bedognetti D, Maccalli C, Bader SB, Marincola FM, Seliger B. Checkpoint inhibitors and their application in breast cancer. Breast Care (Basel). 2016;11:108–15.

57. Emens LA. Breast cancer immunotherapy: facts and hopes. Clin Cancer Res. 2018;24(3):511–20.

58. Ancevski Hunter K, Socinski MA, Villaruz LC. PD-L1 testing in guiding patient selection for PD-1/PD-L1 inhibitor therapy in lung cancer. Mol Diagn Ther. 2018;22(1):1–10.

59. Voong KR, Feliciano J, Becker D, Levy B. Beyond PD-L1 testing-emerging biomarkers for immunotherapy in non-small cell lung cancer. Ann Transl Med. 2017;5:376.

60. Yaziji H, Taylor CR. PD-L1 assessment for targeted therapy testing in cancer: urgent need for realistic economic and practice expectations. Appl Immunohistochem Mol Morphol. 2017;25:1–3.

61. Li X, Wetherilt CS, Krishnamurti U, Yang J, Ma Y, Styblo TM, et al. Stromal PD-L1 expression is associated with better disease-free survival in triple-negative breast cancer. Am J Clin Pathol. 2016;146:496–502.

62. Botti G, Collina F, Scognamiglio G, Rao F, Peluso V, De Cecio R, et al. Programmed death ligand 1 (PD-L1) tumor expression is associated with a better prognosis and diabetic disease in triple negative breast cancer patients. Int J Mol Sci. 2017;18(2):E459.

63. Emens LA, Braiteh FS, Cassier P, Delord J-P, Eder JP, Fasso M, et al. Abstract 2859: inhibition of PD-L1 by MPDL3280A leads to clinical activity in patients with metastatic triple-negative breast cancer (TNBC) [abstract]. Cancer Res. 2015;75(15 Suppl):2859.

64. Mehnert JM, Monjazeb AM, Beerthuijzen JMT, Collyar D, Rubinstein L, Harris LN. The challenge for development of valuable immuno-oncology biomarkers. Clin Cancer Res. 2017;23:4970–9.

65. Salgado R, Denkert C, Demaria S, Sirtaine N, Klauschen F, Pruneri G, et al. The evaluation of tumor-infiltrating lymphocytes (TILs) in breast cancer: recommendations by an international TILs working group 2014. Ann Oncol. 2015;26:259–71.

66. Savas P, Salgado R, Denkert C, Sotiriou C, Darcy PK, Smyth MJ, et al. Clinical relevance of host immunity in breast cancer: from TILs to the clinic. Nat Rev Clin Oncol. 2016;13:228–41.

67. Vonderheide RH, LoRusso PM, Khalil M, Gartner EM, Khaira D, Soulieres D, et al. Tremelimumab in combination with exemestane in patients with advanced breast cancer and treatment-associated modulation of inducible costimulator expression on patient T cells. Clin Cancer Res. 2010;16:3485–94.

68. Ribas A, Kefford R, Marshall MA, Punt CJ, Haanen JB, Marmol M, et al. Phase III randomized clinical trial comparing tremelimumab with standard-of-care chemotherapy in patients with advanced melanoma. J Clin Oncol. 2013;31:616–22.

69. Loi S, Michiels S, Salgado R, Sirtaine N, Jose V, Fumagalli D, et al. Tumor infiltrating lymphocytes are prognostic in triple negative breast cancer and predictive for trastuzumab benefit in early breast cancer: results from the FinHER trial. Ann Oncol. 2014;25:1544–50.

70. Schumacher TN, Schreiber RD. Neoantigens in cancer immunotherapy. Science. 2015;348:69–74.

71. Chen L, Han X. Anti-PD-1/PD-L1 therapy of human cancer: past, present, and future. J Clin Invest. 2015;125:3384–91.

72. Shi Y, Liu CH, Roberts AI, Das J, Xu G, Ren G, et al. Granulocyte-macrophage colony-stimulating factor (GM-CSF) and T-cell responses: what we do and don't know. Cell Res. 2006;16:126–33.

73. Byrne AT, Alferez DG, Amant F, Annibali D, Arribas J, Biankin AV, et al. Interrogating open issues in cancer precision medicine with patient-derived xenografts. Nat Rev Cancer. 2017;17:254–68.

13

Vitamin D, DNA methylation, and breast cancer

Katie M. O'Brien[1,2]* ⓘ, Dale P. Sandler[2], Zongli Xu[2], H. Karimi Kinyamu[3], Jack A. Taylor[2†] and Clarice R. Weinberg[1†]

Abstract

Background: Vitamin D has anticarcinogenic and immune-related properties and may protect against some diseases, including breast cancer. Vitamin D affects gene transcription and may influence DNA methylation.

Methods: We studied the relationships between serum vitamin D, DNA methylation, and breast cancer using a case-cohort sample (1070 cases, 1277 in subcohort) of non-Hispanic white women. For our primary analysis, we used robust linear regression to examine the association between serum 25-hydroxyvitamin D (25(OH)D) and methylation within a random sample of the cohort ("subcohort"). We focused on 198 CpGs in or near seven vitamin D-related genes. For these 198 candidate CpG loci, we also examined how multiplicative interactions between methylation and 25(OH)D were associated with breast cancer risk. This was done using Cox proportional hazards models and the full case-cohort sample. We additionally conducted an exploratory epigenome-wide association study (EWAS) of the association between 25(OH)D and DNA methylation in the subcohort.

Results: Of the CpGs in vitamin D-related genes, cg21201924 (*RXRA*) had the lowest p value for association with 25(OH)D ($p = 0.0004$). Twenty-two other candidate CpGs were associated with 25(OH)D ($p < 0.05$; *RXRA, NADSYN1/DHCR7, GC,* or *CYP27B1*). We observed an interaction between 25(OH)D and methylation at cg21201924 in relation to breast cancer risk (ratio of hazard ratios = 1.22, 95% confidence interval 1.10–1.34; $p = 7 \times 10^{-5}$), indicating a larger methylation-breast cancer hazard ratio in those with high serum 25(OH)D concentrations. We also observed statistically significant ($p < 0.05$) interactions for six other *RXRA* CpGs and CpGs in *CYP24A1, CYP27B1, NADSYN1/DHCR7,* and *VDR*. In the EWAS of the subcohort, 25(OH)D was associated ($q < 0.05$) with methylation at cg24350360 (*EPHX1*; $p = 3.4 \times 10^{-8}$), cg06177555 (*SPN*; $p = 9.8 \times 10^{-8}$), and cg13243168 (*SMARCD2*; $p = 2.9 \times 10^{-7}$).

Conclusions: 25(OH)D concentrations were associated with DNA methylation of CpGs in several vitamin D-related genes, with potential links to immune function-related genes. Methylation of CpGs in vitamin D-related genes may interact with 25(OH)D to affect the risk of breast cancer.

Keywords: Breast cancer, Vitamin D, 25-Hydroxyvitamin D, DNA methylation, Epigenome-wide association study

Background

Vitamin D may protect against poor health outcomes, including heart disease, diabetes, certain cancers, and overall mortality [1–5]. Its biological properties include regulation of cell proliferation and immune function, as well as increased cell differentiation and apoptosis [6–10]. These mechanisms are controlled by the active metabolite 1,25-dihydroxyvitamin D (1,25(OH)$_2$D) and the vitamin D receptor (VDR), often in conjunction with retinoid X receptor alpha (RXRA) [11]. This 1,25(OH)$_2$D-VDR-RXRA complex binds to vitamin D response elements that can activate or repress gene transcription [12].

Circulating vitamin D levels could affect DNA methylation via transcriptional regulation or other mechanisms [13]. In mammals, DNA methylation is an epigenetic process by which a methyl group is transferred onto the C5 position of a cytosine, forming 5-methylcytosine. Increased methylation at CpG sites in promoter regions is associated with gene inactivation and transcriptional

---

* Correspondence: obrienkm2@niehs.nih.gov
[†]Jack A. Taylor and Clarice R. Weinberg contributed equally to this work.
[1]Biostatistics and Computational Biology Branch, National Institute of Environmental Health Sciences, National Institutes of Health, Research Triangle Park, NC 27709, USA
[2]Epidemiology Branch, National Institute of Environmental Health Sciences, National Institutes of Health, Research Triangle Park, NC 27709, USA
Full list of author information is available at the end of the article

repression, while increased methylation at CpGs in gene bodies is associated with actively transcribed genes [14, 15]. Examples of other environmental exposures associated with methylation changes include smoking (for both smokers [16] and their offspring [17–19]), as well as body mass index (BMI) [20, 21], alcohol consumption [22], and nutrients such as folate, vitamin B12, and retinoic acid [23–27].

Some empirical evidence supports a link between vitamin D exposure and DNA methylation. Candidate gene approaches have observed that vitamin D is associated with methylation of *CYP24A1* [28, 29], *BMP2* [30], *PTEN* [31], and *DKK1* [32]. Additionally, one epigenome-wide association study (EWAS) conducted among adolescent African-American males identified two sites (cg16317961 (*MAPRE2*) and cg04623955 (*DIO3*)) that were significantly associated with serum levels of the stable precursor to $1,25(OH)_2D$, 25-hydroxyvitamin D (25(OH)D) [33]. However, those findings did not replicate in a subsequent EWAS conducted among Caucasian men, nor did that subsequent EWAS identify any novel associations [34]. Another EWAS observed no noteworthy associations between maternal 25(OH)D levels and methylation in cord blood [35], and an epigenome-wide in-vitro study identified no detectable methylation changes in blood mononuclear cells treated with vitamin D [36]. Several studies of the association between vitamin D and LINE-1 global methylation levels have also been negative [37–39].

To further investigate a possible link between vitamin D and DNA methylation, we studied the relationship between serum 25(OH)D and CpGs in or near seven vitamin D-related genes (*VDR*, *RXRA*, *CYP2R1*, *CYP24A1*, *GC*, *CYP27B1*, and *DHCR7/NADSYN1*) using a random sample of women from a large prospective cohort ("subcohort"). Based on our previous finding that serum 25(OH)D was associated with a 21% reduction in the hazard of breast cancer over 5 years of follow-up [3], and other research observations that methylation status can modify the responses of individuals to vitamin D treatment [28, 29], we also examined 25(OH)D-methylation interactions in relation to breast cancer risk. We additionally conducted an EWAS of serum 25(OH)D.

Methods
Study sample
The Sister Study is a prospective cohort study of 50,884 US women (2003–2009) [40]. At baseline, participants were 35–74 years old and had a sister who had been diagnosed with breast cancer but who had never had breast cancer themselves. Each completed a computer-assisted telephone interview, with in-home collection of anthropometric measurements and blood samples. Participants remain under active surveillance,

with more than 90% responding to their most recent follow-up request through March 2015 (data release 4.1). When possible, we collected medical records from self-reported breast cancer cases (82%). Among those with medical records available, 99% of self-reported diagnoses were confirmed.

Participants for a DNA methylation substudy were previously sampled using a case-cohort design [41, 42]. To minimize genetic variation due to racial heterogeneity, this sample was limited to non-Hispanic white women, including all such women who had available blood samples and a self-reported diagnosis of invasive breast cancer or ductal carcinoma in situ. The initial methylation sample included 1542 women who developed incident breast cancer between enrollment and March 2015, and a random sample of 1336 women drawn from the full cohort, 74 of whom developed breast cancer by March 2015.

The participants for our previous analysis of serum 25(OH)D and breast cancer [3] were selected to overlap with the case-cohort sample who had DNA methylation data. However, when looking at methylation and 25(OH)D together, we excluded 429 participants who did not have 25(OH)D measured and 102 participants with quality control-related concerns with regard to their DNA methylation (described below). In the end, we had 1070 cases and 1277 in the subcohort (46 of whom were also cases) who had both DNA methylation and serum 25(OH)D data available. All women provided written informed consent and the study was approved by the institutional review boards of the National Institute of Environmental Health Sciences and the Copernicus Group.

Serum 25(OH)D assessment
Baseline serum was stored at –80 °C before being analyzed using liquid chromatography-mass spectrometry (LC/MS) at Heartland Assays, Inc. (Ames, IA). The three 25(OH)D metabolites—$25(OH)D_3$, $25(OH)D_2$, and $3-epi-25(OH)D_3$—were assessed individually, but we summed their concentrations to estimate total 25(OH)D. We adjusted total 25(OH)D values for batch effects using a random effects model and for season of blood draw using LOESS regression. Further details are provided elsewhere [3].

Methylation analysis
We assessed DNA methylation at 485,512 CpGs (450 K HumanMethylation Beadchip; Illumina, Inc.) using whole blood samples collected from case-cohort participants. Briefly, we extracted 1 µg genomic DNA from whole blood and conducted bisulfite-conversion using the EZ DNA Methylation Kit (Zymo Research, Orange County, CA). Methylation analysis was carried out at the

Center for Inherited Disease Research at Johns Hopkins University (Baltimore, MD). Data processing and quality control assessments were completed using the 'ENMIX' package (R v3.2.1) [43], and included correcting fluorescent dye-bias [44], quantile normalization [45], and reduction of background noise. We excluded 102 participants whose sample had > 5% low-quality methylation values, low average bisulfite intensity, or implausible methylation value distributions (final n = 1277 in subcohort and 1024 additional cases, as described above, plus 123 duplicate samples). We excluded CpGs if they were Illumina-designed single nucleotide polymorphism (SNP) probes, on the Y chromosome, had > 5% low-quality data, were within 2 base pairs of a common SNP, or had multimodal distributions. This left us with 423,500 CpGs. For each site, we calculated a β value based on each individual's proportion of unmethylated (U) and methylated (M) sites at a given locus: $\beta = M/(U + M + 100)$.

As interperson variability can be low at some CpGs, we conducted additional screening to better ensure the reliability of our results. We calculated intraclass correlation coefficients (ICCs) to compare the technical variation (within-subject variability, assessed using duplicate samples) to the biologic variation (between-subject variability) [46]. We observed that, for approximately 66% of CpGs, the ICC was less than 0.5, suggesting that there is little interindividual variability and some of the corresponding observed associations may not reflect true biologic differences. We have flagged these CpGs in our results.

Candidate gene selection

Candidate genes included *VDR* and *RXRA*, as well as the vitamin D binding protein gene (*GC*), and genes directly involved in vitamin D metabolism (*DHCR7/NADSYN1*, *CYP24A1*, *CYP27B1*, and *CYP2R1*). We selected any CpGs included on the 450 K HumanMethylation Beadchip (Illumina, Inc.) located within 2000 base pairs from the candidate gene's transcription start and end sites, as defined by University of California Santa Cruz Genome Browser (GRCh37/hg19; RefSeq notation) [47]. We identified 198 eligible CpGs.

Statistical analysis

25(OH)D and methylation of vitamin D-related genes in the subcohort

We assessed the relationship between serum 25(OH)D (continuous, ng/mL) and methylation (continuous, measured as the logit of β) at each of 198 CpGs in or near vitamin D-related genes using robust linear regression with M-estimation. This analysis was limited to the 1270 individuals in the subcohort who had complete information for the following covariates: age at blood draw (continuous), BMI (continuous; kg/m^2), current smoking status (dichotomous), and alcohol use (never/former

drinker, current drinker < 1 drink/day, or current drinker ≥ 1 drink per day). In addition to these covariates, we also adjusted for cell type proportions (CD8 T cells, CD4 T cells, natural killer cells, B cells, monocytes, or granulocytes versus other) [48].

25(OH)D-methylation interaction and breast cancer risk in the case-cohort

Next, we used the case-cohort sample to examine whether interactions between serum 25(OH)D and methylation of vitamin D-related genes were related to breast cancer incidence. This included an assessment of the relationship between methylation at each of the CpG sites in or near vitamin D-related genes and risk of breast cancer. For both sets of analyses, we used Cox proportional hazards models to account for the case-cohort design [41, 42]. We adjusted for age at blood draw, BMI, smoking status, alcohol use, and cell type proportions, as well as education, current hormone therapy use and type, current hormonal birth control use, menopausal status, usual physical activity, history of osteoporosis, parity, and a BMI-menopausal status interaction term. For these candidate CpG locus analyses, we considered p < 0.05 to be statistically significant.

For the interaction analysis, the effect measures of interest were ratios of hazard ratios (RHRs). Here, the numerator of the RHR is the hazard ratio (HR) for the association between methylation (measured as 0.1 increments of logit(β)) and breast cancer among those with 25(OH)D levels > 38.0 ng/mL, and the denominator of the RHR is the HR for the association between methylation and breast cancer among those with 25(OH)D levels ≤ 38.0 ng/mL). Therefore, RHR values > 1.00 correspond to a higher estimated HR for the methylation-breast cancer association among those with 25(OH)D levels > 38.0 ng/mL and values < 1.00 correspond to a higher estimated methylation-breast cancer HR among those with 25(OH)D levels ≤ 38.0 ng/mL. The 25(OH)D cut-point was selected based on previous evidence that 38.0 ng/mL is relevant for predicting breast cancer risk [3]. These models also included all of the baseline covariates listed above for the methylation-breast cancer association analysis.

Epigenome-wide association study of 25(OH)D in subcohort or cases

We examined the association between serum 25(OH)D and DNA methylation in the subcohort for all 423,500 CpGs from the 450 K panel that passed quality control checks. Here, we corrected for multiple comparisons by calculating false discovery rate q values [49], considering those with q < 0.05 to be likely to be true positives.

We next assessed the relationship between 25(OH)D and DNA methylation in an independent sample of participants who developed breast cancer within 5 years of enrollment, who were not part of the subcohort, and had the required covariate information ("cases"; $n = 1024$). Here, our goal was to identify CpGs where the 25(OH)D-methylation association differed by future breast cancer status. We compared the subcohort and case results by plotting the $-\log_{10}$ p values multiplied by the direction of each tested association. We then calculated critical values for a test of the combined p values based on Fisher's method [50]. CpGs that had combined p values below identified thresholds were included in additional interaction analyses using the methods described above.

Results
Women who developed breast cancer during the 5-year follow-up period were slightly older than those in the subcohort (58.7 years versus 55.7 years) and had lower prediagnosis 25(OH)D levels (32.3 versus 32.7 ng/mL). Cases were more likely to have more than one first-degree relative with breast cancer, to be

postmenopausal, to be obese, or to be currently taking hormone therapy (Additional file 1: Table S1).

25(OH)D and methylation of vitamin D-related genes in the subcohort
Of the 198 CpGs from vitamin D-related genes, cg21201924 (*RXRA*) had the lowest p value for association with 25(OH)D in the subcohort ($p = 0.0004$; Table 1 and Additional file 1: Table S2). Twenty-two other candidate CpGs were significantly associated with 25(OH)D, all but one of which were located in *RXRA*, *NADSYN1/ DHCR7*, or *GC*. The large overall contrast between our results and those expected by chance is illustrated by a quantile-quantile plot (Fig. 1a).

25(OH)D-methylation interaction and breast cancer risk in the case-cohort
Eighteen of the 198 candidate CpGs showed evidence of interacting with 25(OH)D to affect breast cancer risk in

Table 1 CpGs in vitamin D-related genes with statistically significant ($p < 0.05$) associations with 25(OH)D; Sister Study subcohort ($n = 1270$)

Rank	CpG	Gene / location type	Chromosome: position	Mean methylation level (SD)	Association with 25(OH)D[a]	
					β	p value
1	cg21201924	RXRA / body	9: 137251825	0.76 (0.042)	−0.020	0.0004
2	cg02127980	RXRA / body	9: 137252116	0.40 (0.067)	−0.015	0.0004
3	cg17559402[b]	NADSYN1 / body	11: 71187890	0.97 (0.006)	−0.017	0.003
4	cg02059519	RXRA / body	9: 137250935	0.83 (0.026)	−0.012	0.003
5	cg09997530	GC / body	4: 72636217	0.91 (0.017)	0.015	0.005
6	cg04329455[b]	RXRA	9: 137215364	0.96 (0.008)	0.014	0.007
7	cg00268518[b]	NADSYN1 / TSS200	11: 71164106	0.01 (0.001)	0.011	0.008
8	cg03146219	NADSYN1 / body	11: 71189514	0.47 (0.097)	−0.012	0.009
9	cg13510651[b]	RXRA / body	9: 137227772	0.94 (0.008)	−0.010	0.01
10	cg03490288[b]	DHCR7 / body	11: 71146658	0.97 (0.006)	0.015	0.01
11	cg05785753	NADSYN1 / body	11: 71189490	0.59 (0.074)	−0.010	0.01
12	cg13687497	RXRA / body	9: 137249839	0.80 (0.023)	−0.010	0.01
13	cg07793224[b]	NADSYN1 / body	11: 71183180	0.97 (0.008)	0.017	0.02
14	cg26044621[b]	DHCR7 / 3′ UTR	11: 71145665	0.94 (0.011)	0.012	002
15	cg04837494	GC / 3′ UTR	4: 72608149	0.85 (0.033)	0.013	0.03
16	cg14236758	RXRA / body	9: 137252129	0.48 (0.066)	−0.009	0.03
17	cg04774822	NADSYN1 / body	11: 71165839	0.78 (0.033)	−0.009	0.03
18	cg16151558[b]	DHCR7 / TSS1500	11: 71159853	0.02 (0.066)	0.013	0.04
19	cg20372759[b]	CYP27B1 / TSS1500	12: 58162287	0.97 (0.006)	−0.010	0.04
20	cg24806812	GC / body	4: 72635202	0.93 (0.018)	0.012	0.04
21	cg14154547[b]	RXRA / body	9: 137293309	0.92 (0.010)	−0.007	0.04
22	cg07099121[b]	DHCR7 / 3′ UTR	11: 71146096	0.98 (0.004)	−0.010	004
23	cg16910670[b]	NADSYN1	11: 71215361	0.97 (0.005)	−0.011	0.05

TSS200 within 200 basepairs upstream of the transcription start site, *TSS1500* within 1500 basepairs upstream of the transcription start site, *UTR* untranslated region

[a]Estimated change in methylation (logit(β)) per 10 ng/mL change in serum 25-hydroxyvitamin D (25(OH)D)

[b]Intraclass correlation coefficient < 0.5

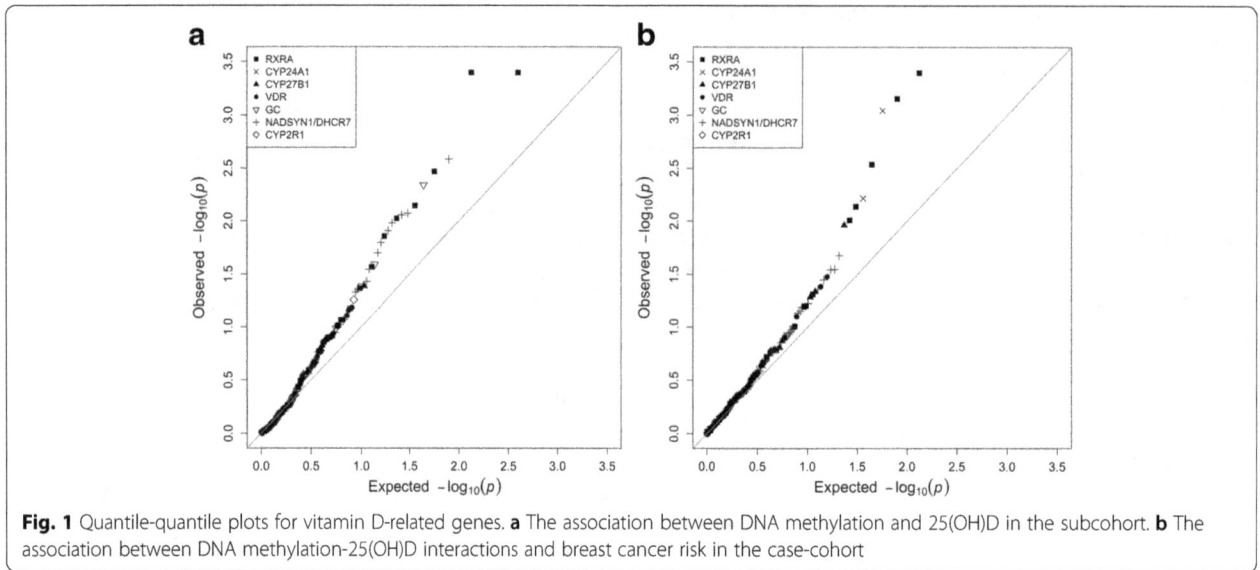

Fig. 1 Quantile-quantile plots for vitamin D-related genes. **a** The association between DNA methylation and 25(OH)D in the subcohort. **b** The association between DNA methylation-25(OH)D interactions and breast cancer risk in the case-cohort

the case-cohort sample ($p < 0.05$; Table 2 and Additional file 1: Table S3). This is more than expected by chance, as illustrated by the quantile-quantile plot (Fig. 1b). Nine of the eighteen had ICCs > 0.5. Only one was directly associated with breast cancer risk (cg10592901 in *VDR*, HR = 1.04, 95% confidence interval (CI) 1.01–1.07).

The CpG with the smallest p value for the 25(OH)D-methylation interaction analysis was cg21201924 (*RXRA*). Among women with 25(OH)D levels > 38.0 ng/mL, each 0.1 change in logit(β) was associated with an 18% increase in the breast cancer hazard (HR = 1.18, 95% CI 1.08–1.29). By contrast, among women with 25(OH)D levels ≤ 38.0 ng/mL, each 0.1 change in logit(β) was associated with a 3% lower hazard of developing breast cancer (HR = 0.97, 95% CI 0.93–1.01). The corresponding RHR was 1.22 (95% CI 1.10–1.29; $p = 7.0 \times 10^{-5}$).

Six other *RXRA* CpGs (cg13786567, cg02127980, cg14154547, cg13510651, cg14236758, and cg13941235) also showed evidence of interacting with 25(OH)D to affect breast cancer risk. Other statistically significant sites included cg12978433 and cg18956481 in *CYP24A1*, cg09253762 and cg16984335 in *CYP27B1*, cg18482822, cg05072492, cg11035813, cg25588697, and cg12474705 in *NADSYN1/DHCR7*, and cg14854850 and cg10592901 in *VDR*. As we have previously reported that the protective association between 25(OH)D and breast cancer appears to be limited to postmenopausal women [3], we present postmenopause-specific analyses in Additional file 1: Tables S4 and S5 and Figure S1.The results were largely consistent with the analyses that included all breast cancers.

Epigenome-wide association study of 25(OH)D in subcohort or cases

Within the subcohort, 25(OH)D was associated with methylation levels at three CpGs at $q < 0.05$ (Fig. 2a and

Table 3). The CpG with the smallest p value was cg24350360 (*EPHX1*; $p = 3.4 \times 10^{-8}$), followed by cg06177555 (*SPN*; $p = 9.8 \times 10^{-8}$) and cg1324316 (*SMARCD2*; $p = 2.9 \times 10^{-7}$). Two other CpGs had $q < 0.10$: cg23761815 (*SLC29A3*; $p = 5.1 \times 10^{-7}$) and cg10401362 (*DNAJB6*; $p = 1.0 \times 10^{-6}$). The quantile-quantile plot (Fig. 2b) demonstrates that the observed p values systematically deviated from what was expected under the null hypothesis. For all five CpGs with $q < 0.10$, increases in serum 25(OH)D were associated with decreased methylation (Table 3; Additional file 1: Figure S2). All except cg24350360 (*EPHX1*) had ICCs > 0.5.

No CpGs were associated with 25(OH)D in case-only analyses (Additional file 1: Figure S3). When we compared the results of 25(OH)D-methylation association tests for the subcohort versus breast cancer cases (Fig. 3), no CpGs had a combined $p < 1.2 \times 10^{-7}$, the Bonferroni-corrected cut-point for significance. Sixteen CpGs with combined p values < 1.0×10^{-5} were deemed worthy of further investigation; all but two of which had ICCs > 0.5 (Table 4). Of the sixteen, nine had RHR p values < 0.05. Three of the latter nine were associated with 25(OH)D at $q < 0.10$ in the initial EWAS: cg13243168 (*SMARCD2*), cg23761815 (*SLC29A3*), and cg24350360 (*EPHX1*). Most of the CpGs with small Fisher combined p values were inversely associated with 25(OH)D in both cases and the subcohort.

Discussion

Among our a priori candidate loci, we found that methylation levels at CpGs in or near *RXRA*, *NADSYN1/DHCR7*, and *GC* were associated with serum 25(OH)D levels. In our larger EWAS analysis, CpGs in *EPHX1*, *SPN*, and *SMARCD2* had epigenome-wide significant associations with serum 25(OH)D. To our knowledge, we are the first

Table 2 Interacting effects of 25(OH)D and methylation at CpG sites in vitamin D-related genes on the 5-year risk of breast cancer (1024 cases, 1270 from subcohort, including 46 additional cases[a]): ratio of hazard ratios and 95% confidence intervals for CpGs with statistically significant interactions ($p < 0.05$)

Rank	CpG site	Gene / location type	HR (95% CI) for methylation-breast cancer association	HR (95% CI) for methylation-breast cancer association, if 25(OH)D ≤ 38.0 ng/mL	HR (95% CI) for methylation-breast cancer association, if 25(OH)D > 38.0 ng/mL	Ratio of Hazard Ratios (95% CI)[b]	Interaction p value
1	cg21201924	RXRA / body	1.00 (0.96–1.04)	0.97 (0.93–1.01)	1.18 (1.08–1.29)	1.22 (1.10–1.34)	7.0×10^{-5}
2	cg13786567	RXRA / body	1.01 (0.94–1.08)	0.94 (0.87–1.02)	1.34 (1.12–1.60)	1.42 (1.17–1.73)	4.0×10^{-4}
3	cg02127980	RXRA / body	1.00 (0.94–1.06)	0.95 (0.88–1.01)	1.22 (1.07–1.38)	1.29 (1.11–1.49)	7.0×10^{-4}
4	cg12978433	CYP24A1 / 1st exon	1.01 (0.98–1.04)	1.04 (1.00–1.07)	0.93 (0.88–0.98)	0.90 (0.84–0.96)	9.0×10^{-4}
5	cg14154547[c]	RXRA / body	0.96 (0.90–1.03)	0.91 (0.84–0.98)	1.17 (1.01–1.36)	1.29 (1.09–1.53)	0.003
6	cg18956481[c]	CYP24A1 / 5′ UTR	0.99 (0.97–1.02)	1.01 (0.99–1.04)	0.93 (0.88–0.98)	0.92 (0.86–0.98)	0.006
7	cg13510651[c]	RXRA / body	0.99 (0.93–1.06)	0.95 (0.88–1.02)	1.18 (1.03–1.35)	1.24 (1.06–1.45)	0.007
8	cg14236758	RXRA / body	1.00 (0.94–1.06)	0.96 (0.90–1.03)	1.19 (1.03–1.37)	1.23 (1.05–1.44)	0.01
9	cg09253762	CYP27B1 / TSS1500	0.99 (0.95–1.04)	0.96 (0.91–1.01)	1.12 (1.01–1.24)	1.16 (1.04–1.31)	0.01
10	cg18482822[c]	DHCR7 / body	1.02 (0.97–1.06)	0.99 (0.93–1.04)	1.13 (1.02–1.24)	1.14 (1.02–1.27)	0.02
11	cg05072492[c]	NADSYN1 / TSS1500	1.01 (0.96–1.06)	0.97 (0.92–1.03)	1.11 (1.00–1.24)	1.15 (1.01–1.29)	0.03
12	cg11035813[c]	DHCR7 / TSS1500	1.02 (0.98–1.07)	1.00 (0.95–1.05)	1.13 (1.02–1.24)	1.13 (1.01–1.26)	0.03
13	cg14854850	VDR / 3′ UTR	0.99 (0.94–1.03)	1.02 (0.97–1.07)	0.90 (0.82–0.99)	0.89 (0.79–0.99)	0.03
14	cg25588697[c]	DHCR7 / body	1.01 (0.95–1.08)	0.96 (0.89–1.05)	1.14 (1.00–1.30)	1.18 (1.01–1.38)	0.04
15	cg10592901	VDR / body	1.04 (1.01–1.07)	1.06 (1.03–1.10)	0.98 (0.92–1.05)	0.92 (0.86–1.00)	0.04
16	cg12474705[c]	NADSYN1 / body	0.96 (0.92–1.01)	0.99 (0.94–1.05)	0.88 (0.80–0.98)	0.89 (0.79–1.00)	0.04
17	cg16984335[c]	CYP27B1 / body	1.00 (0.96–1.04)	1.02 (0.97–1.06)	0.92 (0.83–1.00)	0.90 (0.81–1.00)	0.05
18	cg13941235	RXRA / body	1.00 (0.97–1.02)	0.98 (0.95–1.01)	1.04 (0.99–1.10)	1.06 (1.00–1.13)	0.05

CI confidence interval, *HR* hazard ratio, *TSS1500* within 1500 basepairs upstream of the transcription start site, *UTR* Untranslated region

[a]After excluding those with missing covariate information

[b]Change in the methylation-breast cancer association for being in the 4th quartile of 25-hydroxyvitamin D (25(OH)D) (≥ 38.0 ng/mL) versus the first three (< 38.0 ng/mL)—a value > 1.00 indicates that the estimated HR for the methylation-breast cancer association is higher among those with higher 25(OH)D levels; similarly, an RHR < 1.00 indicates that the estimated HR for the methylation-breast cancer association is higher among those with lower 25(OH)D levels

[c]Intraclass correlation coefficient < 0.5

to report a link between these three genes and 25(OH)D and the first to study methylation-25(OH)D interactions in relation to breast cancer risk.

For candidate CpG analyses, the top hit for both the methylation-25(OH)D association analysis and the breast cancer interaction analyses was cg21201924, located in the gene body of *RXRA*. As previously noted, RXRA acts as a transcription factor with $1,25(OH)_2D$ and VDR and changes to the gene's expression and methylation levels could have widespread biological impacts. Changes in expression or methylation of *GC*, *NADSYN1/DHCR7*, and the other candidate genes may have less pervasive biological effects, but our findings support the hypothesis that these vitamin D-related genes and proteins may interact with circulating vitamin D levels to influence breast cancer risk.

Of the CpGs in or near vitamin D-related genes, most of those that were either associated with 25(OH)D or that showed evidence of interacting with 25(OH)D to affect breast cancer risk were located within gene bodies. Higher 25(OH)D levels tended to be associated with higher methylation, but there was no clear pattern linking CpG locations to the direction of the RHR in the interaction analysis.

None of the candidate CpGs from the vitamin D-related genes met the stringent criterion for statistical significance in the EWAS analysis, and thus there was no overlap between the genes identified in our EWAS and those reported previously to be associated with serum vitamin D levels. One of the two hits reported by Zhu et al. [33] (cg04623955 near *DIO3*) was also assessed in our sample, but we found no evidence of an association ($p = 0.78$). Other CpGs identified in their sample also failed to replicate, including cg23492043 ($p = 0.64$), cg00864867 ($p = 0.15$), and cg16826718 ($p = 0.62$). Eight CpGs reported by Florath et al. [34] were also assessed in our sample, but none were significantly associated with 25(OH)D (p values 0.09–0.85). These discrepancies could be related to differences in race, sex, or study design, but could also be the result of sampling variation.

As previously noted, vitamin D plays a role in immune response, including regulation of innate and adaptive

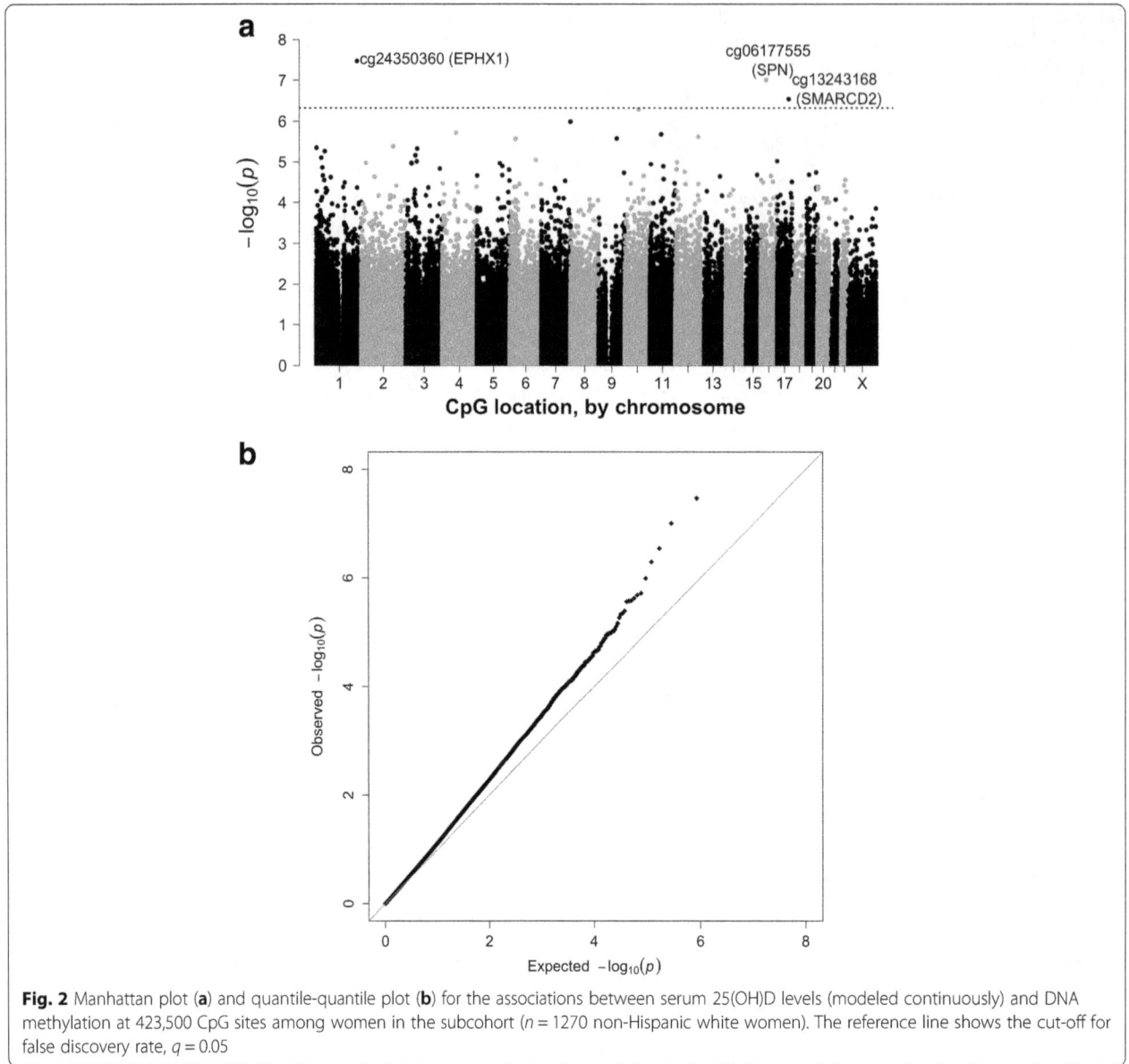

Fig. 2 Manhattan plot (**a**) and quantile-quantile plot (**b**) for the associations between serum 25(OH)D levels (modeled continuously) and DNA methylation at 423,500 CpG sites among women in the subcohort ($n = 1270$ non-Hispanic white women). The reference line shows the cut-off for false discovery rate, $q = 0.05$

Table 3 CpG sites associated with serum 25(OH)D levels in subcohort ($q < 0.10$)

CpG site	Location (Chr:position)	Location type	Gene	Effect estimate[a] (95% CI)	p value	q value
cg24350360	1:225997662[b]	TSS200	EPHX1	−0.04 (−0.06 to −0.03)	3.4×10^{-8}	0.01
cg06177555	16:29678624	3′ UTR	SPN	−0.02 (−0.03 to −0.01)	9.8×10^{-8}	0.02
cg13243168	17:61915833	Body	SMARCD2	−0.02 (−0.03 to −0.01)	2.9×10^{-7}	0.04
cg23761815	10:73083123	Body	SLC29A3	−0.02 (−0.03 to −0.01)	5.1×10^{-7}	0.05
cg10401362	7:157185402	Body	DNAJB6	−0.02 (−0.03 to −0.01)	1.0×10^{-6}	0.09

CI confidence interval, *TSS200* within 200 basepairs upstream of the transcription start site, *UTR* untranslated region
[a]Estimated change in methylation (logit(β)) per 10 ng/mL change in serum 25-hydroxyvitamin D (25(OH)D)
[b]Intraclass correlation coefficient < 0.5

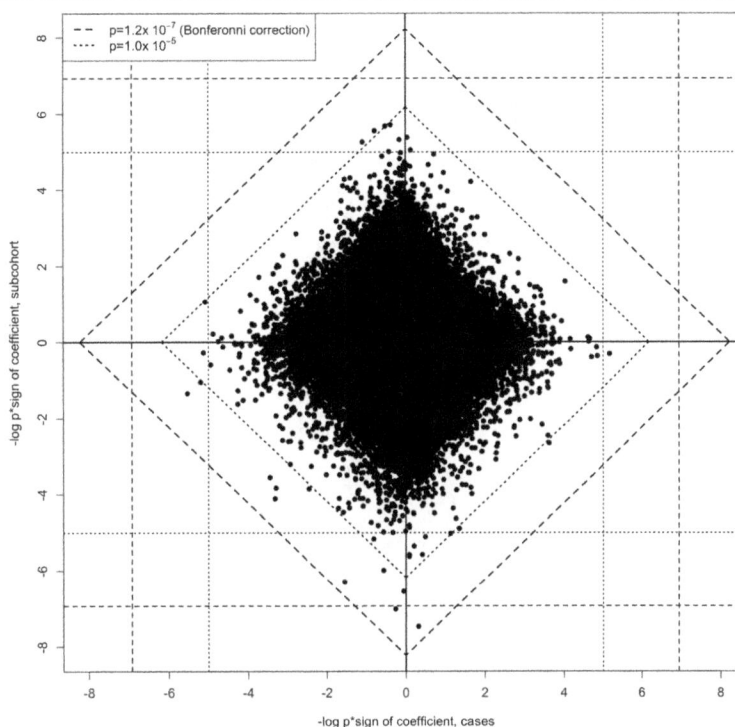

Fig. 3 Diamond plot comparing $-\log_{10} p$ value × sign of coefficient for the estimated association between 25(OH)D and logit(methylation): subcohort ($n = 1270$, including 46 breast cancer cases) versus other breast cancer cases ($n = 1024$). The broken lines show critical values for single (vertical and horizontal grid lines) and Fisher's combined (diagonal lines) p values, based on χ^2 tests with 2 (for single) and 4 (for combined) degrees of freedom

immunity [9, 10], as well as detoxification [51]. Possible mechanisms for these actions could be through the 1,25(OH)$_2$D-VDR-RXRA complex and its effects on gene transcription [12]. Although there is no established link between 25(OH)D or vitamin D metabolism and *SPN*, *SMARCD2*, *SLC29A3*, or *DNAJB6* specifically, the observed associations between these genes and 25(OH)D could be related to VDR or other components of immune function.

EPHX1 encodes epoxide hydrolase, an enzyme that breaks down epoxides from xenobiotic aromatic compounds (e.g., polycyclic aromatic hydrocarbons, benzene) [52]. Further, *EPHX1* regulation of detoxification via CYP450 enzymes has been shown to modulate the immune response in mice [53]. Although the direct mechanisms linking *EPHX1* and vitamin D are unclear, an in-vivo study showed that 1,25(OH)$_2$D$_3$ increased the expression of EPHX1 and other phase I and phase II biotransformation enzymes in the intestinal tissue of vitamin D-deficient rats [54]. There is no known association between *EPHX1* and breast cancer risk [55]. We do note that our results should be interpreted with caution as the *EPHX1* CpG site that was strongly associated with 25(OH)D in our sample had a low ICC (< 0.5), meaning that the within-subject variability was larger than the between-subject variability.

SPN encodes a sialoglycoprotein expressed on leukocytes and platelets. Cell culture models have demonstrated that vitamin A and D metabolites upregulate SPN expression [56, 57]. *SMARCD2* encodes a critical component of the SWItch/Sucrose Non-Fermentable (SWI/SNF) chromatin remodeling complex, which uses ATP-derived energy to unwrap or restructure chromatin [58]. SMARCD subunits serve as a link between the SWI/SNF core complex and transcription regulators, including nuclear receptors such as VDR and RXR [59–61]. Although we found no prior reports of a direct link between these sites and breast cancer risk, recent studies have demonstrated that genes encoding for the SWI/SNF chromatin-remodeling complex are mutated in approximately 20% of all human tumors [62] and are considered to be critical tumor suppressors [58] and epigenetic regulators of tumorigenesis [63].

The effect measures we estimate for the interaction analysis, RHRs, measure the extent to which the hazard ratio for the 25(OH)D-breast cancer association depends on the epigenetics, as measured by methylation at a particular CpG locus. Because methylation and 25(OH)D were measured in the same blood samples, we cannot address the temporality of the identified associations to determine whether 25(OH)D influences methylation, methylation influences 25(OH)D, or a third factor influences both.

Table 4 Ratio of hazard ratios and 95% confidence intervals for the interaction between 25(OH)D and methylation on the risk of breast cancer within 5 years of enrollment (1024 cases, 1270 from subcohort, including 46 additional cases[a]); CpGs with Fisher combined p values $< 1 \times 10^{-5}$ for subcohort combined with case comparison

Rank	CpG	Gene/ Location	25(OH)D-methylation association, subcohort		25(OH)D-methylation association, cases		Fisher combined p value	HR (95% CI) for methylation-breast cancer association	RHRs (95% CI)[c]	Interaction p value
			Cofficient[b]	p value	Cofficient[b]	p value				
1	cg08092930	PPFIA1	−0.03	1.3×10^{-5}	0.02	0.04	8.5×10^{-6}*	1.01 (0.98–1.05)	1.15 (1.06–1.24)	6.3×10^{-4}
2	cg23761815	SLC29A3	−0.02	5.1×10^{-7}	−0.01	0.03	2.7×10^{-7}	1.13 (1.07–1.18)	1.22 (1.08–1.38)	0.002
3	cg13243168	SMARCD2	−0.02	2.9×10^{-7}	-7×10^{-4}	0.87	4.0×10^{-6}	1.05 (0.98–0.91)	1.29 (1.09–1.51)	0.002
4	cg15544721	PPP1R9A	−0.01	0.09	−0.03	6.4×10^{-6}	8.8×10^{-6}	0.98 (0.94–1.03)	0.87 (0.79–0.96)	0.008
5	cg11568290	5p15.1	−0.02	1.4×10^{-4}	−0.01	0.004	7.7×10^{-6}	1.15 (1.08–1.22)	1.23 (1.05–1.44)	0.009
6	cg19420720	P4HB	−0.01	0.002	0.02	2.3×10^{-4}	8.1×10^{-6}*	1.01 (0.94–1.08)	1.27 (1.06–1.52)	0.01
7	cg23839180	FAM49A	−0.02	0.05	−0.05	3.0×10^{-6}	2.3×10^{-6}	0.97 (0.94–1.03)	0.92 (0.86–0.98)	0.01
8	cg15320474[d]	UBD	0.02	2.8×10^{-6}	−0.01	0.16	7.0×10^{-6}*	0.98 (0.83–1.04)	0.87 (0.77–0.99)	0.03
9	cg24350360[d]	EPHX1	−0.04	3.4×10^{-8}	0.01	0.48	3.1×10^{-7}*	1.02 (0.99–1.05)	1.08 (1.01–1.16)	0.04
10	cg22488164	PLBD1	−0.03	1.5×10^{-4}	−0.03	5.0×10^{-4}	1.3×10^{-6}	1.06 (1.02–1.10)	0.93 (0.85–1.01)	0.07
11	cg10401362	DNAJB6	−0.02	1.0×10^{-6}	−0.01	0.27	4.4×10^{-6}	1.02 (0.97–1.07)	1.10 (0.98–1.24)	0.10
12	cg06177555	SPN	−0.02	9.8×10^{-8}	−0.003	0.54	9.3×10^{-7}	0.97 (0.91–1.03)	1.12 (0.98–1.28)	0.10
13	cg11277126	TRPC4AP	−0.02	7.7×10^{-5}	−0.02	4.8×10^{-4}	6.7×10^{-7}	1.04 (0.98–1.11)	1.07 (0.92–1.24)	0.39
14	cg21527411	GLYAT	0.02	2.1×10^{-6}	−0.01	0.30	9.6×10^{-6}*	1.02 (0.97–1.07)	0.95 (0.83–1.08)	0.40
15	cg09914444	DMBX1	0.02	5.4×10^{-6}	−0.01	0.08	6.9×10^{-6}*	1.05 (1.01–1.10)	0.96 (0.87–1.06)	0.44
16	cg23999318	HIPK2	−0.02	2.8×10^{-4}	−0.02	3.5×10^{-4}	1.7×10^{-6}	1.00 (0.94–1.05)	1.00 (0.88–1.14)	1.00

CI confidence interval, *HR* hazard ratio, *RHR* ratio of hazard ratio

[a]After excluding those with missing covariate information

[b]Estimated change in methylation (logit(β)) per 10 ng/mL change in serum 25-hydroxyvitamin D (25(OH)D)

[c]Change in the methylation-breast cancer association for being in the 4th quartile of 25(OH)D (> 38.0 ng/mL) versus the first three (≤ 38.0 ng/mL)—a value > 1.00 indicates that the estimated HR for the methylation-breast cancer association is higher among those with higher 25(OH)D levels; similarly, an RHR < 1.00 indicates that the estimated HR for the methylation-breast cancer association is higher among those with lower 25(OH)D levels

[d]Intraclass correlation coefficient < 0.5

*Effect estimate going in opposing direction for subcohort versus cases

Similarly, we can only assess whether the relationship between methylation and 25(OH)D is different for those who later developed breast cancer, suggesting multiplicative interaction, and not whether 25(OH)D or methylation acts as an effect modifier or mediator. Repeated measures of methylation and 25(OH)D would be needed to address temporality. Future studies could also help to determine the most appropriate cut-point for 25(OH)D levels in gene-by-environment interaction studies. We selected 38.0 ng/mL based on our previous results [3] and other findings supporting a threshold effect of similar magnitude [64], but we cannot be sure what levels have the most biological relevance for breast cancer risk.

We limited our sample to non-Hispanic white women to minimize the influence of genetic ancestry. As such, our results may not be fully generalizable. Our sample is also selective in that all participants had a sister diagnosed with breast cancer, and had, on average, approximately twice the risk of developing breast cancer themselves. Our findings are internally valid, but overrepresented risk factors (e.g., germline genetic or early childhood exposures) may inflate the magnitude of effect estimates if they influence the associations evaluated here.

Conclusions

Serum 25(OH)D concentrations were associated with methylation levels at candidate CpGs in vitamin D-related genes and three genes with links to immune function or regulation of VDR. Methylation levels of some of these CpGs may interact with vitamin D to affect breast cancer risk. These results contribute to our understanding of the relationship between vitamin D and DNA methylation and the impact of vitamin D on breast cancer risk.

Additional file

Additional file 1: Table S1. Characteristics of participants included in the vitamin D and methylation substudy (Sister Study, 2003–2009); only non-Hispanic white women included. **Table S2.** Associations between 25(OH)D and methylation at CpG sites in vitamin D-related genes ($p > 0.05$); Sister Study subcohort ($n = 1270$). **Table S3.** Interaction effects of 25(OH)D and methylation at CpG sites in vitamin D-related genes on the 5-year risk of breast cancer (1024 cases, 1270 from subcohort, including 46 additional cases): ratio of hazard ratios and 95% confidence intervals for CpGs with interaction p values > 0.05. **Table S4.** Interacting effects of 25(OH)D and CpG sites in vitamin D-related genes on the 5-year risk of post-menopausal breast cancer (852 cases, 1026 from subcohort, including 41 additional cases): ratio of hazard ratios and 95% confidence intervals. **Table S5.** Ratio of hazard ratios and 95% confidence intervals for the interaction between 25(OH)D and methylation on the 5-year risk of postmenopausal breast cancer (852 cases, 1026 from subcohort, including 41 additional cases); CpGs with Fisher combined p values < 1×10^{-5} for subcohort versus case comparison. **Figure S1.** Quantile-quantile plot for the association between the epigenetic-by-25(OH)D interaction term and breast cancer risk among postmenopausal women. **Figure S2.** Volcano plot for the associations between serum 25(OH)D levels (modeled continuously) and DNA methylation at 423,500 CpG sites among 1270 non-Hispanic white women randomly selected from the Sister Study cohort (2003–2009). **Figure S3.** Manhattan plot (top) and quantile-quantile plot (bottom) for the association between DNA methylation at 423,500 CpG sites and serum 25(OH)D among non-Hispanic white women with breast cancer ($n = 1024$; excluding those who were selected as part of subcohort). No CpGs were statistically significant at $q < 0.05$. (DOCX 419 kb)

Abbreviations
1,25(OH)$_2$D: 1,25-Dihydroxyvitamin D; 25(OH)D: 25-Hydroxyvitamin D; BMI: Body mass index; CI: Confidence interval; EWAS: Epigenome-wide association study; HR: Hazard ratio; ICC: Intraclass correlation coefficient; LC/MS: Liquid chromatography-mass spectrometry; RHR: Ratio of hazard ratios; RXRA: Retinoid X receptor alpha; SNP: Single nucleotide polymorphism; VDR: Vitamin D receptor

Acknowledgements
The authors would like to thank Drs. Alexandra White and Jacob Kresovich for their comments on an early draft of this paper.

Funding
This work was supported by an Office of Dietary Supplement Research Scholars Program Grant (to KMO) and the Intramural Research Program of the National Institutes of Health, National Institute of Environmental Health Sciences (projects Z01-ES044005 to DPS; Z01-ES102245 to CRW; and Z01-ES049033 to JAT).

Authors' contributions
DPS, JAT, and CRW designed the parent study and acquired the data. ZX and KMO performed statistical analyses. KMO, HKK, JAT, and CRW interpreted the data. KMO drafted the manuscript, with guidance from JAT and CRW and substantial contributions from HKK. All authors critically reviewed the manuscript and approved the final draft.

Competing interests
The authors declare that they have no competing interests.

Author details
[1]Biostatistics and Computational Biology Branch, National Institute of Environmental Health Sciences, National Institutes of Health, Research Triangle Park, NC 27709, USA. [2]Epidemiology Branch, National Institute of Environmental Health Sciences, National Institutes of Health, Research Triangle Park, NC 27709, USA. [3]Chromatin and Gene Expression Section, Epigenetics and Stem Cell Biology Laboratory, National Institute of Environmental Health Sciences, National Institutes of Health, Research Triangle Park, NC 27709, USA.

References
1. Autier P, Boniol M, Pizot C, Mullie P. Vitamin D status and ill health: a systematic review. Lancet Diabetes Endocrinol. 2014;2:76–89.
2. Gandini S, Boniol M, Haukka J, Byrnes G, Cox B, Sneyd MJ, et al. Meta-analysis of observational studies of serum 25-hydroxyvitamin D levels and colorectal, breast and prostate cancer and colorectal adenoma. Int J Cancer. 2011;128:1414–24.
3. O'Brien KM, Sandler DP, Taylor JA, Weinberg CR. Serum vitamin D and risk of breast cancer within five years. Environ Health Perspect. 2017;125:077004.
4. Schöttker B, Jorde R, Peasey A, Thorand B, Jansen EHJM, de GL, et al. Vitamin D and mortality: meta-analysis of individual participant data from a large consortium of cohort studies from Europe and the United States. BMJ. 2014;348:g3656.
5. Kim Y, Je Y. Vitamin D intake, blood 25(OH)D levels, and breast cancer risk or mortality: a meta-analysis. Br J Cancer. 2014;110:2772–84.
6. Holick MF, Herman RH, Award M. Vitamin D: importance in the prevention of cancers, type 1 diabetes, heart disease, and osteoporosis. Am J Clin Nutr. 2004;79:362–71.
7. Trump DL, Hershberger PA, Bernardi RJ, Ahmed S, Muindi J, Fakih M, et al. Anti-tumor activity of calcitriol: pre-clinical and clinical studies. J Steroid Biochem Mol Biol. 2004;89–90:519–26.
8. Welsh J, Wietzke JA, Zinser GM, Byrne B, Smith K, Narvaez CJ. Vitamin D-3 receptor as a target for breast cancer prevention. J Nutr. 2003;133:2425S–33S.
9. Wei R, Christakos S. Mechanisms underlying the regulation of innate and adaptive immunity by vitamin D. Nutrients. 2015;7:8251–60.
10. Prietl B, Treiber G, Pieber TR, Amrein K. Vitamin D and immune function. Nutrients. 2013;5:2502–21.
11. Cheskis B, Freedman LP. Ligand modulates the conversion of DNA-bound vitamin D3 receptor (VDR) homodimers into VDR-retinoid X receptor heterodimers. Mol Cell Biol. 1994;14:3329–38.
12. Goeman F, De Nicola F, De Meo PDO, Pallocca M, Elmi B, Castrignano T, et al. VDR primary targets by genome-wide transcriptional profiling. J Steroid Biochem Mol Biol. Elsevier Ltd. 2014;143:348–56.
13. Fetahu IS, Höbaus J, Kállay EO. Vitamin D and the epigenome. Front Physiol. 2014;5:164.
14. Jjingo D, Conley AB, Yi SV, Lunyak VV, Jordan IK. On the presence and role of human gene-body DNA methylation. Oncotarget. 2012;3:462–74.
15. Lee KWK, Pausova Z. Cigarette smoking and DNA methylation. Front Genet. 2013;4:1–11.
16. Harlid S, Xu Z, Panduri V, Sandler DP, Taylor JA. CpG sites associated with cigarette smoking: analysis of epigenome-wide data from the sister study. Env Heal Perspect. 2014;122:673–8.
17. Joubert BR, Felix JF, Yousefi P, Bakulski KM, Just AC, Breton C, et al. DNA methylation in newborns and maternal smoking in pregnancy: genome-wide consortium meta-analysis. Am J Hum Genet. 2016;98:680–96.
18. Joehanes R, Just AC, Marioni RE, Pilling LC, Reynolds LM, Mandaviya PR, et al. Epigenetic signatures of cigarette smoking. Circ Cardiovasc Genet. 2016;9:436–47.
19. Markunas CA, Xu Z, Harlid S, Wade PA, Lie RT, Taylor JA, et al. Identification of DNA methylation changes in newborns related to maternal smoking during pregnancy. Environ Health Perspect. 2014;122:1147–53.
20. Wilson LE, Harlid S, Xu Z, Sandler DP, Taylor JA. An epigenome-wide study of body mass index and DNA methylation in blood using participants from the sister study cohort. Int J Obes. 2016;41:194–9.
21. Hair BY, Xu Z, Kirk EL, Harlid S, Sandhu R, Robinson WR, et al. Body mass index associated with genome-wide methylation in breast tissue. Breast Cancer Res Treat. 2015;151:453–63.

22. Vaissière T, Hung RJ, Zaridze D, Moukeria A, Cuenin C, Fasolo V, et al. Quantitative analysis of DNA methylation profiles in lung cancer identifies aberrant DNA methylation of specific genes and its association with gender and cancer risk factors. Cancer Res. 2009;69:243–52.

23. Friso S, Udali S, De Santis D, Choi S-W. One-carbon metabolism and epigenetics. Mol Aspects Med. 2016;54:28–36.

24. Steegers-Theunissen RP, Obermann-Borst SA, Kremer D, Lindemans J, Siebel C, Steegers EA, et al. Periconceptional maternal folic acid use of 400 μg per day is related to increased methylation of the IGF2 gene in the very young child. PLoS One. 2009;4:1–5.

25. Chang S, Wang L, Guan Y, Shangguan S, Du Q, Wang Y, et al. Long interspersed nucleotide element-1 hypomethylation in folate-deficient mouse embryonic stem cells. J Cell Biochem. 2013;114:1549–58.

26. Choi SW, Friso S, Ghandour H, Bagley PJ, Selhub J, Mason JB. Vitamin B-12 deficiency induces anomalies of base substitution and methylation in the DNA of rat colonic epithelium. J Nutr. 2004;134:750–5.

27. Cheong HS, Lee HC, Park BL, Kim H, Jang MJ, Han YM, et al. Epigenetic modification of retinoic acid-treated human embryonic stem cells. BMB Rep. 2010;43:830–5.

28. Chung I, Karpf AR, Muindi JR, Conroy JM, Nowak NJ, Johnson CS, et al. Epigenetic silencing of CYP24 in tumor-derived endothelial cells contributes to selective growth inhibition by calcitriol. J Biol Chem. 2007;282:8704–14.

29. Johnson CS, Chung I, Trump DL. Epigenetic silencing of CYP24 in the tumor microenvironment. J Steroid Biochem Mol Biol. 2010;121:338–42.

30. Fu B, Wang H, Wang J, Barouhas I, Liu W, Shuboy A, et al. Epigenetic regulation of BMP2 by 1,25-dihydroxyvitamin D3 through DNA methylation and histone modification. PLoS One. 2013;8:1–10.

31. Stefanska B, Salamé P, Bednarek A, Fabianowska-Majewska K. Comparative effects of retinoic acid, vitamin D and resveratrol alone and in combination with adenosine analogues on methylation and expression of phosphatase and tensin homologue tumour suppressor gene in breast cancer cells. Br J Nutr. 2012;107:781–90.

32. Rawson JB, Sun Z, Dicks E, Daftary D, Parfrey PS, Green RC, et al. Vitamin D intake is negatively associated with promoter methylation of the Wnt antagonist gene DKK1 in a large group of colorectal cancer patients. Nutr Cancer. 2012;64:919–28.

33. Zhu H, Wang X, Shi H, Su S, Harshfield GA, Gutin B, et al. A genome-wide methylation study of severe vitamin D deficiency in African American adolescents. J Pediatr. 2013;162:1004–9.

34. Florath I, Schöttker B, Butterbach K, Bewerunge-Hudler M, Brenner H, Schottker B, et al. Epigenome-wide search for association of serum 25-hydroxyvitamin D concentration with leukocyte DNA methylation in a large cohort of older men. Epigenomics. 2016;8:487–99.

35. Suderman M, Stene LC, Bohlin J, Page CM, Holvik K, Parr CL, et al. 25-hydroxyvitamin D in pregnancy and genome wide cord blood DNA methylation in two pregnancy cohorts (MoBa and ALSPAC). J Steroid Biochem Mol Biol. 2016;159:102–9.

36. Chavez Valencia RA, Martino DJ, Saffery R, Ellis JA. In vitro exposure of human blood mononuclear cells to active vitamin D does not induce substantial change to DNA methylation on a genome-scale. J Steroid Biochem Mol Biol. 2014;141:144–9.

37. Hübner U, Geisel JJJ, Kirsch SH, Kruse V, Bodis M, Klein C, et al. Effect of 1 year B and D vitamin supplementation on LINE-1 repetitive element methylation in older subjects. Clin Chem Lab Med. 2013;51:649–55.

38. Nair-Shalliker V, Dhillon V, Clements M, Armstrong BK, Fenech M. The association between personal sun exposure, serum vitamin D and global methylation in human lymphocytes in a population of healthy adults in South Australia. Mutat Res. 2014;765:6–10.

39. Zhu H, Bhagatwala J, Huang Y, Pollock NK, Parikh S, Raed A, et al. Race/ethnicity-specific association of vitamin D and global DNA methylation: cross-sectional and interventional findings. PLoS One. 2016;11:e0152849.

40. Sandler DP, Hodgson ME, Deming-Halverson SL, Juras PJ, D'Aloisio AD, Suarez L, et al. The sister study: baseline methods and participant characteristics. Env Heal Perspect 2017;In press.

41. Prentice RL. A case-cohort design for epidemiologic cohort studies and disease prevention trials. Biometrika. 1986;73:1–11.

42. Barlow WE, Ichikawa L, Rosner D, Izumi S. Analysis of case-cohort designs. J Clin Epidemiol. 1999;52:1165–72.

43. Xu Z, Niu L, Li L, Taylor JA. ENmix: a novel background correction method for Illumina HumanMethylation450 BeadChip. Nucleic Acids Res. 2015;44:e20.

44. Xu Z, Langie SAS, De Boever P, Taylor JA, Niu LRELIC. A novel dye-bias correction method for Illumina methylation BeadChip. BMC Genomics. 2017;18:1–7.

45. Niu L, Xu Z, Taylor JA. RCP: a novel probe design bias correction method for Illumina methylation BeadChip. Bioinformatics. 2016;32:2659–63.

46. Chen J, Just AC, Schwartz J, Hou L, Jafari N, Sun Z, et al. CpGFilter: model-based CpG probe filtering with replicates for epigenome-wide association studies. Bioinformatics. 2015;32:469–71.

47. University of California Santa Cruz, Genome Browser. Available from: http://genome.ucsc.edu/. [cited 2017 Mar 15]

48. Houseman EA, Kelsey KT, Wiencke JK, Marsit CJ. Cell-composition effects in the analysis of DNA methylation array data: a mathematical perspective. BMC Bioinformatics. 2015;16:95.

49. Benjamini Y, Hochberg Y. Controlling the false discovery rate: a practical and powerful approach to multiple testing. J R Stat Soc B. 1995;57:289–300.

50. Fisher RA. Statistical methods for research workers. Edinburgh: Oliver and Boyd; 1925.

51. Haussler MR, Whitfield GK, Kaneko I, Haussler CA, Hsieh D, Hsieh JC, et al. Molecular mechanisms of vitamin D action. Calcif Tissue Int. 2013;92:77–98.

52. Decker M, Arand M, Cronin A. Mammalian epoxide hydrolases in xenobiotic metabolism and signalling. Arch Toxicol. 2009;83:297–318.

53. Gilroy DW, Edin ML, De Maeyer RPH, Bystrom J, Newson J, Lih FB, et al. CYP450-derived oxylipins mediate inflammatory resolution. Proc Natl Acad Sci. 2016;113:E3240–9.

54. Kutuzova GD, DeLuca HF. 1,25-Dihydroxyvitamin D3 regulates genes responsible for detoxification in intestine. Toxicol Appl Pharmacol. 2007;218:37–44.

55. Tan X, Wang YY, Chen XY, Xian L, Guo JJ, Liang GB, et al. Quantitative assessment of the effects of the EPHX1 Tyr113His polymorphism on lung and breast cancer. Genet Mol Res. 2014;13:7437–46.

56. Babina M, Weber S, Henz BM. CD43 (leukosialin, sialophorin) expression is differentially regulated by retinoic acids. Eur J Immunol. 1997;27:1147–51.

57. Turzová M, Hunáková L, Duraj J, Speiser P, Sedlák J, Chorváth B. Modulation of leukosialin (sialophorin, CD43 antigen) on the cell surface of human hematopoietic cell lines induced by cytokins, retinoic acid and 1,25(OH)2-vitamin D3. Neoplasma. 1993;40:9–13.

58. Wilson BG, Roberts CWM. SWI/SNF nucleosome remodellers and cancer. Nat Rev Cancer. 2011;11:481–92.

59. Hsiao P-W, Fryer CJ, Trotter KW, Wang W, Archer TK. BAF60a mediates critical interactions between nuclear receptors and the BRG1 chromatin-remodeling complex for transactivation. Mol Cell Biol. 2003;23:6210–20.

60. Koszewski NJ, Henry KW, Lubert EJ, Gravatte H, Noonan DJ. Use of a modified yeast one-hybrid screen to identify BAF60a interactions with the vitamin D receptor heterodimer. J Steroid Biochem Mol Biol. 2003;87:223–31.

61. Flajollet S, Lefebvre B, Cudejko C, Staels B, Lefebvre P. The core component of the mammalian SWI/SNF complex SMARCD3/BAF60c is a coactivator for the nuclear retinoic acid receptor. Mol Cell Endocrinol. 2007;270:23–32.

62. Kadoch C, Hargreaves DC, Hodges C, Elias L, Ho L, Ranish J, et al. Proteomic and bioinformatic analysis of mammalian SWI/SNF complexes identifies extensive roles in human malignancy. Nat Genet. 2013;45:592–601.

63. Masliah-Planchon J, Bièche I, Guinebretière J-M, Bourdeaut F, Delattre O. SWI/SNF chromatin remodeling and human malignancies. Annu Rev Pathol Mech Dis. 2015;10:145–71.

64. Bauer SR, Hankinson SE, Bertone-Johnson ER, Ding EL. Plasma vitamin D levels, menopause, and risk of breast cancer: dose-response meta-analysis of prospective studies. Med. 2013;92:123–31.

14

Identifying an early treatment window for predicting breast cancer response to neoadjuvant chemotherapy using immunohistopathology and hemoglobin parameters

Quing Zhu[1*], Susan Tannenbaum[2], Scott H. Kurtzman[3], Patricia DeFusco[4], Andrew Ricci Jr[4], Hamed Vavadi[5], Feifei Zhou[5], Chen Xu[6], Alex Merkulov[2], Poornima Hegde[2], Mark Kane[2], Liqun Wang[7] and Kert Sabbath[3]

Abstract

Background: Breast cancer pathologic complete response (pCR) to neoadjuvant chemotherapy (NAC) varies with tumor subtype. The purpose of this study was to identify an early treatment window for predicting pCR based on tumor subtype, pretreatment total hemoglobin (tHb) level, and early changes in tHb following NAC.

Methods: Twenty-two patients (mean age 56 years, range 34–74 years) were assessed using a near-infrared imager coupled with an Ultrasound system prior to treatment, 7 days after the first treatment, at the end of each of the first three cycles, and before their definitive surgery. Pathologic responses were dichotomized by the Miller-Payne system. Tumor vascularity was assessed from tHb; vascularity changes during NAC were assessed from a percentage tHb normalized to the pretreatment level (%tHb). After training the logistic prediction models using the previous study data, we assessed the early treatment window for predicting pathological response according to their tumor subtype (human epidermal growth factor receptor 2 (HER2), estrogen receptor (ER), triple-negative (TN)) based on tHb, and %tHb measured at different cycles and evaluated by the area under the receiver operating characteristic (ROC) curve (AUC).

Results: In the new study cohort, maximum pretreatment tHb and %tHb changes after cycles 1, 2, and 3 were significantly higher in responder Miller-Payne 4–5 tumors ($n = 13$) than non-or partial responder Miller-Payne 1–3 tumors ($n = 9$). However, no significance was found at day 7. The AUC of the predictive power of pretreatment tHb in the cohort was 0.75, which was similar to the performance of the HER2 subtype as a single predictor (AUC of 0.78). A greater predictive power of pretreatment tHb was found within each subtype, with AUCs of 0.88, 0.69, and 0.72, in the HER2, ER, and TN subtypes, respectively. Using pretreatment tHb and cycle 1 %tHb, AUC reached 0.96, 0.91, and 0.90 in HER2, ER, and TN subtypes, respectively, and 0.95 regardless of subtype. Additional cycle 2 %tHb measurements moderately improved prediction for the HER2 subtype but did not improve prediction for the ER and TN subtypes.

Conclusions: By combining tumor subtypes with tHb, we predicted the pCR of breast cancer to NAC before treatment. Prediction accuracy can be significantly improved by incorporating cycle 1 and 2 %tHb for the HER2 subtype and cycle 1 %tHb for the ER and TN subtypes.

(Continued on next page)

* Correspondence: zhu.q@wustl.edu
[1]Biomedical Engineering and Radiology, Washington University in St Louis, One Brookings Drive, Mail Box 1097, Whitaker Hall 300D, St. Louis, MO 63130, USA
Full list of author information is available at the end of the article

(Continued from previous page)

Keywords: Predicting neoadjuvant chemotherapy, Personalized medicine, Near infrared imaging, Ultrasound-guided optical imaging,

Background

The increasingly widespread use of neoadjuvant chemotherapy (NAC) in breast cancer patients has improved surgical outcomes by preoperatively downsizing the tumor volume. Since the introduction of NAC, breast-conserving surgery rates have increased [1]. Moreover, patients who have achieved pathological complete response (pCR) show improved survival rates compared with those who did not achieve pCR [2]. This relationship is so strong, in fact, that pCR is becoming a surrogate endpoint for evaluating the effectiveness of newer chemotherapy protocols [3, 4]. Early assessment of the degree of patient response to NAC can have a major impact on individualized treatment management [5].

The ability to identify patients with tumors that have a high likelihood of achieving a pCR before starting NAC could enable targeting a treatment plan to patients with only those tumor types. By eliminating ineffective treatment of patients unlikely to benefit, outcomes would be better, and toxicity would be reduced. Published literature shows that an increased probability of achieving pCR is correlated with high tumor grade, positive human epidermal growth factor receptor 2 (HER2) status, negative estrogen receptor (ER) status, and triple negative (TN) receptor status [6–9]. However, prediction models based on these tumor histopathological characteristics are imperfect; within and among these subgroups, the response to chemotherapy varies widely. Dual HER2 blockade with trastuzumab and pertuzumab in combination with cytotoxic chemotherapy now utilized in many HER2$^+$ patients in the neoadjuvant setting results in a high pCR (16.8–66.2%) [10]. Despite this, there is a significant percentage of HER2$^+$ patients who do not achieve a pCR or near pCR. Additionally, the pCR of ER$^+$/HER2$^-$ cancers is less robust (7.0–16.2%) and the pCR for TN cancers is 33.6–35% [11, 12].

Many ongoing investigations are exploring imaging techniques to monitor response and allow early modification of treatment in order to enhance outcomes [13]. The use of imaging as an early surrogate biomarker of response is appealing because it is noninvasive and might allow for a window of opportunity during which treatment regimens could be altered accordingly, depending on the expected response.

Conventional imaging methods, such as mammography and ultrasound (US), to monitor NAC have not been widely used to date due to their low sensitivity for monitoring NAC-treated tumors [14]. Positron emission tomography (PET)/computed tomography (CT) is more sensitive to tumor metabolic activity which has been shown to be an early indicator of treatment effectiveness for breast cancer in the neoadjuvant setting [15, 16]. Contrast-enhanced magnetic resonance imaging (MRI) is effective in predicting TN or HER2$^+$ cancers, but is inaccurate for ER$^+$/HER2$^-$ breast cancers [17]. Both PET/CT and MRI require the injection of contrast agents and are costly for repeated use during treatment.

Optical tomography and spectroscopy using near infrared (NIR) diffused light have been explored as novel tools to predict and monitor the tumor vasculature response to NAC [18–31]. The NIR technique utilizes the intrinsic biomarker of hemoglobin contrast, which is directly related to tumor angiogenesis. Cost effectiveness, portability, and the absence of the need for contrast agents make NIR systems ideal for repeated use in clinical settings. We have reported the development of US-guided optical tomography using NIR diffused light coupled with a commercial ultrasound system (NIR/US) to improve light localization and quantification accuracy in the diagnosis of breast cancer [32, 33] and in predicting NAC response [20]. The logistic prediction models we developed utilize tumor pretreatment pathological parameters and hemoglobin content measured before NAC to predict pathological response [21]. The present study was designed to identify the best treatment window for predicting pathological response during NAC using breast cancer subtype, the pretreatment biomarker of total hemoglobin (tHb) level, and changes in tHb during early-treatment cycles 1, 2, and 3. Ultimately, effectively predicting the response to NAC by combining information from US-guided NIR with breast cancer subtype could help to individualize treatment.

Methods
Patients

The study protocol was approved by institutional review boards and was HIPAA compliant. Written informed consent was obtained from all patients. From March 2014 to June 2016, 28 patients were recruited at three hospitals. All had been referred for NAC to the one of three medical oncologists (PD, ST, and KS) and agreed to participate in our study. Five patients did not complete the study because of a change in their treatment plan or a desire to withdraw from the study. One patient had technically problematic baseline imaging. Data from these six patients were not included in the analysis. The remaining 22 patients (mean age 55 years, range 34–74 years) were repeatedly imaged by NIR/US prior to initiation of NAC, at the end of the first three treatment cycles during chemotherapy, and prior to definitive surgery. Of the 22 patients (Table 1), 11 were HER2$^+$ of which eight were also ER$^+$; six were ER$^+$/HER2$^-$, and five were TN. Of the 22 patients, 12 had T2 tumors, five had T1, and five had T3 tumors. Patients were treated with regimens based on their tumor biomarkers according to current clinical practice. For ER$^+$/HER2$^-$ tumors, patients were treated with dose-dense doxorubicin/cyclophosphamide every 2 weeks for four cycles followed by paclitaxel every 2 weeks for four cycles (ACT). The NIR/US cycle 1 to 3 measurements were performed at the end of the first three cycles before the paclitaxel started. For HER2$^+$ tumors, all patients were treated with trastuzumab, pertuzumab, and docetaxel or paclitaxel with or without carboplatin (TPT) every 3 weeks for six cycles and one patient had two additional cycles of 5-flurouracil, epirubicin, and cyclophosphamide (FEC). The NIR/US cycle 1 to 3 measurements were performed at the end of the first three treatment cycles when TPT was given. For TN tumors, three were treated with ACT, the same as ER$^+$/HER2$^-$ patients, and two were treated with carboplatin and paclitaxel every 3 weeks for six cycles because of their BRCA1 gene mutation. One elderly ER$^+$/HER2$^-$ patient was treated with cyclophosphamide/docetaxel without doxorubicin (TC) every 3 weeks for four cycles.

The HER2$^+$ cohort was monitored at an additional time point of 7 days after the first treatment, and one TN and four ER$^+$/HER2$^-$ patients were also monitored

Table 1 Patient information, tumor characteristics, Miller-Payne Grade, initial tumor size (MRI/PET and US), and treatment regimen

Age	Tumor type	NS	Mitotic count/10 HPF	TN	HER2/ER	Miller-Payne grade	Tumor size (MRI/PET)	Tumor size (US)	Treatment regimen
59	IDC	6	2	–	–/+	3	2.7	1.7	ACT
55	ILC	6	1	–	–/+	4	8.6	–a	ACT
33	IDC	4	2	–	–/+	3	1.6	1.5	ACT
61	IDC/ILC	6	1	+	–/–	1	3.3	1.9	ACT
59	IDC	6	5	–	–/+	2	5.6	2.2	ACT
68	IDC	6	3	–	–/+	3	7.6	2.2	ACT
51	IDC	9	40	+	–/–	5	3.6	2.2	ACT
53	IDC	9	62	+	–/–	3	PET: 3.7	4.3	ACT
									TPT
51	IDC	7	15	–	+/+	5	N/A	1.2	TPT
74	IDC	8	8	–	+/–	5	6.2	–a	TPT
57	IDC	9	16	–	+/–	4	6.9	–b	TPT&FEC
									TPT
51	IDC	9	14	–	+/–	5	3.0	1.9	TPT
59	IDC	7	1	–	+/+	5	N/A	0.6	TPT
61	IDC	4	3	–	+/+c	5	2.0	1.4	TPT
37	IDC/ILC	8	9	–	+/+	4	3.6	1.9	TPT
54	IDC	8	20	–	+/+	5	2.9	2.3	TPT
40	IDC	8	15	–	+/+	5	2.2	2.1	TPT
62	IDC	9	12	–	+/+	3	PET: 1.8	1.2	TPT
37	IDC	8	42	–	+/+c	5	1.5	1.6	TPT
72	IDC	9	42	–	–/+	3	4.3	2.3	TC
57	IDC	9	14	+	–/–	5	2.3	1.3	Carbo/T
41	IDC	9	8	+	–/–	3	4.0	4.0	Carbo/T

aNot US visible

bMuch larger than the size of the US transducer

cER showed a weak positive result

ACT, dose-dense doxorubicin/cyclophosphamide and paclitaxel; *Carbo/T*, carboplatin and paclitaxel, *ER* estrogen receptor, *FEC* 5flurouracil, epirubicin, and cyclophosphamide, *HER2* human epidermal growth factor receptor 2, *IDC* invasive ductal carcinoma, *ILC* invasive lobular carcinoma, *MRI* magnetic resonance imaging, *N/A* not available, *NS* Nottingham Score (out of 9), *PET* positron emission tomography, *TC* cyclophosphamide and docetaxel, *TN* triple negative, *TPT* TP and taxane-based therapy—trastuzumab, pertuzumab and docetaxel or paclitaxel with or without carboplatin, *TPT&FEC* trastuzumab, pertuzumab, paclitaxel; 5flurouracil, epirubicin, cyclophosphamide, *US* ultrasound

at an optional time point of 7 days after the first treatment. The median from 7 days was 0 with a range of 0 to 2 days. Moreover, four TN and five ER$^+$/HER2$^-$ patients were monitored at an additional time point at the end of cycle 5. Thus, a total of 16 patients had an additional time point at 7 days after the first treatment and nine patients had an additional time point at the end of cycle 5.

All 22 patients were studied after their diagnostic core biopsy with an average interval of 28 days (median 26 days, range 7–56 days). Among the 22 patients, one had pretreatment NIR measurements 7 days after biopsy and the remaining patients had the NIR measurements more than 10 days after biopsy. All patients received the first cycle of NAC after the initial NIR/US study (median 2 days, range 0–10 days). The average interval between post-treatment NIR/US and surgery was 19 days (median 15 days, range 2–67 days). During the treatment, the NIR/US scans were performed before their scheduled chemotherapy (median 0 days, range 0–5 days). Among the 22 patients, 18 patients had pretreatment MRI and 12 patients had post-treatment MRI. Two patients had pretreatment PET.

The histologic type of 19 patients was invasive ductal carcinoma; one patient had invasive lobular carcinoma, and the other two patients had invasive mammary carcinoma with mixed ductal and lobular features. One of the 22 patients had two distinct tumor masses in the same breast, adjacent to each other and with the same histologic characteristics. For this patient, one of the two masses was used for data analysis. Invasive carcinoma within the pretreatment core biopsies was graded using the Nottingham histologic score (NS). ER, progesterone receptor (PR), and HER-2/neu (c-erbB-2) immunohistochemistry was performed on formalin-fixed, paraffin-embedded core biopsy tissue. The ER and PR were scored by a modified San Antonio scoring system [34], where the total score ranges from 0 to 8 (scores 0–2 are negative, a score of 3 is equivocal and scores ≥ 4 are positive). Testing for the HER2 gene was performed by immunohistochemistry and by gene amplification utilizing the fluorescence in situ hybridization (FISH) technique, and the results were reported in accordance with 2014 ASCO/CAP guidelines [35]. Results were reported as equivocal HER2 if there was weak to moderate, incomplete membranous staining in > 10% of cells or if FISH showed a HER2/CEP17 ratio < 2, or if the HER2 copy number was ≥ 4 and < 6. HER2 results were negative if the immunohistochemistry or FISH assays fell below the thresholds for interpretation as equivocal. All assays were performed on pretreatment core biopsy samples.

Pathology assessment

Pathologic response was assessed by applying the Miller-Payne grading criteria to definitive surgery specimens in comparison with initial core biopsies (Table 1). Two breast pathologists (AR and PH) individually evaluated cases from their respective hospitals and additional cases from the third hospital. The Miller-Payne system [36] divides pathologic response into five grades based on a comparison of tumor cellularity between the pretreatment core biopsy and the definitive surgical specimen. Grade 1 indicates no change or some minor alteration in individual malignant cells but no reduction in overall cellularity; this is a pathological nonresponse (pNR). Grade 2 indicates a minor loss of tumor cells (up to 30%) but with overall cellularity still high; this is a partial pathologic response (pPR). Grade 3 indicates an estimated 30–90% reduction in tumor cells (pPR). Grade 4 indicates a marked disappearance of tumor cells (> 90%), with only small clusters or widely dispersed individual cells remaining (almost pCR). Grade 5 indicates that no malignant cells are identifiable in sections from the tumor bed (pCR). Grade 5 may show that necrosis, granulation tissue, histiocytes, and vascular fibroelastotic stroma remains, often containing macrophages. Residual ductal carcinoma in situ (DCIS) is acceptable for Miller-Payne grade 5.

US and NIR system and imaging

Ultrasound examinations were performed using a commercial ultrasound system (Phillips IU22 or GE Logiq 5) at the corresponding hospital. Three NIR systems with identical designs were used at the three hospitals, and the details have been given previously [24]. Briefly, the NIR/US probe consists of the commercial US transducer located centrally, with source and detector light guides (optical fibers) distributed around the periphery of the NIR/US probe. Four laser diodes of 740 nm, 780 nm, 808 nm, and 830 nm optical wavelengths were sequentially switched to nine positions on the probe, while the reflected light was coupled by the light guides to 14 parallel detectors. The entire NIR data acquisition interval was less than 5 s. For each patient, US images and optical measurements were acquired simultaneously in the cancer region and a normal region within the contralateral breast in the same quadrant as the cancer. At each cancer and normal region, multiple datasets were acquired. The optical data acquired from the normal contralateral breast was used as a reference for calculating the background optical absorption and reduced scattering coefficients that were used in the image reconstruction of the lesions.

Details of the optical imaging reconstruction algorithm with experimental validation have been described elsewhere [37]. Briefly, the NIR reconstruction takes advantages of the ultrasound localization of lesions to segment the imaging volume into a region of interest (ROI) and background nonlesion regions. Since the spatial resolution of diffused light is poorer than that of US, the ROI is chosen to be at least two to three times larger than the tumor size measured by coregistered US in x to y dimensions. In addition, because the depth localization of diffused light is very poor, a tighter ROI in the depth dimension is set by using coregistered US. For each patient, the same size of ROI as that obtained from the pretreatment US is used for processing all datasets obtained at different treatment cycles. Therefore, the changes in tumor size seen by US during treatment have no major effect on the NIR image reconstruction. Among the 22 patients, two patients had initially palpable tumors with ill-defined and heterogeneous pretreatment ultrasound images. For these patients, tumor sizes estimated from pretreatment MRI measurements were used to assist in determining the US ROI in the x to y dimensions. The ROI in the depth dimension was typically set from the top border of the ill-defined tissue pattern to the chest wall as seen by US.

The optical absorption distribution at each wavelength was reconstructed and the tHb concentration, oxygenated hemoglobin (oxyHb) concentration, and deoxygenated hemoglobin (deoxyHb) concentration maps were computed from absorption maps at the four wavelengths [38]. The maximum values of tHb, oxyHb, and deoxyHb were measured for each set of hemoglobin maps. For each patient imaged at each time point, an average maximum that was obtained from 5 to 10 quality NIR images at the tumor location was used to characterize the tumor. Data with patient motion as evaluated by using two coregistered US images before and after each NIR measurement were excluded from averaging. To assess the response of each patient, the tHb obtained before treatment was taken as the baseline and the percentage normalized to the baseline (%tHb) was used to quantitatively evaluate the remaining tumor vascular fraction during chemotherapy.

MRI and US imaging and measurements

Nineteen patients had well-defined tumors visible by US. Tumor sizes were measured by US technologists under direct supervision of attending radiologists. The percentage ratio (%US) of the largest dimension of each posttreatment measurement over the largest dimension of pretreatment measurement was used to evaluate the morphological change during NAC. One patient had a much larger tumor size than the US transducer, and the baseline US measurement was not accurate. The initial tumor mass of this patient measured by MRI was 6. 9 cm. US scans performed from both medial lateral and cranial-caudal directions using the 5-cm US transducer were used to estimate the approximate mass center. Then the combined probe of 10-cm diameter was placed at the estimated mass center for NIR data acquisition.

This procedure had minimal effect on NIR reconstruction. For the two patients with initially palpable but ill-defined and heterogeneous US images, the tumor location at each measurement was tracked using previous US images as references. The tumor clock position, distance of the tumor from the nipple, and depth below the skin were documented for each case. Additionally, the tumor posterior shadowing and surrounding tissue structures, as well as the metal clip position, were also reviewed and used to help identify the tumor for each subsequent measurement. If an MRI was ordered for clinical reasons, the MRI measurements were obtained from the medical records of the patients.

Prediction models

We have previously developed a logistic regression model to predict the NAC response of a patient using pretreatment tumor clinicopathologic variables, tumor subtype, and baseline tHb values [21]. Briefly, logistic regression is a statistical modeling approach that can be used to describe the relationship of several predictor variables $X_1, X_2... X_k$ to a dichotomous response variable Y, where Y is coded 1 (responder) or 0 (nonresponder) for its two possible categories [39]. The model can be written in the form of the conditional probability of the occurrence of one of the two possible outcomes of Y, as follows:

$$pr(Y = 1 \mid X1, X2, ...Xk)$$
$$= \frac{1}{1 + \exp\left(-\left(\beta 0 + \sum_{n=1}^{k} \beta n Xn\right)\right)} \quad (1)$$

The estimated outputs (probability) for each set of predictor variables range from 0 to 1. Given the data on Y, X_1, ... X_k, the unknown parameters βn, n = 0, 1, ..., k, n = 0, 1, ...k can be estimated using the maximum likelihood method.

In this study, we used the data from 32 patients obtained from an earlier study as a training set [20] to estimate a total of four groups of logistic models, and validated these models using the new dataset reported in this study as a testing dataset. The earlier data obtained from 2008 to 2011 were acquired from almost identical NIR systems with the same data processing and image reconstruction procedures as reported in this study.

To validate that the early data and new data are generated from the same population, we have introduced a dummy variable X_{k+1} in Eq. 1 which is coded as 0 for early data and 1 as new data [40, 41]. We have estimated the model with this dummy variable along with the eight predictor variables using the combined datasets. The estimate on β_{k+1} ($P = 0.214$) is statistically insignificant.

Therefore, we can assume both datasets come from the same patient population.

The Matlab (version 2016a) logistic regression function glmfit was used to estimate the coefficients $\beta_n \beta n$, $n = 0, 1, ..., k$, and glmval was used to calculate the receiver operating characteristic (ROC) with these coefficients for the training set. The same coefficients obtained from the training set were used to predict the response for the testing set.

Evaluation of prediction models

We also assessed the overall performance of the prediction models through the ROC curves and the area under the curves (AUCs) for each pair of training and testing sets of each prediction model. The early data used for training had 20 ER$^+$/HER2$^-$ patients, six TN patients, five HER2$^+$ patients, and one ER$^-$/PR$^+$/HER2$^-$ patient [20]. Similar to the new patient cohort, ER$^+$/HER$^-$ ($n = 14$) and TN ($n = 6$) tumors were treated with ACT every 2 weeks for eight cycles. Six ER$^+$/HER2$^-$ tumors and one ER$^-$/PR$^+$/HER2$^-$ tumor were treated with ACT ($n = 3$) or TC ($n = 4$) every 3 weeks for six cycles. HER2$^+$ tumors ($n = 5$) were treated with trastuzumab and docetaxel or paclitaxel with or without carboplatin (TPT) every 3 weeks for six cycles.

Since the early data did not contain any patients treated with dual HER2 blockade, we have randomly selected six HER2$^+$ patients treated with this regimen from the current study and added these six datasets to the training data. For each random selection, the total of patients in training was 38 (32 from the early data and 6 from this study) and testing was 16 from this study. A total of 6 out of 11 random selections result in 462 combinations of paired training and testing datasets for each group of predictors, and the mean of 462 AUC values was used to evaluate the training and testing results of each prediction model. Each pair of training and testing ROCs was generated using a threshold of 0.5. This was used to separate responders (> 0.5) and nonresponders (≤ 0.5) for each prediction model output. We also used the 462 AUC values to construct the 95% confidence interval (CI) for the mean AUC for each model using a binomial formula. These confidence intervals can provide summary information on comparisons of the different models

in terms of their AUC values. For example, if model I has a higher mean AUC than model II, and if their corresponding confidence intervals do not overlap, then this is an indication that model I may have a higher prediction power than the model II in terms of the AUC criterion. However, this interpretation should be understood with the caveat that the 462 values are not true random samples.

Selection of predictors

To select the independent predictors, Spearman's rho was evaluated between each predictor and Miller-Payne grade and between each pair of predictors. Spearman's rho is more appropriate for assessing the relationship for both continuous and discrete variables. Note that both training and testing data were combined to assess the predictors and the Spearman's rhos reported in this section are from the entire cohort of both earlier and new data (Table 2). To compute rho, the tumor HER2, ER, and TN status were coded as: 1 for TN and 0 for otherwise; 1 for HER2$^+$ and 0 for HER2$^-$; and 0 for ER$^+$ and 1 for ER$^-$. Note that 1 presents increased probability of achieving pCR and 0 otherwise.

Both HER2 and ER are highly correlated with Miller-Payne grade (rho = 0.45, $P < 0.001$; rho = 0.29, $P = 0.035$) and are independent of each other (rho = 0.01, $P = 0.928$); thus, they were selected as predictors. TN tumors did not have a significant correlation with Miller-Payne grade (rho = 0.124, $P = 0.362$). However, TN was selected as a predictor because it is used clinically to characterize this group of patients. Among tumor pathological parameters, NS is a traditional pathological variable used by oncologists to predict response. NS is highly correlated with mitotic counts (rho = 0.82, $P < 0.001$). Thus, only NS was selected as an independent pathological predictor and used in each HER2, ER, and TN subtypes to predict response. Baseline tHb and %tHb changes measured during first three treatment cycles are highly correlated with Miller-Payne grade (see Table 2) and were selected to assess the optimal time window to predict response.

Statistical analysis

A two-sample two-sided t test was used to calculate the statistical significance for comparisons between responder

Table 2 Spearman's rho correlation coefficient and P value between Miller-Payne grade and tumor pathological variables (MC, NS), tumor subtype (HER2, ER, TN), tHb, and %tHb measured at the end of cycles 1 to 3

	NS	MC	HER2	ER	TN	tHb	%tHb cycle 1	%tHb cycle 2	%tHb cycle 3
rho	0.42	0.45	0.45	0.29	0.12	0.48	0.50	0.52	0.69
P	$P = 0.001$	$P < 0.001$	$P < 0.001$	$P = 0.035$	$P = 0.364$	$P < 0.001$	$P < 0.001$	$P < 0.001$	$P < 0.001$

Data are from [20] and this study ($n = 54$ patients)
ER estrogen receptor, *HER2* human epidermal growth factor 2, *MC* mitotic count, *NS* Nottingham score, *tHb* total hemoglobin, *TN* triple negative

groups, and a difference with a *P* value of 0.05 was considered significant. The *t* test was also used to test the difference between AUCs of different prediction models when their 95% CIs overlapped. Minitab 17 software (Minitab, State College, PA) was used for statistical calculations.

Results

There were nine Miller-Payne grade 1–3 tumors and 13 grade 4–5 tumors. For grade 4–5 tumors, the pretreatment mean maximum tHb was 84.8 ± 11.3 μmol/L (mean ± standard deviation), whereas for grade 1–3 tumors the pretreatment mean maximum tHb was 67.9 ± 16.2 μmol/L ($P = 0.018$). The mean difference of the maximum tHb was 16.9 μmol/L and the 95% CI was 3.5–3.04 μmol/L. However, no statistical significance was found at day 7 and at the end of treatment cycles 1, 2, and 3 as the mean tHb level was reduced in grade 4–5 tumors but the mean level did not change in grade 1–3 tumors (Fig. 1).

The pretreatment oxyHb was not significantly different between grade 4–5 and grade 1–3 tumors ($P = 0.083$); however, the deoxyHb difference was significant ($P = 0.028$) (Fig. 2). In subsequent measurements, no significant difference was observed in either oxyHb or deoxyHb.

The %tHb (percentage fraction from baseline) was calculated and the results for the two groups are given in Fig. 3. No statistical significance between the two groups was found at day 7 ($P = 0.238$). Statistical significance was achieved at the end of cycle 1. For Miller-Payne grade 1–3 tumors %tHb was 102 ± 12%, whereas for grade 4–5 tumors %tHb was 72 ± 22%. The mean difference was 30% ($P = 0.001$), and the 95% CI was 14.6–45.

0%. The significance remained high at the end of cycles 2 and 3, with mean differences of 26% ($P = 0.018$) and 95% CI 5.1–46.4%, and 25% ($P = 0.012$) and 95% CI 6.4–43.7%, respectively.

In this new cohort, Spearman's rhos calculated between Miller-Payne grade and pretreatment tHb, oxyHb, and deoxyHb, as well as %tHb measured at different cycles, reveal that the pretreatment maximum tHb and maximum deoxyHb have achieved statistical significance ($P = 0.049$ and 0.030; Table 3). The %tHb values measured at the end of cycles 1, 2, and 3 are highly predictive ($P = 0.002$, $P = 0.006$, and $P = 0.048$, respectively), while %tHb measured at day 7, the end of cycle 5, and before operation are not predictive ($P = 0.321$, $P = 0.321$, and $P = 0.202$, respectively).

There is no correlation between the pretreatment tumor size measured by MRI ($n = 18$, $P = 0.150$) and US ($n = 19$, $P = 0.152$) and the Miller-Payne grade.

An example of a pCR is shown in an HER2-positive tumor (Fig. 4) in a 51-year-old woman with a high-grade invasive ductal carcinoma treated with TPT every 3 weeks for six cycles. US images obtained at pretreatment, day 7, at the completion of cycle 1, and before surgery are shown in the left panel. The tumor was well defined and seen by US before treatment and at day 7, was barely visible at the completion of cycle 1, and was not visible at the completion of cycles 2 (data not shown) and 3 (data not shown), and before surgery. tHb concentration maps obtained at the corresponding time points are shown in the right panel. The tHb reduced from 85.8 μmol/L measured before treatment to 69.4, 36.3, and 21.8 μmol/L measured at day 7, before the completion of cycle 1, and before surgery, respectively. tHb measured at the completion of cycles 2 and 3 were

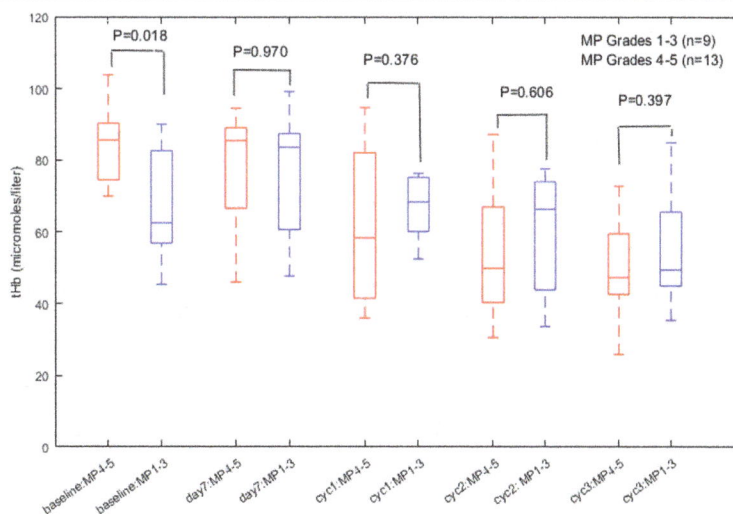

Fig. 1 Box plot of mean maximum total hemoglobin (tHb; μmol/L) of two responder groups of Miller-Payne (MP) 4–5 and MP 1–3 measured at baseline, day 7, and at the end of cycles (cyc) 1, 2, and 3 of NAC

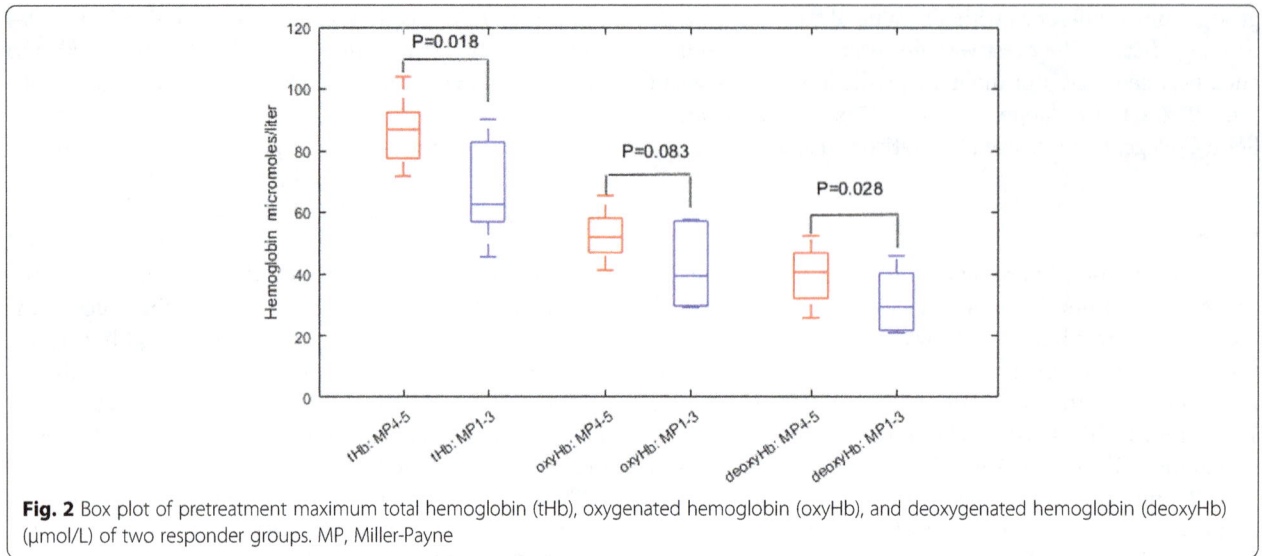

Fig. 2 Box plot of pretreatment maximum total hemoglobin (tHb), oxygenated hemoglobin (oxyHb), and deoxygenated hemoglobin (deoxyHb) (μmol/L) of two responder groups. MP, Miller-Payne

41.8 and 28.7 μmol/L, respectively (data not shown). A dramatic tHb reduction occurred at the end of cycle 1 (%tHb = 42%). This patient had a complete pathologic response with no residual tumor (Miller-Payne grade 5).

An example of a partial responder is shown in a high-grade ER-positive/HER2-negative tumor (Fig. 5). A 72-year-old woman had a locally recurrent invasive ductal carcinoma. She was treated with TC every 3 weeks for four cycles before surgery. US images at the four time points pretreatment, day 7, at the completion of cycle 1, and before surgery are shown in the left panel. The tumor was ill-defined with unclear boundary seen by US. tHb concentration maps obtained at the corresponding time points are shown in the right panel. tHbs

of 90.2, 99.3, 108.8, 105.0 (data not shown), 85.0 (data not shown), and 69.0 μmol/L were measured at pretreatment, day 7, at the completions of cycles 1 to 3, and before surgery, respectively. The patient had a partial response with a residual invasive carcinoma of 2.8 cm (Miller-Payne grade 3).

Based on tumor biomarkers and hemoglobin measurements, predictors are grouped into four categories:1) HER2 status with hemoglobin predictors; 2) ER with hemoglobin predictors; 3) TN with hemoglobin predictors; and 4) hemoglobin predictors (see Table 4). ROCs of validation or testing of these four groups are given in Fig. 6 and Table 4. Note that predictor groups that achieve higher training AUCs do not necessarily

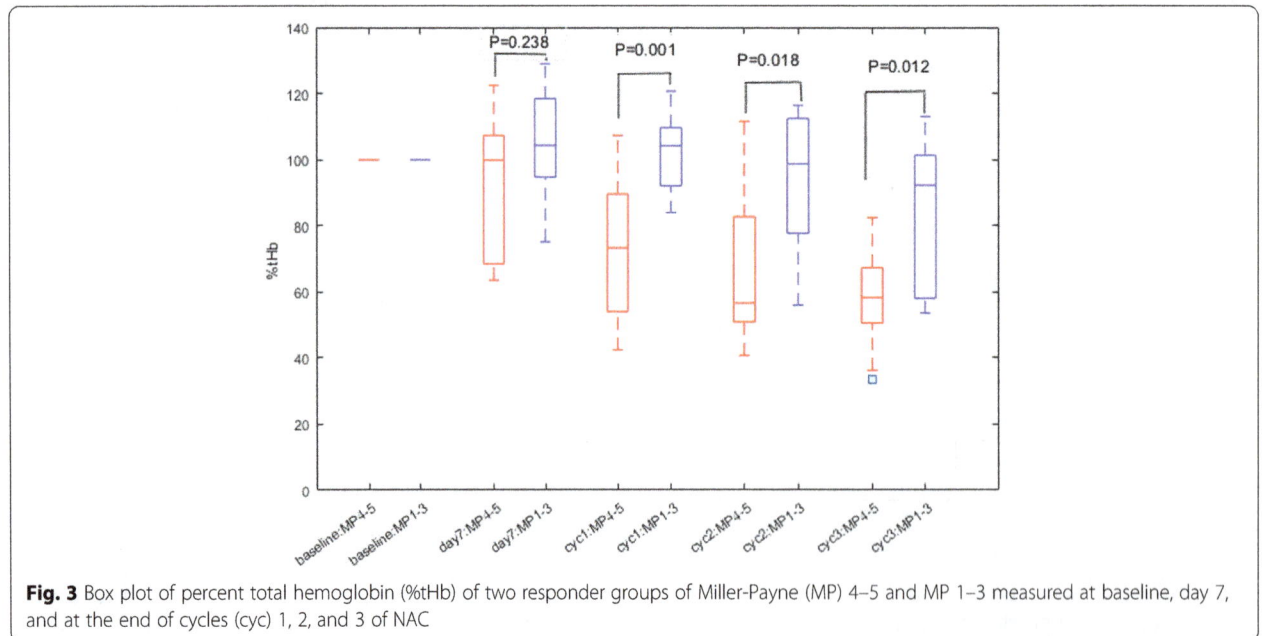

Fig. 3 Box plot of percent total hemoglobin (%tHb) of two responder groups of Miller-Payne (MP) 4–5 and MP 1–3 measured at baseline, day 7, and at the end of cycles (cyc) 1, 2, and 3 of NAC

Table 3 Spearman's rho correlation coefficient and P value between Miller-Payne grade and pretreatment tHb (maximum), oxyHb (maximum), deoxyHb (maximum), %tHb at day 7, and at the end of cycles 1, 2, 3, and 5, and before surgery

	tHb (max)	oxyHb (max)	deoxyHb (max)	%tHb day7	%tHb cycle 1	%tHb cycle 2	%tHb cycle 3	%tHb Cycle 5	%tHb before surgery
rho	0.43	0.28	0.46	0.26	0.61	0.57	0.43	0.26	0.29
P	$P = 0.049$	$P = 0.205$	$P = 0.030$	$P = 0.321$	$P = 0.002$	$P = 0.006$	$P = 0.048$	$P = 0.321$	$P = 0.202$

Data are from the new cohort ($n = 22$ patients)

deoxyHb deoxygenated hemoglobin, *oxyHb* oxygenated hemoglobin, *tHb* total hemoglobin

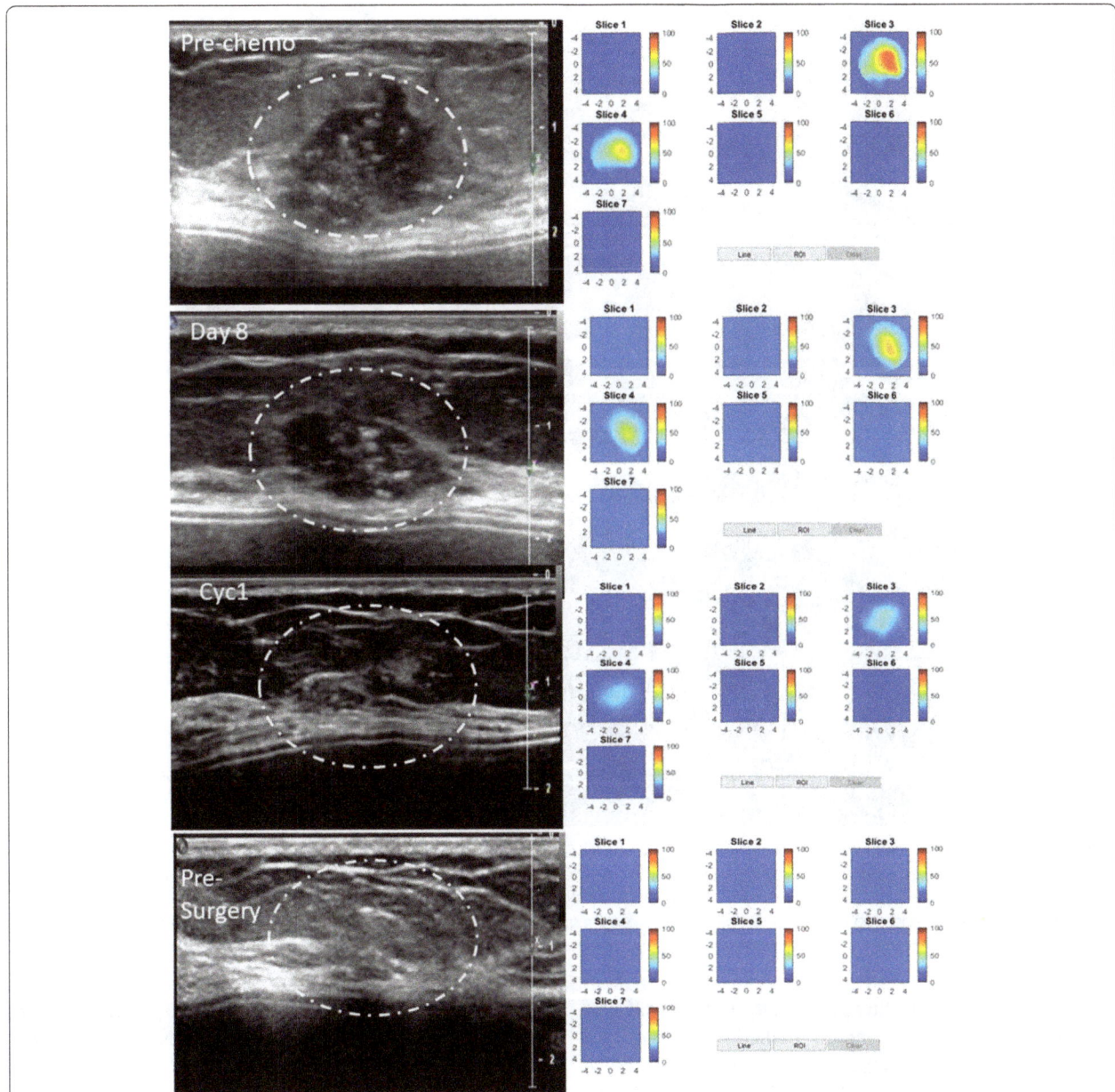

Fig. 4 pCR in an HER2-positive tumor in a 51-year-old woman with a high-grade invasive ductal carcinoma treated with TPT every 3 weeks for six cycles. Left panel: US images obtained at pretreatment, at day 7, at the completion of cycle 1, and before surgery. Right panel: tHb concentration maps obtained at the corresponding time points. Each map shows seven subimages marked as slice 1 to 7, and each subimage shows spatial x and y distribution of tHb concentration reconstructed from 0.5 cm to 3.5 cm below the skin surface. The depth spacing between the subimages in depth is 0.5 cm. The color bar is tHb in micromoles per liter. This patient had a complete pathologic response with no residual tumor, Miller-Payne grade 5

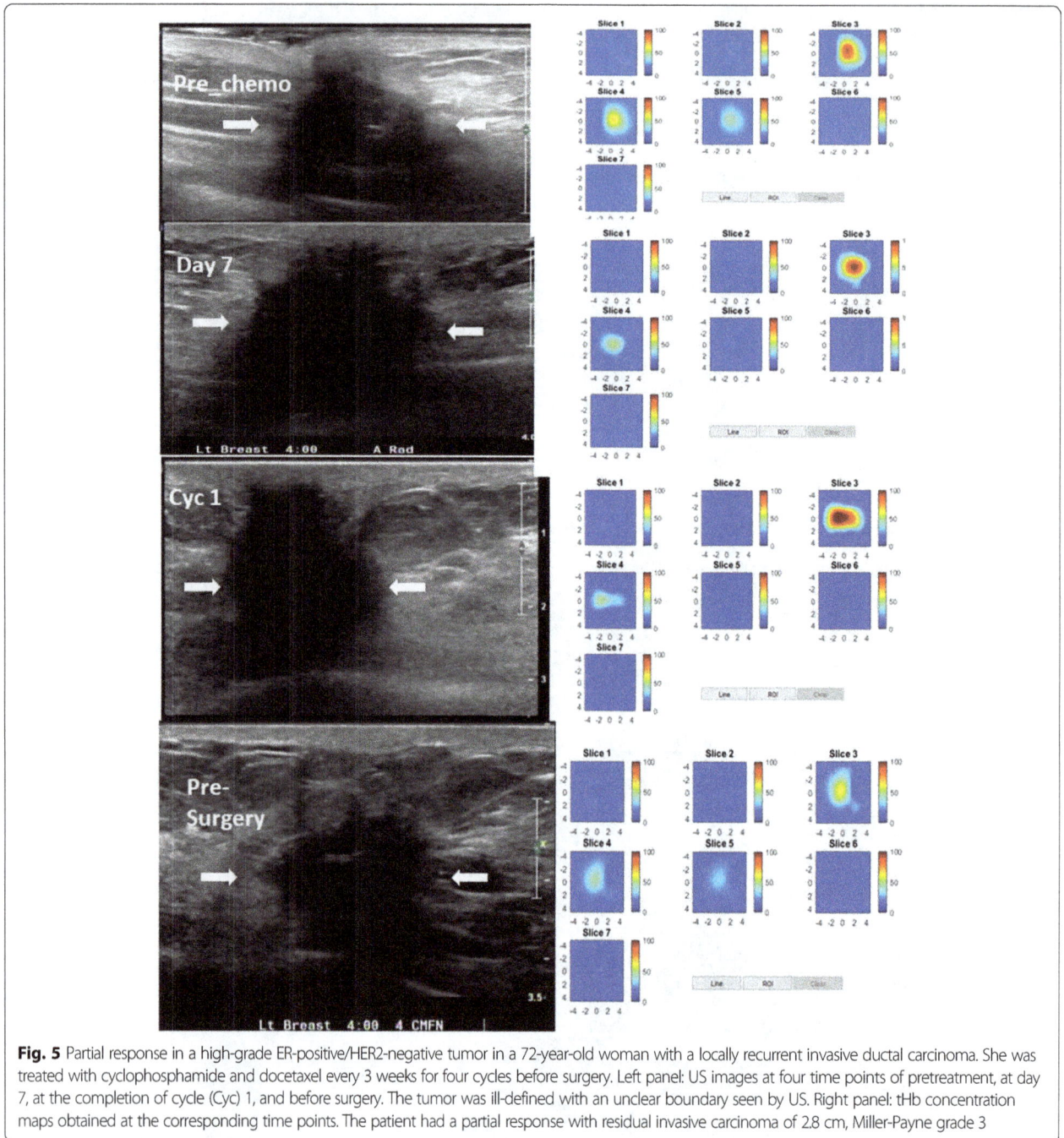

Fig. 5 Partial response in a high-grade ER-positive/HER2-negative tumor in a 72-year-old woman with a locally recurrent invasive ductal carcinoma. She was treated with cyclophosphamide and docetaxel every 3 weeks for four cycles before surgery. Left panel: US images at four time points of pretreatment, at day 7, at the completion of cycle (Cyc) 1, and before surgery. The tumor was ill-defined with an unclear boundary seen by US. Right panel: tHb concentration maps obtained at the corresponding time points. The patient had a partial response with residual invasive carcinoma of 2.8 cm, Miller-Payne grade 3

translate into higher testing AUCs, and higher AUCs of testing data are used to compare prediction models.

For HER2 group 1, HER2 used alone can achieve an AUC of 0.78 (95% CI 0.74–0.81). When HER2 and tHb are used together, the AUC reached 0.88 (95% CI 0.85–0.91). The addition of ER or NS essentially produces similar AUCs of 0.87 (95% CI 0.84–0.90) and 0.85 (0.82–0.88). However, the statistical significance of HER2 and tHb is higher than HER2, tHb, and ER ($P = 0.016$) and HER2, tHb, and NS ($P < 0.001$). This suggests that HER2 and tHb are the best pretreatment predictors regardless of ER or NS. The highest AUC of 0.96 (95% CI 0.95–0.98) is achieved when %tHb measured at the end of cycle 1 is added to HER2 and tHb. This was further modestly improved to 0.97 (95% CI 0.96–0.99) when %tHb measured at end of cycles 1 and 2 are used together with HER2 and tHb. Thus, the optimal time window with an accurate prediction of pathologic response in the HER2 subtype is at the end of cycle 2.

Table 4 Four groups of logistic regression models based on tumor subtype and hemoglobin parameters, AUC of training data, and AUC of testing data

Tumor subtypes	Training AUC (95% CI)	Testing AUC (95% CI)
Group 1 (HER2 subtype)		
Her2	0.71 (0.66–0.75)	0.78 (0.74–0.81)
Her2, tHb	0.88 (0.85–0.91)	0.88 (0.85–0.91)
Her2, tHb, ER	0.91 (0.89–0/94)	0.87 (0.84–0.90)
Her2, tHb, NS	0.91 (0.88–0.94)	0.85 (0.82–0.88)
Her2, tHb, %tHb_cyc1	0.89 (0.87–0.92)	**0.96 (0.95–0.98)**
Her2, tHb, %tHb_cyc2	0.89 (0.86–0.91)	0.94 (0.92–0.96)
Her2, tHb, %tHb_cyc3	0.96 (0.94–0/97)	0.89 (0.86–0.92)
Her2, tHb, %tHb_cyc1, %tHb_cyc2	0.90 (0.87–0.93)	**0.97 (0.96–0.99)**
Her2, tHb, %tHb_cyc1, %tHb_cyc3	0.96 (0.94–0.97)	0.88 (0.85–0.91)
Her2, tHb, %tHb_cyc2, %tHb_cyc3	0.96 (0.94–0.98)	0.88 (0.85–0.91)
Her2, tHb, %tHb_cyc1, %tHb_cyc2, %tHb_cyc3	0.96 (0.94–0.98)	0.88 (0.86–0.92)
Group 2 (ER subtype)		
ER	0.67 (0.63–0.72)	0.55 (0.50–0.59)
ER, tHb	0.81 (0.77–0.85)	0.69 (0.64–0.73)
ER, tHb, NS	0.83 (0.80–0.87)	0.69 (0.65–0.73)
ER, tHb, %tHb_cyc1	0.85 (0.82–0.89)	**0.91 (0.88–0.93)**
ER, tHb, %tHb_cyc2	0.86 (0.83–0.89)	0.79 (0.75–0.83)
ER, tHb, %tHb_cyc3	0.97 (0.95–0.98)	0.77 (0.73–0.81)
ER, tHb, %tHb_cyc1, %tHb_cyc2	0.88 (0.85–0.91)	0.86 (0.83–0.89)
ER, tHb, %tHb_cyc1, %tHb_cyc3	0.96 (0.95–0.98)	0.76 (0.73–0.80)
ER, tHb, %tHb_cyc2, %tHb_cyc3	0.97 (0.95–0.98)	0.77 (0.73–0.81)
Group 3 (TN subtype)		
TN	0.55 (0.51–0.56)	0.46 (0.41–0.50)
TN, tHb	0.77 (0.74–0.81)	0.72 (0.68–0.76)
TN, tHb, NS	0.81 (0.78–0.85)	0.69 (0.65–0.75)
TN, tHb, %tHb_cyc1	0.84 (0.81–0.87)	**0.90 (0.87–0.93)**
TN, tHb, %tHb_cyc2	0.85 (0.82–0.88)	0.84 (0.81–0.88)
TN, tHb, %tHb_cyc3	0.96 (0.94–0.98)	0.76 (0.72–0.80)
TN, tHb, %tHb_cyc1, %tHb_cyc2	0.85 (0.82–0.88)	0.90 (0.87–0.93)
TN, tHb, %tHb_cyc1, %tHb_cyc3	0.96 (0.94–0.98)	0.75 (0.71–0.79)
TN, tHb, %tHb_cyc2, %tHb_cyc3	0.96 (0.94–0.98)	0.75 (0.71–0.79)
Group 4 (tHb and %tHb, all patients)		
tHb	0.77 (0.73–0.81)	0.75 (0.71–0.79)
tHb, %tHb_cyc1	0.83 (0.80–0.87)	**0.95 (0.93–0.97)**
tHb, %tHb_cyc2	0.84 (0.80–0.86)	0.87 (0.84–0.90)
tHb, %tHb_cyc3	0.94 (0.92–0.97)	0.80 (0.76–0.84)
tHb, %tHb_cyc1, %tHb_cyc2	0.84 (0.81–0.88)	0.92 (0.90–0.95)
tHb, %tHb_cyc1, %tHb_cyc2, %tHb_cyc3	0.94 (0.92–0.96)	0.80 (0.76–0.84)
%tHb_cyc1	0.79 (0.75–0.83)	0.89 (0.86–0.92)
%tHb_cyc2	0.83 (0.80–0.86)	0.81 (0.78–0.85)
%tHb_cyc3	0.94 (0.92–0.96)	0.82 (0.78–0.85)
%tHb_cyc1, %tHb_cyc2	0.82 (0.78–0.87)	0.87 (0.83–0.90)

Table 4 Four groups of logistic regression models based on tumor subtype and hemoglobin parameters, AUC of training data, and AUC of testing data *(Continued)*

Tumor subtypes	Training AUC (95% CI)	Testing AUC (95% CI)
%tHb_cyc1, %tHb_cyc2, %tHb_cyc3	0.94 (0.92–0.96)	0.82 (0.79–0.86)

Bold entries indicate the best set of predictors in each group

AUC area under the curve, *CI* confidence interval, *ER* estrogen receptor, *HER2* human epidermal growth factor receptor 2, *NS* Nottingham score, *tHb* total hemoglobin, *TN* triple negative

For ER group 2, ER used alone can achieve an AUC of 0.55 (95% CI 0.50–0.59). ER and tHb achieve AUC of 0.69 (95% CI 0.64–0.73), and ER, tHb, and NS achieve AUC of 0.69 (95% CI 0.65–0.73). NS does not add any value to predicting the response of the ER patient group. The addition of %tHb measured at the end of cycle 1 improves the AUC of ER and tHb to 0.91 (95% CI 0.88–0.93). For TN group 3, TN used alone can achieve an AUC of 0.46 (95% CI 0.40–0.50). TN and tHb achieve an AUC of 0.72 (95% CI 0.68–0.76), and TN, tHb, and NS achieve an AUC of 0.69 (95% CI 0.65–0.75). NS does not add any value to predicting the response of the TN patient group. The addition of %tHb measured at cycle 1 improves the AUC to 0.90 (95% CI 0.87–0.93). For both ER and TN subtypes, %tHbs measured at the end of cycles 2 and 3 do not significantly improve prediction (Table 4). Thus, the optimal time window for assessing response in ER or TN subtypes is at the end of cycle 1.

For group 4, tHb used alone can achieve an AUC of 0.75 (95% CI 0.71–0.79), and %tHb cycle 1 used alone can achieve an AUC of 0.89 (95% CI 0.86–0.92). tHb and %tHb cycle 1 achieve an AUC of 0.95 (95% CI 0.93–0.97), which is significantly higher compared with the ER or TN subtype groups ($P < 0.001$). %tHbs measured at the end of cycles 2 and 3 do not significantly improve prediction (Table 4). Therefore, for ER and TN subtypes, tHb and %tHb are the best predictors and the early window for prediction is at the end of cycle 1.

The sensitivity, specificity, positive predictive value (PPV), and negative predictive values (NPV) of the best groups of predictors are shown in Table 5.

The %US ratio, the largest dimensions of post-treatment US measurements normalized to the pretreatment, of grade 1–3 and 4–5 tumors were calculated for 19 patients with well-defined US images. For grade 1–3 tumors ($n = 9$), %USs were 90.1 ± 9.8%, 84.9 ± 17.3%,

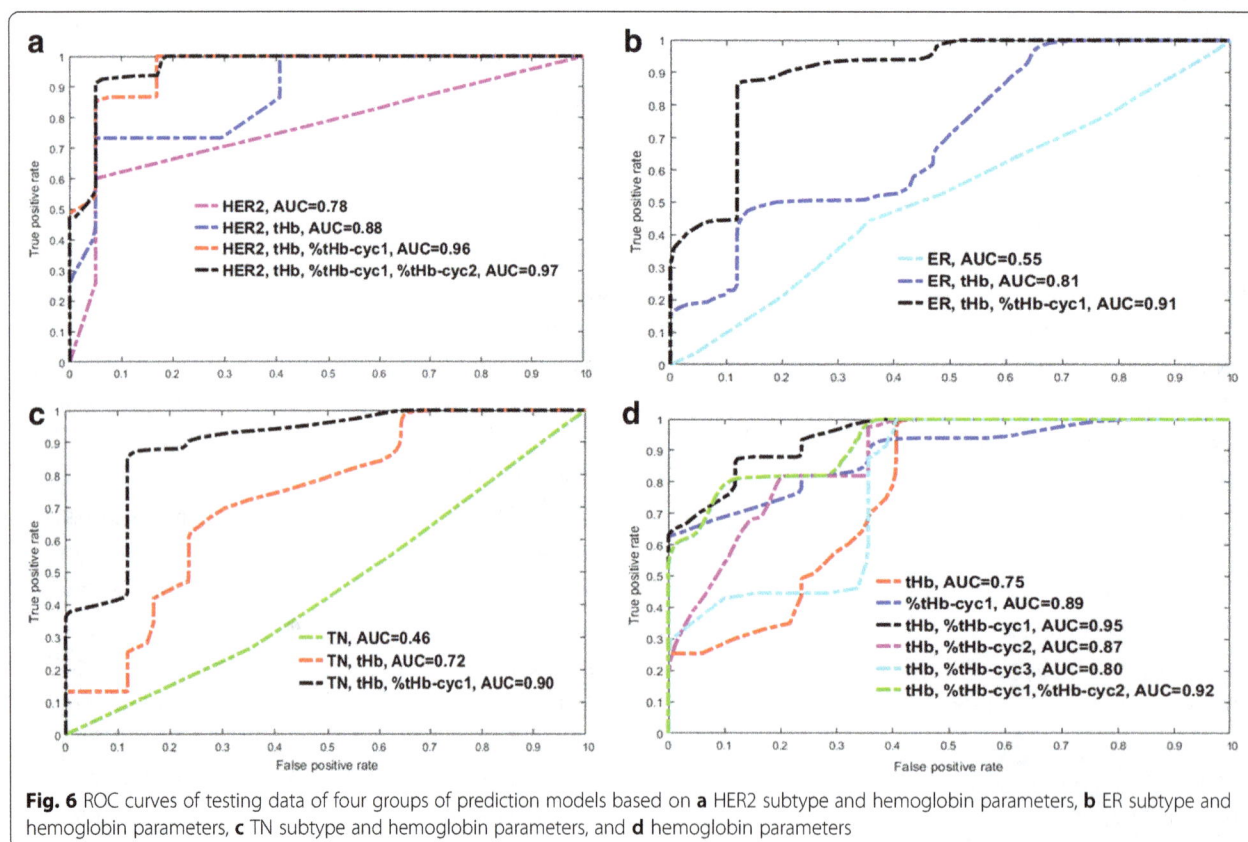

Fig. 6 ROC curves of testing data of four groups of prediction models based on **a** HER2 subtype and hemoglobin parameters, **b** ER subtype and hemoglobin parameters, **c** TN subtype and hemoglobin parameters, and **d** hemoglobin parameters

Table 5 Sensitivity, specificity, PPV, NPV, and AUC of the best set of predictors based on tumor subtype and hemoglobin parameters of the testing data

	Sensitivity	Specificity	PPV	NPV	AUC
Her2, tHb, %tHb_cyc1	73.7	94.9	92.4	84.8	0.96
Her, tHb, %tHb_cyc1, %tHb_cyc2	82.4	94.9	92.5	86.7	0.97
ER, tHb, %tHb_cyc1	81.8	88.1	85.8	85.1	0.90
TN, tHb, %tHb_cyc1	82.0	88.1	85.9	85.1	0.90
tHb, %tHb_cyc1	83.8	88.1	86.1	86.5	0.95

AUC area under the curve, *ER* estrogen receptor, *HER2* human epidermal growth factor receptor 2, *NPV* negative predictive value, *PPV* positive predictive value, *tHb* total hemoglobin, *TN* triple negative

and $77.0 \pm 20\%$ measured at end of cycles 1 to 3, respectively, whereas for grade 4–5 tumors ($n = 11$), %USs were $61.2 \pm 18.0\%$, $52.3 \pm 15.6\%$, and $42.8 \pm 13.7\%$, respectively. Statistical significance was achieved at all cycles ($P < 0.001$, $P < 0.001$, and $P = 0.001$, respectively).

Discussion

The clinical inclination to select patients for NAC who are more likely to be good responders accounts for the large number (11/22, 50%) of HER2$^+$ tumors in this study, especially with the ability to utilize dual HER2 blockade in this setting. In the HER2$^+$ group, there were Miller-Payne grade 4 and 5 responses in 91% despite the large number of cases that coexpressed ER. This apparent anomaly of HER2/ER coexpression is partially explained by the relatively low-level ER expression in two of the eight HER2$^+$/ER$^+$ cases. The remaining patients were either ER$^+$/HER2$^-$ or TN and had Miller-Payne 4 or 5 responses of 17% and 40%, respectively.

In our previous work, we dichotomized our comparison groups as pCR and near pCR (Miller-Payne grades 4–5) versus "other" (Miller-Payne grades 1–3). Our rationale for using these same comparison groups in this report is further supported as follows. In the original study by Ogston [36], the Miller-Payne 5 and 4 groups tended to track together with regard to 5-year disease-free survival after NAC and surgery (85% and 72%) versus 66%, 60%, and 55% for Miller-Payne 1–3, respectively. Later, Zhao et al. [42] while evaluating the Miller-Payne system using a different dataset found very similar 5-year distant disease-free survival and local recurrence-free survival rates for Miller-Payne 4–5 versus Miller-Payne 1–3. Finally, Symmans et al. [43] using the residual cancer burden (RCB) system and another separate dataset for evaluating tumor response after NAC also found that pCR and near-pCR had very similar survival curves after surgery (their categories RCB-0 and RCB-1 compared with RCB-2 (partial response) and RCB-3 (chemoresistant)).

In studies published to date, diffused optical tomography and diffused optical spectroscopy have demonstrated the potential for predicting breast cancer pathological response. Studies have shown that accurate predictions were made in the neoadjuvant setting by utilizing pretreatment hemoglobin levels or blood oxygen saturations (SO$_2$) [20, 21, 23, 31], or by monitoring early changes of hemoglobin content and SO$_2$ at 1 day or 1 week [19, 27], or after the first two cycles of NAC [20, 22, 23]. In this study, we have developed prediction models and have shown that the best pretreatment predictors are HER2 and tHb (AUC = 0.88). The pretreatment predictors based on ER and tHb, and TN and tHb predict response with moderate AUC accuracies of AUC 0.69 and 0.72, which are about the same as for the single predictor tHb (AUC = 0.75). For the HER2 subtype, the best window to accurately predict response is at the completion of the first two cycles of NAC. For ER or TN subtypes, the best window is at the completion of the first cycle of NAC and the best predictors are tHb and %tHb.

In our earlier study of 32 patients [21], the testing data obtained from cross-validations showed that the addition of the pretreatment tHb to pathological variables and biomarkers significantly improved the prediction (AUC 0.92 (95%CI 79.4–99.8)) compared with using these variables alone (AUC 0.84 (95% CI 57.2–99.0). The best pretreatment predictors of HER2, ER, and tHb reported in this study using the new cohort data as the testing set has achieved similar results of AUC 0.87 (95% CI 0.84–0.90).

NIR/US measurements obtained at the end of the first three treatment cycles were used for development and validation of the prediction models. Chemotherapy treatments are delivered generally in specific cycles. These schedules are based on maximal tumor cell kill and allowance of recovery of normal tissues (http://chemocare.com/chemotherapy/what-is-chemotherapy/cancer-cells-chemotherapy.aspx). Some cycles are given every 2 weeks and others every 3 weeks. Tumor responses by imaging studies occur after a specified number of treatment cycles, and not by specific times. Because treatments vary for HER2-positive disease compared with ER-positive or TN disease, the drugs utilized and schedules vary. The effects of the treatments are studied by equivalent treatment cycles. The goal was to give guideline-based treatments and to measure the maximal effect of each of these treatments before the next cycle is given. When combining all patients together, the measurements points were different in terms of weeks but not by cycles—they were consistent. The results show that pretreatment tHb and first cycle %tHb can achieve an accuracy of AUC 0.96 in the HER2 subtype, and AUCs of 0.91 in ER and 0.90 in TN subtypes, and AUC of 0.95 regardless of subtype. Thus, it is the ultimate effect of the drug on the tumor vascularity that is being assessed by near infrared functional parameters.

Baseline tHb measures tumor angiogenesis and correlates with tumor aggressiveness as evaluated by Spearman's rhos with Nottingham score (rho = 0.355, $P = 0.007$) in the combined training and testing data of 54 patients. Aggressive tumors have high proliferative rates and respond quickly to chemotherapy, as shown by PET/CT which detects pretreatment and early changes in tumor metabolic activity after one or two cycles of NAC [44] and predicts pCR. As expected from log cell-kill kinetics of cytotoxic drugs, a given dose kills a constant proportion of a tumor cell population rather than a constant number of cells (https://bajan.files.wordpress.com/2010/09/principles-of-cancer-chemotherapy.pdf). Therefore, for chemosensitive tumors, there are more total cells killed in the first cycle of treatment and more tumor neovasculature damage that may cause a significant decrease in tumor hemoglobin measured by the NIR system. For HER2+ responders, the cycle 1 %tHb is lower (mean %tHb = 77%) and more predictive than that of ER+/HER2− and TN responders (mean %tHb =84%) because trastuzumab has been demonstrated to have a strong antiangiogenic effect [45].

Our study has substantial implications for the combined use of tumor subtypes and NIR-measured tumor hemoglobin content in predicting pathological response even before therapy has begun. If a decision is made to initiate therapy, modification of the treatment can be implemented as soon as cycles 1 and 2 are completed, allowing for personalized treatment. This ability will be of even greater value as our armamentarium of interventions increases and responses can more effectively tailor the agents selected.

In this new cohort of patients, 86% of the tumors were visible on US compared with 65% in our earlier study [20]. This difference could be due to a greater representation of HER2-positive tumors in which US has been shown to be more accurate in measuring tumor size [46]. Pretreatment US does not predict response. However, %US of this cohort demonstrated statistical significance between responders and nonresponders at the early treatment cycles 1 to 3, while the earlier study group [20] showed no statistical significance at the end

of cycles 1 and 2 ($P = 0.437$ and $P = 0.172$) between these two responder groups. Significance was achieved at the end of cycle 3. Additionally, earlier data showed no correlation between %US measured at the end of cycles 1 to 3 and Miller-Payne grade (rho = 0.27, $P = 0.211$; rho = 0.25, $P = 0.257$; and rho = 0.36, $P = 0.106$), respectively. With more patient data, the %US measure will be assessed on its role in predicting response.

There are some limitations to this study. First, all patients were referred for NAC after core biopsy, and hence the baseline NIR/US imaging was performed after the initial biopsy. Bruise or hematoma due to prior biopsy could have some effect on pretreatment NIR measurements. However, 21 patients had the pretreatment NIR measurements more than 10 days and one patient 7 days after biopsy. Based on the literature, the pretreatment NIR measurements 1 week after core biopsy were not affected by the biopsy [47]. However, another study followed a patient before and after biopsy and showed a 10% increase in diffuse optical spectroscopy (DOS)-measured deoxygenated hemoglobin after 9 days following biopsy [48]. Our study patient who imaged 7 days following biopsy had a pCR of Miller-Payne grade 5, and her cycle 1 %tHb was 58%, or a reduction of 42%. This level of %tHb change is too large to be counted as a biopsy effect. Secondly, this new pool of 22 patients had 50% HER2+ tumors and were treated with the dual HER2 blockade regimen which was not available in the training data obtained from 2008 to 2011. We have randomly selected data from 6 out of 11 patients from this study and added these 6 patients' data to the training set to train the prediction models using all combinations. The testing data includes 73% from this study, with adequate samples of all subtypes. Thirdly, the training and testing datasets are still small and overfitting can occur when the training dataset is limited [21]. We have selected the minimal number of independent predictors for each prediction model, performed partial cross-validation, and used fairly high amounts (16/54, 30%) of the patient data for testing. The performances of the prediction models based on respective training and testing datasets are similar with no obvious pattern of higher AUC values for training data and much lower AUCs for testing data, which would be expected if there were problem of overfitting. With more patients recruited to the study, we will be able to establish a large database to validate prediction models with more input predictors.

The technical limitations of the US-guided NIR technique include the accuracy of the reconstructed optical absorption coefficients, the longitudinal repeatability of the measurements, and SO_2 estimation. For a large high-contrast phantom of 3–5 cm in size, about 60–70% reconstruction accuracy in target absorption can be achieved [38]. Because the average pretreatment tumor sizes of the two responder groups were similar, any under-reconstruction should affect the light quantification of both groups similarly. Therefore, the comparison of pretreatment and early treatment hemoglobin levels between the two responder groups should be minimally affected. Additionally, because the same sized ROI obtained from the pretreatment US of each patient is used for reconstructions at all subsequent treatment cycles for the same patient, under-reconstruction should have a minimal effect on the %tHb, which is normalized to the pretreatment level. The longitudinal repeatability of the reconstructed phantom absorption coefficient is about 5–10%, which is obtained by repeatedly imaging solid absorbers embedded in the same concentration of Intralipid over a 1- to 2-year period. This level of change is much smaller than the changes seen in patients who responded to treatments. Finally, SO_2 estimated from DOS has been reported as a good pretreatment predictor [31]. However, SO_2 distribution = oxyHb distribution/tHb distribution is not as robust as tHb, oxyHb, and deoxyHb when the tHb values reconstructed from tomography are lower in some voxels, especially when the tumor is large and distribution is heterogeneous.

Conclusions

In conclusion, our findings indicate that the breast tumor biomarkers (HER2, TN, and ER) combined with the pretreatment tumor total hemoglobin content are strong predictors of the response to NAC. The optimal treatment window to identify patients destined to have complete or near-complete responses is after the completion of the first two treatment cycles for HER2 tumors and the first treatment cycle for ER or TN tumors, when the assessment of total hemoglobin change is further predictive. This technology could be a valuable tool in personalizing treatments by response. These initial results remain to be validated with a larger trial of more patients.

Abbreviations

AUC: Area under the ROC curve; CI: Confidence interval; CT: Computed tomography; deoxyHb: Deoxygenated hemoglobin; DOS: Diffuse optical spectroscopy; ER: Estrogen receptor; FISH: Fluorescence in situ hybridization; HER2: Human epidermal growth factor receptor 2; MRI: Magnetic resonance imaging; NAC: Neoadjuvant chemotherapy; NIR: Near infrared; NPV: Negative predictive value; NS: Nottingham histologic score; oxyHb: Oxygenated hemoglobin; pCR: Pathological complete response; PET: Positron emission tomography; PPV: Positive predictive value; PR: Progesterone receptor; RCB: Residual cancer burden; ROC: Receiver operating characteristic; ROI: Region of interest; SO_2: Oxygen saturation; tHb: Total hemoglobin; TN: triple negative; US: Ultrasound

Acknowledgements

The authors thank the clinical trial office of Hartford Hospital for helping with patient consenting and scheduling. The authors appreciate the help of Jadwiga Jerman, MD, of Waterbury Hospital, and Ali Quratulain of UCONN Cancer Center for patient consenting and scheduling.

Funding

The authors thank the funding support of this work from the National Institute of Health (R01EB002136) and Connecticut Bioscience Innovation Fund (CBIF) Award #513.

Authors' contributions

QZ: designed and conducted all aspects of the ultrasound-guided tomography data acquisition, image reconstruction and data analysis, and contributed to the manuscript preparation and literature review. ST: recruited neoadjuvant chemotherapy patients at UConn Health Center, coordinated all aspects of the study at UCONN Health Center, and contributed to the manuscript preparation and literature review. SHK: coordinated all aspects of the clinical study at Waterbury Hospital and contributed to the manuscript preparation. PD: recruited neoadjuvant chemotherapy patients at Hartford Hospital and coordinated all aspects of the study at Hartford Hospital. AR: assessed and interpreted all histopathologic data of the breast tissue samples of patients recruited from Hartford Hospital and Waterbury Hospital, and contributed to the manuscript preparation and literature review. HV, FZ, and CX: contributed to the near-infrared system development, testing and calibration, and data acquisition. AM and MK: contributed to the US evaluations of the neoadjuvant chemotherapy patients and manuscript review. PH: assessed and interpreted all histopathologic data of the breast tissue samples of patients recruited from UConn Health Center and Waterbury Hospital. LW: contributed to the statistical analysis and manuscript preparation. KS: recruited neoadjuvant chemotherapy patients at Waterbury Hospital and coordinated oncological aspects of the study at Waterbury Hospital. All authors read and approved the final manuscript.

Competing interests

QZ is the inventor of patents related to ultrasound-guided near-infrared tomography technologies and patents owned by the University of Connecticut. The remaining authors declare that they have no competing interests.

Author details

[1]Biomedical Engineering and Radiology, Washington University in St Louis, One Brookings Drive, Mail Box 1097, Whitaker Hall 300D, St. Louis, MO 63130, USA. [2]University of Connecticut Health Center, Farmington, CT 06030, USA. [3]Waterbury Hospital, Waterbury, CT 6708, USA. [4]Hartford Hospital, Hartford, CT 06102, USA. [5]University of Connecticut, Storrs, CT 06269, USA. [6]New York City College of Technology, City University of New York (CUNY), New York, USA. [7]Department of Statistics, University of Manitoba, 186 Dysart Road, Winnipeg, Manitoba R3T 2N2, Canada.

References

1. Kaufmann M, von Minckwitz G, Mamounas EP, Cameron D, Carey LA, Cristofanilli M, Denkert C, Eiermann W, Gnant M, Harris JR, Karn T, Liedtke C, Mauri D, Rouzier R, Ruckhaeberle E, Semiglazov V, Symmans WF, Tutt A, Pusztai L. Recommendations from an international consensus conference on the current status and future of neoadjuvant systemic therapy in primary breast cancer. Ann Surg Oncol. 2012;19(5):1508–16.

2. Cortazar P, Geyer CE Jr. Pathological complete response in neoadjuvant treatment of breast cancer. Ann Surg Oncol. 2015;22(5):1441–6. https://doi.org/10.1245/s10434-015-4404-8.

3. Hennessy BT, Hortobagyi GN, Rouzier R, Kuerer H, Sneige N, Buzdar AU, Kau SW, Fornage B, Sahin A, Broglio K, Singletary SE, Valero V. Outcome after pathologic complete eradication of cytologically proven breast cancer axillary node metastases following primary chemotherapy. J Clin Oncol. 2005;23(36):9304–11.

4. Gianni L, Eiermann W, Semiglazov V, Manikhas A, Lluch A, Tjulandin S, Zambetti M, Vazquez F, Byakhow M, Lichinitser M, Climent MA, Ciruelos E, Ojeda B, Mansutti M, Bozhok A, Baronio R, Feyereislova A, Barton C, Valagussa P, Baselga J. Neoadjuvant chemotherapy with trastuzumab followed by adjuvant trastuzumab versus neoadjuvant chemotherapy alone, in patients with HER2-positive locally advanced breast cancer (the NOAH trial): a randomised controlled superiority trial with a parallel HER2-negative cohort. Lancet. 2010;375(9712):377–84. https://doi.org/10.1016/S0140-6736(09)61964-4.

5. von Minckwitz G, Blohmer JU, Costa SD, Denkert C, Eidtmann H, Eiermann W, Gerber B, Hanusch C, Hilfrich J, Huober J, Jackisch C, Kaufmann M, Kümmel S, Paepke S, Schneeweiss A, Untch M, Zahm DM, Mehta K, Loibl S. Response-guided neoadjuvant chemotherapy for breast cancer. J Clin Oncol. 2013;31(29):3623–30. https://doi.org/10.1200/JCO.2012.45.0940. Epub 2013 Sep 3

6. Wang J, Buchholz TA, Middleton LP, Allred DC, Tucker SL, Kuerer HM, Esteva FJ, Hortobagyi GN, Sahin AA. Assessment of histologic features and expression of biomarkers in predicting pathologic response to anthracycline-based neoadjuvant chemotherapy in patients with breast carcinoma. Cancer. 2002;94(12):3107–14.

7. Lips EH, Mulder L, de Ronde JJ, Mandjes IA, Koolen BB, Wessels LF, Rodenhuis S, Wesseling J. Breast cancer subtyping by immunohistochemistry and histological grade outperforms breast cancer intrinsic subtypes in predicting neoadjuvant chemotherapy response. Breast Cancer Res Treat. 2013;140(1):63–71. https://doi.org/10.1007/s10549-013-2620-0.

8. Liedtke C, Mazouni C, Hess KR, Andre F, Tordai A, Mejia JA, Symmans WF, Gonzalez-Angulo AM, Hennessy B, Green M, Cristofanilli M, Hortobagyi GN, Pusztai L. Response to neoadjuvant therapy and long-term survival in patients with triple-negative breast cancer. J Clin Oncol. 2008;26(8):1275–81. https://doi.org/10.1200/JCO.2007.14.4147.

9. von Minckwitz G, Untch M, Nuesch E, Loibl S, Kaufmann M, Kummel S, Fasching PA, Eiermann W, Blohmer JU, Costa SD, Mehta K, Hilfrich J, Jackisch C, Gerber B, du Bois A, Huober J, Hanusch C, Konecny G, Fett W, Stickeler E, Harbeck N, Muller V, Juni P. Impact of treatment characteristics on response of different breast cancer phenotypes: pooled analysis of the German neo-adjuvant chemotherapy trials. Breast Cancer Res Treat. 2011;125(1):145–56. https://doi.org/10.1007/s10549-010-1228-x.

10. Zardavas D, Piccart M. Neoadjuvant therapy for breast cancer. Annu Rev Med. 2015;66:31–48. https://doi.org/10.1146/annurev-med-051413-024741.

11. Cortazar P, Zhang L, Untch M, Mehta K, Costantino JP, Wolmark N, Bonnefoi H, Cameron D, Gianni L, Valagussa P, et al. Pathological complete response and long-term clinical benefit in breast cancer: the CTNeoBC pooled analysis. Lancet. 2014;384(9938):164–72. https://doi.org/10.1016/S0140-6736(13)62422-8.

12. Straver ME, Rutgers EJ, Rodenhuis S, Linn SC, Loo CE, Wesseling J, Russell NS, Oldenburg HS, Antonini N, Vrancken Peeters MT. The relevance of breast cancer subtypes in the outcome of neoadjuvant chemotherapy. Ann Surg Oncol. 2010;17(9):2411–8. https://doi.org/10.1245/s10434-010-1008-1.

13. Harry VN, Semple SI, Parkin DE, Gilbert FJ. Use of new imaging techniques to predict tumour response to therapy. Lancet Oncol. 2010;11(1):92–102.

14. Yeh E, Slanetz P, Kopans DB, Rafferty E, Georgian-Smith D, Moy L, Halpern E, Moore R, Kuter I, Taghian A. Prospective comparison of mammography, sonography, and MRI in patients undergoing neoadjuvant chemotherapy for palpable breast cancer. AJR Am J Roentgenol. 2005;184(3):868–77.

15. Humbert O, Riedinger JM, Vrigneaud JM, Kanoun S, Dygai-Cochet I, Berriolo-Riedinger A, Toubeau M, Depardon E, Lassere M, Tisserand S, Fumoleau P, Brunotte F, Cochet A. 18F-FDG PET-derived tumor blood flow changes after 1 cycle of neoadjuvant chemotherapy predicts outcome in triple-negative breast cancer. J Nucl Med. 2016;57(11):1707–12.

16. Avril S, Muzic RF Jr, Plecha D, Traughber BJ, Vinayak S, Avril N. 18F-FDG PET/CT for monitoring of treatment response in breast cancer. J Nucl Med. 2016;57(Suppl 1):34S–9S. https://doi.org/10.2967/jnumed.115.157875. Review

17. Loo CE, Straver ME, Rodenhuis S, Muller SH, Wesseling J, Vrancken Peeters MJ, Gilhuijs KG. Magnetic resonance imaging response monitoring of breast cancer during neoadjuvant chemotherapy: relevance of breast cancer subtype. J Clin Oncol. 2011;29(6):660–6. https://doi.org/10.1200/JCO.2010.31.1258. Epub 2011 Jan 10

18. Tromberg BJ, Zhang Z, Leproux A, O'Sullivan TD, Cerussi AE, Carpenter PM, Mehta RS, Roblyer D, Yang W, Paulsen KD, Pogue BW, Jiang S, Kaufman PA, Yodh AG, Chung SH, Schnall M, Snyder BS, Hylton N, Boas DA, Carp SA, Isakoff SJ, Mankoff D. ACRIN 6691 investigators. predicting responses to neoadjuvant chemotherapy in breast cancer: ACRIN 6691 trial of diffuse optical spectroscopic imaging. Cancer Res. 2016;76(20):5933–44. Epub 2016 Aug 15.

19. Tran WT, Childs C, Chin L, Slodkowska E, Sannachi L, Tadayyon H, Watkins E, Wong SL, Curpen B, El Kaffas A, Al-Mahrouki A, Sadeghi-Naini A, Czarnota GJ. Multiparametric monitoring of chemotherapy treatment response in locally advanced breast cancer using quantitative ultrasound and diffuse optical spectroscopy. Oncotarget. 2016;7(15):19762–80. https://doi.org/10.18632/oncotarget.7844.

20. Zhu Q, DeFusco PA, Ricci A Jr, Cronin EB, Hegde PU, Kane M, Tavakoli B, Xu Y, Hart J, Tannenbaum SH. Breast cancer: assessing response to neoadjuvant chemotherapy by using US-guided near-infrared tomography. Radiology. 2013;266(2):433–42. https://doi.org/10.1148/radiol.12112415. Epub 2012 Dec 21

21. Zhu Q, Wang L, Tannenbaum S, Ricci A Jr, DeFusco P, Hegde P. Pathologic response prediction to neoadjuvant chemotherapy utilizing pretreatment near-infrared imaging parameters and tumor pathologic criteria. Breast Cancer Res. 2014;16(5):456. https://doi.org/10.1186/s13058-014-0456-0.

22. Ueda S, Yoshizawa N, Shigekawa T, Takeuchi H, Ogura H, Osaki A, Saeki T, Ueda Y, Yamane T, Kuji I, Sakahara H. Near-infrared diffuse optical imaging for early prediction of breast cancer response to neoadjuvant chemotherapy: a comparative study using 18F-FDG PET/CT. J Nucl Med. 2016;57(8):1189–95. https://doi.org/10.2967/jnumed.115.167320. Epub 2016 Mar 3

23. Jiang S, Pogue BW, Kaufman PA, Gui J, Jermyn M, Frazee TE, Poplack SP, DiFlorio-Alexander R, Wells WA, Paulsen KD. Predicting breast tumor response to neoadjuvant chemotherapy with diffuse optical spectroscopic tomography prior to treatment. Clin Cancer Res. 2014;20(23):6006–15. https://doi.org/10.1158/1078-0432.CCR-14-1415. Epub 2014 Oct 7

24. Xu C, Vavadi H, Merkulov A, Li H, Erfanzadeh M, Mostafa A, Gong Y, Salehi H, Tannenbaum S, Zhu Q. Ultrasound-guided diffuse optical tomography for predicting and monitoring neoadjuvant chemotherapy of breast cancers: recent progress. Ultrason Imaging. 2016;38(1):5–18. https://doi.org/10.1177/0161734615580280. Epub 2015 Apr 16

25. Sajjadi AY, Isakoff SJ, Deng B, Singh B, Wanyo CM, Fang Q, Specht MC, Schapira L, Moy B, Bardia A, Boas DA, Carp SA. Normalization of compression-induced hemodynamics in patients responding to neoadjuvant chemotherapy monitored by dynamic tomographic optical breast imaging (DTOBI). Biomed Opt Express. 2017;8(2):555–69. https://doi.org/10.1364/BOE.8.000555. eCollection 2017 Jan 4.

26. Busch DR, Choe R, Rosen MA, Guo W, Durduran T, Feldman MD, Mies C, Czerniecki BJ, Tchou J, Demichele A, Schnall MD, Yodh AG. Optical malignancy parameters for monitoring progression of breast cancer neoadjuvant chemotherapy. Biomed Opt Express. 2013;4(1):105–21. https://doi.org/10.1364/BOE.4.000105. Epub 2012 Dec 14

27. Roblyer D, Ueda S, Cerussi A, Tanamai W, Durkin A, Mehta R, Hsiang D, Butler JA, McLaren C, Chen WP, Tromberg B. Optical imaging of breast cancer oxyhemoglobin flare correlates with neoadjuvant chemotherapy response one day after starting treatment. Proc Natl Acad Sci USA. 2011;108:14626–31.

28. Enfield LC, Gibson AP, Hebden JC, Douek M. Optical tomography of breast cancer-monitoring response to primary medical therapy. Target Oncol. 2009;4(3):219–33. https://doi.org/10.1007/s11523-009-0115-z. Epub 2009 Sep.

29. Zhu Q, Tannenbaum S, Hegde P, Kane M, Xu C, Kurtzman SH. Noninvasive monitoring of breast cancer during neoadjuvant chemotherapy using optical tomography with ultrasound localization. Neoplasia. 2008;10(10):1028–40.

30. Cerussi A, Hsiang D, Shah N, Mehta R, Durkin A, Butler J, Tromberg BJ. Predicting response to breast cancer neoadjuvant chemotherapy using diffuse optical spectroscopy. Proc Natl Acad Sci U S A. 2007;104(10):4014–9. Epub 2007 Feb 28

31. Ueda S, Roblyer D, Cerussi A, Durkin A, Leproux A, Santoro Y, Xu S, O'Sullivan TD, Hsiang D, Mehta R, Butler J, Tromberg BJ. Baseline tumor oxygen saturation correlates with a pathologic complete response in breast cancer patients undergoing neoadjuvant chemotherapy. Cancer Res. 2012;72(17):4318–28. https://doi.org/10.1158/0008-5472.CAN-12-0056. Epub 2012 Jul 9

32. Zhu Q, Ricci A Jr, Hegde P, Kane M, Cronin E, Merkulov A, Xu Y, Tavakoli B, Tannenbaum S. Assessment of functional differences in malignant and benign breast lesions and improvement of diagnostic accuracy by using US-guided diffuse optical tomography in conjunction with conventional US. Radiology. 2016;280(2):387–97. https://doi.org/10.1148/radiol.2016151097. Epub 2016 Mar 2

33. Zhu Q, Hegde PU, Ricci A Jr, Kane M, Cronin EB, Ardeshirpour Y, Xu C, Aguirre A, Kurtzman SH, Deckers PJ, Tannenbaum SH. Early-stage invasive breast cancers: potential role of optical tomography with US localization in assisting diagnosis. Radiology. 2010;256(2):367–78. https://doi.org/10.1148/radiol.10091237. Epub 2010 Jun 22

34. Harvey JM, Clark GM, Osborne CK, Allred DC. Estrogen receptor status by immunohistochemistry is superior to the ligand-binding assay for predicting response to adjuvant endocrine therapy in breast cancer. J Clin Oncol. 1999; 17(5):1474–81.

35. Wolff AC, Hammond ME, Hicks DG, Dowsett M, LM MS, Allison KH, Allred DC, Bartlett JM, Bilous M, Fitzgibbons P, Hanna W, Jenkins RB, Mangu PB, Paik S, Perez EA, Press MF, Spears PA, Vance GH, Viale G, Hayes DF. Recommendations for human epidermal growth factor receptor 2 testing in breast cancer: American Society of Clinical Oncology/College of American Pathologists clinical practice guideline update. Am Soc Clin Oncol. 2014; 138(2):241–56. https://doi.org/10.5858/arpa.2013-0953-SA. Epub 2013 Oct 7

36. Ogston KN, Miller ID, Payne S, et al. A new histologic grading system to assess response of breast cancers to primary chemotherapy; prognostic significance and survival. Breast. 2003;12:320–7.

37. Zhu Q, Chen N, Kurtzman SH. Imaging tumor angiogenesis by use of combined near-infrared diffusive light and ultrasound. Opt Lett. 2003;28(5):337–9.

38. Zhu Q, Xu C, Guo P, Aguirre A, Yuan B, Huang F, Castilo D, Gamelin J, Tannenbaum S, Kane M, Hegde P, Kurtzman S. Optimal probing of optical contrast of breast lesions of different size located at different depths by US localization. Technol Cancer Res Treat. 2006;5(4):365–80.

39. Kleinbaum D, Kupper L, Muller K, Nizam A. Applied regression analysis and other multivariable methods. 3rd ed. Belmont: Duxbury Press; 1998.

40. Agresti A. Categorical data analysis. 2nd ed: Wiley; (Section 5.3.2). Somerset, NJ, USA: Wiley; 2002.

41. Pindyck RS, Rubinfeld DL. Econometric models and economic forecasts. 4th ed. (Section 5.2). 2 Pennsylvania Plaza, NY, USA: Irwin/McGraw-Hill; 1998.

42. Zhao Y, Dong X, Li R, Ma X, Song J, Li Y, Zhan D. Evaluation of the pathological response and prognosis following neoadjuvant chemotherapy in molecular subtypes of breast cancer. Onco Targets Ther. 2015;8:1511–21.

43. Symmans WF, Peintinger F, Hatzis C, et al. Measurement of residual breast cancer burden to predict survival after neoadjuvant chemotherapy. J Clin Oncol. 2007;25:4414–22.

44. Humbert O, Lasserre M, Bertaut A, Fumoleau P, Coutant C, Brunotte F, Cochet A. Pattern of breast cancer blood flow and metabolism assessed using dual-acquisition 18FDGPET: correlation with tumor phenotypic features and pathological response to neoadjuvant chemotherapy. J Nucl Med. 2018; https://doi.org/10.2967/jnumed.117.203075. Epub ahead of print

45. Isumin Y, Xu L, di Tomaso E, Fukumura D, Jain RK. Tumor biology: herceptin acts as an anti-angiogenic cocktail. Nature. 2002;416:279–80.

46. Tanamai W, Chen C, Siavoshi S, Cerussi A, Hsiang D, Butler J, Tromberg B. Diffuse optical spectroscopy measurements of healing in breast tissue after core biopsy: case study. J Biomed Opt. 2009;14(1):014024.

47. Stein RG, Wollschläger D, Kreienberg R, Janni W, Wischnewsky M, Diessner J, Stüber T, Bartmann C, Krockenberger M, Wischhusen J, Wöckel A, Blettner M, Schwentner L, BRENDA Study Group. The impact of breast cancer biological subtyping on tumor size assessment by ultrasound and mammography—a retrospective multicenter cohort study of 6543 primary breast cancer patients. BMC Cancer. 2016;16:459. https://doi.org/10.1186/s12885-016-2426-7.

48. Choe R, Konecky SD, Corlu A, Lee K, Durduran T, Busch DR, Pathak S, Czerniecki BJ, Tchou J, Fraker DL, Demichele A, Chance B, Arridge SR, Schweiger M, Culver JP, Schnall MD, Putt ME, Rosen MA, Yodh AG. Differentiation of benign and malignant breast tumors by in-vivo three-dimensional parallel-plate diffuse optical tomography. J Biomed Opt. 2009; 14(2):024020.

15

A phase II clinical trial of the Aurora and angiogenic kinase inhibitor ENMD-2076 for previously treated, advanced, or metastatic triple-negative breast cancer

Jennifer R. Diamond[1,4]* (iD), S. G. Eckhardt[2], Todd M. Pitts[1], Adrie van Bokhoven[1], Dara Aisner[1], Daniel L. Gustafson[1], Anna Capasso[2], Sharon Sams[1], Peter Kabos[1], Kathryn Zolman[1], Tiffany Colvin[1], Anthony D. Elias[1], Anna M. Storniolo[3], Bryan P. Schneider[3], Dexiang Gao[1], John J. Tentler[1], Virginia F. Borges[1] and Kathy D. Miller[3]

Abstract

Background: Triple-negative breast cancer (TNBC) remains an aggressive breast cancer subtype with limited treatment options. ENMD-2076 is a small-molecule inhibitor of Aurora and angiogenic kinases with proapoptotic and antiproliferative activity in preclinical models of TNBC.

Methods: This dual-institution, single-arm, two-stage, phase II clinical trial enrolled patients with locally advanced or metastatic TNBC previously treated with one to three prior lines of chemotherapy in the advanced setting. Patients were treated with ENMD-2076 250 mg orally once daily with continuous dosing in 4-week cycles until disease progression or unacceptable toxicity occurred. The primary endpoint was 6-month clinical benefit rate (CBR), and secondary endpoints included progression-free survival, pharmacokinetic profile, safety, and biologic correlates in archival and fresh serial tumor biopsies in a subset of patients.

Results: Forty-one patients were enrolled. The 6-month CBR was 16.7% (95% CI, 6–32.8%) and included two partial responses. The 4-month CBR was 27.8% (95% CI, 14–45.2%), and the average duration of benefit was 6.5 cycles. Common adverse events included hypertension, fatigue, diarrhea, and nausea. Treatment with ENMD-2076 resulted in a decrease in cellular proliferation and microvessel density and an increase in p53 and p73 expression, consistent with preclinical observations.

Conclusions: Single-agent ENMD-2076 treatment resulted in partial response or clinical benefit lasting more than 6 months in 16.7% of patients with pretreated, advanced, or metastatic TNBC. These results support the development of predictive biomarkers using archival and fresh tumor tissue, as well as consideration of mechanism-based combination strategies.

Keywords: Breast cancer, ENMD-2076, Aurora kinase inhibitor, Triple negative

* Correspondence: jennifer.diamond@ucdenver.edu
[1]University of Colorado Cancer Center, Aurora, CO, USA
[4]Division of Medical Oncology, University of Colorado Anschutz Medical Campus, University of Colorado Cancer Center, 12801 East 17th Avenue, Mailstop 8117, Aurora, CO 80045, USA
Full list of author information is available at the end of the article

Background

Triple-negative breast cancer (TNBC) is an aggressive breast cancer subtype defined by a lack of expression of the estrogen receptor (ER), progesterone receptor, and human epidermal growth factor receptor 2 (HER2) [1]. TNBC accounts for 10–15% of all newly diagnosed breast cancer and is associated with an increased risk of distant metastasis and death compared with other breast cancer subtypes [1–3]. The median duration of first-line therapy for metastatic TNBC is approximately 12 weeks, and the median survival for patients with metastatic disease is 10–13 months [2, 4]. Despite the characterization of biologic subtypes within TNBC, this disease remains critically in need of effective targeted systemic therapies [5].

ENMD-2076 is an orally bioavailable small-molecule inhibitor of angiogenic and mitotic kinases. The antiangiogenic activity of ENMD-2076 is mediated through the inhibition of vascular endothelial growth factor receptors (VEGFRs) and fibroblast growth factor receptors (FGFRs), whereas antiproliferative activity occurs via inhibition of mitotic kinases, including Aurora kinase A (Aur A) [6]. ENMD-2076 is active against preclinical TNBC models, including p53-mutated cancer cell lines and patient-derived tumor xenograft (PDX) models [7, 8]. The purpose of this study was to evaluate the anticancer activity of ENMD-2076 in patients with previously treated locally advanced or metastatic TNBC, to further characterize the side effect profile, and to explore pharmacodynamic changes in serial tumor biopsies.

Methods

Study design

This phase II clinical trial was a dual-institution, single-arm, Simon two-stage study of single-agent ENMD-2076 administered orally once daily with continuous dosing (ClinicalTrials.gov identifier NCT01639248). The primary objective of the study was to determine the 6-month clinical benefit rate (CBR), defined as patients with complete response, partial response (PR), or stable disease (SD) lasting for ≥ 24 weeks based on Response Evaluation Criteria in Solid Tumors (RECIST version 1.1) [9]. Secondary objectives included progression-free survival (PFS), objective response rate, safety, and pharmacokinetics (PK). Exploratory objectives included evaluation of p53 mutation status on archival tumor tissue and pharmacodynamic effects of ENMD-2076 in serial tumor tissue samples obtained in a subset of patients. This protocol was approved by the institutional review boards of both institutions, and informed consent was obtained from all patients prior to performing study-related procedures in accordance with federal and institutional guidelines.

Eligibility criteria

Eligible patients had locally advanced or metastatic TNBC previously treated with one to three prior lines of chemotherapy in the advanced setting. For the purpose of this study, locally advanced breast cancer was defined as unresectable local or regional disease. TNBC was defined as negative for estrogen and progesterone receptor by local pathology report, Allred score ≤ 2, or < 5% weak positive staining. Negative HER2 testing was defined as IHC score 0 or 1+ or fluorescence in situ hybridization ratio < 2.0. Patients were required to have measurable disease by RECIST 1.1 [9], Eastern Cooperative Oncology Group (ECOG) Performance Status of 0–1, and archival tumor tissue available for analysis. Patients also had to be aged 18 years or older and to have adequate hematopoietic, hepatic, and kidney function, defined as hemoglobin ≥ 9 g/dl, absolute neutrophil count ≥ 1500/μl, platelets ≥ 100,000/μl, total bilirubin < 1.5 times the institutional upper limit of normal (ULN), aspartate aminotransferase/alanine aminotransferase and ≤ 2.5 times the ULN or < 5 times the ULN if hepatic metastases were present, and creatinine ≤ 1.5 times the ULN. Brain magnetic resonance imaging (MRI) was required to exclude brain metastasis. For patients undergoing the optional serial tumor biopsies, prothrombin time and activated partial thromboplastin time were required to be within the normal range. Patients were recovered from the expected toxicity of prior treatments and did not require therapeutic doses of any anticoagulant or have any significant cardiac problems.

Pretreatment evaluation

Prior to the initiation of study treatment, all patients underwent clinical history and physical examination, ECOG Performance Status assessment, vital signs, complete blood count, chemistries, urinalysis, serum pregnancy test (if applicable), coagulation parameters (for patients undergoing tumor biopsies), echocardiogram or multigated acquisition, and baseline tumor assessment with imaging. Archival tissue was submitted for correlative analysis for all enrolled patients. Additionally, serial tumor biopsies were performed for correlative analysis in a subset of patients, with the first occurring before the initiation of study treatment.

Treatment and dose modifications

Patients were treated with ENMD-2076 250 mg oral once daily with continuous dosing in 4-week cycles until disease progression or unacceptable toxicity occurred. The dose of study drug was selected on the basis of tolerability of ENMD-2076 in a phase II clinical trial in patients with recurrent, platinum-resistant ovarian cancer where the initial ENMD-2076 dose was 325 mg oral once daily for patients with a body surface area (BSA) ≥ 1.65 m² and 275 mg/d for patients with a BSA ≤ 1.64 m² [10]. Due to higher-than-expected rates of treatment-related toxicity resulting in dose delays in that study, the starting dose was reduced to 275 mg/d and 250 mg/d for the two BSA groups, respectively. Taking into account this tolerability data for ENMD-2076 administered on a once-daily continuous dosing schedule, a flat dose of 250 mg/d was selected as the starting dose for this study.

Restaging was performed every two cycles (8 weeks) according to RECIST 1.1. Blood pressure was monitored weekly during the first cycle, every 2 weeks during cycle 2, and every 4 weeks during cycles 3 and beyond. Complete blood count and chemistries were performed every 2 weeks during cycles 1 and 2, then every 4 weeks. Urinalysis was performed every 4 weeks, and if 2+ proteinuria was observed, a spot urine protein/creatinine ratio was calculated and a 24-hour urine sample was collected for quantification of protein. Patients were allowed to continue treatment if the spot urine/protein ratio was ≤ 1 and the 24-hour urine showed ≤ 3.5 g protein/24 h. If the 24-hour urine protein was > 3.5 g, treatment was withheld until a repeat study was ≤ 3.5 g protein/24 h. Thyroid-stimulating hormone was tested on cycle 3, day 1 and subsequently as clinically indicated.

Dosing delays of up to 2 weeks were permitted to allow for recovery from treatment-related toxicities or other intercurrent illness. Longer delays were also allowed in patients experiencing clinical benefit from ENMD-2076 treatment. Two dose reductions were allowed for treatment-related toxicity (dose − 1 was 225 mg/d and dose − 2 was 150 mg/d). The protocol did not dictate specific management strategies for ENMD-2076-related treatment toxicities, including hypertension. The treatment management strategy was at the discretion of the treating physician.

Pharmacokinetic sampling and assay
Blood samples were collected in sodium heparin tubes prior to the first dose on cycle 1, day 1 and then 4 hours following dosing. Samples were obtained prior to dosing on cycle 2, day 1 and on the day of tumor biopsy. Plasma concentrations of ENMD-2076 and its active metabolite, ENMD-2060, were determined using a validated LC-MS/MS method. The lower limits of quantification were 2.5 ng/ml for ENMD-2076 and 1 ng/ml for ENMD-2060.

Correlative studies using archival tumor tissue and serial tumor biopsies
Archival tumor tissue was requested from all eligible patients and subject to evaluation for p53 mutation and IHC expression. If multiple samples were available, the most recent tumor tissue was selected for testing unless it was quantitatively insufficient. Microdissection was performed using a stereotactic microscope with

hematoxylin-stained slides, and DNA was isolated for sequencing of *TP53* exons 5–8 and 10. Briefly, following microdissection, samples were purified using the QIAamp DSP FFPE Tissue Kit (Qiagen, Valencia, CA, USA). Exons 5–8 and 10 were PCR-amplified followed by Sanger sequencing using the Applied Biosystems BigDye system (Life Technologies, Carlsbad, CA, USA), and capillary electrophoresis was performed on an ABI 3500xL instrument (Applied Biosystems/Thermo Fisher Scientific, Foster City, CA, USA). Sequence analysis was performed using MutationSurveyor software (SoftGenetics, State College, PA, USA). *TP53* alterations were assessed for pathogenicity by first determining whether they represented population polymorphisms using the Exome Aggregation Consortium database (exac.broadinstitute.org). Any alteration with a population minor allele frequency > 1% was excluded from further analysis. All remaining identified alterations were examined for pathogenicity on the basis of classification by the International Agency for Research on Cancer TP53 Database (p53.iarc.fr), and all alterations classified as "deleterious" by this database were considered mutations for the purposes of subsequent analysis.

Serial tumor biopsies were performed in a subset of patients during the first cycle prior to day 1 and at days 14–16. An additional biopsy was obtained at the time of progression in patients responding to treatment. Formalin-fixed, paraffin-embedded samples were analyzed by IHC for Ki-67 (30-9; Ventana Medical Systems, Inc., Tucson, AZ, USA), cleaved caspase 3 (Cell Signaling Technology, Danvers, MA, USA), p53 (Cell Marque, Rocklin, CA, USA), and CD34 (Abcam, Cambridge, MA, USA). Following antigen retrieval and primary antibody incubation, IHC stains were visualized with the UltraView Universal DAB Detection Kit (Ki-67 and p53; Ventana Medical Systems, Inc.) or ImmPRESS HRP Antirabbit IgG (CD34 and cleaved caspase 3; Vector Laboratories, Burlingame, CA, USA). IHC for Ki-67 was scored as follows: low proliferative index ≤ 15% positive cells, intermediate 16–30%, and high > 30%. IHC for p53 was scored as low ≤ 15% positive cells, intermediate 16–30%, and high > 30%. The average number of vessels from three × 20 magnification fields was used as the microvessel density (MVD) score. The cleaved caspase 3 score was determined by evaluating the percentage of stained tumor cells.

Immunofluorescence (IF) was performed in a subset of biopsy samples for 4′,6-diamidino-2-phenylindole (DAPI), p53, p73, and BAX as previously described [8]. In brief, samples were freshly collected, placed into individual cryomolds (Sakura Finetek, Torrance, CA, USA) and embedded in Tissue-Tek optimum cutting compound (Sakura Finetek). Cryomold blocks were frozen in liquid nitrogen and individually cut into 5-μm-thick sections by the University of Colorado Cancer Center Tissue Biobanking and Histology Shared Resource. Slides were fixed in a 1:1 ratio in a solution of methanol and acetone at − 20 °C for 10 minutes, blocked, and incubated with primary antibodies (p53, Cell Signaling Technology; p73, Abcam). Slides were washed three times in 1 × PBS and incubated with secondary antibodies (Alexa Fluor 555 or Alexa Fluor 488; Life Technologies) and counterstained with 300 nM DAPI. Slides were mounted, and images were acquired using the FLUOVIEW FV1000 confocal microscope (Olympus America, Center Valley, PA, USA) at × 60 magnification.

Statistical methods

The primary endpoint of the study was the 6-month CBR, defined as the sum of patients who experienced complete response, PR, and/or stable disease (SD) for ≥ 24 weeks by RECIST version 1.1. The sample size was determined using a null hypothesis of 10% [11, 12] and an alternate hypothesis of interest to continue single-agent studies in the patient population of 30%. The sample size of 35 yielded a power of 90% to detect this difference with an alpha of 0.05 (one--sided). Patients were considered evaluable for the primary endpoint if they received at least one cycle of therapy and underwent repeat disease assessment. Patients who came off study during the first cycle for toxicity or patient preference without disease progression were not considered evaluable for the primary endpoint. This study used a two-stage study design. The interim analysis (stage 1) was performed after enrollment of 18 patients. If 2 or fewer of the first 18 patients experienced a "success", then it would be concluded that the treatment does not have sufficient activity for further investigation, and accrual would be terminated. If 3 or more of these 18 patients experienced a "success," enrollment would continue to 17 additional evaluable patients.

Descriptive statistics were used for PK and toxicity parameters. Fisher's exact test was used to assess the correlation between p53 mutation and response to treatment.

Results
Patients

Between July 2012 and October 2016, 65 patients were consented, and 41 patients were enrolled at the University of Colorado Cancer Center (Aurora, CO, USA) and the Indiana University Melvin and Bren Simon Cancer Center (Indianapolis, IN, USA). This included 18 patients enrolled in stage 1 and 23 patients in stage 2 (Fig. 1). A total of 24 patients were consented and excluded prior to starting treatment, most commonly for not meeting the eligibility criteria owing to asymptomatic brain metastasis detected on required screening brain MRI or abnormal liver function tests.

The median age of patients was 54 years (range, 30–73 years); 40 were female, and 1 was male. Patients received, on average, 1.7 prior lines of chemotherapy for locally advanced unresectable or metastatic disease, and 80.5% underwent prior neoadjuvant or adjuvant chemotherapy for localized disease. In addition, 48.8% of patients received prior systemic targeted anticancer therapies, and 85.4% received prior radiation therapy. ECOG Performance Status was 1 in 53.7% of patients and 0 in 46.3% of patients. BRCA1/2 germline mutation status was collected if known; 9.8% had known

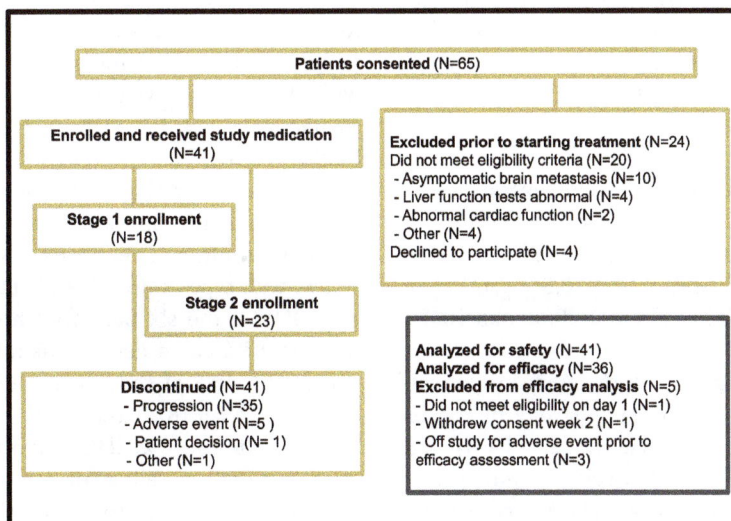

Fig. 1 Trial profile and study design

deleterious mutations, 46.3% were known wild type, and status was unknown in 43.9% of patients. Additional baseline patient characteristics and demographics can be found in Table 1.

Efficacy

Thirty-six patients were evaluable per protocol for the primary efficacy analysis. Five patients (12.2%) were not included in the efficacy analysis owing to adverse events leading to discontinuation prior to objective efficacy assessment ($n = 3$), not meeting eligibility criteria on day 1 ($n = 1$), and withdrawal of consent in cycle 1 ($n = 1$) (Fig. 1). The study proceeded to the second stage of enrollment based on observing three 6-month CBR events in stage 1 ($n = 18$ patients). The 6-month CBR in the overall trial was 16.7% (exact 95% CI, 6–32.8%), and the 4-month CBR was 27.8% (exact 95% CI, 14–45.2%) (Table 2). Two patients achieved partial response to treatment, and no complete responses were observed. The average duration of response for patients achieving clinical benefit for 4 months was 6.5 cycles ($n = 10$) (Fig. 2). The median PFS for all patients treated with ENMD-2076 ($n = 41$) was 1.84 months (95% CI, 1.81–3.68) (Fig. 2). The median PFS for all patients evaluable for the efficacy analysis ($n = 36$) was 1.86 months (95% CI, 1.73–3.73).

Safety profile

The most common treatment-related adverse events were hypertension (66%), fatigue (54%), diarrhea (54%), and nausea (49%). Table 3 lists all treatment-related adverse events occurring in 10% or more of patients. Dose reduction occurred in eight patients (20%) for fatigue, hypertension, and proteinuria. The most common grade 3 treatment-related adverse events were hypertension (37.5%) and fatigue (10%). One patient experienced grade 4 hypertension. Five patients (12.2%) discontinued treatment owing to a treatment-related adverse event (Fig. 1).

Pharmacokinetics

The mean steady-state plasma concentration of ENMD-2076 at cycle 2, day 1 was 441 ± 394 ng/ml. The mean steady-state concentration of its active metabolite, ENMD-2060, was 43.3 ± 10.3 ng/ml. The mean ratio of ENMD-2076 to ENMD-2060 was 10.3 ± 4.9.

Additional PK sampling was performed in patients undergoing serial tumor biopsies on the day of the biopsy. This was performed at cycle 1, days 14–16. PK sampling data was available for ten subjects undergoing serial tumor biopsy, and the mean plasma concentrations of ENMD-2076 and ENMD-2060 were 441 ± 275 ng/ml and 40.1 ± 22.9 ng/ml, respectively.

Correlative analysis of serial tumor biopsies and archival tumor tissue

A total of 15 patients underwent at least one tumor biopsy analysis. Eight patients had predose and postdose samples (days 14–16) with sufficient tissue for IHC analysis. One patient underwent an additional biopsy at the time of disease progression following treatment for ten cycles.

Analysis of serial tumor biopsies prior to and following 2 weeks of ENMD-2076 ($n = 8$ patients) demonstrated a treatment-induced decrease in cellular proliferation (Ki-67) (Fig. 3a) and MVD (CD34) (Fig. 3b) as assessed by IHC. This was a trend observed in patients regardless of tumor response to treatment by RECIST 1.1. An increase in cleaved caspase 3 as a marker of apoptosis was only observed in association with response to treatment and not in nonresponders (Figs. 3c and d). The posttreatment decrease in Ki-67 and increase in cleaved caspase 3 observed in patient 01-028 (Fig. 3c, responder) was lost at the time of progression at day 280 of treatment, consistent with preclinical modeling of ENMD-2076 activity in TNBC PDX models [8]. An increase in MVD was not observed at the time of acquired progression in this patient's tumor sample.

On the basis of emerging preclinical data, the final two patients undergoing serial tumor biopsies had their samples processed for IF to investigate changes in p53, p21, p73, BAX, and senescence-associated β-galactosidase (SA-β-gal) following treatment [8]. One patient had sufficient tissue obtained from the pretreatment and posttreatment samples for IF and SA-β-gal. In this patient, an increase in p53 and p73 expression was observed (Fig. 3e), in combination with an increase in SA-β-gal staining. DNA mutational testing of p53 revealed the presence of an R273S mutation in this patient's tumor, and the patient had SD for three cycles on study followed by progression. An increase in p53 family member expression following treatment is consistent with changes observed in preclinical TNBC PDX models treated with ENMD-2076 and other Aurora kinase inhibitors [8, 13].

Archival tumor tissue was obtained from all enrolled patients, and p53 mutation testing revealed deleterious missense mutations in 38.9%, frameshift mutations in 13.9%, wild type in 36.1%, and status unknown for 11.1% (Fig. 3f). Of the six patients who had PR or SD for > 6 months, 83% had a deleterious mutation in p53, as compared with 46% of those who did not meet that efficacy endpoint ($p = 0.18$). Archival tumor tissue samples were also subjected to p53 IHC. High p53 expression was defined as > 30% of cells expressing p53. High p53 expression was present in 16 (50%) patients who had tissue available for analysis ($n = 32$), and high p53 expression plus p53 mutation was present in 11 of 32 (34.4%). High

Table 1 Baseline demographics and patient characteristics

Characteristic	Number of patients (N = 41)
Age, years	
Median (range)	54 (30–73)
Sex	
Male	1 (2.4%)
Female	40 (97.6%)
Race	
White	33 (80.5%)
Black or African American	5 (12.2%)
Unknown	3 (7.3%)
Ethnicity	
Hispanic or Latino	6 (14.6%)
Not Hispanic or Latino	30 (73.2%)
Unknown	5 (12.2%)
ECOG Performance Status	
0	19 (46.3%)
1	22 (53.7%)
Prior lines of systemic therapy	
(locally advanced unresectable or metastatic disease) Mean	1.7
1	21 (51.2%)
2	10 (24.4%)
3	10 (24.4%)
Prior neoadjuvant or adjuvant chemotherapy	
Yes	33 (80.5%)
No	8 (19.5%)
Prior targeted systemic anticancer therapy	
Yes	20 (48.8%)
No	21 (51.2%)
Prior radiation therapy	
Yes	35 (85.4%)
No	6 (14.6%)
BRCA1/2 germline deleterious mutation status	
Mutated	4 (9.8%)
Wildtype	19 (46.3%)
Unknown	18 (43.9%)
Number of metastatic sites	
1	16 (39.0%)
2	14 (34.1%)
≥ 3	11 (26.8%)
Sites of metastasis	
Lung	15 (24.4%)
Lymph nodes	20 (48.8%)
Liver	15 (24.4%)

Table 1 Baseline demographics and patient characteristics (Continued)

Characteristic	Number of patients (N = 41)
Bone	16 (39.0%)
Chest wall	8 (19.5%)
Other	6 (14.6%)

ECOG Eastern Cooperative Oncology Group

p53 expression was observed in 50% of patients meeting the 6-month CBR endpoint and those not meeting this efficacy endpoint, showing no correlation between high expression of p53 by IHC and efficacy.

Discussion

This study demonstrates that ENMD-2076 has durable clinical activity in a subset of patients with previously treated metastatic TNBC. We observed 27.8% and 16.7% of patients achieving prolonged clinical benefit at 4 and 6 months, respectively. The average duration of response for patients achieving clinical benefit for 4 months was 6.5 cycles. The prolonged benefit observed in a subset of patients is meaningful, given the aggressive nature of TNBC and low response rates to single-agent chemotherapies used in clinical practice. In a retrospective multicenter review of 111 patients with metastatic TNBC treated with standard-of-care chemotherapy, Kassam et al. found the median duration of therapy to be 9 weeks in the second-line setting and just 4 weeks in the third-line setting. Only 50% of patients went on to receive third-line therapy [4]. In a more recent analysis of the comparative effectiveness of eribulin, capecitabine, gemcitabine, and navelbine in metastatic previously treated TNBC, Dranitsaris et al. reported a median duration of therapy of 1.6–2 months for these agents [14]. There remains a critical unmet need for effective, targeted therapies to treat TNBC, and to achieve this will likely require patient selection strategies to identify a responding population for new therapies.

ENMD-2076 treatment resulted in mechanism-based toxicities, most commonly hypertension, fatigue, and diarrhea, consistent with prior clinical trials in solid

Table 2 Efficacy analysis

Efficacy response	Number of patients (N = 36)
Complete response	0 (0%)
Partial response	2 (5.6%)
Stable disease	14 (38.9%)
Progressive disease	20 (55.6%)
4-Month clinical benefit rate (4-CBR)	10 (27.8%)
6-Month clinical benefit rate (6-CBR)	6 (16.7%)

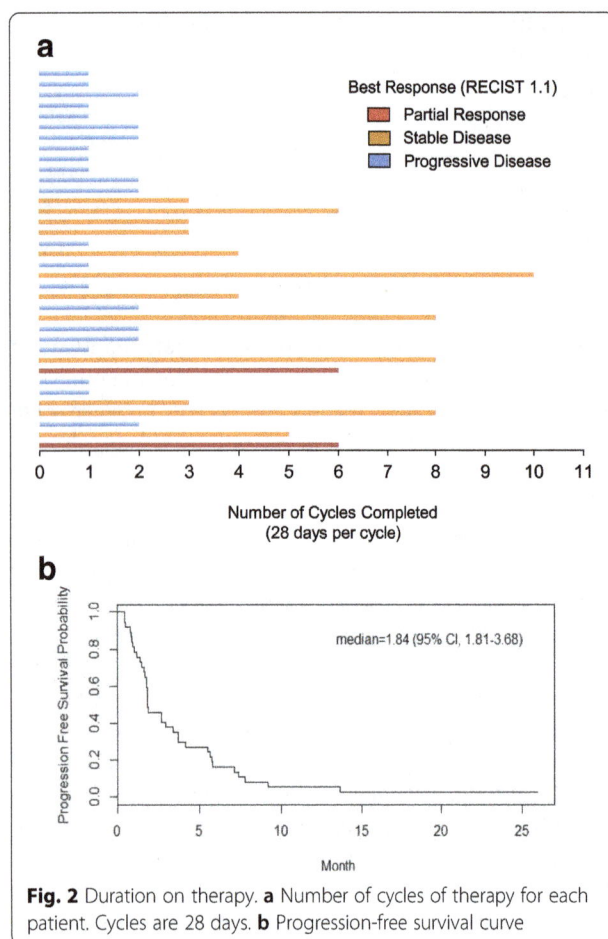

Fig. 2 Duration on therapy. **a** Number of cycles of therapy for each patient. Cycles are 28 days. **b** Progression-free survival curve

Table 3 Treatment-related adverse events occurring in 10% or more of patients

Adverse event	No. of patients (N = 41)	
	All grades	Grade ≥ 3
Hypertension	27 (66%)	16 (39%)
Fatigue	22 (54%)	4 (10%)
Diarrhea	22 (54%)	1 (2%)
Nausea	20 (49%)	0 (0%)
Constipation	10 (24%)	0 (0%)
Headaches	10 (24%)	0 (0%)
Vomiting	9 (22%)	1 (2%)
Mucositis	6 (15%)	0 (0%)
Proteinuria	6 (15%)	3 (7%)
Dysgeusia	5 (12%)	0 (0%)
GERD	5 (12%)	0 (0%)
Anorexia	4 (10%)	0 (0%)

GERD Gastroesophageal reflux disease

tumor patients [10, 15]. Hematologic toxicity was not common in this study. The majority of patients (66%) experienced hypertension, and for 39% it was grade 3 or higher. This incidence and severity are similar to rates observed in prior studies of ENMD-2076 in patients with cancer and is likely related to VEGFR2 inhibition [10, 15]. In most cases, hypertension was easily controlled with antihypertensive agents, most commonly a dihydropyridine calcium channel blocker or an angiotensin-converting enzyme inhibitor. Close monitoring of blood pressure and careful management of hypertension should continue to be required in future studies of ENMD-2076.

Despite lowering the starting dose in this trial from that used in the phase II ovarian cancer trial, dose reduction was required in 20% of patients, and 12.2% of patients discontinued treatment owing to treatment-related toxicity [10]. These rates of toxicity and dose modification are similar to those for other approved multitarget tyrosine kinase inhibitors, including sorafenib [16]. Limited PK analysis performed in this study demonstrated a mean steady-state plasma concentration of ENMD-2076 at cycle 2, day 1 of 441 ± 394 ng/ml, which is similar to 356 ng/ml observed in patients with ovarian cancer [10]. The toxicity observed in this trial should be considered in the design of future studies of ENMD-2076, and the incorporation of standard toxicity management algorithms may assist in the management of hypertension.

This trial incorporated archival tumor tissue analysis for p53 mutation and protein expression, as well as serial tumor biopsies in a subset of patients. These correlative studies were designed to further delineate the mechanism of action of this multitarget drug using human tumor samples and to explore a potential relationship between deleterious p53 mutations and ENMD-2076 activity in TNBC. Although these studies are exploratory in nature owing to a limited sample size, analysis can be performed in the context of previously published preclinical studies [7, 8, 13].

As expected, ENMD-2076 was antiangiogenic, as evidenced by a decrease in blood vessel formation in tumor tissue following 2 weeks of treatment. ENMD-2076 is a potent inhibitor of the angiogenic kinases VEGFR2 (half-maximal inhibitory concentration [IC_{50}], 58 nM), VEGFR3 (IC_{50}, 16 nM), FGFR1/2 (IC_{50}, 71 and 93 nM, respectively), and platelet-derived growth factor receptor-α (IC_{50}, 56 nM) [7]. We previously demonstrated in vivo that administration of ENMD-2076 treatment results in a decrease in MVD, as well as vascular permeability and perfusion, as measured by dynamic contrast-enhanced MRI [17]. TNBC commonly overexpresses vascular endothelial growth factor, which acts to promote angiogenesis and early metastatic potential

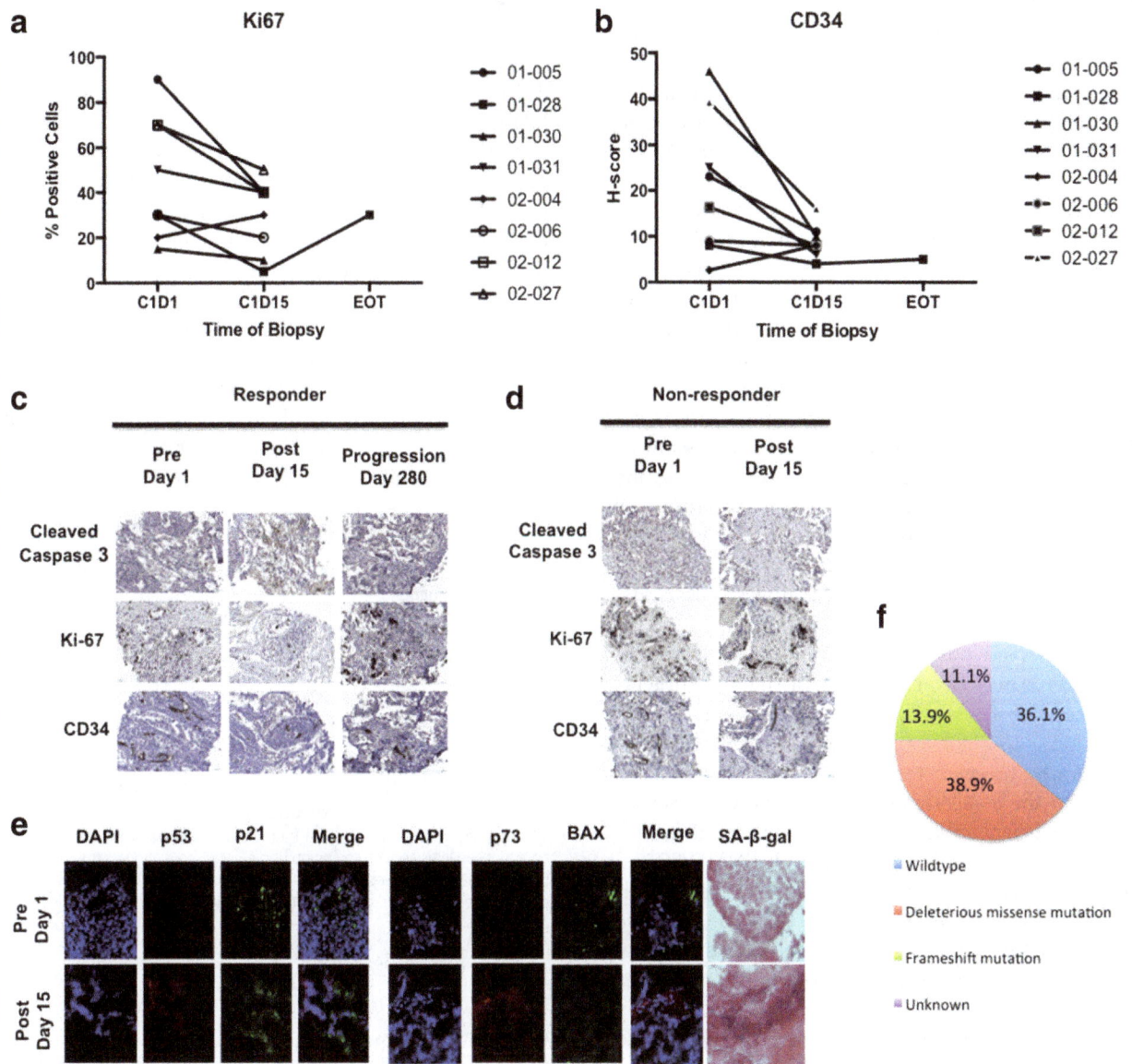

Fig. 3 Effects of ENMD-2076 on pharmacodynamic markers in serial tumor biopsies obtained in a subset of patients. **a** Paired samples were available for eight patients at baseline prior to dosing (C1D1) and postdose on days 14–16 (C1D15). An additional sample was obtained in one patient who experienced stable disease for ten cycles followed by progression (end of treatment [EOT]). Tissue was analyzed by IHC for Ki-67 as a marker of cellular proliferation. **b** Nonresponder. Staining was performed as in panel **a**. Note that there is no decrease in proliferation or increase in apoptosis in the nonresponder following ENMD-2076 treatment. Samples were analyzed by IHC for CD34 expression as a marker of microvessel density. Changes were independent of tumor response and clinical benefit to ENMD-2076 treatment. Patients 01-005, 01-030, 02-004, 02-006, 02-012, and 02-027 had progressive disease (PD) at first imaging assessment following two cycles; 01-028 had stable disease (SD) for ten cycles; and 01-031 had SD for four cycles. **c** Immunoflurorescence analysis of tumor biopsies for 4′,6-diamidino-2-phenylindole (DAPI), p53, and p73 in a patient who had stable disease by Response Evaluation Criteria in Solid Tumors (RECIST version 1.1) after two cycles of treatment and then progressed after cycle 3. Patient has a p53 mutation R273S. Note an increase in p53 and p73 following treatment, which is consistent with preclinical findings in patient-derived tumor xenograft models. IHC images from 01-028 responder. Cleaved caspase 3, Ki-67, and CD34 on serial tumor biopsies were used to assess apoptosis, proliferation, and microvessel density, respectively, in a patient responding to ENMD-2076 treatment with prolonged stable disease for ten cycles. Biopsies were obtained prior to treatment, 15 days after treatment, and at the time of disease progression day 280. Formalin-fixed, paraffin-embedded tissue sections were stained with the indicated antibodies, and representative images were obtained at ×20 magnification. Note an increase in cleaved caspase 3 and a decrease in Ki-67 and CD34 in the posttreatment biopsy. At the time of disease progression, these changes were reversed. Changes in (**d**) Ki-67 and (**e**) CD34 (microvessel density) in serial tumor biopsies. Baseline and day 15 samples were available for eight patients. An additional sample was obtained from one patient at the time of progression following prolonged stable disease. Ki-67 and CD34 were assessed using IHC. *SA-β-gal* Senescence-associated β-galactosidase

[18, 19]. Similar to other trials, this study did not demonstrate a correlation between a decrease in MVD and clinical benefit. This highlights the multifaceted mechanisms of cancer progression and that inhibiting angiogenesis alone is unlikely to be sufficient to lead to durable tumor response in TNBC.

A decrease in cellular proliferation that was also independent of response to therapy was observed and is likely a result of Aurora kinase inhibition. ENMD-2076 is more selective for Aur A than Aurora kinase B (IC_{50}, 14 nM and 350 nM, respectively); however, inhibition of both is likely in tumor tissue, based on the drug exposure observed in this study. The early time point selected for the on-treatment biopsy may have resulted in capturing a decrease in cellular proliferation that occurred early and was lost quickly with tumor progression at the 2-month repeat imaging time point. As expected, induction of apoptosis was observed only in association with a favorable response to treatment, consistent with preclinical models [13]. ENMD-2076 treatment-emergent increases in p53 and p73 expression were observed, also consistent with preclinical data.

We observed p53 mutations in the majority of patients, as expected on the basis of the known genomic landscape of TNBC [20]. Deleterious mutations in p53 were more common in patients with clinical benefit for > 6 months; however, this was not statistically significant, owing to the small sample size. An increased sensitivity of p53-deficient models to Aurora kinase inhibitors, including AZD1152, AMG 900, and ENMD-2076, has been previously reported [7, 21, 22]. This is likely related to an impaired p53-dependent cell cycle checkpoint, which results in cells continuing to cycle through aberrant mitoses following drug exposure, ultimately resulting in cell death.

In this study, we observed a relatively high incidence of asymptomatic brain metastasis. Approximately 15% (10 of 65 patients consented) of patients in this trial had asymptomatic brain metastasis detected on the required screening brain MRI. Patients with TNBC are more likely than patients with hormone receptor-positive, HER2-negative breast cancer to develop brain metastasis. Approximately 50% of patients with metastatic TNBC will develop brain metastasis over the course of their disease [23–26]. These patients were not eligible for enrollment in this trial, owing to concerns regarding the risk of hemorrhagic events at the time of trial conception; however, data are now available to support the safety of antiangiogenics in asymptomatic brain metastasis [27]. Patients with stable, asymptomatic brain metastasis previously treated with radiation therapy could be considered for future trials of ENMD-2076. The propensity for asymptomatic brain metastasis should be considered in the design of future metastatic TNBC trials.

Conclusions

ENMD-2076 has meaningful clinical benefit in a small subset of patients with previously treated metastatic TNBC. Future studies should continue to evaluate the relationship between p53 and response to treatment with a focus on the development of a patient selection strategy. Currently ongoing studies include a phase II clinical trial of ENMD-2076 in patients with metastatic previously treated TNBC in Asia, and biomarker development work is ongoing. This trial demonstrates the feasibility of performing serial tumor biopsies in multisite trials in metastatic TNBC and highlights the importance of these studies in confirming data generated in preclinical models. Combination therapies with immunotherapy and mammalian target of rapamycin pathway inhibitors are also under investigation based on ongoing preclinical work [8].

Acknowledgements
The University of Colorado Cancer Center Biobanking and Histology Shared Resource and Molecular Pathology Shared Resource were used for this project.

Funding
This work was supported by the National Institutes of Health (NIH) and the National Cancer Institute (NCI) through grants 5P30CA046934-25 (University of Colorado Cancer Center Support Grant), 1R21CA164617-01A1 (to JRD), and 1K23CA172691-01A1 (to JRD). This funding was used for study design and collection, analysis and interpretation of data, and the writing of the manuscript. Support was also received from CASI Pharmaceuticals in the form of provision of study medication and coverage of some clinical care costs for enrolled patients.

Authors' contributions
JRD led development of the concept and design of the trial, data acquisition, analysis, and manuscript writing. SGE contributed to trial design and data analysis. TMP and JJT designed the correlative study sample acquisition protocol and did biomarker data analysis. DA and AvB contributed to trial design and data analysis for molecular studies and performed microdissection, DNA isolation, and p53 sequencing. DLG contributed to trial design, data acquisition, and analysis for pharmacokinetic analysis. AC performed correlative studies on biopsy samples and analyzed data for correlative studies. SS performed IHC analysis and scoring and interpretation of data. PK, ADE, VFB, and KDM contributed to trial concept and design as well as data acquisition, patient enrollment, and interpretation of clinical trial data. KZ and TC contributed to the trial design, acquisition of data, and analysis of data. DG developed the statistical design of the study and performed the final statistical analysis. AMS and BPS contributed to acquisition of data, patient enrollment, and analysis/interpretation of clinical trial data. All authors read and approved the final manuscript.

Competing interests
Scientific consulting (to SGE) and research funding (to JRD) were provided by CASI Pharmaceuticals.

Author details

[1]University of Colorado Cancer Center, Aurora, CO, USA. [2]Department of Oncology, University of Texas at Austin, Dell Medical School, Austin, TX, USA. [3]Indiana University Melvin and Bren Simon Cancer Center, Indianapolis, IN, USA. [4]Division of Medical Oncology, University of Colorado Anschutz Medical Campus, University of Colorado Cancer Center, 12801 East 17th Avenue, Mailstop 8117, Aurora, CO 80045, USA.

References

1. Carey L, Winer E, Viale G, Cameron D, Gianni L. Triple-negative breast cancer: disease entity or title of convenience? Nat Rev Clin Oncol. 2010;7: 683–92.
2. Anders CK, Carey LA. Biology, metastatic patterns, and treatment of patients with triple-negative breast cancer. Clin Breast Cancer. 2009; 9(Suppl 2):S73–81.
3. Perou CM, Sorlie T, Eisen MB, van de Rijn M, Jeffrey SS, Rees CA, et al. Molecular portraits of human breast tumours. Nature. 2000;406:747–52.
4. Kassam F, Enright K, Dent R, Dranitsaris G, Myers J, Flynn C, et al. Survival outcomes for patients with metastatic triple-negative breast cancer: implications for clinical practice and trial design. Clin Breast Cancer. 2009;9: 29–33.
5. Lehmann BD, Bauer JA, Chen X, Sanders ME, Chakravarthy AB, Shyr Y, et al. Identification of human triple-negative breast cancer subtypes and preclinical models for selection of targeted therapies. J Clin Invest. 2011;121: 2750–67.
6. Fletcher GC, Brokx RD, Denny TA, Hembrough TA, Plum SM, Fogler WE, et al. ENMD-2076 is an orally active kinase inhibitor with antiangiogenic and antiproliferative mechanisms of action. Mol Cancer Ther. 2011;10:126–37.
7. Diamond JR, Eckhardt SG, Tan AC, Newton TP, Selby HM, Brunkow KL, et al. Predictive biomarkers of sensitivity to the Aurora and angiogenic kinase inhibitor ENMD-2076 in preclinical breast cancer models. Clin Cancer Res. 2013;19:291–303.
8. Ionkina AA, Tentler JJ, Kim J, Capasso A, Pitts TM, Ryall KA, et al. Efficacy and molecular mechanisms of differentiated response to the Aurora and angiogenic kinase inhibitor ENMD-2076 in preclinical models of p53-mutated triple-negative breast cancer. Front Oncol. 2017;7:94.
9. Therasse P, Arbuck SG, Eisenhauer EA, Wanders J, Kaplan RS, Rubinstein L, et al. New guidelines to evaluate the response to treatment in solid tumors. J Natl Cancer Inst. 2000;92:205–16.
10. Matulonis UA, Lee J, Lasonde B, Tew WP, Yehwalashet A, Matei D, et al. ENMD-2076, an oral inhibitor of angiogenic and proliferation kinases, has activity in recurrent, platinum resistant ovarian cancer. Eur J Cancer. 2013;49: 121–31.
11. Martín M. Platinum compounds in the treatment of advanced breast cancer. Clin Breast Cancer. 2001;2:190–208. discussion 209
12. Finn RS, Bengala C, Ibrahim N, Roche H, Sparano J, Strauss LC, et al. Dasatinib as a single agent in triple-negative breast cancer: results of an open-label phase 2 study. Clin Cancer Res. 2011;17:6905–13.
13. Tentler JJ, Ionkina A, Tan AC, Newton TP, Pitts TM, Glogowska MJ, et al. p53 family members regulate phenotypic response to Aurora kinase A inhibition in triple-negative breast cancer. Mol Cancer Ther. 2015;14:1117–29.
14. Dranitsaris G, Gluck S, Faria C, Cox D, Rugo H. Comparative effectiveness analysis of monotherapy with cytotoxic agents in triple-negative metastatic breast cancer in a community setting. Clin Ther. 2015;37:134–44.
15. Diamond JR, Bastos BR, Hansen RJ, Gustafson DL, Eckhardt SG, Kwak EL, et al. Phase I safety, pharmacokinetic, and pharmacodynamic study of ENMD-2076, a novel angiogenic and Aurora kinase inhibitor, in patients with advanced solid tumors. Clin Cancer Res. 2011;17:849–60.
16. Li Y, Gao ZH, Qu XJ. The adverse effects of sorafenib in patients with advanced cancers. Basic Clin Pharmacol Toxicol. 2015;116:216–21.
17. Tentler JJ, Bradshaw-Pierce EL, Serkova NJ, Hasebroock KM, Pitts TM, Diamond JR, et al. Assessment of the in vivo antitumor effects of ENMD-2076, a novel multitargeted kinase inhibitor, against primary and cell line-derived human colorectal cancer xenograft models. Clin Cancer Res. 2010; 16:2989–98.
18. Greenberg S, Rugo HS. Triple-negative breast cancer: role of antiangiogenic agents. Cancer J. 2010;16:33–8.
19. Andre F, Job B, Dessen P, Tordai A, Michiels S, Liedtke C, et al. Molecular characterization of breast cancer with high-resolution oligonucleotide comparative genomic hybridization array. Clin Cancer Res. 2009;15:441–51.
20. Pareja F, Geyer FC, Marchio C, Burke KA, Weigelt B, Reis-Filho JS. Triple-negative breast cancer: the importance of molecular and histologic subtyping, and recognition of low-grade variants. NPJ Breast Cancer. 2016;2:16036.
21. Kalous O, Conklin D, Desai AJ, Dering J, Goldstein J, Ginther C, et al. AMG 900, pan-Aurora kinase inhibitor, preferentially inhibits the proliferation of breast cancer cell lines with dysfunctional p53. Breast Cancer Res Treat. 2013;141:397–408.
22. Tao Y, Zhang P, Girdler F, Frascogna V, Castedo M, Bourhis J, et al. Enhancement of radiation response in p53-deficient cancer cells by the Aurora-B kinase inhibitor AZD1152. Oncogene. 2008;27:3244–55.
23. Lin NU, Claus E, Sohl J, Razzak AR, Arnaout A, Winer EP. Sites of distant recurrence and clinical outcomes in patients with metastatic triple-negative breast cancer: high incidence of central nervous system metastases. Cancer. 2008;113:2638–45.
24. Matsuo S, Watanabe J, Mitsuya K, Hayashi N, Nakasu Y, Hayashi M. Brain metastasis in patients with metastatic breast cancer in the real world: a single-institution, retrospective review of 12-year follow-up. Breast Cancer Res Treat. 2017;162:169–79.
25. Molnar IA, Molnar BA, Vizkeleti L, Fekete K, Tamas J, Deak P, et al. Breast carcinoma subtypes show different patterns of metastatic behavior. Virchows Arch. 2017;470:275–83.
26. Saraf A, Grubb CS, Hwang ME, Tai CH, Wu CC, Jani A, et al. Breast cancer subtype and stage are prognostic of time from breast cancer diagnosis to brain metastasis development. J Neurooncol. 2017;134:453–63.
27. Besse B, Le Moulec S, Mazieres J, Senellart H, Barlesi F, Chouaid C, et al. Bevacizumab in patients with nonsquamous non-small cell lung cancer and asymptomatic, untreated brain metastases (BRAIN): a nonrandomized, phase II study. Clin Cancer Res. 2015;21:1896–903.

16

Longitudinal enumeration and cluster evaluation of circulating tumor cells improve prognostication for patients with newly diagnosed metastatic breast cancer in a prospective observational trial

Anna-Maria Larsson[1,2†], Sara Jansson[1†], Pär-Ola Bendahl[1], Charlotte Levin Tykjaer Jörgensen[1], Niklas Loman[1,2], Cecilia Graffman[2], Lotta Lundgren[1,2], Kristina Aaltonen[1] and Lisa Rydén[3,4*]

Abstract

Background: Circulating tumor cells (CTCs) carry independent prognostic information in patients with metastatic breast cancer (MBC) on different lines of therapy. Moreover, CTC clusters are suggested to add prognostic information to CTC enumeration alone but their significance is unknown in patients with newly diagnosed MBC. We aimed to evaluate whether longitudinal enumeration of circulating tumor cells (CTCs) and CTC clusters could improve prognostication and monitoring of patients with metastatic breast cancer (MBC) starting first-line therapy.

Methods: This prospective study included 156 women with newly diagnosed MBC. CTCs and CTC clusters were detected using CellSearch technology at baseline (BL) and after 1, 3, and 6 months of systemic therapy. The primary end point was progression-free survival (PFS) and the secondary end point overall survival (OS). Median follow-up time was 25 (7–69) months.

Results: There were 79 (52%) and 30 (20%) patients with ≥ 5 CTCs and ≥ 1 CTC cluster at baseline, respectively; both factors were significantly associated with impaired survival. Landmark analyses based on follow-up measurements revealed increasing prognostic hazard ratios for ≥ 5 CTCs and CTC clusters during treatment, predicting worse PFS and OS. Both factors added value to a prognostic model based on clinicopathological variables at all time points and ≥ 5 CTCs and presence of CTC clusters enhanced the model's C-index to > 0.80 at 1, 3, and 6 months. Importantly, changes in CTCs during treatment were significantly correlated with survival and patients with a decline from ≥ 5 CTCs at BL to < 5 CTCs at 1 month had a similar odds ratio for progression to patients with < 5 CTCs at BL and 1 month. Stratification of patients based on CTC count and CTC clusters into four groups (0 CTCs, 1–4 CTCs, ≥ 5 CTCs, and ≥ 1 CTC + CTC clusters) demonstrated that patients with CTC clusters had significantly worse survival compared to patients without clusters.

(Continued on next page)

* Correspondence: lisa.ryden@med.lu.se
†Anna-Maria Larsson and Sara Jansson contributed equally to this work.
[3]Department of Clinical Sciences Lund, Division of Surgery, Lund University, Medicon Village, SE-223 81 Lund, Sweden
[4]Department of Surgery and Gastroenterology, Skåne University Hospital, Malmö, Sweden
Full list of author information is available at the end of the article

(Continued from previous page)

Conclusions: Longitudinal evaluation of CTC and CTC clusters improves prognostication and monitoring in patients with MBC starting first-line systemic therapy. The prognostic value increases over time, suggesting that changes in CTC count are clinically relevant. The presence of CTC clusters adds significant prognostic value to CTC enumeration alone.

Keywords: Metastatic breast cancer, Circulating tumor cells (CTCs), Enumeration, Cluster, Prognosis

Background

The prognostic value of circulating tumor cell (CTC) enumeration was first shown in patients with metastatic breast cancer (MBC) assessed by the CellSearch system in 2004 [1]. Since then, several studies have been published in support of these results [2–14] and in 2014 a pooled analysis of data from 1944 patients confirmed that a CTC count of ≥ 5 cells per 7.5 mL blood is an independent predictor of worse progression-free survival (PFS) and overall survival (OS) in patients with MBC [15]. The authors of the pooled analysis developed a clinicopathological prognostication model that included CTC count in addition to other clinically relevant variables, and concluded that CTC-based survival prognostication models should be considered as optimum prognostic models for counselling of patients [15]. Recently, a meta-analysis demonstrated that CTC status can be applied in monitoring the effectiveness of systemic therapy for MBC, since a shift in CTC status between two time points was prognostic [16]. Thus far, most individual studies evaluating CTC count in MBC included patients regardless of prior lines of systemic therapy and baseline CTC was measured in a heterogeneous population of patients on different lines of treatment. The focus of these studies has primarily been on CTC evaluation before starting a new line of treatment or at the first post-treatment evaluation, but no studies have conclusively evaluated long-term monitoring of CTC dynamics. Hence, the presence and dynamics of CTCs during first-line systemic treatment in patients with MBC and its clinical relevance have yet to be fully elucidated. Furthermore, recent studies have shown that detection of CTC clusters in patients with MBC adds prognostic value to CTC enumeration alone [12, 13, 17], but limited data are available on the prognostic value of CTC clusters in previously untreated patients with MBC before and during treatment [18].

The aim of this prospective study was to evaluate longitudinal CTC count ≥ 5 cells/7.5 mL blood and CTC clusters using the CellSearch system as a prognostic instrument in women with newly diagnosed MBC from baseline to 6 months, and examine how these relate to progression-free survival (PFS) and overall survival (OS).

A secondary aim was to evaluate if early changes in CTC status can predict response at the first radiological evaluation at 3 months.

Methods
Patients and study design

Patients diagnosed with MBC and scheduled for first-line systemic treatment at Skåne University Hospital and Halmstad County Hospital, Sweden, were enrolled into a prospective monitoring trial (ClinicalTrials.gov NCT01322893) conducted by the Department of Oncology and Pathology at Lund University, Sweden. The study was approved by the Lund University Ethics Committee (LU 2010/135). Inclusion criteria were age ≥ 18 years, Eastern Cooperative Oncology Group (ECOG) performance status score 0–2, and predicted life expectancy of > 2 months. Exclusion criteria were prior systemic therapy for metastatic disease, inability to understand the study information, and other malignant disease in the preceding 5 years. After selection, the participating patients started first-line systemic therapy for MBC according to national guidelines; the treating physicians were blind to the CTC results. Patients underwent structured clinical and radiological evaluation every 3 months or at the discretion of the treating physician. Progression versus non-progression was defined according to clinical practice based on clinical and radiological evaluation using the modified Response Evaluation Criteria In Solid Tumors (RECIST) 1.1 [19]. Using this approach progression was defined as progressive disease (PD), whilst non-progression was defined as stable disease (SD), partial response (PR) or complete response (CR).

Samples of whole blood and serum were collected at baseline and after approximately 1, 3, and 6 months of treatment. The serum marker CA15-3 was analyzed at the Department of Clinical Chemistry at Skåne University Hospital with an accredited method used in clinical practice (CA15-3 on Cobas, NPU01449). Twenty-three of the participating patients experienced treatment failure within 6 months of commencement; therefore, they were started on second-line therapy, for which blood sampling was repeated (at baseline after treatment failure (baseline 2) and after 1, 3, and 6 months).

Detection of CTCs and CTC clusters

Blood samples were collected in 10 mL CellSave Preservation tubes (Menarini Silicon Biosystems, Bologna, Italy), stored between 15 and 30 °C and processed within 96 h of collection. CTCs were isolated and enumerated using the Food and Drug Administration (FDA)-approved CellSearch system (Menarini Silicon Biosystems) as has been described in detail previously [1, 20]. Two investigators certified in the CellSearch technology independently evaluated all images within the generated galleries for events. Any event for which the assessment differed between the investigators was re-evaluated until consensus was reached.

CTC clusters were defined as groups consisting of ≥ 2 CTCs clustered together and with non-overlapping nuclei. Presence of other cell types in addition to CTCs was not documented. Two independent assessors evaluated CTC clusters in CTC galleries exported from the CellTracks Analyzer II system, as described previously [17]. No additional staining of CTCs was performed after the CellSearch analysis was completed. CTC enumeration and CTC clusters were evaluated at baseline and during treatment at 1, 3, and 6 months. A blood sample was considered positive for CTC clusters if ≥ 1 CTC cluster was detected.

Statistical analysis

Statistical power calculations based on estimated PFS, fraction of patients with a CTC count above the predefined threshold (≥ 5 CTCs), the inclusion period, and the estimated follow-up time determined the required study sample size to be 154 patients (Additional file 1). An additional threshold of ≥ 20 CTCs proposed by Botteri et al. [21] was applied to explore the relationship between the number of CTCs and the presence of CTC clusters.

Categorical or categorized characteristics of the patients, tumors, and CTCs at different time points were compared using Pearson's chi-squared test or if counts were lower than expected in one or more of the cells, Fisher's exact test was used. Ordinal data were compared using Pearson's chi-squared test for trend and variables measured on a continuous scale by the Mann-Whitney U test or, if there were more than two categories, the Kruskal Wallis test.

The primary end point was PFS and the secondary end points were OS and progression versus non-progression at first evaluation, in relation to changes in numbers of CTCs and/or presence of CTC clusters. The study was in accordance with the Reporting Recommendations for Tumor Marker (REMARK) criteria [22]. Time from the date of the blood draw to progression or death from any cause was calculated. If an outcome was not reached the time variables were censored at the last follow up. Kaplan-Meier plots and the log-rank test were used to illustrate and compare survival between subgroups. Survival analysis of variables measured at 1, 3, and 6 months was performed by landmark analysis. Univariable and multivariable hazard ratios (HRs) for selected potential predictors of PFS and OS were determined by Cox proportional hazards regression. Proportional hazards assumptions were checked graphically. Model fit was measured using Harrell's C-index, and the fit of nested prognostic models was compared using likelihood ratio (LR) tests.

In addition, Cox models with time-dependent covariates were used to estimate the effects of the longitudinally measured binary variables ≥ 5 CTCs and CTC clusters on OS. Briefly, the follow up of each patient was split into multiple non-overlapping episodes for which each of the two covariates were constant. The number of such episodes per patient varied between 1 and 6: 1 episode was sufficient for patients with the same CTC and CTC-cluster status at BL and all follow-up visits. With three follow-up visits (1, 3, and 6 months), change in one or both of these variables can be observed up to three times for patients staying on first-line treatment. Patients who switched to second-line treatment within 6 months from BL can have up to three additional episodes with change in one or both variables. Missing values at follow-up visits were imputed using the principle of last observation carried forward. For example, the HR for ≥ 5 CTCs in models of this kind should be interpreted as the ratio of the mortality during episodes with ≥ 5 CTCs to that of episodes with < 5 CTCs. The method of last observation carried forward is reportedly less prone to selection bias than deletion by list [23], but it is not state of the art within the field of imputation. However, in the light of the low fraction of missing data and the exploratory nature of these analyses, we judge the method reliable.

The association between CTC count and the outcome of the first evaluation was assessed by logistic regression. The value added of CTC count and CTC clusters to a prognostic clinicopathological model was evaluated using LR statistics in Cox regression models, based on a model previously described by Bidard et al. [15]. P values in the exploratory analyses were not adjusted for multiple testing and should therefore not be compared to the 5% cutoff. Statistical analysis was with IBM SPSS Statistics (version 24.0, IBM, Armonk, NY, USA) and STATA (version 15.0, StataCorp. College Station, TX, USA).

Results

Patient characteristics

In total, 156 patients with newly diagnosed MBC were enrolled in the study between April 2011 and June 2016. There were 31 patients with stage IV disease at initial diagnosis and 125 patients were diagnosed with distant recurrence. Patient and tumor characteristics are summarized in Table 1. The median follow-up time from baseline was

Table 1 Baseline patient and tumor characteristics stratified by CTC count and CTC clusters

	All patients (n = 156)	Baseline CTC < 5 (n = 73)	Baseline CTC ≥5 (n = 79)	P value	Baseline clusters absent (n = 122)	Baseline clusters ≥ 1 (n = 30)	P value
Age MBC, median (range)	65 (40–90)	65 (40–84)	65 (41–90)	0.71[a]	67 (40–90)	60 (42–72)	0.002[a]
Baseline ECOG							
0	91	48 (53)	43 (47)	0.07[b]	76 (84)	15 (16)	0.32[b]
1	37	17 (46)	20 (54)		29 (78)	8 (22)	
2	22	6 (30)	14 (70)		15 (75)	5 (25)	
Unknown	6						
PT NHG							
I	13	9 (69)	4 (31)	0.58[b]	12 (92)	1 (8)	0.85[b]
II	65	26 (41)	38 (59)		47 (73)	17 (27)	
III	46	22 (49)	23 (51)		38 (84)	7 (16)	
Unknown	32						
PT tumor size							
T1	57	30 (55)	25 (45)	0.16[b]	49 (89)	6 (11)	0.07[b]
T2	51	25 (49)	26 (51)		39 (76)	12 (24)	
T3	20	8 (40)	12 (60)		15 (75)	5 (25)	
T4	19	7 (39)	11 (61)		13 (72)	5 (28)	
Unknown	9						
PT node status							
Negative	44	27 (61)	17 (39)	0.04[c]	39 (89)	5 (11)	0.10[c]
Positive	92	38 (42)	52 (58)		69 (77)	21 (23)	
Unknown	20						
Breast cancer subtype[d]							
ER+ HER2-	105	46 (44)	58 (56)	0.52[c]	86 (83)	18 (17)	0.34[c]
HER2+	20	11 (58)	8 (42)		14 (74)	5 (26)	
ER- HER2-	26	12 (50)	12 (50)		17 (71)	7 (29)	
Unknown	5						
Metastasis-free interval (years)							
0	31	14 (47)	16 (53)	0.57[b]	24 (80)	6 (20)	0.97[b]
> 0-3	28	11 (41)	16 (59)		22 (81)	5 (19)	
> 3	97	48 (51)	47 (49)		76 (80)	19 (20)	
Metastatic sites, number							
< 3	109	58 (54)	49 (46)	0.02[c]	88 (82)	19 (18)	0.34[c]
≥ 3	47	15 (33)	30 (67)		34 (76)	11 (24)	
Site of metastasis							
Non-visceral	65	29 (45)	35 (55)	0.57[c]	47 (73)	17 (27)	0.07[c]
Visceral[e]	91	44 (50)	44 (50)		75 (85)	13 (15)	
1st line treatment for MBC[f]							
Endocrine	58	31 (53)	27 (47)	0.28[c]	56 (97)	2 (3)	< 0.001[c]
Chemotherapy	71	29 (42)	40 (58)		48 (70)	21 (30)	
HER2-targeted	15	9 (60)	6 (40)		11 (73)	4 (27)	

Table 1 Baseline patient and tumor characteristics stratified by CTC count and CTC clusters *(Continued)*

	All patients	Baseline CTC < 5	Baseline CTC ≥5	P value	Baseline clusters absent	Baseline clusters ≥ 1	P value
	(n = 156)	(n = 73)	(n = 79)		(n = 122)	(n = 30)	
One or more clusters of ≥ 2 CTCs at baseline[g]							
No	122	73 (60)	49 (40)	< 0.001[c]			
Yes	30	0	30 (100)				

Abbreviations: CTC circulating tumor cell, *MBC* metastatic breast cancer, *ECOG* Eastern Cooperative Oncology Group, *NHG* Nottingham histological grade, *PT* primary tumor, *ER* estrogen receptor, *HER2* human epidermal growth factor receptor 2
[a]*P* value from Mann-Whitney test
[b]*P* value from Pearson's chi-squared test for trend
[c]*P* value from Pearson's chi-squared test
[d]Breast cancer subtype was primarily derived from immunohistochemical staining of the metastasis (*n* = 114). If no information was available from the metastasis, the subtype was derived by staining of the primary tumor (*n* = 36)
[e]Visceral metastasis defined as lung, liver, brain, peritoneal, and/or pleural involvement
[f]A total of 12 patients died and/or treatment was ended before the first structured clinical follow up at 3 months post treatment initiation and consequently no data are available for these patients
[g]Four patients had no baseline sample and thus had no data on CTCs and CTC clusters

25 months (range 7–69) for patients alive at the last medical visit before the cutoff date of 31 May 2017. The median age at MBC diagnosis was 65 years (range 40–90) and the median metastasis-free interval for patients with recurrent disease was 5.8 years (range 0.4–36.3). Breast cancer subtype was determined in metastases in 114 patients and in primary tumors in 126 patients. There were 105 patients (70%) with estrogen receptor-positive (ER+) tumors, 20 (13%) had human epidermal growth factor receptor 2 positive (HER2+) tumors, and 26 (17%) had triple-negative breast cancer (TNBC), determined primarily from metastatic data, and secondarily from primary tumor data. Visceral metastases (defined as lung, liver, brain, peritoneal, and/or pleural involvement) were present in 91 patients (58%): 36 patients (23%) had bone metastasis only. First-line systemic therapy included endocrine treatment in 58 patients (40%), chemotherapy in 71 patients (49%) and HER2-directed agents in combination with chemotherapy or endocrine therapy in 15 patients (10%).

CTC count and CTC clusters

Blood samples from 115 patients at all time-points (baseline, 1, 3 and 6 months) were analyzed. In total, 591 blood samples were collected and analyzed; two sampling errors and four technical errors were encountered. At baseline, 79 (52%) of 152 evaluable patients had ≥ 5 CTCs (predefined cutoff). The fraction of patients with ≥ 5 CTCs decreased during first-line treatment from baseline to 1, 3, and 6 months, and patients receiving subsequent second-line systemic therapy had on average higher CTC counts at all time points, as depicted in Fig. 1. Applying a cut point of ≥ 20 CTCs, the corresponding numbers for patients with CTCs ≥ 20 were 54/152 (36%), 27/137 (20%), 11/121 (9%), and 8/104 (8%) at baseline, 1, 3, and 6 months, respectively. There were no significant differences in CTC counts between breast cancer subtypes at baseline.

There were 30 patients with CTC clusters at baseline. During first-line systemic therapy, 39 patients had CTC clusters at any time point (baseline, 1, 3 and/or 6 months) and during second-line therapy, 10 patients had CTC clusters (Fig. 1). The presence of CTC clusters was associated with CTC count at all time points and patients with clusters more frequently had ≥ 20 CTCs (Additional file 2). However, there were some patients with clusters and a low CTC count (2–4 CTCs) and half of the patients with a high CTC count (≥ 20 CTCs) did not have any CTC clusters in the sample (Additional file 2). There was no association between breast cancer subtype and presence of CTC clusters.

Prediction of outcome in relation to CTCs and CTC clusters

Patients with ≥ 5 CTCs at baseline had inferior PFS (HR$_{PFS}$ 1.68; 95% confidence interval (CI) 1.17–2.42; *P* = 0.005) and OS (HR$_{OS}$ 2.52; 95% CI 1.58–4.01; *P* < 0.001) (Fig. 2a-b). These results remained significant in multivariable analysis even when adjusting for other prognostic factors (Table 2).

HRs increased time-dependently during treatment in longitudinal landmark analysis of CTC count, predicting worse PFS and OS from all follow-up sample time points in patients with CTCs ≥ 5 in the sample (Table 2). A reduction in CTC count during systemic therapy from ≥ 5 CTCs at baseline to < 5 CTCs at follow up (at 1, 3, and 6 months) was also significantly associated with improved survival, in comparison to patients with persistent CTCs ≥ 5 at 1, 3, and 6 months (Fig. 2c-h). Univariable Cox regression analysis of OS with time-varying covariates confirmed the poor prognosis in patients with high CTC count, and the mortality in patients with CTCs ≥ 5 was 5.74 (95% CI 3.48–9.48) times higher than in those with CTCs < 5. The corresponding mortality ratio after adjustment for clinicopathological variables

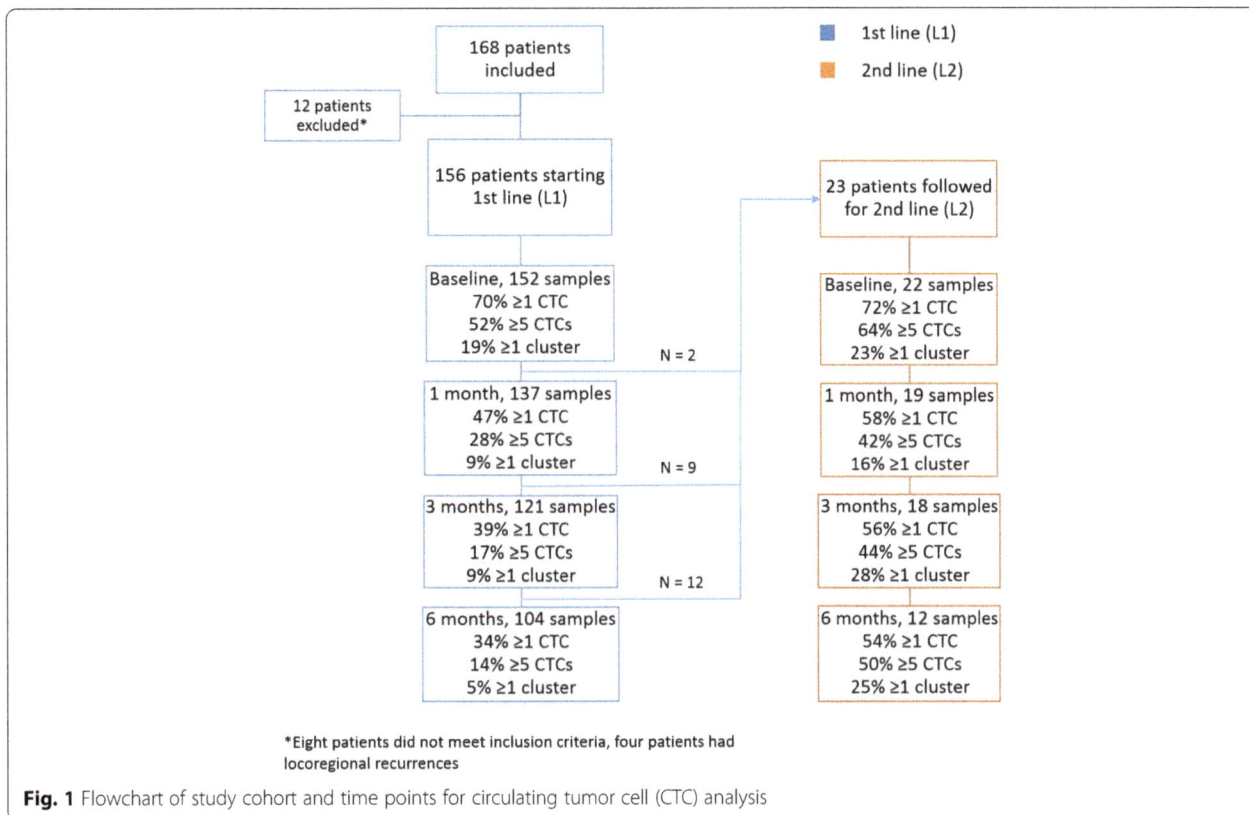

Fig. 1 Flowchart of study cohort and time points for circulating tumor cell (CTC) analysis

(listed in Additional file 3) was 9.01 (95% CI 4.70–17.2). When applying the threshold of ≥ 20 CTCs in relation to outcome (Additional file 4), the HRs for progression or death were higher at all time points compared to analysis with the predefined cutoff of ≥ 5 CTCs, shown in Table 2.

Patients with presence of ≥ 1 CTC cluster at baseline had inferior OS and PFS compared to patients without CTC clusters (Table 2). HRs for presence versus absence of CTC clusters increased during systemic treatment for both PFS and OS (Table 2). For CTC count, on Cox regression with time-dependent covariates there was significantly higher mortality in episodes with CTC clusters compared to episodes without CTC clusters (univariable HR 5.14; 95% CI 2.86–9.24; multivariable HR 6.23; 95% CI 3.56–13.50). In a bivariate Cox model including CTCs ≥ 5 and CTC clusters, mortality was 7.79 times higher during episodes where both factors were unfavorable compared to episodes where both factors were favorable. The corresponding HR for mortality was 11.5 in a model adjusted for clinico-pathological variables.

Stratifying patients based on CTC count and presence of CTC clusters revealed four risk groups (0 CTC; 1–4 CTCs, 0 clusters; ≥ 5 CTCs, 0 clusters; and ≥ 1 CTC, ≥ 1 cluster) where patients with CTC clusters had the worst PFS and OS from all evaluated time points (Fig. 3a-h). When applying the cutoff of ≥ 20 CTCs, presence of CTC clusters was no longer significantly prognostic (data not shown).

To evaluate CTCs as an early predictor of progression in MBC, changes in CTC count from baseline to 1 month or 3 months were analyzed in relation to the outcome of the first evaluation at 3 months (progression versus non-progression). In logistic regression models, patients with a rapid decrease in CTC count (from baseline to 1 month) had an odds of progression that did not differ significantly compared to patients with a consistently low (< 5) CTC count (odds ratio (OR) 1.27; $P = 0.7$, Additional file 5), supporting the notion that a rapid decrease in CTCs is important. In contrast, patients with a high CTC count at 1 month, in addition to those with a high CTC count at 3 months, had significantly higher odds of progression at the 3-month evaluation when compared to patients with low CTC count at baseline and at 1 and 3 months (ORs, 4.21 and 9.16, respectively; Additional file 5). Furthermore, compared to the reference group with persistent low CTC count at baseline and 3 months, patients with a decrease in CTCs from baseline to 3 months had 3.56 times higher odds of progression (9 patients with progression and 36 with non-progressions compared to 4 with progression and 57 with non-progression; OR = (9/36)/(4/57); Additional file 5).

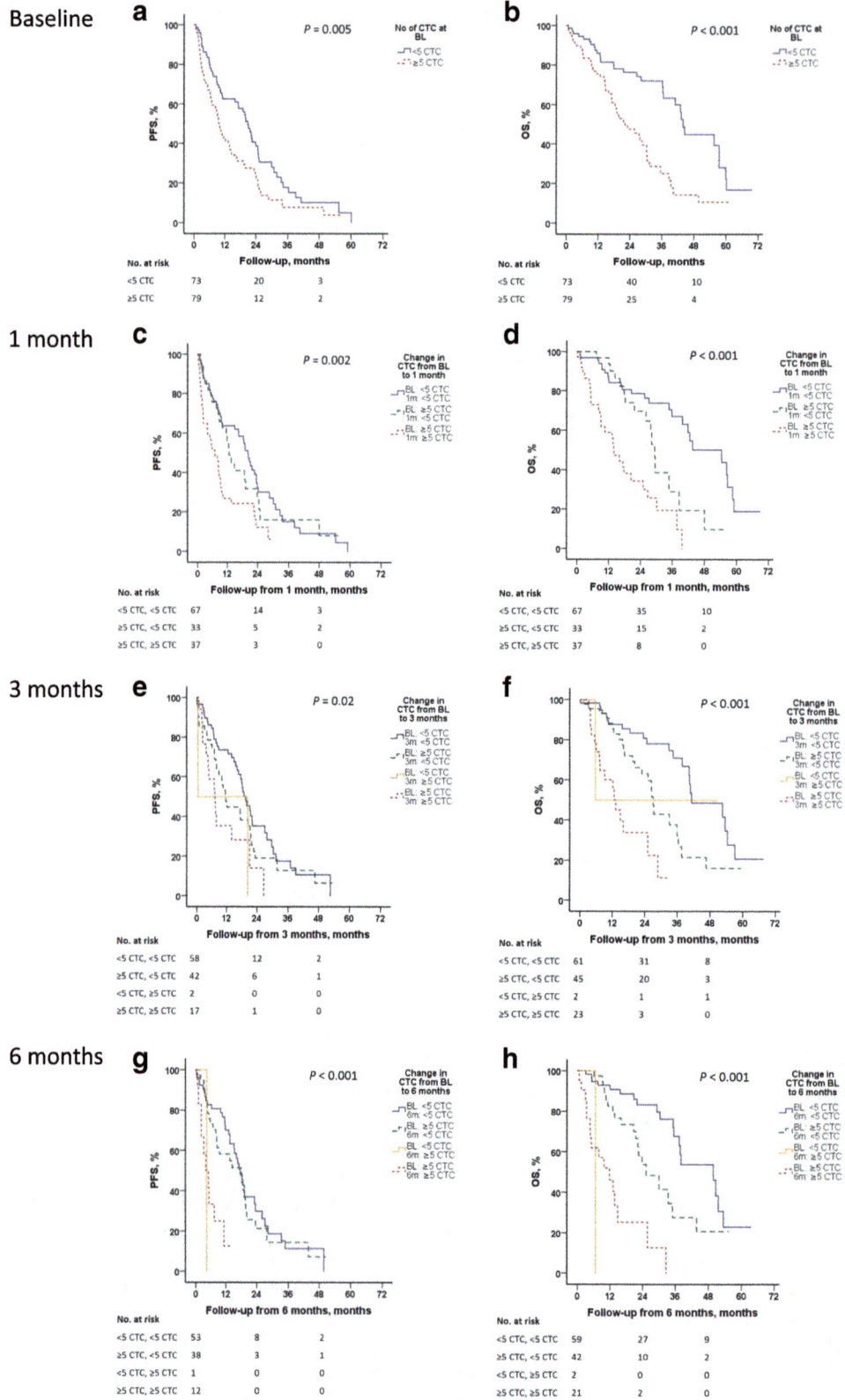

Fig. 2 (See legend on next page.)

(See figure on previous page.)

Fig. 2 Progression-free survival (PFS) and overall survival (OS) by circulating tumor cell (CTC) count. Kaplan-Meier curves displaying PFS and OS by baseline (BL) CTC count (≥ 5 CTCs) (**a-b**), by CTC count at BL and 1 month (**c-d**), by CTC count at BL and 3 months (**e-f**) and by CTC count at BL and 6 months (**g-h**) during the first 6 months of systemic therapy for MBC. Analyses at 1, 3, and 6 months were performed using landmark analysis, in which the follow-up time was recalculated with a new starting date from the 1, 3, and 6-month sample, respectively

Prognostication by a clinicopathological model including CTC count and CTC clusters

To evaluate the value added by CTC count and CTC clusters compared to the currently used clinical prognostic variables, we built a prognostic model based on the previously published model by Bidard et al. [15]. The baseline model included clinicopathological variables reported by Bidard et al. to have significant prognostic value in pooled analysis and included breast cancer subtype, histologic grade, ECOG performance status, age, metastasis-free interval, and visceral metastases (Additional file 3). In addition, the number of metastatic locations was included in our model since this was a significant prognostic marker in univariable analysis in the present cohort. The commonly used serum marker CA15-3 did not show prognostic value in our

Table 2 Cox regression hazard ratios for CTC count ≥ 5 versus < 5, and presence versus absence of CTC clusters

	PFS	P value	OS	P value
	HR (95% CI)		HR (95% CI)	
Baseline				
Unadjusted				
CTC ≥ 5	1.68 (1.17–2.42)	0.005	2.52 (1.58–4.01)	< 0.001
Clusters present	1.54 (1.00–2.40)	0.05	2.23 (1.35–3.69)	0.002
Adjusted[a]				
CTC ≥ 5	2.30 (1.43–3.71)	0.001	3.92 (2.09–7.36)	< 0.001
Clusters present	2.64 (1.46–4.78)	0.001	4.07 (1.99–8.31)	< 0.001
One month[b]				
Unadjusted				
CTC ≥ 5	2.17 (1.43–3.30)	< 0.001	4.38 (2.63–7.30)	< 0.001
Clusters present	3.23 (1.70–-6.14)	< 0.001	4.52 (2.24–9.15)	< 0.001
Adjusted[c]				
CTC ≥ 5	2.30 (1.23–4.32)	0.009	4.39 (2.04–9.43)	< 0.001
Clusters present	3.37 (1.51–7.55)	0.003	5.67 (2.30–13.95)	< 0.001
Three months[b]				
Unadjusted				
CTC ≥ 5	2.24 (1.24–4.03)	0.07	3.28 (1.76–6.12)	< 0.001
Clusters present	3.16 (1.60–6.22)	0.001	3.35 (1.68–6.68)	0.001
Adjusted[c]				
CTC ≥ 5	2.95 (1.44–6.06)	0.003	5.93 (2.62–13.42)	< 0.001
Clusters present	3.04 (1.35–6.84)	0.007	3.55 (1.44–8.77)	0.006
Six months[b]				
Unadjusted				
CTC ≥ 5	4.33 (2.10–8.93)	< 0.001	7.74 (3.52–16.99)	< 0.001
Clusters present	6.48 (2.26–18.56)	0.001	9.92 (3.30–29.78)	< 0.001
Adjusted[c]				
CTC ≥ 5	6.43 (2.30–17.94)	< 0.001	15.72 (3.79–65.17)	< 0.001
Clusters present	7.17 (2.03–25.36)	0.002	21.65 (5.06–92.63)	< 0.001

Abbreviations: PFS progression-free survival, *OS* overall survival, *HR* hazard ratio, *CTC* circulating tumor cell
[a]Adjusted for the variables included in the clinicopathological model (Additional file 3)
[b]Assessed by landmark analysis
[c]Adjusted for the variables included in the clinicopathological model (Additional file 3) and for baseline CTC count (< 5 vs ≥ 5)

Baseline

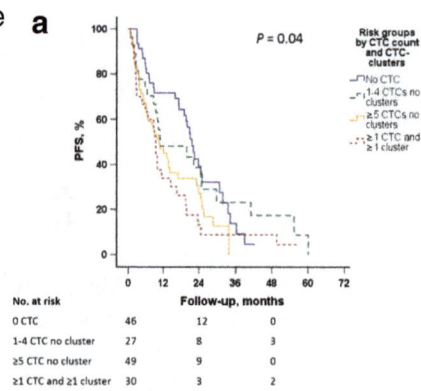

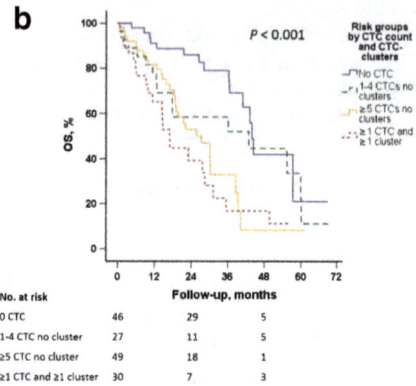

1 month

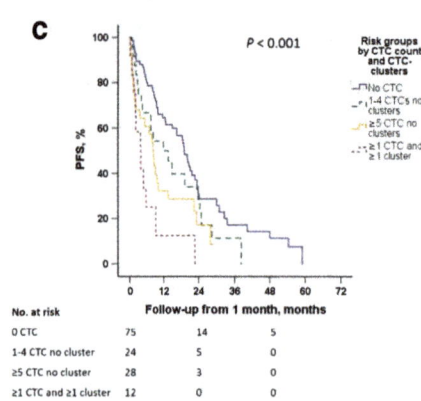

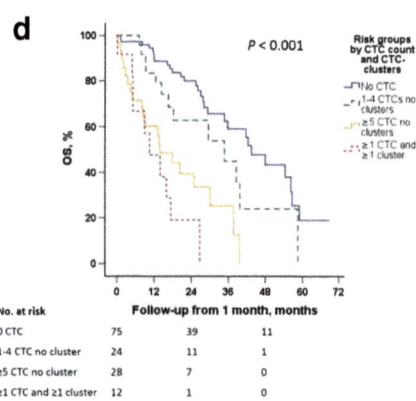

3 months

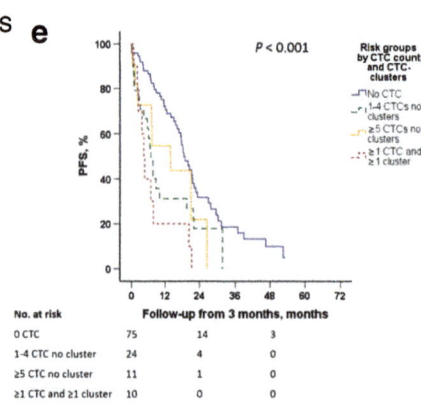

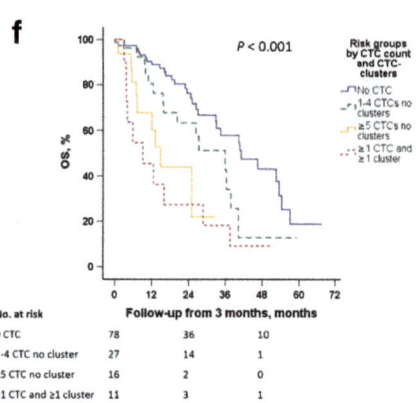

6 months

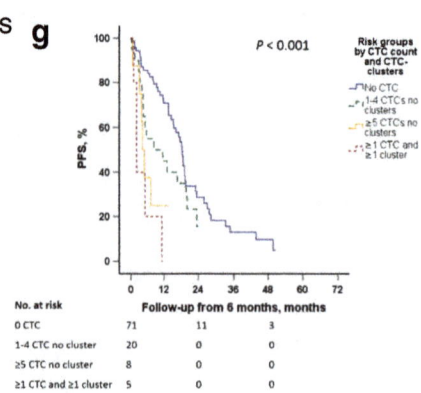

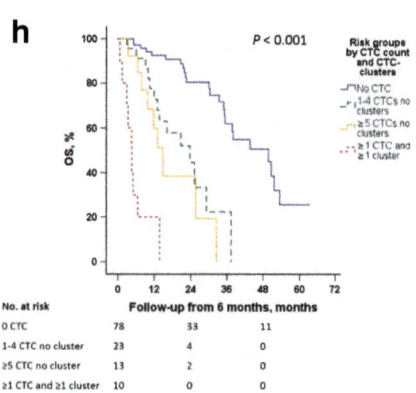

Fig. 3 (See legend on next page.)

(See figure on previous page.)
Fig. 3 Progression-free survival (PFS) and overall survival (OS) by circulating tumor cell (CTC) count and CTC cluster detection. Kaplan-Meier curves displaying PFS and OS by four groups including CTC count and CTC cluster detection at baseline (**a-b**) at 1 month (**c-d**), 3 months (**e-f**) and 6 months (**g-h**). The four groups were patients with no CTCs, patients with 1–4 CTCs and no clusters, patients with ≥ 5 CTCs and no clusters, and patients with > 1 CTC and clusters. Analyses at 1, 3, and 6 months were performed with landmark analysis where the follow-up time was recalculated with a new starting date from the 1, 3, and 6-month samples, respectively

univariable analysis and was therefore not included in the model (Additional file 6).

The addition of baseline CTC count (CTC_{BL}, cutoff ≥ 5 CTCs) and baseline CTC clusters (CTC cluster$_{BL}$, cutoff ≥ 1 cluster of ≥ 2 CTCs) to the baseline clinicopathological model constructed in this cohort, revealed a significant improvement in survival prognostication for both PFS and OS when the variables were added separately (Table 3). Follow-up samples from 1, 3, and 6 months were also evaluated in the prognostic model to assess the value added by CTC count and detection of CTC clusters during treatment. This demonstrated that both CTC count ≥ 5 cells and presence of CTC clusters improved the model at all time points and onwards for both PFS and OS. Notably, the improvement in prognostication was stronger for OS from all follow-up time points (compared to baseline) where CTCs and CTC cluster presence enhanced the model C-index to > 0.80 at 3 and 6 months (Table 3).

Discussion

In this study, we showed that longitudinal evaluation of CTC and CTC cluster dynamics for 6 months improves prognostication and treatment monitoring in patients with MBC who are starting first-line systemic therapy. Elevated CTC count ≥ 5 CTCs and detection of CTC clusters were prognostic from all investigated time points, and independently added significant value to a prognostic clinicopathological model at baseline and during follow up. Importantly, changes in CTC count throughout treatment significantly correlated with survival and the prognostic value was more prominent at later time points. To the best of our knowledge, this is the first study to describe the longitudinal dynamics and independent prognostic value of CTCs and CTC clusters within a prospective cohort of patients newly diagnosed with MBC and starting first-line systemic therapy.

The prognostic value of CTC count in patients with MBC has been confirmed at the highest level of evidence [15] in a pooled analysis; however, previous studies evaluating CTC enumeration in patients with newly diagnosed MBC are sparse and have mainly focused on its prognostic value at baseline [12] or first follow up [9]. Few studies have addressed the value added by detection of CTC clusters [12, 13, 17], and the ones that have, were mostly performed in mixed populations and were not focused on patients starting first-line systemic

therapy. Furthermore, the study design was often retrospective [2, 3, 7] and/or they included only patients fulfilling certain pre-specified criteria such as a specific subtype [14] or type of systemic therapy [6].

During first-line systemic therapy in the present study, CTC count decreased rapidly in most patients indicating systemic treatment efficacy. In contrast, patients who switched to second-line systemic therapy more often had ≥ 5 CTCs and did not experience a similar decline in CTC count during treatment (Fig. 1). A change in CTC count from baseline to follow up at 1, 3, and 6 months was prognostic at all time points, and patients with persistent CTCs ≥ 5 had worse PFS and OS compared to patients with ≥ 5 CTCs at baseline but < 5 CTCs in follow-up samples. This is in accordance with previous studies in cohorts that were more heterogeneous [15, 24] and with a recently published meta-analysis reporting that CTC status predicts treatment response in patients with MBC [16]. In addition, these results support findings in the recent SWOG S0500 trial suggesting that patients with persistent CTCs ≥ 5 during systemic treatment may harbor cancers that are more resistant to chemotherapy [11]. However, CTC enumeration alone is not able to elucidate the molecular mechanisms responsible for therapy resistance, nor provide guidance on the selection of systemic therapy. Further molecular characterization of CTCs is important for this purpose, and might provide a basis for modification of future treatment based on CTC molecular subtyping.

The persistent presence of ≥ 5 CTCs at baseline, 1, and 3 months significantly increased the OR for progression at the first-response evaluation. Interestingly, we found that patients who had a decrease in CTCs from ≥ 5 at baseline to < 5 at 1 month had the same probability of progression at first evaluation as those with consistently low CTC count. The usefulness of CTC count in prediction of treatment efficacy has been shown [16, 25, 26], and our results support the application of CTCs as a marker of therapy response in women with MBC receiving systemic therapy. Our results show that CTC enumeration and CTC clusters are promising candidates for evaluation of therapy efficacy in MBC and provide reliable prognostication during follow up.

This study is one of the largest to evaluate CTC clusters in patients with MBC on first-line systemic therapy during long-term follow up. The results convincingly

Table 3 Prognostic information of CTC count and CTC clusters in a clinicopathological model

Model 1	Model 1 C-index	Model 2	Model 2 C-index	LRχ^2	df	P value
PFS at baseline[a]						
CP	0.690	CP + CTC$_{BL}$	0.707	11.46	1	0.0007
CP	0.690	CP + cluster	0.706	9.47	1	0.0021
CP	0.690	CP + CTC$_{BL}$ + cluster	0.714	14.46	2	0.0007
OS at baseline[a]						
CP	0.752	CP + CTC$_{BL}$	0.786	18.96	1	< 0.0001
CP	0.752	CP + cluster$_{BL}$	0.777	13.16	1	0.0003
CP	0.752	CP + CTC$_{BL}$ + cluster$_{BL}$	0.799	23.54	2	< 0.0001
PFS at 1 month[b]						
CP + CTC$_{BL}$	0.697	CP + CTC$_{BL}$ + CTC$_{1M}$	0.709	6.69	1	0.0097
CP + CTC$_{BL}$	0.697	CP + CTC$_{BL}$ + cluster$_{1M}$	0.712	7.56	1	0.0060
CP + CTC$_{BL}$	0.697	CP + CTC$_{BL}$ + CTC$_{1M}$+cluster$_{1M}$	0.713	10.56	2	0.0051
OS at 1 month[b]						
CP + CTC$_{BL}$	0.766	CP + CTC$_{BL}$ + CTC$_{1M}$	0.812	15.73	1	0.0001
CP + CTC$_{BL}$	0.766	CP + CTC$_{BL}$ + cluster$_{1M}$	0.788	12.01	1	0.0005
CP + CTC$_{BL}$	0.766	CP + CTC$_{BL}$ + CTC$_{1M}$+cluster$_{1M}$	0.817	20.57	2	< 0.0001
PFS at 3 months[b]						
CP + CTC$_{BL}$	0.695	CP + CTC$_{BL}$ + CTC$_{3M}$	0.701	7.31	1	0.0068
CP + CTC$_{BL}$	0.695	CP + CTC$_{BL}$ + cluster$_{3M}$	0.711	6.22	1	0.0126
CP + CTC$_{BL}$	0.695	CP + CTC$_{BL}$ + CTC$_{3M}$+cluster$_{3M}$	0.710	9.01	2	0.0110
OS at 3 months[b]						
CP + CTC$_{BL}$	0.774	CP + CTC$_{BL}$ + CTC$_{3M}$	0.806	14.76	1	0.0001
CP + CTC$_{BL}$	0.774	CP + CTC$_{BL}$ + cluster$_{3M}$	0.806	7.02	1	0.0081
CP + CTC$_{BL}$	0.774	CP + CTC$_{BL}$ + CTC$_{3M}$+cluster$_{3M}$	0.806	15.16	2	0.0005
PFS at 6 months[b]						
CP + CTC$_{BL}$	0.694	CP + CTC$_{BL}$ + CTC$_{6M}$	0.732	11.14	1	0.0008
CP + CTC$_{BL}$	0.694	CP + CTC$_{BL}$ + cluster$_{6M}$	0.709	7.14	1	0.0075
CP + CTC$_{BL}$	0.694	CP + CTC$_{BL}$ + CTC$_{6M}$+cluster$_{6M}$	0.727	12.14	2	0.0023
OS at 6 months[b]						
CP + CTC$_{BL}$	0.758	CP + CTC$_{BL}$ + CTC$_{6M}$	0.804	15.88	1	0.0001
CP + CTC$_{BL}$	0.758	CP + CTC$_{BL}$ + cluster$_{6M}$	0.813	13.24	1	0.0003
CP + CTC$_{BL}$	0.758	CP + CTC$_{BL}$ + CTC$_{6M}$+cluster$_{6M}$	0.818	20.66	2	< 0.0001

Abbreviations: BL baseline, 3M 3 months, 6M 6 months, df degrees of freedom, LRχ^2 likelihood ratio chi-square, CP clinicopathological model, CTC circulating tumor cell, PFS progression-free survival, OS overall survival
[a]Adjusted for subtype, histologic grade, performance status (Eastern Cooperative Oncology Group (ECOG)), age, metastasis-free interval (MFI), visceral metastases, and number of metastatic locations
[b]Adjusted for baseline CTC count ≥ 5, subtype, histologic grade, performance status (ECOG), age, MFI, visceral metastases, and number of metastatic locations. Analyses at 1, 3, and 6 months were performed by landmark analysis

showed that the presence of CTC clusters was significantly and independently prognostic at all investigated time points and could identify patients with worse prognosis than those with ≥ 5 CTCs alone. This is in line with our previous results [17] and other recently published studies showing that CTC clusters add prognostic value to CTC enumeration in women with MBC [12, 13]. Incorporating CTC counts and CTC clusters into the clinicopathologic prognostication model proposed by Bidard et al. revealed that these factors significantly improved prognostication at all time points for both PFS and OS. Cox regression analysis of OS with time-varying covariates showed that mortality was increased for episodes with concomitant presence of CTCs ≥ 5 and CTC clusters (HRs, 5.7 and 5.1, respectively), thus confirming the poor prognosis over time in patients with high CTC count and presence of CTC clusters. For patients with both high CTC count (CTCs ≥ 5) and presence of CTC clusters, the mortality was 11 times higher than in patients without these factors when adjusting for standard clinicopathological variables. However, presence of ≥ 20 CTCs was strongly associated with the presence of CTC clusters, and thus CTC clusters did not add any significant prognostic information after adjustment for a high CTC count ≥ 20. Notably, half of patients with ≥ 20 CTCs did not have CTC clusters, and some patients with a CTC count < 5 did have CTC clusters. There were few patients with a high CTC count without clusters and a low CTC count and presence of CTC clusters (Additional file 2), therefore it would not have been meaningful to perform survival analyses for these subgroups. These results further support the use of CTC count and CTC cluster presence to improve prognostication in patients with MBC at baseline and during follow-up.

The presence of CTC clusters added significant value independently of CTC count ≥ 5 CTCs, which underlines the importance of future research focusing on the biological significance of CTC clusters in patients with MBC. Previous studies have shown that CTC clusters have a higher metastatic potential than single CTCs [27–30] and CTC cluster-mediated metastasis has emerged as an alternative model of metastatic seeding along with epithelial-mesenchymal transition (EMT) [18]. Others hypothesize that clusters shed into the circulation as an entity composed of several tumor cells [27] and sometimes with platelets and/or leukocytes. This is in contrast to the EMT model in which single cells enter the bloodstream after transformation into a mesenchymal phenotype. Clearly, the clusters are tumor cells with an improved capacity to survive in the circulation and can avoid clearance by sheer force. Several studies have shown that none or very few CTCs within clusters are apoptotic, whereas a relatively large number of single CTCs are [14, 17, 31]. The widely used CellSearch system easily identifies CTC clusters and thus it would be feasible to assess them in all centers that possess this technology.

Survival analysis was performed including patients with 1–4 CTCs (normally considered low risk and grouped with patients with no CTCs) as a separate group to further explore CTC count and CTC cluster detection. This revealed that 6 months after therapy initiation, patients with 1–4 CTCs had PFS and OS closer to patients with ≥ 5 CTCs than to patients with no CTCs, indicating that even a small number of CTCs in addition to the predefined prognostic cutoff ≥ 5 CTCs [1, 15] might be informative at later follow-up time points. In early breast cancer, a prognostic CTC cutoff ≥ 1 CTC has been proposed [32], and in a metastatic setting this has also been suggested as an alternative cutoff [33]. Furthermore, a threshold of ≥20 CTCs was linked to higher incidence of progression and death at all time points, compared to when the predefined cutoff ≥ 5 CTCs was applied. This study was not powered to evaluate cutoffs other than the predefined cutoff ≥ 5 CTCs and our results support the prognostic value of this cutoff. However, our findings also suggest that the threshold for CTC number needs to be interpreted with care (Fig. 3a-h), particularly during follow up. CTC dynamics over time seem to be essential for estimating prognosis, especially in patients with a reduction in CTCs during treatment for whom the estimated prognosis improves.

A strength of this study is the prospective design of serial CTC and CTC cluster evaluation over 6 months in women with newly diagnosed MBC, including sampling before the start of first-line systemic therapy and structured evaluation at pre-specified intervals. The median follow-up time from baseline was 25 (range 7–69) months and the follow-up data were extensive as few patients terminated the study prematurely. Molecular data to determine breast cancer subtype were available from metastasis biopsies from 73% of patients. Furthermore, the treating physicians were blinded to the CTC results, which avoided treatment bias. This study thus enabled investigation of the presence and dynamics of CTCs and CTC clusters during the first 6 months of treatment, and we applied structured monitoring and blood sampling at predefined time points. A potential weakness of this study is the long inclusion period related to the strict inclusion criteria that included only newly diagnosed cases of MBC before the start of first-line therapy and ECOG performance status score between 0 and 2. Moreover, we included patients irrespective of type of systemic therapy and thus we can draw no conclusion on treatment response related to a specific type of therapy.

Conclusion

The results of this study support the clinical utility of longitudinal CTC and CTC cluster evaluation for prognostication and treatment monitoring in patients with MBC, who are starting first-line systemic therapy. The prognostic value of CTC count ≥ 5 CTCs and CTC cluster evaluation increased over time, suggesting that the dynamic changes in CTCs and CTC clusters are more relevant to prognosis than a single baseline enumeration. Presence of CTC clusters added significant prognostic value to CTC enumeration alone and standard clinicopathological characteristics at all time points and could identify a subgroup of patients with a notably worse prognosis. These findings are highly relevant for improving prognostication in MBC and in helping clinicians monitor patients with MBC during systemic therapy.

Additional files

> **Additional file 1:** Supplementary information: power calculation performed before initiation of the study. (PDF 483 kb)
>
> **Additional file 2: Figure S1.** CTC count as a continuous variable in relation to presence of CTC clusters. (PDF 182 kb)
>
> **Additional file 3: Table S1.** Multivariable Cox regression analysis of prognostic variables. (PDF 426 kb)
>
> **Additional file 4: Table S2.** Unadjusted Cox regression HRs for CTC count ≥ 5 vs < 5 CTCs, and CTC count ≥ 20 vs < 20 CTCs. (PDF 114 kb)
>
> **Additional file 5: Table S3.** Change in CTC count in relation to progression versus non-progression at first radiological evaluation. (PDF 131 kb)
>
> **Additional file 6: Table S4.** Unadjusted Cox regression analyses of patient and tumor characteristics at baseline. (PDF 146 kb)

Abbreviations

BL: Baseline; CI: Confidence interval; CK: Cytokeratin; CR: Complete response; CTC: Circulating tumor cell; ECOG: Eastern Cooperative Oncology Group; EMT: Epithelial-mesenchymal transition; EpCAM: Epithelial cell adhesion molecule; ER: Estrogen receptor; FU: Follow-up; HER2: Human epidermal growth factor receptor 2; HR: Hazard ratio; KM: Kaplan-Meier; LR: Likelihood ratio; MBC: Metastatic breast cancer; OR: Odds ratio; OS: Overall survival; PFS: Progression-free survival; PgR: Progesterone receptor; PR: Partial response; RECIST: Response Evaluation Criteria in Solid Tumors; REMARK: Reporting recommendations for tumor marker; SD: Stable disease; TNBC: Triple-negative breast cancer

Acknowledgements

We thank the research nurses Anette Ahlin-Gullers, Jessica Åkesson, Emma Edvik, Lina Zander, and Petra Andersson, and the clinical oncologists at Skåne University Hospital and Halmstad County Hospital for their invaluable work in the inclusion of patients during the study period.
We thank the laboratory technicians Kristina Lövgren, Anna Ebbesson, Sara Baker, and Charlotte Welinder, PhD, for skilled technical assistance in the CellSearch analysis.

Funding

Anna-Maria Larsson and Lisa Rydén: Governmental Funding of Clinical Research within the National Health Services. Lisa Rydén: BioCARE, a Strategic Research Program at Lund University, Mrs. Bertha Kamprad Foundation BKS 44/2015 and FBKS 2017-39, Crafoord Foundation 20150961 and 20170702, The Swedish Cancer Society 2010/1234 2013/533, 2016/563, Swedish Research Council 2015-02516, Skåne University Hospital Funds 2017-92502.

Authors' contributions

A-ML and SJ were involved in conception and design of the study, took part in acquisition of data, analysis and interpretation of data, and drafting and reviewing of the manuscript. P-OB was engaged in conception and design of the study, was responsible for data analysis, and was involved in interpretation of data, and drafting and reviewing of the manuscript. CLTJ, NL, CG, and LL were involved in acquisition of data and reviewed the manuscript. KA was involved in conception and design of the study, development of methodology, interpretation of data, and reviewing the manuscript. LR was responsible for conception and design, development of methodology, and acquisition and analysis of data, and was involved in drafting and reviewing of the manuscript. All authors approved the final version of the manuscript. A-ML and SJ contributed equally to the work.

Competing interests

The authors declare that they have no competing interests.

Author details

[1]Department of Clinical Sciences Lund, Division of Oncology and Pathology, Lund University, Lund, Sweden. [2]Department of Hematology, Oncology and Radiation Physics, Skåne University Hospital, Lund, Sweden. [3]Department of Clinical Sciences Lund, Division of Surgery, Lund University, Medicon Village, SE-223 81 Lund, Sweden. [4]Department of Surgery and Gastroenterology, Skåne University Hospital, Malmö, Sweden.

References

1. Cristofanilli M, Budd GT, Ellis MJ, Stopeck A, Matera J, Miller MC, Reuben JM, Doyle GV, Allard WJ, Terstappen LW, et al. Circulating tumor cells, disease progression, and survival in metastatic breast cancer. N Engl J Med. 2004;351(8):781–91.
2. Cristofanilli M, Broglio KR, Guarneri V, Jackson S, Fritsche HA, Islam R, Dawood S, Reuben JM, Kau SW, Lara JM, et al. Circulating tumor cells in metastatic breast cancer: biologic staging beyond tumor burden. Clin Breast Cancer. 2007;7(6):471–9.
3. Dawood S, Broglio K, Valero V, Reuben J, Handy B, Islam R, Jackson S, Hortobagyi GN, Fritsche H, Cristofanilli M. Circulating tumor cells in metastatic breast cancer: from prognostic stratification to modification of the staging system? Cancer. 2008;113(9):2422–30.
4. Nole F, Munzone E, Zorzino L, Minchella I, Salvatici M, Botteri E, Medici M, Verri E, Adamoli L, Rotmensz N, et al. Variation of circulating tumor cell levels during treatment of metastatic breast cancer: prognostic and therapeutic implications. Ann Oncol. 2008; 19(5):891–7.
5. Nakamura S, Yagata H, Ohno S, Yamaguchi H, Iwata H, Tsunoda N, Ito Y, Tokudome N, Toi M, Kuroi K, et al. Multi-center study evaluating circulating tumor cells as a surrogate for response to treatment and overall survival in metastatic breast cancer. Breast Cancer. 2010;17(3):199–204.
6. Hartkopf AD, Wagner P, Wallwiener D, Fehm T, Rothmund R. Changing levels of circulating tumor cells in monitoring chemotherapy response in patients with metastatic breast cancer. Anticancer Res. 2011;31(3):979–84.
7. Giuliano M, Giordano A, Jackson S, Hess KR, De Giorgi U, Mego M, Handy BC, Ueno NT, Alvarez RH, De Laurentiis M, et al. Circulating tumor cells as prognostic and predictive markers in metastatic breast cancer patients receiving first-line systemic treatment. Breast Cancer Res. 2011;13(3):R67.
8. Pierga JY, Hajage D, Bachelot T, Delaloge S, Brain E, Campone M, Dieras V, Rolland E, Mignot L, Mathiot C, et al. High independent prognostic and predictive value of circulating tumor cells compared with serum tumor markers in a large prospective trial in first-line chemotherapy for metastatic breast cancer patients. Ann Oncol. 2012;23(3):618–24.
9. Martin M, Custodio S, de Las Casas ML, Garcia-Saenz JA, de la Torre JC, Bellon-Cano JM, Lopez-Tarruella S, Vidaurreta-Lazaro M, de la Orden V, Jerez Y, et al. Circulating tumor cells following first chemotherapy cycle: an early and strong predictor of outcome in patients with metastatic breast cancer. Oncologist. 2013;18(8):917–23.
10. Wallwiener M, Riethdorf S, Hartkopf AD, Modugno C, Nees J, Madhavan D, Sprick MR, Schott S, Domschke C, Baccelli I, et al. Serial enumeration of circulating tumor cells predicts treatment response and prognosis in metastatic breast cancer: a prospective study in 393 patients. BMC Cancer. 2014;14:512.
11. Smerage JB, Barlow WE, Hortobagyi GN, Winer EP, Leyland-Jones B, Srkalovic G, Tejwani S, Schott AF, O'Rourke MA, Lew DL, et al. Circulating tumor cells and response to chemotherapy in metastatic breast cancer: SWOG S0500. J Clin Oncol. 2014;32(31):3483–9.
12. Mu Z, Wang C, Ye Z, Austin L, Civan J, Hyslop T, Palazzo JP, Jaslow R, Li B, Myers RE, et al. Prospective assessment of the prognostic value of circulating tumor cells and their clusters in patients with advanced-stage breast cancer. Breast Cancer Res Treat. 2015;154(3):563–71.

13. Wang C, Mu Z, Chervoneva I, Austin L, Ye Z, Rossi G, Palazzo JP, Sun C, Abu-Khalaf M, Myers RE, et al. Longitudinally collected CTCs and CTC-clusters and clinical outcomes of metastatic breast cancer. Breast Cancer Res Treat. 2017;161(1):83–94.

14. Paoletti C, Li Y, Muniz MC, Kidwell KM, Aung K, Thomas DG, Brown ME, Abramson VG, Irvin WJ Jr, Lin NU, et al. Significance of circulating tumor cells in metastatic triple-negative breast cancer patients within a randomized, phase II trial: TBCRC 019. Clin Cancer Res. 2015;21(12):2771–9.

15. Bidard FC, Peeters DJ, Fehm T, Nole F, Gisbert-Criado R, Mavroudis D, Grisanti S, Generali D, Garcia-Saenz JA, Stebbing J, et al. Clinical validity of circulating tumour cells in patients with metastatic breast cancer: a pooled analysis of individual patient data. Lancet Oncol. 2014;15(4):406–14.

16. Yan WT, Cui X, Chen Q, Li YF, Cui YH, Wang Y, Jiang J. Circulating tumor cell status monitors the treatment responses in breast cancer patients: a meta-analysis. Sci Rep. 2017;7:43464. https://doi.org/10.1038/srep43464.

17. Jansson S, Bendahl PO, Larsson AM, Aaltonen KE, Ryden L. Prognostic impact of circulating tumor cell apoptosis and clusters in serial blood samples from patients with metastatic breast cancer in a prospective observational cohort. BMC Cancer. 2016;16:433.

18. Fabisiewicz A, Grzybowska E. CTC clusters in cancer progression and metastasis. Med Oncol. 2017;34(1):12. https://doi.org/10.1007/s12032-016-0875-0.

19. Eisenhauer EA, Therasse P, Bogaerts J, Schwartz LH, Sargent D, Ford R, Dancey J, Arbuck S, Gwyther S, Mooney M, et al. New response evaluation criteria in solid tumours: revised RECIST guideline (version 1.1). Eur J Cancer. 2009;45(2):228–47.

20. Allard WJ, Matera J, Miller MC, Repollet M, Connelly MC, Rao C, Tibbe AG, Uhr JW, Terstappen LW. Tumor cells circulate in the peripheral blood of all major carcinomas but not in healthy subjects or patients with nonmalignant diseases. Clin Cancer Res. 2004;10(20):6897–904.

21. Botteri E, Sandri MT, Bagnardi V, Munzone E, Zorzino L, Rotmensz N, Casadio C, Cassatella MC, Esposito A, Curigliano G, et al. Modeling the relationship between circulating tumour cells number and prognosis of metastatic breast cancer. Breast Cancer Res Treat. 2010;122(1):211–7.

22. McShane LM, Altman DG, Sauerbrei W, Taube SE, Gion M, Clark GM. Reporting recommendations for tumor marker prognostic studies (REMARK). J Natl Cancer Inst. 2005;97(16):1180–4.

23. Molenberghs G, Kenward MG. Missing data in clinical studies, 1st edition. Chichester: Wiley; 2007.

24. Hayes DF, Cristofanilli M, Budd GT, Ellis MJ, Stopeck A, Miller MC, Matera J, Allard WJ, Doyle GV, Terstappen LW. Circulating tumor cells at each follow-up time point during therapy of metastatic breast cancer patients predict progression-free and overall survival. Clin Cancer Res. 2006;12(14 Pt 1):4218–24.

25. Budd GT, Cristofanilli M, Ellis MJ, Stopeck A, Borden E, Miller MC, Matera J, Repollet M, Doyle GV, Terstappen LW, et al. Circulating tumor cells versus imaging–predicting overall survival in metastatic breast cancer. Clin Cancer Res. 2006;12(21):6403–9.

26. Liu MC, Shields PG, Warren RD, Cohen P, Wilkinson M, Ottaviano YL, Rao SB, Eng-Wong J, Seillier-Moiseiwitsch F, Noone AM, et al. Circulating tumor cells: a useful predictor of treatment efficacy in metastatic breast cancer. J Clin Oncol. 2009;27(31):5153–9.

27. Aceto N, Bardia A, Miyamoto DT, Donaldson MC, Wittner BS, Spencer JA. Yu M, Pely A, Engstrom A, Zhu H et al: Circulating tumor cell clusters are oligoclonal precursors of breast cancer metastasis. Cell. 2014;158(5):1110–22.

28. Watanabe S. The metastasizability of tumor cells. Cancer. 1954;7(2):215–23.

29. Fidler IJ. The relationship of embolic homogeneity, number, size and viability to the incidence of experimental metastasis. Eur J Cancer. 1973;9(3):223–7.

30. Liotta LA, Saidel MG, Kleinerman J. The significance of hematogenous tumor cell clumps in the metastatic process. Cancer Res. 1976;36(3):889–94.

31. Hou JM, Krebs MG, Lancashire L, Sloane R, Backen A, Swain RK, Priest LJ, Greystoke A, Zhou C, Morris K, et al. Clinical significance and molecular characteristics of circulating tumor cells and circulating tumor microemboli in patients with small-cell lung cancer. J Clin Oncol. 2012;30(5):525–32.

32. Rack B, Schindlbeck C, Juckstock J, Andergassen U, Hepp P, Zwingers T, Friedl TW, Lorenz R, Tesch H, Fasching PA, et al. Circulating tumor cells predict survival in early average-to-high risk breast cancer patients. J Natl Cancer Inst. 2014;106(5):1-11. https://doi.org/10.1093/jnci/dju273.

33. Shiomi-Mouri Y, Kousaka J, Ando T, Tetsuka R, Nakano S, Yoshida M, Fujii K, Akizuki M, Imai T, Fukutomi T, et al. Clinical significance of circulating tumor cells (CTCs) with respect to optimal cut-off value and tumor markers in advanced/metastatic breast cancer. Breast Cancer. 2016;23(1):120–7.

17

Foxf2 plays a dual role during transforming growth factor beta-induced epithelial to mesenchymal transition by promoting apoptosis yet enabling cell junction dissolution and migration

Nathalie Meyer-Schaller[1,2†], Chantal Heck[1,3†], Stefanie Tiede[1], Mahmut Yilmaz[1,4] and Gerhard Christofori[1*] (iD)

Abstract

Background: The most life-threatening step during malignant tumor progression is reached when cancer cells leave the primary tumor mass and seed metastasis in distant organs. To infiltrate the surrounding tissue and disseminate throughout the body, single motile tumor cells leave the tumor mass by breaking down cell-cell contacts in a process called epithelial to mesenchymal transition (EMT). An EMT is a complex molecular and cellular program enabling epithelial cells to abandon their differentiated phenotype, including cell-cell adhesion and cell polarity, and to acquire mesenchymal features and invasive properties.

Methods: We employed gene expression profiling and functional experiments to study transcriptional control of transforming growth factor (TGF)β-induced EMT in normal murine mammary gland epithelial (NMuMG) cells.

Results: We identified that expression of the transcription factor forkhead box protein F2 (Foxf2) is upregulated during the EMT process. Although it is not required to gain mesenchymal markers, Foxf2 is essential for the disruption of cell junctions and the downregulation of epithelial markers in NMuMG cells treated with TGFβ. Foxf2 is critical for the downregulation of E-cadherin by promoting the expression of the transcriptional repressors of E-cadherin, Zeb1 and Zeb2, while repressing expression of the epithelial maintenance factor Id2 and miRNA 200 family members. Moreover, Foxf2 is required for TGFβ-mediated apoptosis during EMT by the transcriptional activation of the proapoptotic BH3-only protein Noxa and by the negative regulation of epidermal growth factor receptor (EGFR)-mediated survival signaling through direct repression of its ligands betacellulin and amphiregulin. The dual function of Foxf2 during EMT is underscored by the finding that high Foxf2 expression correlates with good prognosis in patients with early noninvasive stages of breast cancer, but with poor prognosis in advanced breast cancer.

Conclusions: Our data identify the transcription factor Foxf2 as one of the important regulators of EMT, displaying a dual function in promoting tumor cell apoptosis as well as tumor cell migration.

Keywords: Apoptosis, Breast cancer, Cell migration, E-cadherin, EGFR, EMT, Foxf2, Noxa

* Correspondence: gerhard.christofori@unibas.ch
†Nathalie Meyer-Schaller and Chantal Heck contributed equally to this work.
[1]Department of Biomedicine, University of Basel, Mattenstrasse 28, 4058 Basel, Switzerland
Full list of author information is available at the end of the article

Background

The process of epithelial to mesenchymal transition (EMT) describes a complex molecular and cellular program by which epithelial cells abandon their differentiated features and acquire mesenchymal characteristics, including motility, invasiveness, and increased resistance to apoptosis [1–5]. EMT has been implicated in several physiological as well as pathological processes. While it is a critical mechanism for embryonic development, EMT is re-engaged in adults during wound healing, tissue regeneration, organ fibrosis, and cancer progression and metastasis [2]. Recent studies implicate that primary tumors displaying an EMT-like gene expression profile are more likely to be associated with distant metastasis formation and a worse prognosis for overall survival [6–8]. In contradiction to these findings are the observations that distant metastases frequently exhibit an epithelial phenotype highly similar to the primary tumor [9, 10]. Explaining this observation, it has been shown that disseminated mesenchymal cancer cells undergo the reverse process (mesenchymal to epithelial transition (MET)) after metastatic spread and colonization and revert to a differentiated, epithelial cell state enabling them to establish in the distant location [11–13]. However, the contribution of EMT to the metastatic process is debated. Recent lineage tracing experiments have suggested that EMT is required for the development of drug resistance but not for metastasis [14, 15]. However, these reports have been met with great skepticism and data questioning these results [16–18]. In summary, overwhelming evidence supports the conclusion that EMT and its reverse process MET are pivotal regulators of cell plasticity in malignant tumor progression and play important roles in drug resistance, relapse, and metastatic progression [19].

Recently, a number of transcription factors have been identified that play critical roles in the initiation and execution of an EMT and in the metastatic process, including Snail (Snail), Snai2 (Slug), Zeb1 (δEF1), Zeb2 (Sip1), E47, Twist, goosecoid, Foxc2, Dlx2, RBPjκ, Yap/Taz, Sox4 and 9, Klf4, and NFκB [3, 19–22]. We have previously established a list of genes that change in their expression during the consecutive morphological states of transforming growth factor (TGF)β-induced EMT in normal murine mammary gland (NMuMG) epithelial cells [20, 23]. This analysis identified forkhead box protein F2 (Foxf2) as a transcription factor that is upregulated in its expression during EMT in NMuMG cells and in several other experimental EMT systems. The family of Forkhead box (Fox) genes are defined by a conserved DNA binding domain of a winged helix structure acting as transcription factors, which have been found to serve as key regulators in embryogenesis, signal transduction, maintenance of differentiated cell states, and tumorigenesis [24]. There are three families of Fox genes, Foxc, Foxf, and Foxl1, that form paralogous clusters in the genome and that are extensively expressed in mesodermal tissue [25, 26]. One of the best characterized members of this family is Foxc2, which has been implicated in the regulation of EMT by interacting with Smad proteins and to be a key player in metastasis [27, 28]. Moreover, Foxc1 and Foxc2 are highly expressed in the claudin-low metaplastic breast cancer subtype, which is associated with EMT and cancer stemness [29]. Furthermore, the overexpression of Foxm1 in pancreatic cancer cells leads to the acquisition of an EMT phenotype via upregulation of Zeb1 and Zeb2 as well as stem cell-like characteristics [30].

Foxf2 (also known as Freac-2 or Fkhl6) is a widely expressed protein in various mesenchymal tissues and was first identified as a transcriptional activator containing a forkhead domain for nuclear localization and two independent C-terminal activation domains [31]. Foxf2 interacts with TBP and TFIIB, two components of the general transcriptional activator complex binding a specific DNA motif [32, 33]. Expression of several Fox family genes, including Foxf1 and Foxf2, is specifically regulated by sonic hedgehog (Shh) signaling in a crosstalk with Notch, epidermal growth factor (EGF)/fibroblast growth factor (FGF), and TGFβ signaling [34, 35]. Indeed, TGFβ-induced EMT is one of the mechanisms strongly involved in regulating fusion of the palatal cleft, and Foxf2 levels are high in the mesenchyme of the secondary palate and in the mesenchyme of the lung and gut [36, 37]. Accordingly, Foxf2-deficient mice die shortly after birth due to cleft palate and abnormal tongue and gut development, indicating an essential role of Foxf2 in this EMT-associated developmental process [38, 39]. Epithelial cells of Foxf2-deficient mice show typical signs of depolarization, and the subcellular localization of adherens junctions, normally confined to lateral membranes, expands into the basal and apical membranes.

In many cancer types, the expression of Foxf2 is repressed by promoter hypermethylation or by oncogenic microRNAs (miRNAs), such as miR-301, which promotes breast cancer cell proliferation, invasion, and tumor growth [40, 41], indicating that Foxf2 may act as a tumor suppressor. However, other studies have reported a protumorigenic role of Foxf2 in other cancer types (reviewed in [41]), for example by repressing intestinal stem cells and preventing adenoma formation by inhibiting Wnt signaling [42]. Furthermore, low Foxf2 expression has been reported to correlate with early-onset metastasis and poor prognosis in breast cancer patients [43], and loss of Foxf2 expression promotes an EMT and metastasis of experimental cancer [44, 45]. These conflicting results seem to mirror a double-sided role for Foxf2 in maintaining tissue homeostasis, in regulating an EMT, and in breast cancer progression [46].

Here, we have employed a TGFβ-induced EMT in NMuMG cells and in murine and human breast cancer cells to demonstrate a critical role of Foxf2 during an EMT by concomitantly regulating an EMT, cell survival, and apoptosis. The mechanistic insights into Foxf2 functions also support a dual role of Foxf2 in breast cancer progression and metastasis, on one hand by affecting cell junction homeostasis, and by regulating cell proliferation and survival on the other hand.

Methods

Reagents and antibodies
See Additional file 1.

Cell culture and cell lines
All reagents used for cell culture were obtained from Sigma/Fluka (Basel, Switzerland) if not otherwise mentioned. All cells were cultured at 37 °C with 5% CO_2 in Dulbecco's modified Eagle's medium (DMEM) supplemented with glutamine (2 mM), penicillin (100 U), streptomycin (0.2 mg/l) and 10% fetal bovine serum (FBS). The subclone NMuMG/E9 (hereafter called NMuMG) is expressing E-cadherin and has previously been described [47]. MTΔEcad and MCF7-shEcad have been described previously [23]. NMuMG-shSmad4 and NMuMG-shCtr were obtained from P. ten Dijke (Leiden University Medical Center, The Netherlands) [48]. Py2T breast cancer cells were established from a tumor of the MMTV-PyMT mouse model of breast cancer as previously described [49]. NMuMG cells were treated with TGFβ (2 ng/ml) without serum deprivation, and TGFβ was replenished every 2 days. siRNA transfections with lipofectamine RNAiMAX (Invitrogen) were performed according to the manufacturer's protocol 24 h before treatment with TGFβ.

Generation of lentivirus
A cDNA encoding Foxf2 (kindly provided by Leif Lundh, Goteborg University, Sweden) [50] was tagged N-terminally with HA-tag and cloned into the lentiviral expression vector pLenti-CMV-Puro (kindly provided by Matthias Kaeser, Bern). Lentiviral particles were produced by transfecting HEK293T cells with the lentiviral expression vectors in combination with the packaging vector pR8.91 and the envelope encoding vector pVSV using Fugene HD (Roche). After 2 days, the virus-containing HEK293T supernatant was harvested, filtered (0.45 μm), supplemented with polybrene (8 ng/ml), and used for target cell infection. Infections were performed twice a day on 2 consecutive days.

Growth curves
One day before t_0, 1.6×10^4 NMuMG cells were seeded in triplicate into 24-well plates and transfected with the indicated siRNA. After 24 h the cells were treated with TGFβ and cell numbers were determined using a Neubauer counting chamber.

Migration assay
NMuMG cells (2×10^4/well) pretreated for 18 days with TGFβ were seeded in DMEM, 2% FBS, and TGFβ into the upper chamber of a cell culture insert (pore size 8 μm; Falcon BD, Franklin Lakes, NJ). The lower chamber was filled with DMEM, 20% FBS, and TGFβ. After 16 h incubation at 37 °C and 5% CO_2, the cells that had traversed the membrane were fixed in 4% paraformaldehyde/phosphate-buffered saline (PBS) (15 min at room temperature), stained with DAPI (0.5 μg/ml), and counted using a fluorescence microscope.

Quantitative real-time polymerase chain reaction (RT-PCR)
Total RNA was prepared using Tri Reagent (Sigma-Aldrich), reverse transcribed with ImProm-II Reverse Transcriptase (Promega) and transcription levels were quantified using SYBR-green PCR Mastermix (Eurogentec) in a real-time PCR system (Step One Plus, Applied Biosystems). Human or mouse riboprotein L19 primers were used for normalization. PCR assays were performed in duplicate and the fold induction was calculated against control-treated cells using the comparative Ct method ($\Delta\Delta C_t$). To quantify miRNA levels, RNA was isolated with the miRNeasy kit (Qiagen) followed by poly-adenylation and reverse transcription using QuantiMir RT kit (BioCat). Primers are listed in Additional file 1.

Immunoblotting and immunofluorescence staining
See Additional file 1.

Apoptosis assay
Cells were washed twice in ice-cold PBS and suspended in 1× Annexin-V binding buffer (0.01 M HEPES, pH 7.4, 0.14 M NaCl, 2.5 mM $CaCl_2$,) at a concentration of 1×10^6 cells/ml; 5 μl of Cy5 Annexin-V was added to 1×10^5 cells and incubated for 15 min on ice in the dark. Stained cells were filtered through a 40-μm mesh and analyzed on a FACSCanto II using DIVA Software (Becton Dickinson). Cell debris and duplets were excluded by a combination of light scatter and forward scatter plus width.

Cell cycle analysis
Cells were incubated with 10 μM BrdU for 2 h at 37 °C and 5% CO_2. The cells were then fixed in 70% ice-cold ethanol and lysed by incubating first with 2 N HCl and 0.5% Triton X-100 for 30 min and then in 0.1 M $Na_2B_4O_7$, pH 8.5, for 2 min at room temperature. Nuclei were washed with 0.5% Tween-20, 1% bovine serum albumin (BSA)/PBS and incubated with FITC-labeled anti-BrdU antibody (#347583, Beckton Dickinson) for

30 min at room temperature. Nuclei were stained for DNA content by incubating with 5 µg/ml propidium iodide (PI) for a minimum of 1 h at room temperature. Stained cells were filtered through a 40-µm mesh and analyzed on a FACSCanto II using DIVA Software (Becton Dickinson).

Chromatin immunoprecipitation

Chromatin immunoprecipitation (ChIP) experiments were performed as previously described with some modifications [51]. In brief, cells were crosslinked either with 1% formaldehyde or in combination with 2 mM EGS (ethylene glycol bis(succinimidyl succinate); Thermo-Fisher, 21,565). Crosslinked chromatin was sonicated to receive an average fragment size of 500 bp. ChIP was performed with 100 µg of chromatin and 2.5–5 µg HA-tag antibody per IP, and 1% of ChIP material or input material was used for quantitative RT-PCR using specific primers covering Foxf2 binding sites in promoter regions of *Btc* (−450 to −253 from TSS), of *Ereg* (−851 to −654 from TSS), of *Areg* exon2 (+1086 to 1210 from TSS), and of *Noxa* (−696 to −499 from TSS). Primers covering an intergenic region were used as control, and the amplification efficiencies were normalized between the primer pairs. Enrichment of IP/input over IgG background control was calculated and the specificity measured as fold change to an unspecific intergenic region.

Transcriptome, survival, and metastasis correlation analysis

See Additional file 1.

Statistical analysis

Statistical analysis and graphs were generated using the GraphPad Prism software (GraphPad Software Inc., San Diego CA). All statistical analyses were performed as indicated by paired or unpaired two-sided *t* test.

Results

Foxf2 expression is induced during EMT

We screened for changes in gene expression by DNA oligonucleotide microarray analysis during an EMT in three independent in vitro model systems. First, MTflE-cad cells have been derived from a breast tumor of MMTV-Neu transgenic mice [52] in which both E-cadherin alleles were flanked by LoxP recombination sites [53]. Genetic ablation of E-cadherin was achieved by the transient expression of Cre-recombinase (MTΔE-cad) [23]. Second, EMT was induced in the human breast cancer cell line MCF7 by downregulation of E-cadherin using stable expression of shRNA [23] and, thirdly, EMT was induced in normal murine mammary epithelial (NMuMG) cells by treatment with TGFβ [54] (Additional file 1: Figure S1A). The forkhead transcription factor Foxf2 was identified as a commonly

upregulated gene during EMT in all three experimental systems (Additional file 1: Figure S1B, C). To assess whether Foxf2 is a target of canonical or noncanonical TGFβ signaling, we monitored Foxf2 expression in NMuMG cells stably depleted of Smad4 expression (NMuMG-shSmad4) [48]. Foxf2 mRNA expression levels were significantly reduced in TGFβ-treated NMuMG-shSmad4 cells compared with control cells, indicating that Foxf2 is regulated via canonical Smad4-dependent TGFβ signaling (Additional file 1: Figure S1D).

Foxf2 is partially required for EMT

We first assessed whether the expression of Foxf2 is able to induce an EMT by infecting NMuMG cells with lentiviral particles encoding HA-tagged human Foxf2. Although the cells expressed Foxf2 in their nuclei, the cells did not gain an EMT-like phenotype (data not shown). Conversely, to investigate whether the upregulation of Foxf2 expression is required for an EMT, we stably infected NMuMG cells with lentiviral particles expressing two different shRNAs against murine Foxf2 (shFoxf2 #703, shFoxf2 #704). NMuMG-shFoxf2 cells treated with TGFβ apparently changed to a mesenchymal cell morphology, comparable to TGFβ-treated NMuMG-shCtrl cells. However, NMuMG-shFoxf2 cells did not completely lose their tight cell-cell contacts, a key step during an EMT (Fig. 1a). Indeed, quantitative RT-PCR (Fig. 1b, c) and immunoblotting (Fig. 1d) analysis revealed that the shRNA-mediated ablation of Foxf2 expression resulted in a sustained expression of the epithelial adherens and tight junction molecules E-cadherin and ZO-1, whereas the increased expression of the mesenchymal markers fibronectin, Ncam1, and N-cadherin remained unaffected.

To investigate whether the shRNA-mediated depletion of Foxf2 expression affects EMT-associated changes in cell adhesion, cell junctions, and/or cytoskeletal composition, we performed immunofluorescence microscopy analysis for the cell adhesion proteins E-cadherin, N-cadherin, and Ncam1, the tight junction protein ZO-1, the focal adhesion protein paxillin, and actin stress fibers (phalloidin). NMuMG-shFoxf2 cells did not show a classical cadherin switch when treated with TGFβ. In Foxf2-ablated cells, a normal upregulation of the mesenchymal marker N-cadherin was observed, but the expression of the epithelial markers E-cadherin and ZO-1 was partially maintained at the cell membrane, in contrast to shCtrl-expressing cells which showed a bona-fide EMT (Additional file 1: Figure S2A, B). Upregulated expression of Foxf2 during an EMT was also not required for the EMT-associated cytoskeletal reorganization of cortical actin into actin stress fibers, for the

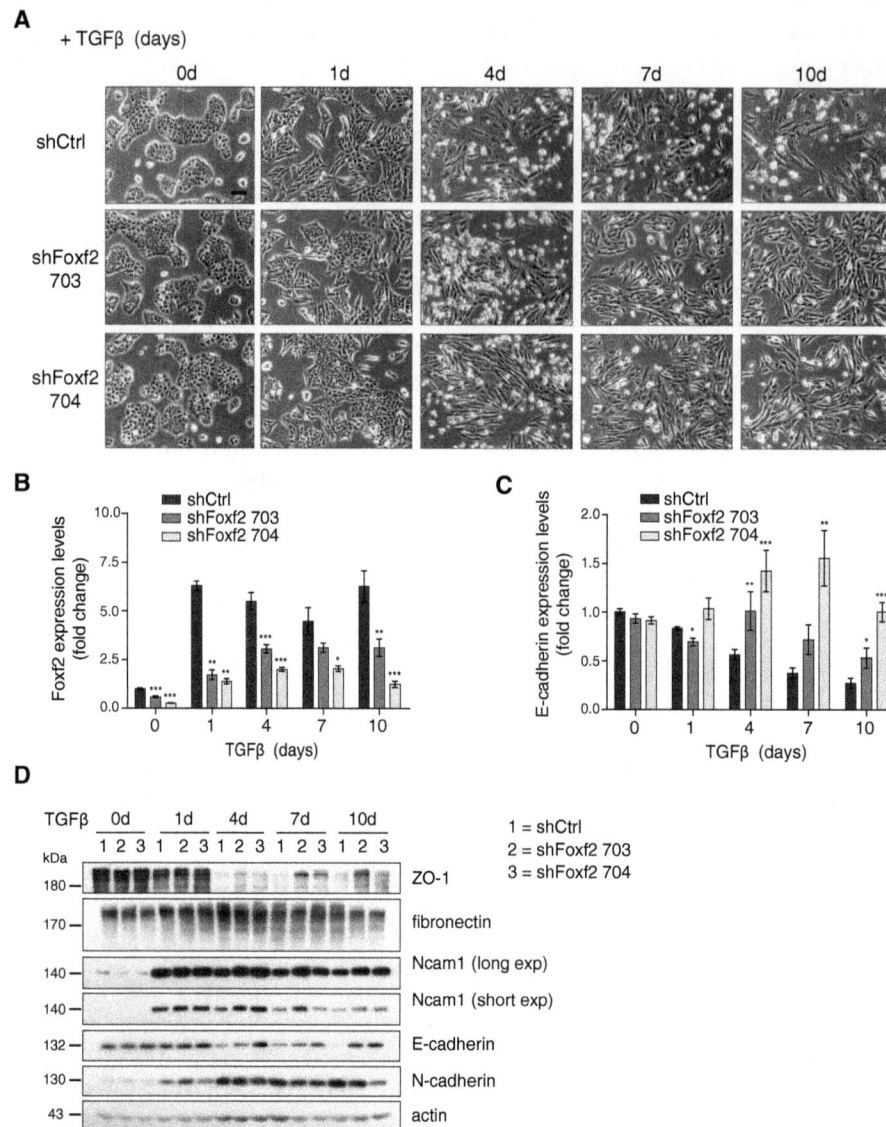

Fig. 1 Downregulation of Foxf2 attenuates TGFβ-induced EMT. **a** Phase-contrast micrographs of NMuMG cells stably expressing a control shRNA (shCtrl) or shRNAs against Foxf2 (shFoxf2 703, shFoxf2 704) treated with transforming growth factor (TGF)β for the times indicated. Scale bar = 100μm. **b** Foxf2 knockdown efficiency was determined by quantitative RT-PCR in NMuMG cells stably infected with shCtrl, shFoxf2 703, or shFoxf2 704 and treated with TGFβ for the times indicated. Values were normalized to RPL19 and presented as fold changes compared with untreated shCtrl NMuMG cells. **c** Loss of E-cadherin expression during TGFβ-induced EMT depends on Foxf2. E-cadherin mRNA levels in shFoxf2 and shCtrl-transfected NMuMG cells were determined by quantitative RT-PCR. Values were normalized to RPL19 and reported as fold changes compared with untreated shCtrl NMuMG cells. **d** Knocking down Foxf2 leads to a sustained expression of cell junction components. Immunoblotting analysis for the epithelial markers E-cadherin and ZO-1 as well as the mesenchymal markers Ncam1, N-cadherin, and fibronectin in shFoxf2 knockdown and shCtrl NMuMG cells treated with TGFβ for the times indicated. Actin was used as a loading control. Data are shown as mean ± SEM of three independent experiments. Statistical values were calculated using a paired two-tailed t test. *$p \leq 0.05$; **$p \leq 0.01$; ***$p \leq 0.001$

upregulation of the mesenchymal marker Ncam1, or for the formation of focal adhesions shown by paxillin staining (Additional file 1: Figure S2B, C). Together, these results indicate that Foxf2 is required for the disruption of cell-cell junctions but not for the induction of a mesenchymal cellular phenotype and mesenchymal marker expression.

Foxf2 regulates EMT transcriptional regulators and cell migration

The maintenance of an epithelial morphology and E-cadherin expression in Foxf2-depleted NMuMG cells became even more apparent when treated for 19 to 20 days with TGFβ, a time frame necessary for control NMuMG cells to acquire an EMT stage associated with cellular migration (Fig. 2a–d). Since Foxf2 appeared essential for the loss of E-cadherin expression and the disruption of cell-cell junctions, we assessed whether the loss of Foxf2 expression affected the migratory capabilities of cells. Transwell migration assays revealed a decrease in motility for cells stably expressing shRNAs against murine Foxf2 compared with NMuMG cells expressing control shRNA (Fig. 2e).

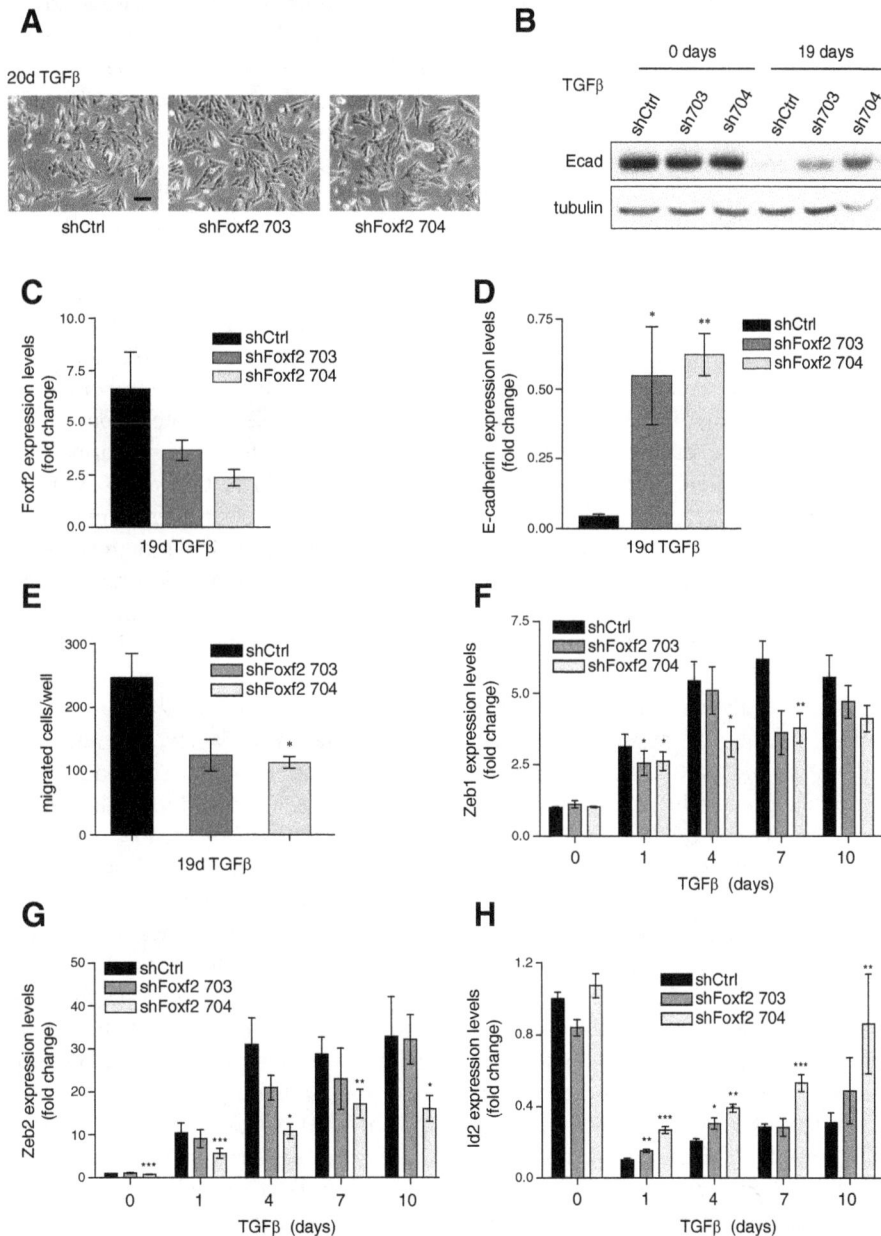

Fig. 2 Foxf2 regulates cell migration and the expression of E-cadherin transcriptional repressors. **a** Phase-contrast micrographs of NMuMG cells stably expressing a control shRNA (shCtrl) or a Foxf2-specific shRNA (shFoxf2 703, 704) treated with transforming growth factor (TGF)β for 20 days. Scale bar = 100μm. **b** shRNA-mediated ablation of Foxf2 leads to sustained E-cadherin expression after 19 days of TGFβ treatment shown by immunoblotting analysis in shFoxf2 and shCtrl NMuMG cells. Tubulin was used as a loading control. **c** Foxf2 and **d** E-cadherin mRNA levels were determined by quantitative RT-PCR in shFoxf2 and shCtrl NMuMG cells treated with TGFβ for 19 days. Values were normalized to RPL19 and reported as fold changes compared with untreated shCtrl NMuMG cells. **e** Depletion of Foxf2 leads to reduced cell migration of NMuMG cells treated for 19 days with TGFβ through transwell filters compared with control cells (shCtrl). mRNA levels of **f** Zeb1, **g** Zeb2, and **h** Id2 were determined by quantitative RT-PCR in shFoxf2- and shCtrl-transfected NMuMG cells. Values were normalized to RPL19 and reported as fold changes compared with untreated shCtrl NMuMG cells. Data are shown as mean ± SEM of three independent experiments. Statistical values were calculated using a paired two-tailed t test between shCtrl and shFoxf2 cells. *$p \leq 0.05$; **$p \leq 0.01$; ***$p \leq 0.001$

The loss of E-cadherin is often attributed to transcriptional dysregulation. Several transcription factors have been identified that are able to repress E-cadherin gene expression, among them the zinc-finger-homeodomain transcription factors Zeb1 and Zeb2 [55–57]. Quantitative RT-PCR analysis revealed that shRNA-mediated ablation of Foxf2 expression during a TGFβ-induced EMT in NMuMG cells attenuated the upregulation of Zeb1 and Zeb2 expression observed in shCtrl-transfected cells (Fig. 2f, g). Inhibitors of differentiation (Ids) act as positive regulators of proliferation and as negative regulators of differentiation. The Id proteins lack a DNA-binding motif and inhibit, for example, E2A-dependent suppression of the E-cadherin promoter [58]. Consistent with the sustained expression of E-cadherin, ablation of Foxf2 in TGFβ-treated NMuMG cells interfered with the downregulation of Id2 expression during an EMT (Fig. 2h).

The loss of Foxf2 maintained E-cadherin expression during a TGFβ-induced EMT in NMuMG cells in a similar manner as the loss of the major transcriptional repressor of E-cadherin expression, Zeb1 (Additional file 1: Figure S3A, B). Also comparable to the siRNA-mediated ablation of Zeb1 expression, loss of Foxf2 expression resulted in the upregulated expression of the miR-200 family members miR-200a-3p, miR-200b-3p, and miR-429-3p (Additional file 1: Figure S3C). On the other hand, both Foxf2 and Zeb1 are predicted targets of miR-200 family members, and ectopic expression of the miR-200 family members miR-200b-3p, miR-200c-3p, and miR-429-3p downregulated both transcription factors (Additional file 1: Figure S3D, E). Consistent with a regulatory role of Foxf2 on the expression of Zeb family proteins, Foxf2 upregulation after 1 day of TGFβ treatment of NMuMG cells was followed by the induction of Zeb1 and Zeb2 expression, leading to a continuous downregulation of E-cadherin (Additional file 1: Figure S3F). These results indicate tight control of E-cadherin expression by a double-negative feedback loop between Foxf2 and miR-200 family members, as well as regulation of the expression of known targets of miR200 family members and transcriptional repressors of E-cadherin expression, such as Zeb1, Zeb2, and Id2. Similarly, Foxf2 is essential for the proper downregulation of E-cadherin and the regulation of Zeb2 and Id2 during a TGFβ-induced EMT of Py2T murine breast cancer cells that have been derived from a tumor of the MMTV-PyMT mouse model of breast cancer (Additional file 1: Figure S3G).

In conclusion, the upregulation of Foxf2 in NMuMG cells undergoing an EMT is essential for the transcriptional repression of E-cadherin, for the disruption of cell-cell adhesions, and for EMT-associated cell migration, yet has only minor effects on the induction of mesenchymal marker expression.

Foxf2 regulates cell death and survival pathways

To identify the actual genes and signaling pathways that are regulated by Foxf2 during an EMT, we performed gene expression profiling by RNA sequencing of NMuMG cells that were transfected with control siRNA (siCtrl; epithelial state) or with siCtrl or siRNA targeting Foxf2 (siFoxf2) in the presence of TGFβ for 4 days (mesenchymal state). We found 1789 genes to be differentially expressed at least twofold upon Foxf2 knockdown compared with siRNA control at 4 days of TGFβ treatment, and 2689 genes were significantly changed upon induction of EMT comparing siCtrl in the absence or presence of TGFβ (siCtrl 0 days vs 4 days TGFβ; EMT). In total, 792 genes were commonly regulated by the loss of Foxf2 expression and by the induction of an EMT with TGFβ (Fig. 3a; Additional file 1: Table S1). Unsupervised hierarchical clustering revealed that Foxf2-deficient cells treated with TGFβ more closely resembled the mesenchymal state of TGFβ-treated control cells, however they formed a separate clustering arm (Fig. 3b). To study in more detail which transcripts were specifically altered compared with the mesenchymal and epithelial control states, gene expression signatures were generated using weighted gene coexpression network analysis (WGCNA). Six different gene expression signatures were extracted, with the yellow and the brown signatures summarizing genes from an intermediate mesenchymal state (Fig. 3b; Additional file 1: Table S2). The EMT-induced expression of the genes in the yellow signature was strongly reduced by the ablation of Foxf2 knockdown. Conversely, the EMT-repressed expression of the genes in the brown signature was blocked by the loss of Foxf2 (Fig. 3c).

Pathway enrichment analysis using ingenuity pathway analysis (IPA) revealed major functions of the yellow signature-associated genes in cellular movement and cell-cell signaling and interaction, functions that can be attributed to the loss of E-cadherin expression as described above (Fig. 3d). On the other hand, the brown signature was found to be associated with molecular transport and metabolism (lipid, vitamin, and mineral metabolism) pathways (Fig. 3d). Interestingly, both up- and downregulated EMT signatures that are also affected by Foxf2 knockdown (brown and yellow signatures) were enriched in pathways describing cell death and survival, indicating a regulatory role of Foxf2 in these processes (Fig. 3d). Indeed, NMuMG cells stably expressing shRNA against Foxf2 showed significantly less TGFβ-mediated growth inhibition compared with shCtrl-transfected cells, and the cell number increased significantly compared with shCtrl-expressing cells (Fig. 4a).

Foxf2 affects apoptosis by regulating the expression of Noxa

To assess whether the increase in cell numbers was due to increased proliferation or decreased cell death, we

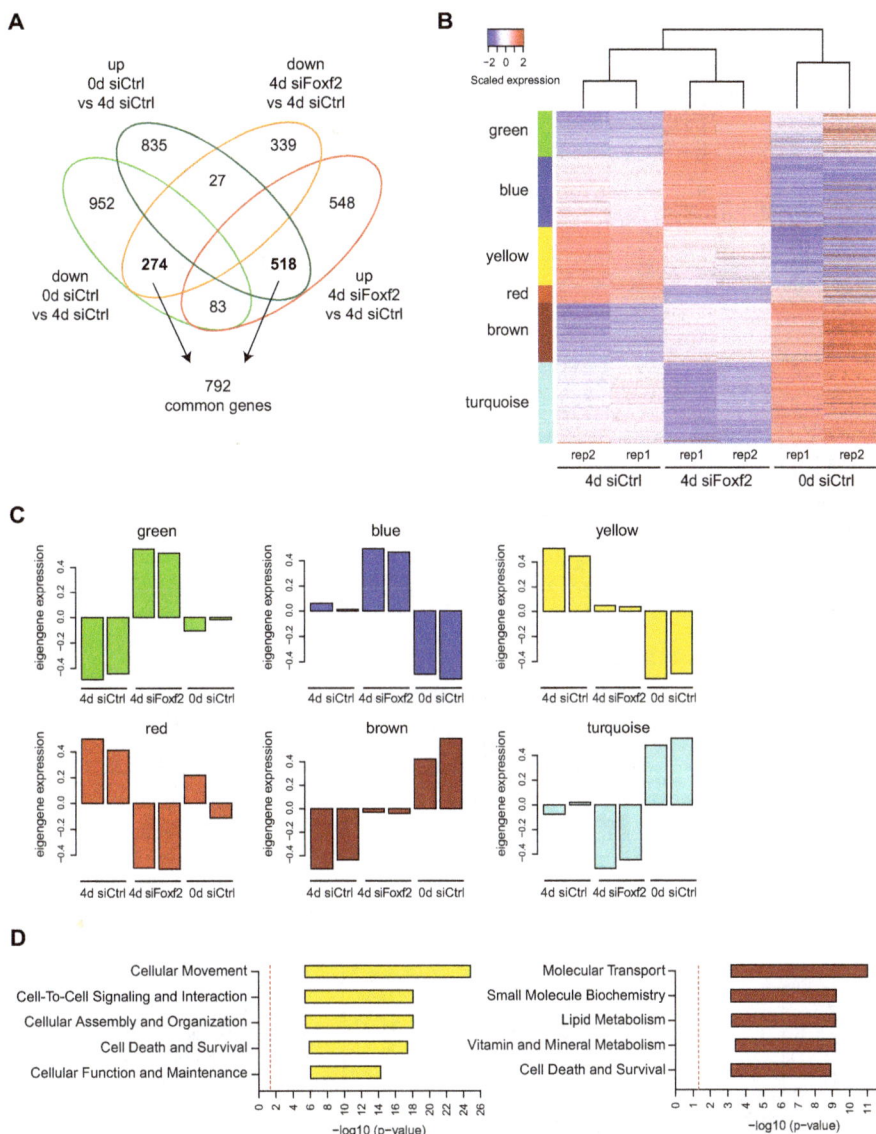

Fig. 3 RNA sequencing analysis of Foxf2-dependent gene expression. **a** Venn diagram illustrating the overlap of significantly differentially expressed genes (p adjusted < 0.05, abs(log2 fold change) ≥ 1) between the epithelial and mesenchymal state (0 days vs 4 days siRNA control (siCtrl)) or for the Foxf2 perturbation (4 days siFoxf2 vs 4 days siCtrl). Highlighted in bold are genes whose change during EMT is reversed by Foxf2 knockdown. **b** Heatmap of gene expression from RNA-sequencing of epithelial control samples (untreated siCtrl NMuMG cells) and of siCtrl- or siFoxf2-treated NMuMG cells in the presence of TGFβ for 4 days. The sample order in the heatmap was obtained from an unsupervised hierarchical clustering, while rows (genes) were arranged according to the gene signatures derived from WGCNA. **c** The eigengene expression of the different gene signatures derived from WGCNA (see **a**) illustrates a general expression trend of all genes belonging to a gene signature. **d** IPA analysis of the brown and yellow gene signature. Shown in the bar plot are the significance ranges of pathways belonging to the most significantly enriched categories. The dotted red line indicates a p value of 0.05. Differential gene expression and gene signature memberships are reported in Additional file 1 (Table S1 and S2, respectively)

compared the rates of apoptosis and proliferation by Annexin-V staining and BrdU incorporation and PI staining, respectively, in NMuMG cells treated with TGFβ and depleted or not for Foxf2 expression. The loss of Foxf2 significantly reduced the levels of apoptosis when compared with control cells (Fig. 4b), while only a moderate difference in the number of cycling cells was observed (Additional file 1: Figure S4A). The lack of Foxf2 reduced caspase-dependent programmed cell death, as the levels of cleaved caspase-3 and its downstream cleavage target poly-(ADP-ribose) polymerase (PARP) were diminished upon knockdown of Foxf2 (Fig. 4c). In summary, the results show that the increased expression of Foxf2 during EMT is critical for promoting TGFβ-induced cell death.

TGFβ has been shown to act as a tumor suppressor in the early stages of tumorigenesis by inducing the expression of cell cycle inhibitors and proapoptotic factors

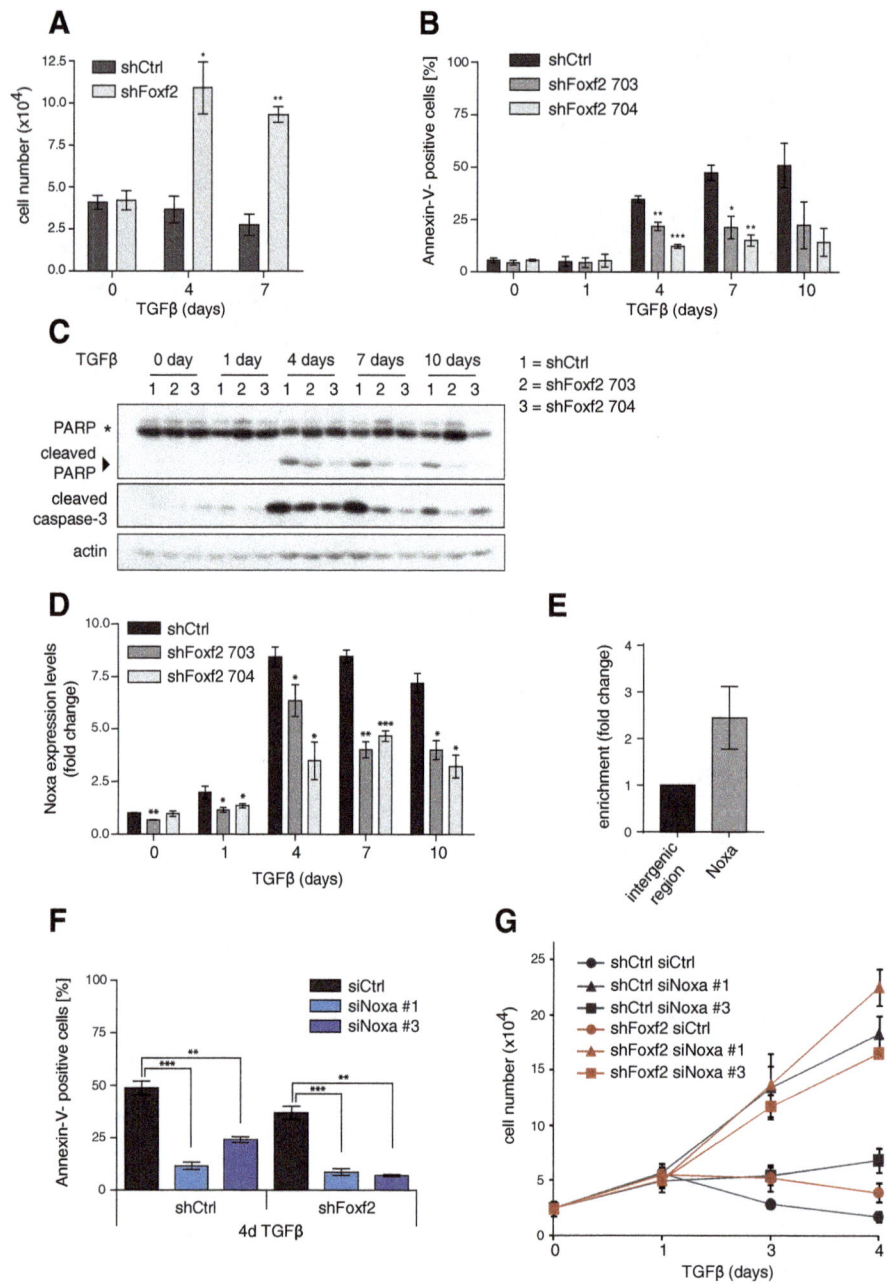

Fig. 4 (See legend on next page.)

(See figure on previous page.)
Fig. 4 Depletion of Foxf2 attenuates TGFβ-induced apoptosis and the expression of the proapoptotic protein Noxa. **a** Downregulation of Foxf2 promotes cell proliferation. shFoxf2- and shCtrl-expressing NMuMG cells were treated with transforming growth factor (TGF)β for the times indicated and counted using a Neubauer chamber. **b** Foxf2 depletion decreases apoptosis during TGFβ-induced EMT. shFoxf2- and shCtrl-expressing NMuMG cells were treated with TGFβ for the times indicated, and apoptosis was detected by Annexin-V staining and flow cytometry analysis. **c** TGFβ induces classical caspase-mediated apoptosis dependent on the upregulation of Foxf2. Immunoblotting analyses of the same experiment as shown in Fig. 1d for cleaved caspase-3 and PARP in shFoxf2- and shCtrl-expressing NMuMG cells treated with TGFβ for the times indicated. Actin was used as a loading control. **d** Knockdown of Foxf2 attenuates the upregulation of Noxa expression. Noxa mRNA levels in shFoxf2- and shCtrl-expressing NMuMG cells treated with TGFβ for the times indicated were determined by quantitative RT-PCR. Values were normalized to RPL19 and presented as fold changes compared with untreated shCtrl NMuMG cells. **e** Foxf2 regulates Noxa expression by direct transcriptional activation. Chromatin immunoprecipitation of HA-tagged Foxf2 was performed either on Foxf2-expressing or control NMuMG cells treated for 2 days with TGFβ. Immunoprecipitated DNA fragments were quantified by quantitative PCR using primers covering base pairs −696 to −499 of the *noxa* promoter region. Enrichment (IP/input) for specific primers was calculated relative to primers covering an intergenic region. **f** Noxa depletion significantly decreases TGFβ-induced apoptosis. shFoxf2- and shCtrl-expressing NMuMG cells were transfected with control siRNA (siCtrl) and two different siRNAs specific for murine Noxa (siNoxa #1, siNoxa #3) and incubated with TGFβ for 4 days. The extent of apoptosis was measured by Annexin-V staining and flow cytometry. **g** The impairment of Noxa expression leads to increased cell proliferation. shFoxf2- and shCtrl-expressing NMuMG cells were transfected with control siRNA (siCtrl) and two different siRNAs specific for murine Noxa (siNoxa #1, siNoxa #3) and incubated with TGFβ for the times indicated. Cell numbers were determined using a Neubauer chamber. Results show the mean ± SEM of three independent experiments. Statistical values were calculated using paired/unpaired two-tailed *t* test. *$p \leq 0.05$; **$p \leq 0.01$; ***$p \leq 0.001$

[59]. Differential gene expression analysis between TGFβ-treated control and Foxf2-deficient NMuMG cells revealed a substantial regulation of the BH3-only factor Noxa by Foxf2, which was confirmed by quantitative RT-PCR analysis (Fig. 4d). ChIP experiments with NMuMG cells expressing HA-tagged Foxf2 treated for 2 days with TGFβ demonstrated a weak direct binding of Foxf2 to the *noxa* gene promoter, suggesting additional indirect regulatory mechanisms (Fig. 4e). As the upregulation of Foxf2 is necessary for TGFβ-induced Noxa expression, we next assessed whether loss of Noxa is sufficient to prevent apoptosis in TGFβ-treated NMuMG cells. Noxa expression in NMuMG cells was ablated by transient transfection of two different siRNAs (siNoxa #1, siNoxa #3) or control siRNA (siCtrl) in shFoxf2- and shCtrl-expressing cells. Following the reduction of Noxa mRNA levels in siNoxa #1- and #3-treated cells (Additional file 1: Figure S4B), apoptosis was attenuated and cell growth inhibition was compensated in TGFβ-treated cells (Fig. 4f, g; Additional file 1: Figure S4C). These results demonstrate that depletion of Noxa is sufficient to protect NMuMG cells from TGFβ-induced apoptosis. Together, these data indicate that Foxf2 mediates TGFβ-induced apoptosis by the transcriptional activation of the proapoptotic protein Noxa.

Foxf2 promotes TGFβ-induced growth arrest by repressing EGF receptor signaling

As well as activating transcription of the *noxa* gene and inducing apoptosis, we investigated whether Foxf2 regulates any prosurvival signaling pathway. EGF receptor (EGFR) family members are known to provide protection from TGFβ-induced cell cycle arrest and apoptosis by activating the PI3K pathway [60, 61]. Indeed, immunoblotting analyses revealed that the levels of activated (tyrosine 1173-phosphorylated) forms of EGFR were higher in Foxf2-depleted NMuMG cells compared with control NMuMG cells when treated with TGFβ (Fig. 5a).

Previously, we have reported that survival of NMuMG cells undergoing a TGFβ-induced EMT depends on activated EGFR signaling [20]. We thus investigated whether inhibition of EGFR signaling impaired the antiapoptotic effect of Foxf2 depletion. Towards this aim, shFoxf2- and shCtrl-transfected NMuMG cells were treated with the EGFR inhibitor (EGFRi) AG1478 during TGFβ treatment, and cell growth and rates of apoptosis were determined. Combined treatment with EGFRi and TGFβ for 4 days led to a significantly reduced growth in shFoxf2-expressing NMuMG cells compared with the solvent (dimethyl sulfoxide (DMSO))-treated shFoxf2-expressing NMuMG cells (Fig. 5b; Additional file 1: Figure S5A). In addition, treatment of shFoxf2-expressing NMuMG cells with AG1478 increased apoptosis to a similar extent as observed in shCtrl-expressing cells (Fig. 5c). The extent of apoptosis thereby correlated with the levels of EGFR inhibition (Fig. 5d). This result indicates that TGFβ-resistant growth of Foxf2 knockdown cells relies on the activation of EGFR survival signaling.

To investigate how Foxf2 influences EGFR activation, we assessed whether the expression of EGFR ligands was affected by the modulation of Foxf2 expression. Gene expression profiling and validation by quantitative RT-PCR revealed that the EGFR-ligands betacellulin (Btc), amphiregulin (Areg), and (moderately) epiregulin (Ereg) showed sustained expression upon knockdown of Foxf2 during an EMT in both NMuMG and Py2T cells (Additional file 1: Figure S5B, C). Promoter binding prediction programs indicated a potential direct binding of Foxf2 to the *Btc* promoter (data not shown). ChIP followed by quantitative PCR of HA-tagged Foxf2 in NMuMG cells during TGFβ-induced EMT revealed a direct binding of Foxf2 to the *Btc* promoter region, to a

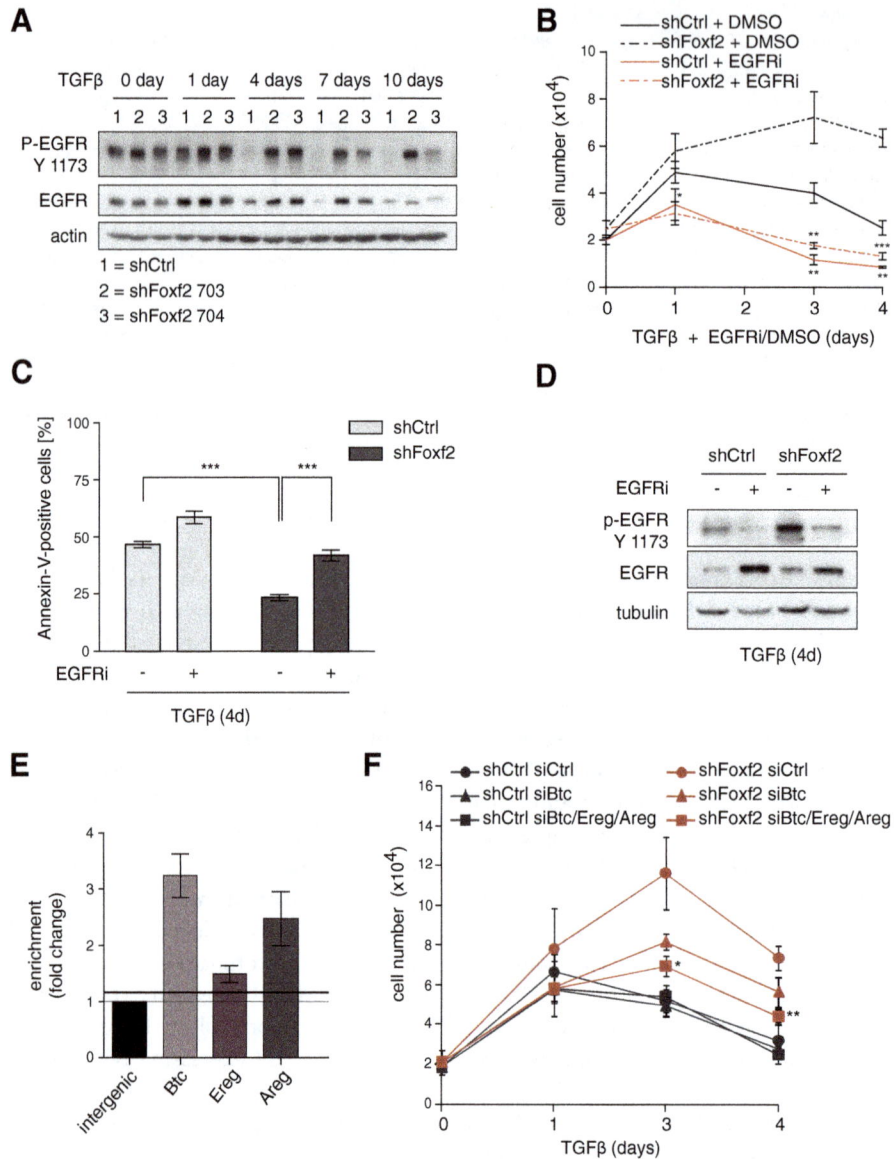

Fig. 5 Inhibition of EGFR signaling increases apoptosis in Foxf2-depleted cells. **a** Depletion of Foxf2 leads to sustained epidermal growth factor receptor (EGFR) activation. Immunoblotting analysis of the phosphorylation status of EGFR and total EGFR protein levels in shFoxf2- and shCtrl-expressing NMuMG cells treated with transforming growth factor (TGF)β for the times indicated. Actin was used as a loading control. **b–d** NMuMG cells expressing shRNA specific for Foxf2 or control shRNA were treated with TGFβ and AG1478 (EGFR inhibitor (EGFRi)) or control solvent (dimethyl sulfoxide (DMSO)) for the indicated times. **b** Cell numbers were determined using a Neubauer chamber. **c** EGFR inhibition significantly increases apoptosis in Foxf2 knockdown cells. Apoptosis was detected by Annexin-V staining and flow cytometry. **d** Treatment with AG1478 decreases EGFR activation in shFoxf2 cells to a similar extent as seen in TGFβ-treated NMuMG cells expressing control shRNA. Immunoblotting analysis for EGFR phosphorylation and total EGFR levels is shown. Tubulin was used as a loading control. **e** Foxf2 regulates the expression of EGFR ligands by direct transcriptional repression. Chromatin immunoprecipitation of Foxf2 was performed either on HA-Foxf2 expressing or control NMuMG cells treated for 2 days with TGFβ. Immunoprecipitated DNA fragments were quantified by quantitative PCR using primers covering base pairs −450 to −253 of the *Btc* promoter region, base pairs −851 to −654 of the *Ereg* promoter, and base pairs +1086 to 1210 of the *Areg* exon 2. Enrichment (IP/input) for specific primers was calculated relative to primers covering an intergenic region. **f** Individual depletion of Btc or combined depletion of betacellulin (Btc), epiregulin (Ereg), and amphiregulin (Areg) reduces cell numbers in shFoxf2- but not in shCtrl-expressing NMuMG cells in the presence of TGFβ for 4 days. Cell numbers were determined using a Neubauer chamber. Data are shown as mean ± SEM of at least three independent experiments. Statistical values were calculated using a paired/unpaired two-tailed t test. $*p \leq 0.05$; $**p \leq 0.01$; $***p \leq 0.001$

regulatory region in exon 2 of the *Areg* gene, and with less efficiency to the *Ereg* promoter region (Fig. 5e).

To assess whether Btc, Areg, or Ereg were responsible for the stimulation of EGFR and increased cell survival of Foxf2-depleted cells, NMuMG cells stably expressing shRNA against Foxf2 or a control shRNA were transiently transfected with siRNAs against Btc or with a mix of siR-NAs against Btc, Areg, and Ereg and treated with TGFβ. The efficiency of Btc or combined Btc/Areg/Ereg ablation was determined by quantitative RT-PCR (Additional file 1: Figure S5D, E). Knockdown of Btc alone or in combination with the other two family members resulted in reduced cell growth in shFoxf2-expressing cells when treated with TGFβ (Fig. 5f). These results indicate that attenuation of EGFR activation by siRNA-mediated depletion of its ligands abrogates the survival benefit of Foxf2 depletion. We conclude that TGFβ-induced Foxf2 expression represses the transcriptional activation of the *Btc* and *Areg* genes, resulting into a reduced expression of these EGFR ligands and a repression of EGFR survival signaling.

Foxf2 expression correlates with poor prognosis in patients

Cancer-associated gene expression profiling has emerged as an appropriate tool to predict the relapse risk and to identify genes that mediate disease progression. To investigate whether Foxf2 expression is predictive for tumor progression or metastasis formation, we analyzed a breast cancer database of the Memorial Sloan-Kettering Cancer Center (MSKCC), published by Minn et al. [62]. This "Minn" database consists of microarray gene expression analysis of tumor samples from 82 patients with advanced breast cancer (T2–T4). The tumors were divided into two groups according to the log expression levels relative to the median expression of the investigated gene. The low and high Foxf2-expressing groups were further stratified for lymph node (LN) metastasis status. Interestingly, low Foxf2 expression significantly correlated with early distant metastasis formation in lymph node-negative (LN⁻) tumors, whereas the opposite tendency was found in tumors of patients that were positive for lymph node metastasis (LN⁺) (Fig. 6a, b).

To further substantiate a potential correlation between Foxf2 expression and patient survival, we analyzed the Netherlands Cancer Institute (NKI295) breast cancer database for Foxf2 expression [63]. The NKI295 database consists of microarray gene expression analysis of tumor samples from 295 patients with early-stage breast cancer (stage I or stage II primary breast carcinomas). Although Foxf2 expression was not predictive for metastasis formation or survival in the total patient pool (Fig. 6c), high expression of Foxf2 correlated with poor overall survival in patients with luminal subtype B breast cancer (Fig. 6d). High expression of Foxf2 in tumors with negative estrogen receptor (ER) status correlated

with high significance of early metastasis onset as well as poor overall survival (Fig. 6e, f). Similarly, in a large tumor collection from the Metabric consortium [64, 65], high Foxf2 expression predicted worse survival in the luminal B breast cancer subtype (Fig. 6g). Interestingly, Foxf2 expression was significantly higher in more aggressive tumor subtypes, such as ER⁻ compared with ER⁺, triple-negative compared with all other subtypes, and in claudin-low tumors (the breast cancer subtype associated with an EMT signature), compared with all others (Fig. 6h).

Together, the expression of Foxf2 in human patient samples and its prediction for clinical outcome reflect the dual function of Foxf2 observed in our in-vitro studies. Foxf2 may function as a tumor suppressor in early cancer development by promoting apoptosis, hence showing a poor prognosis in LN⁻ patients with low Foxf2 expression. More advanced tumors with high Foxf2 expression correlate with shorter metastasis-free survival, supporting a role of Foxf2 in cancer cell invasion and metastasis formation.

Discussion

Overcoming the growth inhibitory effect of TGFβ during the early stages of tumorigenesis as well as the conversion of TGFβ-mediated growth inhibition into TGFβ-induced tumor progression are fundamental processes during primary tumor growth and metastasis formation [1, 66]. Thus, understanding the mechanisms underlying this dual role of TGFβ in cancer progression and the strategies of cancer cells to circumvent TGFβ-induced apoptosis may offer new opportunities for novel cancer therapies.

Here, we have employed nontransformed NMuMG cells and Py2T murine breast cancer cells to delineate the molecular mechanisms underlying a TGFβ-induced EMT, including overcoming TGFβ-induced resistance to apoptosis and the acquisition of invasive properties. We report a dual function of the transcription factor Foxf2, acting as a tumor suppressor by promoting apoptosis and by repressing survival, while exerting protumorigenic activity at later stages of tumor progression, such as a promigratory function by inducing the disruption of cell-cell adhesion. Foxf2 is upregulated via the canonical TGFβ pathway, and gain of function studies in NMuMG cells reveal that its expression is not sufficient to induce an EMT. However, loss of function studies demonstrate that Foxf2 is essential for the disruption of cell junctions and the repression of epithelial marker expression but not for the gain of mesenchymal marker expression. Notably, Foxf2 is crucial for TGFβ-mediated cell death by the transcriptional activation of the *Nox*a gene, encoding for a BH3-only proapoptotic factor, and the subsequent induction of caspase-dependent apoptosis. Moreover, Foxf2 directly represses transcription of the *Btc*

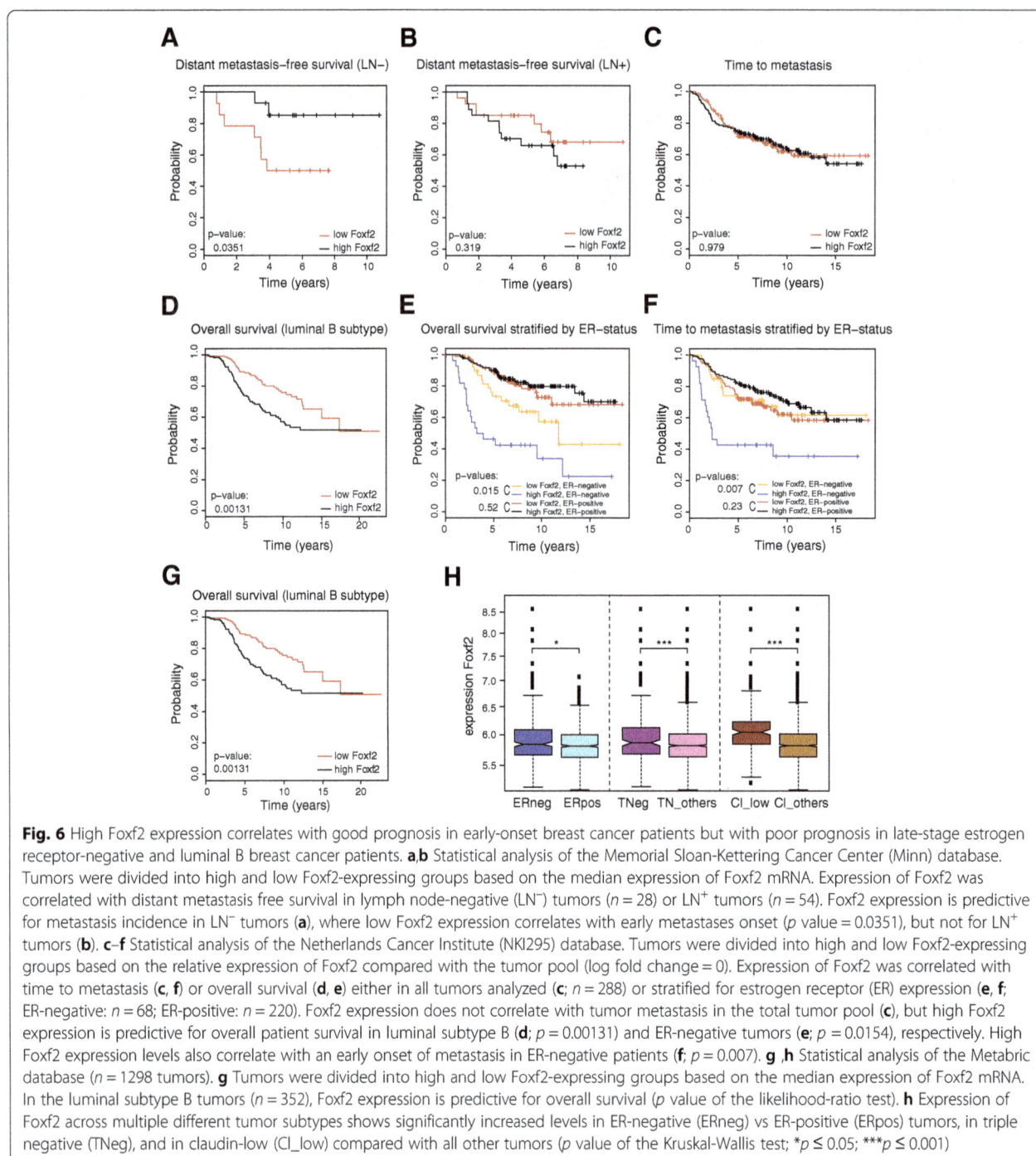

Fig. 6 High Foxf2 expression correlates with good prognosis in early-onset breast cancer patients but with poor prognosis in late-stage estrogen receptor-negative and luminal B breast cancer patients. **a,b** Statistical analysis of the Memorial Sloan-Kettering Cancer Center (Minn) database. Tumors were divided into high and low Foxf2-expressing groups based on the median expression of Foxf2 mRNA. Expression of Foxf2 was correlated with distant metastasis free survival in lymph node-negative (LN⁻) tumors ($n = 28$) or LN⁺ tumors ($n = 54$). Foxf2 expression is predictive for metastasis incidence in LN⁻ tumors (**a**), where low Foxf2 expression correlates with early metastases onset (p value = 0.0351), but not for LN⁺ tumors (**b**). **c–f** Statistical analysis of the Netherlands Cancer Institute (NKI295) database. Tumors were divided into high and low Foxf2-expressing groups based on the relative expression of Foxf2 compared with the tumor pool (log fold change = 0). Expression of Foxf2 was correlated with time to metastasis (**c, f**) or overall survival (**d, e**) either in all tumors analyzed (**c**; $n = 288$) or stratified for estrogen receptor (ER) expression (**e, f**; ER-negative: $n = 68$; ER-positive: $n = 220$). Foxf2 expression does not correlate with tumor metastasis in the total tumor pool (**c**), but high Foxf2 expression is predictive for overall patient survival in luminal subtype B (**d**; $p = 0.00131$) and ER-negative tumors (**e**; $p = 0.0154$), respectively. High Foxf2 expression levels also correlate with an early onset of metastasis in ER-negative patients (**f**; $p = 0.007$). **g ,h** Statistical analysis of the Metabric database ($n = 1298$ tumors). **g** Tumors were divided into high and low Foxf2-expressing groups based on the median expression of Foxf2 mRNA. In the luminal subtype B tumors ($n = 352$), Foxf2 expression is predictive for overall survival (p value of the likelihood-ratio test). **h** Expression of Foxf2 across multiple different tumor subtypes shows significantly increased levels in ER-negative (ERneg) vs ER-positive (ERpos) tumors, in triple negative (TNeg), and in claudin-low (Cl_low) compared with all other tumors (p value of the Kruskal-Wallis test; *$p \leq 0.05$; ***$p \leq 0.001$)

and *Areg* genes, encoding for ligands of EGFR, and thus attenuates EGFR-mediated survival signaling (Fig. 7).

The failure of Foxf2-depleted cells to disrupt tight and adherens junctions exemplifies its indispensable role in the acquisition of an invasive cell morphology. Loss of E-cadherin is an early event during EMT resulting in the disruption of the polarity complex, a prerequisite for the dissociation and invasion of cancer cells [67–69]. Direct

transcriptional repression has emerged as one common regulatory mechanism of E-cadherin expression in various cancer types [70, 71]. Here we demonstrate that, by mediating the TGFβ-induced upregulation of the transcriptional repressors Zeb1 and Zeb2 as well as the repression of Id2, Foxf2 mediates the transcriptional downregulation of E-cadherin and consequently the disruption of cell-cell adhesion. In addition, we show that

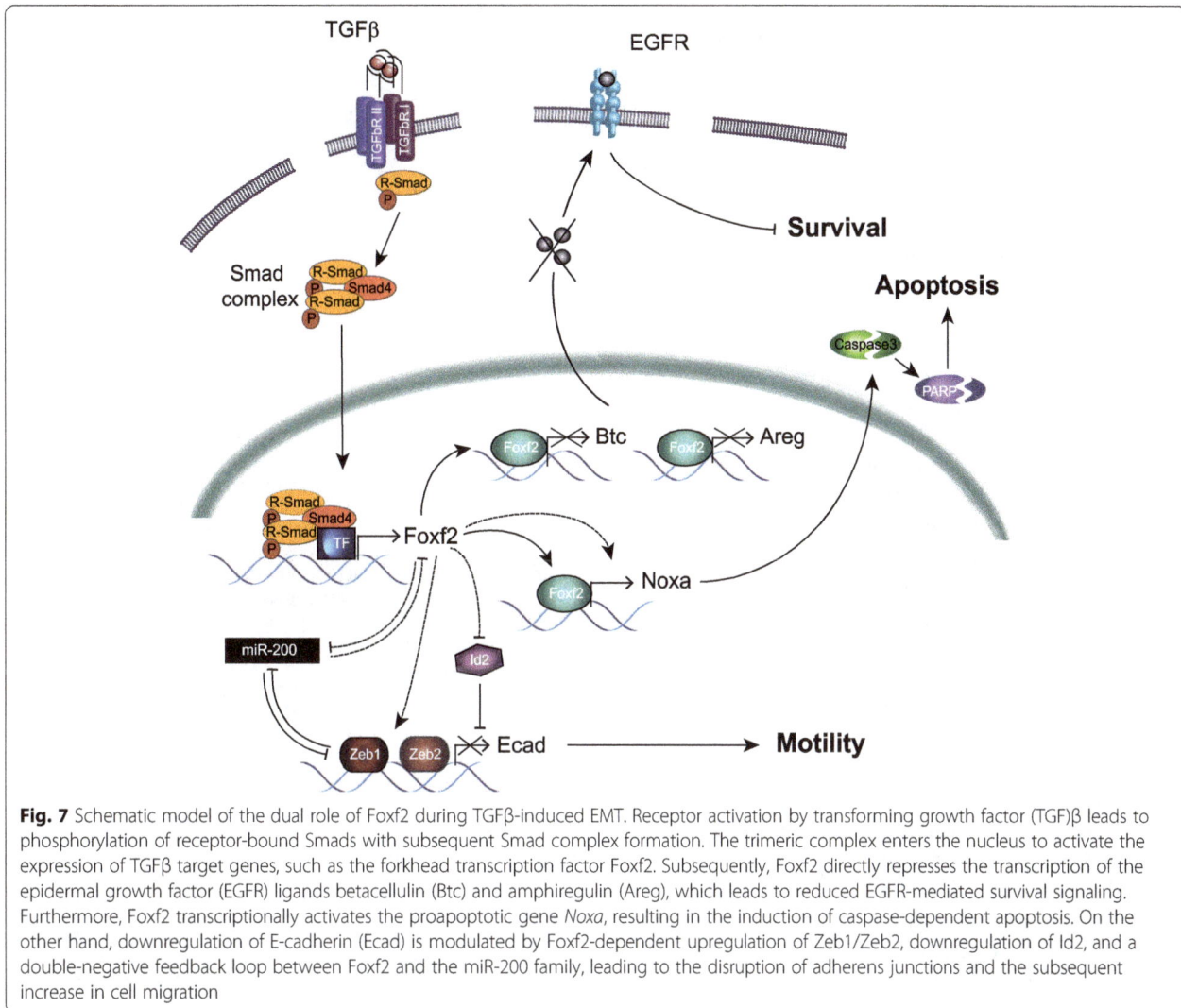

Fig. 7 Schematic model of the dual role of Foxf2 during TGFβ-induced EMT. Receptor activation by transforming growth factor (TGF)β leads to phosphorylation of receptor-bound Smads with subsequent Smad complex formation. The trimeric complex enters the nucleus to activate the expression of TGFβ target genes, such as the forkhead transcription factor Foxf2. Subsequently, Foxf2 directly represses the transcription of the epidermal growth factor (EGFR) ligands betacellulin (Btc) and amphiregulin (Areg), which leads to reduced EGFR-mediated survival signaling. Furthermore, Foxf2 transcriptionally activates the proapoptotic gene *Noxa*, resulting in the induction of caspase-dependent apoptosis. On the other hand, downregulation of E-cadherin (Ecad) is modulated by Foxf2-dependent upregulation of Zeb1/Zeb2, downregulation of Id2, and a double-negative feedback loop between Foxf2 and the miR-200 family, leading to the disruption of adherens junctions and the subsequent increase in cell migration

Foxf2 also affects the expression of the miR-200 family which are potent EMT-repressing noncoding RNAs that target Zeb1 and Zeb2 transcripts [72–74]. Interestingly, the expression of Foxf2 and miR-200 are controlled in a double-negative feedback loop, similar to the well-studied Zeb1-miR200 loop. The mechanism by which Foxf2 regulates the expression of these transcription (co)factors remains elusive, but the presence of putative Foxf2 binding sites in the promoter region of Zeb1 and Zeb2 (data not shown) and data from Kundu et al. [75] in nonsmall-cell lung cancer (NSCLC) cells suggest a direct regulatory mechanism, thus ensuring the downregulation of cell-cell junctions at multiple levels (Fig. 7). Moreover, consistent with our finding that Foxf2 predicts poor survival in a subset of breast cancer patients, our results identify Foxf2 as a promigratory and prometastatic factor (Fig. 7).

Our results also show that Foxf2 is essential for TGFβ-mediated apoptosis. The reduction of TGFβ-induced apoptosis in Foxf2-deficient cells is a consequence of the loss of the transcriptional activation of *Noxa* gene expression. Noxa has been shown to be critical in fine-tuning cell death decisions via degradation of the prosurvival molecule Mcl1 [76]. Noxa has been identified as a primary p53 target gene; however, oncogenic stress, such as irradiation and hypoxia, results in efficient induction of Noxa also in the absence of p53 [77, 78]. Our findings identify Foxf2 as a novel transcriptional activator of the tumor suppressor Noxa (Fig. 7).

Besides triggering apoptosis via regulation of Noxa expression, Foxf2 is also involved in the negative regulation of survival signals by the transcriptional repression of the EGFR ligands betacellulin (Btc), amphiregulin (Areg), and, to a lesser degree, epiregulin (Ereg). Although the regulatory effect of Foxf2 on the transcription level of the individual EGFR ligands is moderate (Additional file 1: Figure S5B, C), a cumulative effect by the simultaneous modulation of Btc, Areg, and Ereg expression enables a significant shift towards less EGFR signaling (Fig. 5a). Reduced EGFR signaling leads to a reduction in EGFR phosphorylation and, hence, reduced PKB activation. Blocking EGFR signaling has been shown to amplify the apoptotic response to TGFβ [61]. Here, we show that both pharmacological receptor inhibition as well as the combined reduction of the expression of the EGFR ligands Btc, Areg, and Ereg increased TGFβ-induced apoptosis in Foxf2-depleted NMuMG cells. These results indicate that, in addition to Noxa regulation, Foxf2 mediates its apoptotic effect by blocking EGFR-mediated survival signaling (Fig. 7).

To support the importance of a Foxf2 function during tumor development and progression, we have performed correlation studies for Foxf2 on three different breast cancer databases [62–64]. Analysis of a lymph node-negative stratified patient subset demonstrates that low Foxf2 expression significantly correlates with early metastasis formation. Comparably, low Foxf2 expression has been recently reported to correlate with early-onset metastasis and poor prognosis in breast cancer patients [43]. Interestingly, the opposite is found in more progressive breast cancers, where high Foxf2 expression correlates with poor prognosis. Stratification for luminal subtype B or for ER status reveals a highly significant correlation of high Foxf2 expression and early metastasis onset, concomitant with reduced overall survival. ER⁻ tumors represent highly aggressive breast cancer subtypes. In addition, Foxf2 transcript levels are increased in more aggressive ER⁻, in triple negative, and in the EMT-like, claudin-low breast cancer subtypes. Together, our findings identify high levels of Foxf2 as a marker for good prognosis in early noninvasive stages of tumor development, but with poor prognosis in malignant stages [79]. These findings substantiate the dual role of Foxf2 in cancer patients.

Conclusions

In our study, we demonstrate a dual role for the transcription factor Foxf2. It induces proapoptotic and represses antiapoptotic genes and, thus, acts as a tumor suppressor, likely with the help of specific cofactors. On the other hand, it induces the expression of EMT-inducing genes and thus exerts prometastatic functions to cells that have overcome the apoptotic crisis and undergone EMT. The role of Foxf2 in pre- and post-EMT cells reflects the well-studied dual role of TGFβ in cancer progression. Our results also substantiate findings in knockout mouse models where Foxf2 was found to play an important role in EMT-associated developmental processes and maintenance of the epithelial-mesenchymal structure in lung and gut tissues

[38, 39]. Hence, fine-tuning of the expression of Foxf2 and its cofactors could be pivotal during carcinogenesis, and insights into its regulation and molecular function are critical for the design of novel therapeutic strategies.

Additional file

Additional file 1: Figure S1. Foxf2 expression is upregulated during EMT via the canonical Smad pathway. The increased expression of Foxf2 during an EMT was assessed in normal murine mammary gland epithelial cells (NMuMG) and in murine and human breast cancer cells. Figure S2. Foxf2 is required for TGFβ-induced disruption of adherens junctions. RNAi-mediated ablation prevents an EMT as visualized by immunofluorescence staining for epithelial and mesenchymal markers. Figure S3. Foxf2 regulates the expression of Zeb1, Zeb2, Id2, and members of the miR-200 family as determined by quantitative RT-PCR of their expression during an EMT in the absence of presence of Foxf2. Figure S4. Foxf2 regulates Noxa expression and thus affects cell proliferation and apoptosis. Foxf2 regulated the expression of Noxa, and siRNA-mediated depletion of Noxa prevented an increase in cell death induced by the loss of Foxf2 expression as assessed by quantitative RT-PCR. Figure S5. EGF ligand-mediated EGF receptor signaling overcomes Foxf2-controlled cell survival. Foxf represses the expression of EGF receptor ligands as assessed by quantitative RT-PCR. Supplementary material and methods. Detailed information is given on the antibodies and reagents, on biochemical and cell biological methods, and on RNA sequencing and bioinformatics analysis used in the study. Table S1. Excel file summarizing the differential expression analysis (siFoxf2 to siCtrl after 4 days TGFβ treatment or siCtrl with vs without TGFβ for 4 days) of all transcripts detected with RNA-sequencing. Table S2. Excel file showing the list of genes belonging to the different gene signatures (modules) and the strength of their modular membership (kME values). (ZIP 14675 kb)

Abbreviations
Areg: Amphiregulin; Btc: Betacellulin; ChIP: Chromatin immunoprecipitation; EGFR: Epidermal growth factor receptor; EGFRi: EGFR inhibitor; EMT: Epithelial to mesenchymal transition; Ereg: Epiregulin; Foxf2: Forkhead box protein F2; Ids: Inhibitors of differentiation; IPA: Ingenuity pathway analysis; MET: Mesenchymal to epithelial transition; NMuMG: Normal murine mammary gland; PARP: Poly-(ADP-ribose) polymerase; TGF: Transforming growth factor; WGCNA: Weighted gene coexpression network analysis

Acknowledgments
We thank Drs. L. Lundh, M. Kaeser, and P. ten Dijke for sharing important reagents. We are grateful to P. Schmidt, H. Antoniadis, I. Galm, U. Schmieder, and R. Jost for excellent technical support. We thank P. Lorentz and the DBM microscopy facility (DBM, University of Basel) for excellent support with microscopy, C. Beisel and the Genomics Facility Basel (D-BSSE) for next generation RNA sequencing, and R. Ivanek and the Bioinformatics Core Facility (DBM, University of Basel) for help with RNA sequencing analysis.

Funding
This research has been supported by the Swiss National Science Foundation, the Swiss Initiative for Systems Biology (RTD Cellplasticity), and the Swiss Cancer League. NM-S was supported by a Marie-Heim Vögtlin grant from the Swiss National Foundation.

Authors' contributions
NM-S, CH, ST, and MY designed and performed the experiments, analyzed the data, and wrote the manuscript. GC designed the experiments, analyzed the data, and wrote the manuscript. All authors read and approved the final manuscript.

Competing interests

The authors declare that they have no competing interests.

Author details

[1]Department of Biomedicine, University of Basel, Mattenstrasse 28, 4058 Basel, Switzerland. [2]Present address: Institute of Pathology, University Hospital of Basel, Basel, Switzerland. [3]Present address: Integra Biosciences AG, Zizers, Switzerland. [4]Present address: Roche Pharma, Basel, Switzerland.

References

1. Yang J, Weinberg RA. Epithelial-mesenchymal transition: at the crossroads of development and tumor metastasis. Dev Cell. 2008;14(6):818–29.
2. Kalluri R. EMT: when epithelial cells decide to become mesenchymal-like cells. J Clin Invest. 2009;119(6):1417–9.
3. Thiery JP, Acloque H, Huang RY, Nieto MA. Epithelial-mesenchymal transitions in development and disease. Cell. 2009;139(5):871–90.
4. Chaffer CL, San Juan BP, Lim E, Weinberg RA. EMT, cell plasticity and metastasis. Cancer Metastasis Rev. 2016;35(4):645–54.
5. Nieto MA. Epithelial plasticity: a common theme in embryonic and cancer cells. Science. 2013;342(6159):1234850.
6. Bloushtain-Qimron N, Yao J, Snyder EL, Shipitsin M, Campbell LL, Mani SA, Hu M, Chen H, Ustyansky V, Antosiewicz JE, et al. Cell type-specific DNA methylation patterns in the human breast. Proc Natl Acad Sci U S A. 2008; 105(37):14076–81.
7. Shipitsin M, Campbell L, Argani P, Weremowicz S, Bloushtain-Qimron N, Yao J, Nikolskaya T, Serebryiskaya T, Beroukhim R, Hu M, et al. Molecular definition of breast tumor heterogeneity. Cancer Cell. 2007;11(3):259–73.
8. Graff JR, Gabrielson E, Fujii H, Baylin SB, Herman JG. Methylation patterns of the E-cadherin 5' CpG island are unstable and reflect the dynamic, heterogeneous loss of E-cadherin expression during metastatic progression. J Biol Chem. 2000;275(4):2727–32.
9. Shipitsin M, Polyak K. The cancer stem cell hypothesis: in search of definitions, markers, and relevance. Lab Invest. 2008;88(5):459–63.
10. Brabletz T, Hlubek F, Spaderna S, Schmalhofer O, Hiendlmeyer E, Jung A, Kirchner T. Invasion and metastasis in colorectal cancer: epithelial-mesenchymal transition, mesenchymal-epithelial transition, stem cells and beta-catenin. Cells Tissues Organs. 2005;179(1–2):56–65.
11. Chaffer C, Thompson E, Williams E. Mesenchymal to epithelial transition in development and disease. Cells Tissues Organs. 2007;185(1–3):7–19.
12. Ocana OH, Corcoles R, Fabra A, Moreno-Bueno G, Acloque H, Vega S, Barrallo-Gimeno A, Cano A, Nieto MA. Metastatic colonization requires the repression of the epithelial-mesenchymal transition inducer Prrx1. Cancer Cell. 2012;22(6):709–24.
13. Tsai JH, Donaher JL, Murphy DA, Chau S, Yang J. Spatiotemporal regulation of epithelial-mesenchymal transition is essential for squamous cell carcinoma metastasis. Cancer Cell. 2012;22(6):725–36.
14. Fischer KR, Durrans A, Lee S, Sheng J, Li F, Wong ST, Choi H, El Rayes T, Ryu S, Troeger J, et al. Epithelial-to-mesenchymal transition is not required for lung metastasis but contributes to chemoresistance. Nature. 2015;527(7579): 472–6.
15. Zheng X, Carstens JL, Kim J, Scheible M, Kaye J, Sugimoto H, Wu CC, LeBleu VS, Kalluri R. Epithelial-to-mesenchymal transition is dispensable for metastasis but induces chemoresistance in pancreatic cancer. Nature. 2015; 527(7579):525–30.
16. Aiello NM, Brabletz T, Kang Y, Nieto MA, Weinberg RA, Stanger BZ. Upholding a role for EMT in pancreatic cancer metastasis. Nature. 2017; 547(7661):E7–8.
17. Ye X, Brabletz T, Kang Y, Longmore GD, Nieto MA, Stanger BZ, Yang J, Weinberg RA. Upholding a role for EMT in breast cancer metastasis. Nature. 2017;547(7661):E1–3.
18. Krebs AM, Mitschke J, Lasierra Losada M, Schmalhofer O, Boerries M, Busch H, Boettcher M, Mougiakakos D, Reichardt W, Bronsert P, et al. The EMT-activator Zeb1 is a key factor for cell plasticity and promotes metastasis in pancreatic cancer. Nat Cell Biol. 2017;19(5):518–29.
19. Polyak K, Weinberg RA. Transitions between epithelial and mesenchymal states: acquisition of malignant and stem cell traits. Nat Rev Cancer. 2009; 9(4):265–73.
20. Yilmaz M, Maass D, Tiwari N, Waldmeier L, Schmidt P, Lehembre F, Christofori G. Transcription factor Dlx2 protects from TGFbeta-induced cell-cycle arrest and apoptosis. EMBO J. 2011;30(21):4489–99.
21. Tiwari N, Meyer-Schaller N, Arnold P, Antoniadis H, Pachkov M, van Nimwegen E, Christofori G. Klf4 is a transcriptional regulator of genes critical for EMT, including Jnk1 (Mapk8). PLoS One. 2013;8(2):e57329.
22. Tiwari N, Tiwari VK, Waldmeier L, Balwierz PJ, Arnold P, Pachkov M, Meyer-Schaller N, Schubeler D, van Nimwegen E, Christofori G. Sox4 is a master regulator of epithelial-mesenchymal transition by controlling Ezh2 expression and epigenetic reprogramming. Cancer Cell. 2013;23(6):768–83.
23. Lehembre F, Yilmaz M, Wicki A, Schomber T, Strittmatter K, Ziegler D, Kren A, Went P, Derksen PW, Berns A, et al. NCAM-induced focal adhesion assembly: a functional switch upon loss of E-cadherin. EMBO J. 2008;27(19): 2603–15.
24. Kaufmann E, Knochel W. Five years on the wings of fork head. Mech Dev. 1996;57(1):3–20.
25. Kaestner KH, Knochel W, Martinez DE. Unified nomenclature for the winged helix/forkhead transcription factors. Genes Dev. 2000;14(2):142–6.
26. Wotton KR, Shimeld SM. Analysis of lamprey clustered fox genes: insight into fox gene evolution and expression in vertebrates. Gene. 2011;489(1):30–40.
27. Fuxe J, Vincent T, Garcia de Herreros A. Transcriptional crosstalk between TGF-beta and stem cell pathways in tumor cell invasion: role of EMT promoting Smad complexes. Cell Cycle. 2010;9(12):2363–74.
28. Mani SA, Yang J, Brooks M, Schwaninger G, Zhou A, Miura N, Kutok JL, Hartwell K, Richardson AL, Weinberg RA. Mesenchyme forkhead 1 (FOXC2) plays a key role in metastasis and is associated with aggressive basal-like breast cancers. Proc Natl Acad Sci U S A. 2007;104(24):10069–74.
29. Taube JH, Herschkowitz JI, Komurov K, Zhou AY, Gupta S, Yang J, Hartwell K, Onder TT, Gupta PB, Evans KW, et al. Core epithelial-to-mesenchymal transition interactome gene-expression signature is associated with claudin-low and metaplastic breast cancer subtypes. Proc Natl Acad Sci U S A. 2010; 107(35):15449–54.
30. Bao B, Wang Z, Ali S, Kong D, Banerjee S, Ahmad A, Li Y, Azmi AS, Miele L, Sarkar FH. Over-expression of FoxM1 leads to epithelial-mesenchymal transition and cancer stem cell phenotype in pancreatic cancer cells. J Cell Biochem. 2011;112(9):2296–306.
31. Aitola M, Carlsson P, Mahlapuu M, Enerback S, Pelto-Huikko M. Forkhead transcription factor FoxF2 is expressed in mesodermal tissues involved in epithelio-mesenchymal interactions. Dev Dyn. 2000;218(1):136–49.
32. Blixt A, Mahlapuu M, Bjursell C, Darnfors C, Johannesson T, Enerback S, Carlsson P. The two-exon gene of the human forkhead transcription factor FREAC-2 (FKHL6) is located at 6p25.3. Genomics. 1998;53(3):387–90.
33. Hellqvist M, Mahlapuu M, Blixt A, Enerback S, Carlsson P. The human forkhead protein FREAC-2 contains two functionally redundant activation domains and interacts with TBP and TFIIB. J Biol Chem. 1998;273(36):23335–43.
34. Lan Y, Jiang R. Sonic hedgehog signaling regulates reciprocal epithelial-mesenchymal interactions controlling palatal outgrowth. Development. 2009;136(8):1387–96.
35. Katoh Y, Katoh M. Hedgehog signaling, epithelial-to-mesenchymal transition and miRNA (review). Int J Mol Med. 2008;22(3):271–5.
36. Yu W, Ruest LB, Svoboda KK. Regulation of epithelial-mesenchymal transition in palatal fusion. Exp Biol Med (Maywood). 2009;234(5):483–91.
37. Wilkie AO, Morriss-Kay GM. Genetics of craniofacial development and malformation. Nat Rev Genet. 2001;2(6):458–68.
38. Wang T, Tamakoshi T, Uezato T, Shu F, Kanzaki-Kato N, Fu Y, Koseki H, Yoshida N, Sugiyama T, Miura N. Forkhead transcription factor Foxf2 (LUN)-deficient mice exhibit abnormal development of secondary palate. Dev Biol. 2003;259(1):83–94.
39. Ormestad M, Astorga J, Landgren H, Wang T, Johansson BR, Miura N, Carlsson P. Foxf1 and Foxf2 control murine gut development by limiting mesenchymal Wnt signaling and promoting extracellular matrix production. Development. 2006;133(5):833–43.

40. Shi W, Gerster K, Alajez NM, Tsang J, Waldron L, Pintilie M, Hui AB, Sykes J, P'ng C, Miller N, et al. MicroRNA-301 mediates proliferation and invasion in human breast cancer. Cancer Res. 2011;71(8):2926–37.

41. Lo HW, Hsu SC, Xia W, Cao X, Shih JY, Wei Y, Abbruzzese JL, Hortobagyi GN, Hung MC. Epidermal growth factor receptor cooperates with signal transducer and activator of transcription 3 to induce epithelial-mesenchymal transition in cancer cells via up-regulation of TWIST gene expression. Cancer Res. 2007;67(19):9066–76.

42. Nik AM, Reyahi A, Ponten F, Carlsson P. Foxf2 in intestinal fibroblasts reduces numbers of Lgr5(+) stem cells and adenoma formation by inhibiting Wnt signaling. Gastroenterology. 2013;144(5):1001–11.

43. Kong PZ, Yang F, Li L, Li XQ, Feng YM. Decreased FOXF2 mRNA expression indicates early-onset metastasis and poor prognosis for breast cancer patients with histological grade II tumor. PLoS One. 2013;8(4):e61591.

44. Cai J, Tian AX, Wang QS, Kong PZ, Du X, Li XQ, Feng YM. FOXF2 suppresses the FOXC2-mediated epithelial-mesenchymal transition and multidrug resistance of basal-like breast cancer. Cancer Lett. 2015;367(2):129–37.

45. Wang QS, Kong PZ, Li XQ, Yang F, Feng YM. FOXF2 deficiency promotes epithelial-mesenchymal transition and metastasis of basal-like breast cancer. Breast Cancer Res. 2015;17:30.

46. Lo PK. The controversial role of forkhead box F2 (FOXF2) transcription factor in breast cancer. PRAS Open. 2017;1.

47. Maeda M, Johnson KR, Wheelock MJ. Cadherin switching: essential for behavioral but not morphological changes during an epithelium-to-mesenchyme transition. J Cell Sci. 2005;118(Pt 5):873–87.

48. Deckers M, van Dinther M, Buijs J, Que I, Lowik C, van der Pluijm G, ten Dijke P. The tumor suppressor Smad4 is required for transforming growth factor beta-induced epithelial to mesenchymal transition and bone metastasis of breast cancer cells. Cancer Res. 2006;66(4):2202–9.

49. Waldmeier L, Meyer-Schaller N, Diepenbruck M, Christofori G. Py2T murine breast cancer cells, a versatile model of TGFbeta-induced EMT in vitro and in vivo. PLoS One. 2012;7(11):e48651.

50. Hellqvist M, Mahlapuu M, Samuelsson L, Enerback S, Carlsson P. Differential activation of lung-specific genes by two forkhead proteins, FREAC-1 and FREAC-2. J Biol Chem. 1996;271(8):4482–90.

51. Weber M, Hellmann I, Stadler MB, Ramos L, Paabo S, Rebhan M, Schubeler D. Distribution, silencing potential and evolutionary impact of promoter DNA methylation in the human genome. Nat Genet. 2007;39(4):457–66.

52. Muller WJ, Sinn E, Pattengale PK, Wallace R, Leder P. Single-step induction of mammary adenocarcinoma in transgenic mice bearing the activated c-neu oncogene. Cell. 1988;54(1):105–15.

53. Derksen PW, Liu X, Saridin F, van der Gulden H, Zevenhoven J, Evers B, van Beijnum JR, Griffioen AW, Vink J, Krimpenfort P, et al. Somatic inactivation of E-cadherin and p53 in mice leads to metastatic lobular mammary carcinoma through induction of anoikis resistance and angiogenesis. Cancer Cell. 2006;10(5):437–49.

54. Piek E, Moustakas A, Kurisaki A, Heldin CH, ten Dijke P. TGF-(beta) type I receptor/ALK-5 and Smad proteins mediate epithelial to mesenchymal transdifferentiation in NMuMG breast epithelial cells. J Cell Sci. 1999;112(Pt 24):4557–68.

55. Brabletz S, Brabletz T. The ZEB/miR-200 feedback loop—a motor of cellular plasticity in development and cancer? EMBO Rep. 2010;11(9):670–7.

56. Caramel J, Ligier M, Puisieux A. Pleiotropic roles for ZEB1 in cancer. Cancer Res. 2018;78(1):30–5.

57. Gheldof A, Hulpiau P, van Roy F, De Craene B, Berx G. Evolutionary functional analysis and molecular regulation of the ZEB transcription factors. Cell Mol Life Sci. 2012;69(15):2527–41.

58. Kondo M, Cubillo E, Tobiume K, Shirakihara T, Fukuda N, Suzuki H, Shimizu K, Takehara K, Cano A, Saitoh M, et al. A role for Id in the regulation of TGF-beta-induced epithelial-mesenchymal transdifferentiation. Cell Death Differ. 2004;11(10):1092–101.

59. Derynck R, Akhurst RJ, Balmain A. TGF-beta signaling in tumor suppression and cancer progression. Nat Genet. 2001;29(2):117–29.

60. Fabregat I, Herrera B, Fernandez M, Alvarez AM, Sanchez A, Roncero C, Ventura JJ, Valverde AM, Benito M. Epidermal growth factor impairs the cytochrome C/caspase-3 apoptotic pathway induced by transforming growth factor beta in rat fetal hepatocytes via a phosphoinositide 3-kinase-dependent pathway. Hepatology. 2000;32(3):528–35.

61. Murillo MM, del Castillo G, Sanchez A, Fernandez M, Fabregat I. Involvement of EGF receptor and c-Src in the survival signals induced by TGF-beta1 in hepatocytes. Oncogene. 2005;24(28):4580–7.

62. Minn A, Gupta G, Siegel P, Bos P, Shu W, Giri D, Viale A, Olshen A, Gerald W, Massague J. Genes that mediate breast cancer metastasis to lung. Nature. 2005;436(7050):518–24.

63. van 't Veer LJ, Dai H, van de Vijver MJ, He YD, Hart AA, Mao M, Peterse HL, van der Kooy K, Marton MJ, Witteveen AT, et al. Gene expression profiling predicts clinical outcome of breast cancer. Nature. 2002;415(6871):530–6.

64. Curtis C, Shah SP, Chin SF, Turashvili G, Rueda OM, Dunning MJ, Speed D, Lynch AG, Samarajiwa S, Yuan Y, et al. The genomic and transcriptomic architecture of 2,000 breast tumours reveals novel subgroups. Nature. 2012; 486(7403):346–52.

65. Dvinge H, Git A, Graf S, Salmon-Divon M, Curtis C, Sottoriva A, Zhao Y, Hirst M, Armisen J, Miska EA, et al. The shaping and functional consequences of the microRNA landscape in breast cancer. Nature. 2013;497(7449):378–82.

66. Thiery JP, Sleeman JP. Complex networks orchestrate epithelial-mesenchymal transitions. Nat Rev Mol Cell Biol. 2006;7(2):131–42.

67. Birchmeier W, Behrens J. Cadherin expression in carcinomas: role in the formation of cell junctions and the prevention of invasiveness. Biochim Biophys Acta. 1994;1198(1):11–26.

68. Christofori G. New signals from the invasive front. Nature. 2006;441(7092):444–50.

69. Kalluri R, Weinberg R. The basics of epithelial-mesenchymal transition. J Clin Invest. 2009;119(6):1420–8.

70. Peinado H, Olmeda D, Cano A. Snail, Zeb and bHLH factors in tumour progression: an alliance against the epithelial phenotype? Nat Rev Cancer. 2007;7(6):415–28.

71. Perk J, Iavarone A, Benezra R. Id family of helix-loop-helix proteins in cancer. Nat Rev Cancer. 2005;5(8):603–14.

72. Park SM, Gaur AB, Lengyel E, Peter ME. The miR-200 family determines the epithelial phenotype of cancer cells by targeting the E-cadherin repressors ZEB1 and ZEB2. Genes Dev. 2008;22(7):894–907.

73. Gregory PA, Bert AG, Paterson EL, Barry SC, Tsykin A, Farshid G, Vadas MA, Khew-Goodall Y, Goodall GJ. The miR-200 family and miR-205 regulate epithelial to mesenchymal transition by targeting ZEB1 and SIP1. Nat Cell Biol. 2008;10(5):593–601.

74. Burk U, Schubert J, Wellner U, Schmalhofer O, Vincan E, Spaderna S, Brabletz T. A reciprocal repression between ZEB1 and members of the miR-200 family promotes EMT and invasion in cancer cells. EMBO Rep. 2008;9(6):582–9.

75. Kundu ST, Byers LA, Peng DH, Roybal JD, Diao L, Wang J, Tong P, Creighton CJ, Gibbons DL. The miR-200 family and the miR-183~96~182 cluster target Foxf2 to inhibit invasion and metastasis in lung cancers. Oncogene. 2016; 35(2):173–86.

76. Willis SN, Chen L, Dewson G, Wei A, Naik E, Fletcher JI, Adams JM, Huang DC. Proapoptotic Bak is sequestered by Mcl-1 and Bcl-xL, but not Bcl-2, until displaced by BH3-only proteins. Genes Dev. 2005;19(11):1294–305.

77. Kim JY, Ahn HJ, Ryu JH, Suk K, Park JH. BH3-only protein Noxa is a mediator of hypoxic cell death induced by hypoxia-inducible factor 1alpha. J Exp Med. 2004;199(1):113–24.

78. Ploner C, Kofler R, Villunger A. Noxa: at the tip of the balance between life and death. Oncogene. 2009;27:S84–92.

79. Dairkee SH, Ljung BM, Smith H, Hackett A. Immunolocalization of a human basal epithelium specific keratin in benign and malignant breast disease. Breast Cancer Res Treat. 1987;10(1):11–20.

18

Evaluation of osteopenia and osteoporosis in younger breast cancer survivors compared with cancer-free women: a prospective cohort study

Cody Ramin[1], Betty J. May[1], Richard B. S. Roden[2], Mikiaila M. Orellana[1], Brenna C. Hogan[1], Michelle S. McCullough[1], Dana Petry[3], Deborah K. Armstrong[2] and Kala Visvanathan[1,2,3*] (iD)

Abstract

Background: Osteoporosis, an indicator of significant bone loss, has been consistently reported among older breast cancer survivors. Data are limited on the incidence of osteopenia, an earlier indicator of bone loss, and osteoporosis in younger breast cancer survivors compared with cancer-free women.

Methods: We prospectively examined bone loss in 211 breast cancer survivors (mean age at breast cancer diagnosis = 47 years) compared with 567 cancer-free women in the same cohort with familial risk for breast cancer. Multivariable-adjusted Cox proportional hazards models were used to estimate HRs and 95% CIs of osteopenia and/or osteoporosis incidence based on physician diagnosis.

Results: During a mean follow-up of 5.8 years, 66% of breast cancer survivors and 53% of cancer-free women reported having a bone density examination, and 112 incident cases of osteopenia and/or osteoporosis were identified. Breast cancer survivors had a 68% higher risk of osteopenia and osteoporosis compared to cancer-free women (HR = 1.68, 95% CI = 1.12–2.50). The association was stronger among recent survivors after only 2 years of follow-up (HR = 2.74, 95% CI = 1.37–5.47). A higher risk of osteopenia and osteoporosis was also observed among survivors aged ≤ 50 years, estrogen receptor-positive tumors, and those treated with aromatase inhibitors alone or chemotherapy plus any hormone therapy relative to cancer-free women.

Conclusions: Younger breast cancer survivors are at higher risk for osteopenia and osteoporosis compared to cancer-free women. Studies are needed to determine effective approaches to minimize bone loss in this population.

Keywords: Osteopenia, Osteoporosis, Bone loss, Breast cancer survivors, Cancer-free women

Introduction

Osteopenia and osteoporosis, both systemic skeletal conditions associated with varying degrees of bone loss, are prevalent among postmenopausal breast cancer survivors, with prior reports of up to 80% experiencing loss in bone density [1]. Untreated bone loss can lead to significant morbidity due to pain and fractures, as well as to death [2]. Osteopenia is diagnosed among individuals with lower-than-average bone density, while osteoporosis is characterized by both low bone density and architectural deterioration of bone tissue [3]. Among breast cancer survivors, cancer-related risk factors for osteopenia and osteoporosis include both treatment and premature menopause [4]. Importantly, the excess risk of osteopenia and osteoporosis among breast cancer survivors, particularly those of a younger age, relative to their cancer-free peers remains unknown.

Osteopenia and osteoporosis are also prevalent in the general population. Among women aged ≥ 50 years in the United States, approximately 15.4% have osteoporosis and 51.4% have low bone density [5]. Furthermore,

* Correspondence: kvisvan1@jhu.edu
[1]Department of Epidemiology, Johns Hopkins Bloomberg School of Public Health, Baltimore, MD 21205, USA
[2]Johns Hopkins Sidney Kimmel Comprehensive Cancer Center, Baltimore, MD, USA
Full list of author information is available at the end of the article

it is estimated that 1 in 2 women will be at risk for an osteoporosis-related fracture during their lifetime [2, 6]. Among cancer-free women, loss in bone density is associated with advancing age, menopause-induced estrogen deficiency, low body weight, lack of physical activity, excess alcohol consumption, family history of bone fracture, cigarette smoking, low calcium intake, and vitamin D deficiency [4, 7]. Loss of bone density in cancer survivors could be due to similar risk factors in addition to treatment-related effects. By comparing cancer survivors with cancer-free individuals, these risk factors can be differentiated.

Few epidemiologic studies have examined osteopenia and osteoporosis in breast cancer survivors relative to cancer-free women within the same cohort [8–10]. One prior study reported significantly lower levels of bone mineral density [8], the gold standard for assessing bone loss, and two other previous studies observed an increased risk of osteopenia and osteoporosis [9, 10] compared with cancer-free women. These studies were primarily conducted among older and long-term breast cancer survivors and did not differentiate based on tumor subtypes and detailed treatment regimens. One reason for the paucity of studies among younger breast cancer survivors is likely the challenge of identifying a comparable cancer-free group, because young cancer-free women do not routinely undergo assessment for bone health. Fortunately, we found this not to be the case in women with familial breast cancer risk, and we were therefore able to prospectively examine the risk of osteopenia and osteoporosis in a familial risk cohort known as the Breast and Ovarian Surveillance Service (BOSS) study.

Methods
Study population
The BOSS study is an ongoing prospective cohort study that includes women and men with familial risk for breast and/or ovarian cancer [11]. Participants were enrolled from 2005 to 2013 primarily from the Clinical Cancer Genetics Program at The Johns Hopkins Sidney Kimmel Comprehensive Cancer Center in Baltimore, MD, USA. Participants were aged ≥ 18 years with either (1) a family history of breast and/or ovarian cancer, (2) a documented *BRCA1/2* mutation, (3) a diagnosis of breast cancer at ≤ 40 years of age without a family history of breast cancer, or (4) a diagnosis of ovarian cancer at any age without a family history of ovarian cancer. Participants completed a baseline questionnaire so that information could be collected on a variety of demographic, lifestyle, and health-related factors, including detailed information on medical history and breast cancer treatment. Subsequent follow-up questionnaires have been completed every 3–4 years thereafter (> 92% have completed at least one follow-up

questionnaire). Completion of the second and third follow-up questionnaires is ongoing.

For the present prospective analysis, women were included if they completed a baseline questionnaire and at least one follow-up questionnaire through September 30, 2017 ($n = 1173$). Women with a physician diagnosis of osteopenia or osteoporosis at baseline ($n = 272$ total; $n = 174$ with osteopenia only; $n = 46$ osteoporosis only) or bisphosphonate use at baseline ($n = 5$) were excluded. We further excluded women with missing responses for osteopenia or osteoporosis on baseline ($n = 1$) or follow-up ($n = 5$) questionnaires. For this analysis, breast cancer survivors were defined as women diagnosed with breast cancer (ductal carcinoma in situ [stage 0] or stages I–III breast cancer) within 5 years prior to enrollment. The comparison group was restricted to women with no prior history of cancer at baseline except nonmelanoma skin cancer or cervical carcinoma in situ. After these exclusions, 778 women (211 breast cancer survivors and 567 cancer-free) became our analytic study population.

Exposure assessment
Cancer diagnoses were self-reported at enrollment, and pathology records were reviewed to confirm all diagnoses (by International Classification of Diseases Codes, Tenth Revision: invasive breast cancer [C50]; ductal carcinoma in situ [D05.1], and lobular carcinoma in situ [D05.0]) as well as stage and hormone receptor status (estrogen receptor [ER] /progesterone receptor [PR] and human epidermal growth factor receptor 2 [HER2]). Breast cancer treatment was reported in baseline questionnaires, and details were confirmed by medical record review (96% confirmed). Treatment information included surgery (none, lumpectomy, mastectomy) and adjuvant therapy (chemotherapy, radiation, and hormone therapy). Detailed information on type of chemotherapy and hormone therapy was also collected. We classified cancer treatment into mutually exclusive categories of surgery only, hormone therapy alone, chemotherapy alone, and chemotherapy plus hormone therapy. Hormone therapy was further classified as tamoxifen or aromatase inhibitor use.

Outcome assessment
Osteopenia and osteoporosis diagnoses were ascertained in baseline and follow-up questionnaires. In each questionnaire, participants were asked to indicate whether they had received a physician's diagnosis of osteopenia or osteoporosis and the date of that diagnosis. Incident cases of osteopenia and osteoporosis were identified on follow-up questionnaires. Our outcome of interest was a composite outcome that included incident osteopenia (i.e., low bone mass) and/or osteoporosis. Participants also reported whether they had ever had a bone density

examination and the year of examination on both base-line and follow-up questionnaires.

Ascertainment of covariates

Information on covariates (age, race, education level, menopausal status, age at menopause, oophorectomy at a young age, body mass index [BMI], physical activity based on metabolic equivalents of task [METs] per week, alcohol intake, smoking status, hormone replacement therapy [HRT] use, current bisphosphonate use, vitamin D supplement use, and calcium supplement use) was available from the baseline questionnaire. Bilateral oophorectomy at a young age was defined as both ovaries removed prior to age 45 years and based on self-report. We calculated age at bilateral oophorectomy from the date that the second ovary was removed. Medical procedures and screening examinations, including mammograms, pap smears, sigmoidoscopy, and colonoscopy, were also reported on both baseline and follow-up questionnaires.

Statistical analysis

Baseline characteristics of breast cancer survivors and cancer-free women were compared with frequency distributions for categorical variables and means (SDs) for continuous variables. We used Cox proportional hazards models with age as the time scale to calculate HRs and 95% CIs. Women contributed person-time from the completion date of the baseline questionnaire to the date of osteopenia or osteoporosis diagnosis or until the end of the last follow-up through September 30, 2017, whichever occurred first. The proportional hazards assumption was assessed with log-log survival plots and Schoenfeld residuals; neither method indicated that the assumption of proportional hazards was violated. Confounders were identified a priori as variables that may be associated with both breast cancer incidence and osteopenia/osteoporosis. Multivariable (MV) models were adjusted for menopausal status (premenopausal, postmenopausal), HRT use (ever, never), BMI (kg/m^2), bilateral oophorectomy at age < 45 years (yes, no), physical activity (MET-h/wk), smoking status (ever, never), and alcohol use (g/d). To account for a small percentage of missing data (< 1% missing) in covariates, we imputed missing data with the most common category for categorical covariates and the median value for continuous covariates among cancer-free women.

To identify whether bone loss differed by subgroups of breast cancer survivors, we examined the risk of osteopenia and osteoporosis in survivors stratified by age at diagnosis, menopausal status at diagnosis, ER tumor status, and breast cancer treatment relative to cancer-free women. For models that stratified breast cancer survivors by ER status, survivors were restricted to invasive breast cancer because ER status was not routinely measured in women with a stage 0 diagnosis. We were unable to

conduct analyses by HER2 status or triple-negative breast cancer, due to small numbers. We additionally conducted analyses by family history of breast cancer (no family history, first-degree relative only, first- and second-degree relatives) and an exploratory analysis by BRCA1/2 carrier status among a subgroup of women with genetic testing.

Finally, to examine whether risk of osteopenia and osteoporosis varied by time since diagnosis, we used time since enrollment as the time metric and restricted survivors to women diagnosed with breast cancer within 1 year prior to enrollment. Models were then stratified by follow-up time (≤ 2 years and > 2 years), and heterogeneity was tested using the likelihood ratio test.

Analyses were conducted using SAS version 9.4 (SAS Institute Inc., Cary, NC, USA) and Stata version 14.0 (StataCorp LP, College Station, TX, USA) software. All statistical tests were two-sided, and p values ≤ 0.05 were considered statistically significant.

Results

Age and age-adjusted baseline characteristics were compared in breast cancer survivors and cancer-free women (Table 1). Compared with cancer-free women, breast cancer survivors were more likely to be slightly older, postmenopausal, and current vitamin D users and less likely to have had a bilateral oophorectomy at a young age and a family history of breast cancer. Both survivors and cancer-free women were predominately white and highly educated (≥ 4 years of college). Among breast cancer survivors, the mean time from diagnosis to enrollment was 1.4 years, and the mean age at diagnosis was 47 years. Over 80% of breast cancer survivors were diagnosed with a first invasive breast cancer, and 76% had ER-positive breast tumors. In addition, all breast cancer survivors received surgery prior to adjuvant therapy; 65% of survivors received hormone therapy (67% tamoxifen, 41% aromatase inhibitors); and 50% of survivors received chemotherapy.

During an average of 5.8 years of follow-up, 66% of breast cancer survivors and 53% of cancer-free women reported having a bone density examination, and there were 112 incident cases of osteopenia and/or osteoporosis (75% osteopenia only). The incidence rates for osteopenia and osteoporosis were 44 cases/1000 person-years among breast cancer survivors and 19 cases/1000 person-years in their cancer-free peers. Overall, breast cancer survivors had a 68% higher risk of osteopenia and osteoporosis than cancer-free women (MV-HR = 1.68, 95% CI = 1.12–2.50) (Table 2). Results were similar when we restricted our analytic population to women who reported having a bone density examination prior to baseline and during follow-up (MV-HR = 1.90, 95% CI = 1.08–3.34; MV-HR = 1.72, 95% CI = 1.14–2.58, respectively). The results were also

Table 1 Age and age-adjusted baseline characteristics of cancer-free women and breast cancer survivors in the BOSS cohort study

Characteristic	Cancer-free (n = 567)	Survivors[a] (n = 211)	p Value
Age[b], years, mean (SD)	44.7 (11.3)	48.1 (10.3)	< 0.001
Race, white, %	88.7	83.3	0.02
Education, ≥ 4 years of college, %	77.6	77.4	0.72
Postmenopausal, %	27.4	51.6	< 0.001
Age at menopause[c], years, mean (SD)	49.6 (4.9)	48.8 (3.4)	0.86
Bilateral oophorectomy at age < 45 years[d], %	49.0	34.3	0.02
BMI, kg/m^2, mean (SD)	26.2 (5.1)	25.9 (3.1)	0.29
Physical activity, MET-h/wk[e], mean (SD)	29.4 (27.9)	26.0 (15.5)	0.29
Alcohol intake, g/d, mean (SD)	5.7 (7.5)	5.7 (4.8)	0.99
Smoking status, %			
Never	58.8	52.5	0.55
Former	36.7	44.8	
Current	4.2	2.7	
Missing	0.3	0.0	
HRT ever use, %	15.1	14.5	0.04
Ever mammogram[f], %	99.5	97.8	0.63
Ever pap smear, %	98.6	99.1	0.15
Current vitamin D supplement use, %	7.8	20.8	< 0.001
Current calcium supplement use, %	25.5	28.1	0.97
Bone density examination, %	28.9	43.0	0.02
Bone density examination in women aged ≥ 45 years, %	51.2	60.0	0.08
Ever broken bone, %	6.4	6.8	0.84
Family history of breast cancer, %			
No family history	14.7	38.9	< 0.001
First-degree relative only	64.8	50.7	
First- and second-degree relatives	17.0	9.0	
Missing	3.5	1.4	
BRCA1/2 status[g], %			
Negative	69.7	73.9	0.33
Positive	27.3	19.4	
Variants of uncertain significance	2.9	6.7	
Age at diagnosis, years, mean (SD)	–	46.8 (10.2)	–
Time from diagnosis to baseline, years, mean (SD)	–	1.4 (1.3)	–
Invasive breast cancer (stage I–III), %	–	82.5	–
Estrogen receptor status[h], %	–		–
Positive	–	75.9	–
Negative	–	23.6	–
Missing/untested	–	< 1.0	–
HER2 status[h], %	–		–
Positive	–	14.4	–
Negative	–	81.6	–
Missing/untested	–	3.5	–
Triple-negative status[h], %	–	19.0	–

Table 1 Age and age-adjusted baseline characteristics of cancer-free women and breast cancer survivors in the BOSS cohort study (*Continued*)

Characteristic	Cancer-free (n = 567)	Survivors[a] (n = 211)	p Value
Breast cancer treatment[i,j], %	–	–	–
Surgery	–	100.0	–
Chemotherapy	–	49.8	–
Hormone therapy, any	–	65.4	–
Hormone therapy, by type[k]	–		–
Tamoxifen	–	67.4	–
Aromatase inhibitor	–	41.3	–

Abbreviations: *BMI* Body mass index, *HER2* Human epidermal growth factor receptor 2, *HRT* Hormone replacement therapy
Values are means (SD) or percentages and are standardized to the age distribution of the study population
[a]Women were diagnosed with stages 0–III breast cancer ≤ 5 years prior to baseline
[b]Value is not age-adjusted
[c]Among postmenopausal women
[d]Among women who had both ovaries removed (n = 86)
[e]Metabolic equivalents from recreational and occupational activity
[f]Among women aged ≥ 50 years
[g]Among women tested for *BRCA* status (n = 414)
[h]Among invasive cases only (n = 174)
[i]Treatment groups are not mutually exclusive
[j]Chemotherapy and hormone therapy are adjuvant
[k]Seven percent of breast cancer survivors received both tamoxifen and aromatase inhibitors (n = 15)

Table 2 Risk of incident osteopenia and osteoporosis among breast cancer survivors compared with cancer-free women

	Events/person-years	Age-adjusted HR (95% CI)	MV-adjusted HR (95% CI)[a]
Overall			
Cancer-free	67/3509	1.00 (reference)	1.00 (reference)
Breast cancer survivors	45/1026	2.01 (1.38–2.94)	1.68 (1.12–2.50)
Excluding women without bone density examinations prior to baseline			
Cancer-free	27/1023	1.00 (reference)	1.00 (reference)
Breast cancer survivors	27/497	1.96 (1.15–3.36)	1.90 (1.08–3.34)
Excluding women without bone density examinations during follow-up			
Cancer-free	63/1890	1.00 (reference)	1.00 (reference)
Breast cancer survivors	45/703	1.89 (1.29–2.78)	1.72 (1.14–2.58)
Excluding early bilateral oophorectomy prior to baseline[b]			
Cancer-free	64/3347	1.00 (reference)	1.00 (reference)
Breast cancer survivors	42/957	1.93 (1.30–2.85)	1.63 (1.08–2.46)
Excluding pre- to postmenopausal during follow-up			
Cancer-free	34/2308	1.00 (reference)	1.00 (reference)
Breast cancer survivors	32/745	2.18 (1.34–3.55)	1.57 (0.93–2.63)
Excluding current vitamin D users[c]			
Cancer-free	60/3263	1.00 (reference)	1.00 (reference)
Breast cancer survivors	36/820	2.03 (1.34–3.08)	1.68 (1.08–2.61)
Excluding current calcium users[c]			
Cancer-free	40/2637	1.00 (reference)	1.00 (reference)
Breast cancer survivors	28/743	2.14 (1.32–3.48)	1.59 (0.95–2.68)

Abbreviations: *MV* Multivariable
[a]Adjusted for age (years), menopausal status (premenopausal, postmenopausal), bilateral oophorectomy at age < 45 years (yes, no), body mass index (kg/m^2), physical activity (MET-h/wk), smoking status (never, ever), alcohol intake (g/d), and hormone replacement therapy (never, ever)
[b]Both ovaries removed prior to age 45 years
[c]Vitamin D and calcium supplement use was ascertained at baseline

similar when we excluded women who had premature menopause secondary to a bilateral oophorectomy at age < 45 years (MV-HR = 1.63, 95% CI = 1.08–2.46) and only slightly attenuated when we restricted our analysis to women with no change in menopausal status during follow-up (MV-HR = 1.57, 95% CI = 0.93–2.63). Finally, the results did not change when we restricted our analytic sample to women without current vitamin D use at baseline (MV-HR = 1.68, 95% CI = 1.08–2.61) and became slightly attenuated among women without current calcium use at baseline (MV-HR = 1.59, 95% CI = 0.95–2.68).

The risk of osteopenia and osteoporosis in breast cancer survivors stratified by age at diagnosis, menopausal status at diagnosis, and ER status was compared with that of cancer-free women (Table 3). Breast cancer survivors diagnosed at age ≤ 50 years had an almost twofold increased risk of osteopenia and osteoporosis compared with cancer-free women (MV-HR = 1.98, 95% CI = 1.21–3.24). Surprisingly, the association was not significant in older women. In addition, breast cancer survivors who were premenopausal at diagnosis had increased risk of osteopenia and osteoporosis relative to their cancer-free peers (MV-HR = 1.76, 95% CI = 1.09–2.84), and this risk was similar but attenuated among women who were postmenopausal at diagnosis (MV-HR = 1.58, 95% CI = 0.86–2.89). Finally, women with ER-positive tumors had an over twofold increased risk of osteopenia and osteoporosis compared with cancer-free women (MV-HR = 2.10; 95% = 1.34–3.29). Although women with ER-negative tumors had a modest increased risk of osteopenia and osteoporosis relative to their cancer-free peers, the association was not statistically significant (MV-HR = 1.26;

95% CI = 0.54–2.94). Results were attenuated but did not differ by family history of breast cancer and BRCA1/2 carrier status (data not shown).

Next, the risk of osteopenia and osteoporosis in breast cancer survivors stratified by treatment compared with cancer-free women was examined (Fig. 1). Breast cancer survivors treated with chemotherapy plus hormone therapy had an over twofold increased risk of osteopenia and osteoporosis compared with cancer-free women (MV-HR = 2.70; 95% CI = 1.56–4.68). No significant association was observed for breast cancer survivors treated with surgery, chemotherapy, or hormone therapy alone compared with cancer-free women. Breast cancer survivors treated with aromatase inhibitors alone and combined chemotherapy plus aromatase inhibitors had a greater than two- and threefold increased risk of osteopenia and osteoporosis compared with cancer-free women (MV-HR = 2.72, 95% CI = 1.31–5.65; MV-HR = 3.83, 95% CI = 1.87–7.83, respectively). In addition, breast cancer survivors treated with chemotherapy plus tamoxifen had a greater than twofold increased risk compared with cancer-free women (MV-HR = 2.48, 95% CI = 1.16–5.30).

Finally, breast cancer survivors diagnosed within 1 year prior to enrollment had a greater than twofold increased risk of osteopenia and osteoporosis compared to their cancer-free peers within the first 2 years of follow-up (MV-HR = 2.74, 95% CI = 1.37–5.47) and a nonsignificant 85% increased risk of osteopenia and osteoporosis after 2 years of follow-up (MV-HR = 1.85, 95% CI = 0.98–3.51), although the p value for heterogeneity was not significant (p = 0.44) (Table 4).

Table 3 Risk of incident osteopenia and osteoporosis among breast cancer survivors compared with cancer-free women, stratified by characteristics at diagnosis

	Events/person-years	Age-adjusted HR (95% CI)	MV-adjusted HR[a] (95% CI)[a]
Age at diagnosis			
Cancer-free	67/3509	1.00 (reference)	1.00 (reference)
≤ 50 years	27/651	2.34 (1.46–3.75)	1.98 (1.21–3.24)
> 50 years	18/375	1.64 (0.93–2.88)	1.34 (0.75–2.40)
Menopausal status at diagnosis			
Cancer-free	67/3509	1.00 (reference)	1.00 (reference)
Premenopausal at diagnosis	27/728	1.97 (1.24–3.12)	1.76 (1.09–2.84)
Postmenopausal at diagnosis	18/298	2.05 (1.15–3.64)	1.58 (0.86–2.89)
ER status[b]			
Cancer-free	67/3509	1.00 (reference)	1.00 (reference)
ER-negative	7/200	1.68 (0.76–3.72)	1.26 (0.54–2.94)
ER-positive	32/611	2.32 (1.52–3.55)	2.10 (1.34–3.29)

Abbreviations: ER Estrogen receptor, MV Multivariable
[a]Adjusted for age (years), menopausal status (premenopausal, postmenopausal), bilateral oophorectomy at age < 45 years (yes, no), body mass index (kg/m^2), physical activity (MET-h/wk), smoking status (never, ever), alcohol intake (g/d), and hormone replacement therapy (never, ever)
[b]Breast cancer survivors were restricted to stages I–III

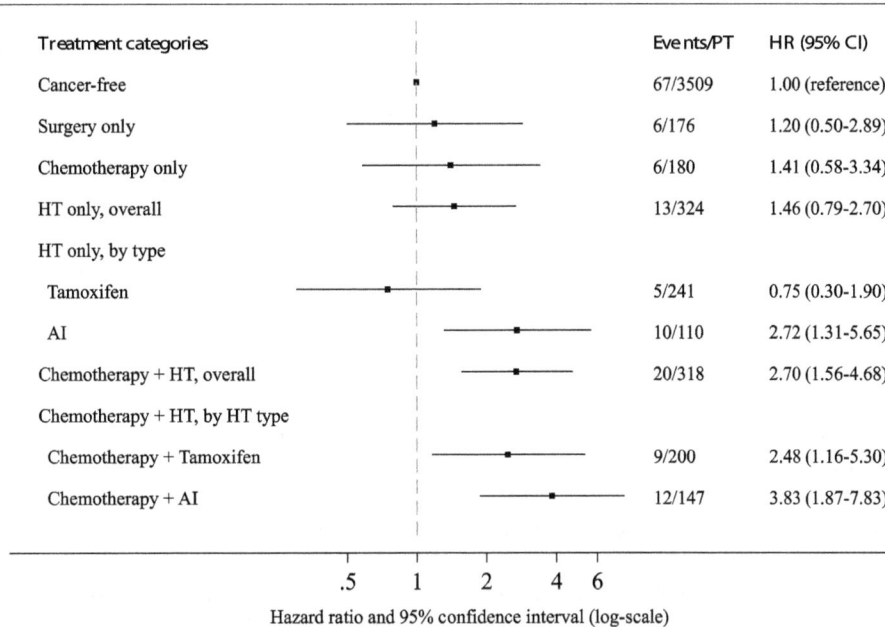

Treatment categories		Events/PT	HR (95% CI)
Cancer-free		67/3509	1.00 (reference)
Surgery only		6/176	1.20 (0.50-2.89)
Chemotherapy only		6/180	1.41 (0.58-3.34)
HT only, overall		13/324	1.46 (0.79-2.70)
HT only, by type			
Tamoxifen		5/241	0.75 (0.30-1.90)
AI		10/110	2.72 (1.31-5.65)
Chemotherapy + HT, overall		20/318	2.70 (1.56-4.68)
Chemotherapy + HT, by HT type			
Chemotherapy + Tamoxifen		9/200	2.48 (1.16-5.30)
Chemotherapy + AI		12/147	3.83 (1.87-7.83)

Hazard ratio and 95% confidence interval (log-scale)

Fig. 1 Abbreviations: Multivariable HRs (95% CIs) for incident osteopenia and osteoporosis among breast cancer survivors, stratified by type of treatment, compared with cancer-free women. Models are adjusted for Data are adjusted for age (years), menopausal status (premenopausal, postmenopausal), bilateral oophorectomy at age < 45 years (yes, no), body mass index (kg/m^2), physical activity (MET-h/wk), smoking status (never, ever), alcohol intake (g/d), and hormone replacement therapy (never, ever). *Abbreviations: AI* Aromatase inhibitor, *HT* Hormone therapy, *PT* Person time in years

Discussion

To our knowledge, this is the first study to prospectively assess risk of osteopenia and osteoporosis in young and recently diagnosed breast cancer survivors compared with their cancer-free peers in a familial high-risk cohort. In this prospective study, the incidence of osteopenia and osteoporosis was almost twofold higher in breast cancer survivors than in cancer-free women over an average of 5.8 years of follow-up. The results were also similar when we excluded women with premature menopause,

suggesting an effect of cancer treatment on bone health that is independent of early menopause. Breast cancer survivors who were younger, had ER-positive tumors, received aromatase inhibitors alone, or received combined chemotherapy with aromatase inhibitors or tamoxifen had a higher risk of osteopenia and osteoporosis than cancer-free women. Importantly, this was after accounting for age, menopause, and other risk factors for bone loss.

The majority of prior studies have examined bone health in breast cancer survivors without a cancer-free

Table 4 Risk of incident osteopenia and osteoporosis among recent breast cancer survivors compared with cancer-free women, stratified by follow-up time[a]

	Events/person-years	Age-adjusted HR (95% CI)	MV-adjusted HR (95% CI)[b]
Overall			
Cancer-free	67/3497	1.00 (reference)	1.00 (reference)
Survivors	27/475	2.49 (1.58–3.91)	2.17 (1.37–3.46)
0–2 years			
Cancer-free	22/1126	1.00 (reference)	1.00 (reference)
Survivors	14/214	3.15 (1.61–6.17)	2.74 (1.37–5.47)
3+ years			
Cancer-free	45/2371	1.00 (reference)	1.00 (reference)
Survivors	13/261	2.07 (1.11–3.85)	1.85 (0.98–3.51)

Abbreviations: *MV* Multivariable
[a]Breast cancer survivors were restricted to women diagnosed within 1 year prior to enrollment
[b]Adjusted for age (years), menopausal status (premenopausal, postmenopausal), bilateral oophorectomy at age < 45 years (yes, no), body mass index (kg/m^2), physical activity (MET-h/wk), smoking status (never, ever), alcohol intake (g/d), and hormone replacement therapy (never, ever)
p(s) for the likelihood ratio test of the interaction between breast cancer status and time was 0.42 for age- and 0.44 for *MV*-adjusted models

comparison group [12–20]. Several studies have found a higher risk of fracture in women diagnosed with breast cancer than in cancer-free women [21–23]; however, results have been inconsistent [24, 25]. Even fewer epidemiologic studies have assessed osteopenia and osteoporosis risk in women with breast cancer compared with their cancer-free peers within the same cohort [8–10]. Furthermore, these studies have included primarily older and long-term survivors. The first of these studies was conducted in the Women's Health Initiative Observational Study (WHI-OS). This study compared the prevalence of osteoporosis and the rate of bone loss in postmenopausal breast cancer survivors compared with cancer-free women [8]. Although the investigators found that breast cancer survivors had a higher prevalence of low bone density and osteoporosis at baseline, they did not have an increased rate of bone loss compared with cancer-free women over follow-up. However, breast cancer survivors were identified from prevalent cases at study enrollment, and the time from breast cancer diagnosis to study enrollment was not reported. Therefore, it is possible that the rate of bone loss may have been assessed to late after cancer diagnosis or treatment cessation, particularly if substantial bone loss occurred shortly after diagnosis or treatment.

The second study was a retrospective registry study in the Cancer Genetics Network conducted to assess early and late effects of cancer treatment [9]. In this study, the authors assessed osteopenia and osteoporosis risk based on self-report in women with and without invasive breast cancer and found a significant positive association for both outcomes (HR = 2.1, 95% CI = 1.8–2.4 for osteopenia; HR = 1.5, 95% CI = 1.2–1.9 for osteoporosis). Although this study included younger women with familial cancer risk, breast cancer survivors were identified from 1990 to 2009, and history of bone health was collected retrospectively in 2009. Among these breast cancer survivors, over 70% were diagnosed ≥ 10 years prior to the assessment of self-reported bone health in 2009, and thus the study was susceptible to substantial recall bias.

The third study was conducted among the U.K. General Practice Research Database to examine long-term health outcomes among older cancer survivors and cancer-free individuals (overall mean age = 66.9 years, SD = 12.3 years) [10]. The authors assessed osteoporosis risk, but not osteopenia, based on medical records among breast cancer survivors and found that survivors had a 26% higher risk of osteoporosis than cancer-free women (HR = 1.26, 95% CI = 1.13–1.40). None of these studies have assessed these associations by tumor subtype or incorporated detailed information on cancer treatment and bone density examination history. In addition, only one study has previously assessed osteopenia risk [9], an earlier indication of bone loss, which is also associated with a high fracture risk.

The most common cause of bone loss in women is menopause and aging. Aging is associated with greater bone resorption and less bone formation, whereas menopause induces accelerated bone loss due to lowering levels of endogenous estrogen [26]. Therefore, a cancer-free comparison of similar age and menopausal status is important when assessing bone loss. Given that we still observed significantly higher bone loss in breast cancer survivors relative to their cancer-free peers after accounting for age and menopause, it is likely that the additional bone loss is due to the effect of treatment on bone formation.

We observed a greater than twofold increased risk of osteopenia and osteoporosis in women diagnosed with ER-positive tumors, which is likely due to hormone therapy rather than to differences in tumor biology. This is supported by the fact that the highest risk of osteopenia and osteoporosis was found among breast cancer survivors treated with aromatase inhibitors alone and chemotherapy plus aromatase inhibitors. These findings are in agreement with the underlying biology of aromatase inhibitors [27], as well as with studies in breast cancer survivors [16–20] and high-risk women in chemoprevention trials [28, 29]. Aromatase inhibitors, prescribed to postmenopausal women with ER-positive tumors, blocks the aromatase enzyme, resulting in a hypoestrogenic state associated with bone loss [27]. We found no association among women with tamoxifen use alone, a group that was primarily premenopausal at baseline (mean age at baseline = 46 years; 76% premenopausal at baseline). However, we did observe an almost twofold increased risk of osteopenia and osteoporosis among women with chemotherapy plus tamoxifen use (mean age at baseline = 43; 50% premenopausal at baseline). Although tamoxifen, a selective ER modulator, is generally thought to be protective against bone loss in postmenopausal women [30], reports suggest that it may cause bone loss among premenopausal women due to premature menopause [13, 31]. Chemotherapy may also cause bone loss due to treament-induced premature menopause in premenopausal women [32] and may have direct toxic effects on bone formation cells [27]. In addition, medications commonly presribed along with chemotherapy (e.g., corticosteroids) have also been associated with bone loss [33]. Therefore, it is biologically plausible that chemotherapy plus hormone therapy might have a joint deleterious effect on bone health early in treatment.

The strengths of this study include the prospective study design, direct comparison with cancer-free women from the same cohort, and detailed information on cancer treatment. There are also several limitations to our analysis. First, our sample size may have limited our power to detect small to moderate associations. Second, osteopenia and osteoporosis incidence was ascertained on the basis of self-reported physician diagnosis and may be susceptible to misclassification. However, 96% of women who reported a diagnosis of osteopenia or osteoporosis also reported receiving a bone density examination. Third, breast cancer survivors may have increased surveillance for bone health and therefore may be more likely than cancer-free women to be diagnosed with osteopenia and osteoporosis. In our cohort, breast cancer survivors were slightly more likely than cancer-free women to have had a bone density examination at baseline (43% vs. 29%; 60% vs. 51% among women aged ≥ 45 years) and in follow-up (66% vs. 53%). However, sensitivity analyses to further reduce the possibility of undetected prevalent or incident cases found that results were similar when restricted to women with bone density examinations prior to baseline (MV-HR = 1.90, 95% CI = 1.08–3.34) and during follow-up (MV-HR = 1.72, 95% CI = 1.14–2.58). Furthermore, both women with and without breast cancer in our cohort underwent close monitoring for their health. Specifically, overall health screening history at baseline was similar in breast cancer survivors compared with cancer-free women (e.g., 99% vs. 99% had ever had a pap smear; 100% vs. 98% had ever had a mammogram among women aged ≥ 50 years). Finally, our results may not be generalizable to other populations, because our study population was composed predominately of white and highly educated women at high risk for breast cancer. However, we believe that the underlying biology of cancer treatment and its effect on bone health are likely similar across ethnicities. The homogeneity of our study population also improves the internal validity of this study because it reduces the influence of potential unmeasured factors.

Conclusions

In summary, our results demonstrate that incident osteopenia and osteoporosis are significantly higher in young breast cancer survivors within a few years of diagnosis than in cancer-free women and that risk varies by cancer treatment. These findings provide support for a baseline evaluation of bone density and fracture risk assessment close to breast cancer diagnosis, particularly among young survivors being treated with combined chemotherapy and hormone therapy, so that prevention strategies and appropriate monitoring can be implemented early. Future studies are needed to address the frequency of monitoring in breast cancer survivors by specific age and treatment groups.

Abbreviations

BMI: Body mass index; BOSS: Breast and Ovarian Surveillance Service; ER: Estrogen receptor; HER2: Human epidural growth factor receptor 2; HRT: Hormone replacement therapy; METs: Metabolic equivalents of tasks

Acknowledgements

The authors thank the State of Maryland, the Maryland Cigarette Restitution Fund, and the National Program of Cancer Registries of the Centers for Disease Control and Prevention for the funds that helped support the collection and availability of the cancer registry data. The Maryland Cancer Registry contributed cancer incidence data to this project. Center for Cancer Prevention and Control, Department of Health and Mental Hygiene, 201 West Preston Street, Room 400, Baltimore, MD 21201; https://phpa.health.maryland.gov/cancer/Pages/mcr_home.aspx, 410-767-4055. The authors also thank the participants and staff of the BOSS cohort study.

Funding

This research was supported in part by the Breast Cancer Research Foundation, the Avon Breast Cancer Research Program Network, and grants from the National Cancer Institute at the National Institutes of Health (T32-CA009314, P50CA098252, and P30CA06973).

Authors' contributions

This analysis was conceived by CR and KV. CR and KV contributed to the design and interpretation of data. Acquisition of data was performed by BJM, MMO, BCH, and MSM, Data analysis was performed by CR and KV. CR, BJM, BSRR, MMO, BCH, MSM, DP, DKA, and KV were involved in critically revising the manuscript for intellectual content. All authors read and approved the final manuscript for publication.

Competing interests

The authors declare that they have no competing interests.

Author details

[1]Department of Epidemiology, Johns Hopkins Bloomberg School of Public Health, Baltimore, MD 21205, USA. [2]Johns Hopkins Sidney Kimmel Comprehensive Cancer Center, Baltimore, MD, USA. [3]The Johns Hopkins School of Medicine, Baltimore, MD, USA.

References

1. Runowicz CD, Leach CR, Henry NL, Henry KS, Mackey HT, Cowens-Alvarado RL, et al. American Cancer Society/American Society of Clinical Oncology breast cancer survivorship care guideline. J Clin Oncol. 2016;34:611–35.
2. Office of the Surgeon General. Bone health and osteoporosis: a report of the Surgeon General. Rockville: U.S. Department of Health and Human Services; 2004.
3. Coleman R, Body JJ, Aapro M, Hadji P, Herrstedt J. Bone health in cancer patients: ESMO Clinical Practice Guidelines. Ann Oncol. 2014;25(Suppl 3): iii124–37.
4. Gralow JR, Biermann JS, Farooki A, Fornier MN, Gagel RF, Kumar R, et al. NCCN Task Force Report: bone health in cancer care. J Natl Compr Cancer Netw. 2013;11(Suppl 3):S1–50.
5. Wright NC, Looker AC, Saag KG, Curtis JR, Delzell ES, Randall S, et al. The recent prevalence of osteoporosis and low bone mass in the United States based on bone mineral density at the femoral neck or lumbar spine. J Bone Miner Res. 2014;29:2520–6.
6. U.S. Preventive Services Task Force. Screening for osteoporosis: U.S. Preventive Services Task Force recommendation statement. Ann Intern Med. 2011;154:356–64.
7. Karaguzel G, Holick MF. Diagnosis and treatment of osteopenia. Rev Endocr Metab Disord. 2010;11:237–51.

8.   Chen Z, Maricic M, Pettinger M, Ritenbaugh C, Lopez AM, Barad DH, et al. Osteoporosis and rate of bone loss among postmenopausal survivors of breast cancer. Cancer. 2005;104:1520–30.

9.   Hill DA, Horick NK, Isaacs C, Domchek SM, Tomlinson GE, Lowery JT, et al. Long-term risk of medical conditions associated with breast cancer treatment. Breast Cancer Res Treat. 2014;145:233–43.

10. Khan NF, Mant D, Carpenter L, Forman D, Rose PW. Long-term health outcomes in a British cohort of breast, colorectal and prostate cancer survivors: a database study. Br J Cancer. 2011;105 Suppl 1:S29–37.

11. Gross AL, May BJ, Axilbund JE, Armstrong DK, Roden RBS, Visvanathan K. Weight change in breast cancer survivors compared to cancer-free women: a prospective study in women at familial risk of breast cancer. Cancer Epidemiol Biomark Prev. 2015;24:1262–9.

12. Love RR, Mazess RB, Barden HS, Epstein S, Newcomb PA, Jordan VC, et al. Effects of tamoxifen on bone mineral density in postmenopausal women with breast cancer. N Engl J Med. 1992;326:852–6.

13. Powles TJ, Hickish T, Kanis JA, Tidy A, Ashley S. Effect of tamoxifen on bone mineral density measured by dual-energy x-ray absorptiometry in healthy premenopausal and postmenopausal women. J Clin Oncol. 1996;14:78–84.

14. Sverrisdóttir Á, Fornander T, Jacobsson H, Schoultz EV, Rutqvist LE. Bone mineral density among premenopausal women with early breast cancer in a randomized trial of adjuvant endocrine therapy. J Clin Oncol. 2004;22: 3694–9.

15. Zaman K, Thürlimann B, Huober J, Schönenberger A, Pagani O, Lüthi J, Simcock M, et al. Bone mineral density in breast cancer patients treated with adjuvant letrozole, tamoxifen, or sequences of letrozole and tamoxifen in the BIG 1-98 study. Ann Oncol. 2012;23:1474–81.

16. Coleman RE, Banks LM, Girgis SI, Kilburn LS, Vrdoljak E, Fox J, et al. Skeletal effects of exemestane on bone-mineral density, bone biomarkers, and fracture incidence in postmenopausal women with early breast cancer participating in the Intergroup Exemestane Study (IES): a randomised controlled study. Lancet Oncol. 2007;8:119–27.

17. Cuzick J, Sestak I, Baum M, Buzdar A, Howell A, Dowsett M, et al. Effect of anastrozole and tamoxifen as adjuvant treatment for early-stage breast cancer: 10-year analysis of the ATAC trial. Lancet Oncol. 2010;11:1135–41.

18. Eastell R, Hannon RA, Cuzick J, Dowsett M, Clack G, Adams JE. Effect of an aromatase inhibitor on BMD and bone turnover markers: 2-year results of the Anastrozole, Tamoxifen, Alone or in Combination (ATAC) trial (18233230). J Bone Miner Res. 2006;21:1215–23.

19. Lønning PE, Geisler J, Krag LE, Erikstein B, Bremnes Y, Hagen AI, et al. Effects of exemestane administered for 2 Years versus placebo on bone mineral density, bone biomarkers, and plasma lipids in patients with surgically resected early breast cancer. J Clin Oncol. 2005;23:5126–37.

20. Perez EA, Josse RG, Pritchard KI, Ingle JN, Martino S, Findlay BP, et al. Effect of letrozole versus placebo on bone mineral density in women with primary breast cancer completing 5 or more years of adjuvant tamoxifen: a companion study to NCIC CTG MA.17. J Clin Oncol. 2006;24:3629–35.

21. Chen Z, Maricic M, Aragaki AK, Mouton C, Arendell L, Lopez AM, et al. Fracture risk increases after diagnosis of breast or other cancers in postmenopausal women: results from the Women's Health Initiative. Osteoporos Int. 2009;20:527–36.

22. Chen Z, Maricic M, Bassford TL, Pettinger M, Ritenbaugh C, Lopez AM, et al. Fracture risk among breast cancer survivors: results from the women's health initiative observational study. Arch Intern Med. 2005;165:552–8.

23. Tsa CH, Muo CH, Tzeng HE, Tang CH, Hsu HC, Sung FC. Fracture in asian women with breast cancer occurs at younger age. PLoS One. 2013;8:e75109.

24. Lamont EB, Lauderdale DS. Low risk of hip fracture among elderly breast cancer survivors. Ann Epidemiol. 2003;13:698–703.

25. Pawloski PA, Geiger AM, Haque R, Kamineni A, Fouayzi H, Ogarek J, et al. Fracture risk in older, long-term survivors of early-stage breast cancer. J Am Geriatr Soc. 2013;61:888–95.

26. Demontiero O, Vidal C, Duque G. Aging and bone loss: new insights for the clinician. Ther Adv Musculoskelet Dis. 2012;4:61–76.

27. Taxel P, Choksi P, Van Poznak C. The management of osteoporosis in breast cancer survivors. Maturitas. 2012;73:275–9.

28. Cheung AM, Tile L, Cardew S, Pruthi S, Robbins J, Tomlinson G, et al. Bone density and structure in healthy postmenopausal women treated with exemestane for the primary prevention of breast cancer: a nested substudy of the MAP.3 randomised controlled trial. Lancet Oncol. 2012;13:275–84.

29. Sestak I, Singh S, Cuzick J, Blake GM, Patel R, Gossiel F, et al. Changes in bone mineral density at 3 years in postmenopausal women receiving anastrozole and risedronate in the IBIS-II bone substudy: an international, double-blind, randomised, placebo-controlled trial. Lancet Oncol. 2014;15: 1460–8.

30. Kristensen B, Ejlertsen B, Dalgaard P, Larsen L, Holmegaard SN, Transbøl I, et al. Tamoxifen and bone metabolism in postmenopausal low-risk breast cancer patients: a randomized study. J Clin Oncol. 1994;12:992–7.

31. Vehmanen L, Elomaa I, Blomqvist C, Saarto T. Tamoxifen treatment after adjuvant chemotherapy has opposite effects on bone mineral density in premenopausal patients depending on menstrual status. J Clin Oncol. 2006; 24:675–80.

32. Shapiro CL, Manola J, Leboff M. Ovarian failure after adjuvant chemotherapy is associated with rapid bone loss in women with early-stage breast cancer. J Clin Oncol. 2001;19:3306–11.

33. Pitts CJD, Kearns AE. Update on medications with adverse skeletal effects. Mayo Clin Proc. 2011;86:338–43.

19

Long-term exposure to road traffic noise and incidence of breast cancer: a cohort study

Zorana Jovanovic Andersen[1,2]* (iD), Jeanette Therming Jørgensen[1], Lea Elsborg[1], Søren Nymand Lophaven[1], Claus Backalarz[3], Jens Elgaard Laursen[3], Torben Holm Pedersen[3], Mette Kildevæld Simonsen[4], Elvira Vaclavik Bräuner[5] and Elsebeth Lynge[2]

Abstract

Background: Exposure to road traffic noise was associated with increased risk of estrogen receptor (ER)-negative (ER-) breast cancer in a previous cohort study, but not with overall or ER-positive (ER+) breast cancer, or breast cancer prognosis. We examined the association between long-term exposure to road traffic noise and incidence of breast cancer, overall and by ER and progesterone receptor (PR) status.

Methods: We used the data from a nationwide Danish Nurse Cohort on 22,466 female nurses (age > 44 years) who at recruitment in 1993 or 1999 reported information on breast cancer risk factors. We obtained data on the incidence of breast cancer from the Danish Cancer Registry, and on breast cancer subtypes by ER and PR status from the Danish Breast Cancer Cooperative Group, up to 31 December 2012. Road traffic noise levels at the nurses' residences were estimated by the Nord2000 method between 1970 and 2013 as annual means of a weighted 24 h average (L_{den}) at the most exposed facade. We used time-varying Cox regression to analyze the associations between the 24-year, 10-year, and 1-year mean of L_{den} and breast cancer, separately for total breast cancer and by ER and PR status.

Results: Of the 22,466 women, 1193 developed breast cancer in total during 353,775 person-years of follow up, of whom 611 had complete information on ER and PR status. For each 10 dB increase in 24-year mean noise levels at their residence, we found a statistically significant 10% (hazard ratio and 95% confidence interval 1.10; 1.00–1.20) increase in total breast cancer incidence and a 17% (1.17; 1.02–1.33) increase in analyses based on 611 breast cancer cases with complete ER and PR information. We found positive, statistically significant association between noise levels and ER+ (1.23; 1.06–1.43, $N = 494$) but not ER- (0.93; 0.70–1.25, $N = 117$) breast cancers, and a stronger association between noise levels and PR+ (1.21; 1.02–1.42, $N = 393$) than between noise levels and PR- (1.10; 0.89–1.37, $N = 218$) breast cancers. Association between noise and ER+ breast cancer was statistically significantly stronger in nurses working night shifts (3.36; 1.48–7.63) than in those not working at night (1.21; 1.02–1.43) (p value for interaction = 0.05).

Conclusion: Long-term exposure to road traffic noise may increase risk of ER+ breast cancer.

Keywords: Road traffic noise, Breast cancer, Estrogen receptor, Progesterone receptor, Nurses, Night shift work

* Correspondence: zorana.andersen@sund.ku.dk
[1]Section of Environmental Health, Department of Public Health, University of Copenhagen, Øster Farimagsgade 5, 1014 Copenhagen, Denmark
[2]Nykøbing F Hospital, University of Copenhagen, Ejegodvej 63, 4800 Nykøbing F, Denmark
Full list of author information is available at the end of the article

Background

Noise from road traffic is a persistent environmental stressor posing a huge and increasing health burden on urban populations. It was estimated in 2012 that environmental noise was responsible for at least one million healthy life years lost per year in Western Europe. [1] Epidemiological studies have shown that exposure to residential road traffic noise can lead to the development of cardiovascular disease and stroke [2], metabolic disease [3, 4], and possibly breast cancer (BC) [5–7].

The proposed mechanism behind the possible association between road traffic noise and BC include a psychological stress pathway, as persistent annoyance from exposure to environmental stressors such as traffic noise can lead to hyper-activation of the hypothalamic-pituitary-adrenal gland and release of stress hormones [8]. Accumulating evidence suggests that psychological stress increases the risk of BC, but the mechanism remains unknown [9]. Exposure to stress hormones (cortisol, catecholamines, etc.) can result in accumulation in DNA damage [10]. Stress hormone glucocorticoid steroid might promote tumor development and progression by inhibiting apoptosis [11]. In a single controlled experimental study in 18 healthy subjects, exposure to residential road traffic noise (48 or 75 dB) has been shown to result in increased levels of gene expression biomarkers of oxidative stress and DNA repair [12]. A recent experimental study found that rats exposed to noise (105 dB) for 30 days had significantly higher serum levels of malondialdehyde (MDA) and lower total antioxidant capacity (TAC), biomarkers of oxidative stress, than nonexposed rats [13]. Oxidative stress promotes BC development and progression [14, 15] and one study suggests that this mechanism is most relevant for estrogen receptor (ER)-positive (ER+) BC [15]. Another mechanism behind the possible link between noise exposure and BC involves sleep disturbance, reduced sleep quality and duration, which have been linked to residential road traffic noise exposure at night [16, 17]. Sleep disturbance and BC have been extensively studied with respect to night shift work, since "shift work that involves circadian disruption" was classified in 2007 as a probable human carcinogen by the International Agency for Research on Cancer (IARC) [18]. However, the epidemiological evidence on the relationship between night shift work and BC is mixed, as some meta-analyses suggest positive [19] and others no association [20, 21]. Similarly, the most recent literature on sleep duration and BC identifies no evidence of association [22, 23]. Finally, exposure to residential road traffic noise may increase the risk of weight gain [24], obesity [25, 26], and type II diabetes mellitus [27], all risk factors for postmenopausal BC [28, 29].

The evidence to date is mixed and there are three epidemiological studies on road traffic noise and BC, two on incidence [5, 7] and one on survival [6]. The study on long-term exposure to residential road traffic and railway noise and BC incidence in 29,875 women from the Danish Diet, Cancer and Health cohort detected a positive association between these exposures and ER-negative (ER-) BC, which comprises 20% of total BC, but found no association between exposure and ER+ or overall BC [5]. A study on BC survival in the same cohort found no association between residential road traffic noise and concurrent breast-cancer-specific mortality [6]. Finally, a case-control study of women living close to Frankfurt airport found no association between residential road traffic or railway noise and BC overall, but found a positive association between aircraft noise and ER- BC [7]. BCs classified by ER or PR expression have different clinical, pathologic, and molecular features and the etiology of these are heterogenous. Still, no study to date has investigated the association between traffic noise exposure and the incidence of BC classified by progesterone (PR) status.

Here we report on the association between exposure to residential road traffic noise over 24 years and the incidence of BC, overall and by subtypes, according to ER status, and for the first time, by PR status.

Methods

The Danish nurse cohort

The Danish Nurse Cohort [30] was inspired by the American Nurses' Health Study to initially investigate the health effects of hormone therapy (HT) in a European population. The cohort was initiated in 1993 by sending a questionnaire to 23,170 female Danish nurses (age > 44 years), members of the Danish Nursing Organization, which included 95% of all nurses in Denmark. In total, 19,898 (86%) nurses replied, and the cohort was reinvestigated in 1999, including an additional 10,534 nurses who turned 45 years in the period 1993–1999 and 2231 non-responders from 1993, of whom 8833 in total (69%) replied. At recruitment, the nurses filled out a questionnaire on working conditions, weight and height, lifestyle (diet, active smoking, alcohol consumption, and leisure time physical activity), parity, age at first birth, age of menarche and menopause, and use of oral contraceptives (OC) and HT. We utilized baseline information from 1993 (19,898) or 1999 (8833) for 28,731 female nurses in total. Using a unique identification number, we linked the cohort participants to the Civil Registration System [31] to obtain vital status as of 31st December 2012 (active, date of death or emigration) and full residential address history since 1970.

Breast cancer definition

We linked the records of 28,731 nurses using the unique identification number to the Danish Cancer Register [32] to extract all cancer diagnoses until the end of 2012. First, we identified nurses with diagnoses for any cancer (other than non-melanoma skin cancer) before baseline (1 April 1993 or 1 April 1999), and excluded these nurses from the analyses. Second, among nurses who were cancer-free at the cohort baseline, we extracted primary invasive BC diagnoses (ICD-10 codes C50), as the main outcome, and any other cancer (other than non-melanoma skin cancer), for censoring purposes, between cohort baseline (1 April 1993 or 1 April 1999) and 31 December 2012. We extracted data on BC subtype by ER and PR status from the clinical database of the Danish BC Cooperative Group [33], and in the subset of cases with available ER and PR status, we defined the following BC subtypes: ER+, ER-, PR+, PR-, ER+/PR+, ER+/PR-, ER-/PR+, and ER-/PR- BCs.

Residential road traffic noise exposure

The road traffic noise levels at the nurses' residential addresses were calculated using the Nord2000 method [34]. The Nord2000 method is the state-of-the-art traffic noise propagation model. It is based on input variables including geocodes of the location, the height of apartments above street level, road lines with information on yearly average daily traffic, traffic composition and speed, road type and properties (e.g. motorway, rural highway, road wider than 6 m, and other roads), building polygons for all surrounding buildings (height of buildings, etc.) and meteorology, including wind speed and direction, air temperature, and cloud cover. The traffic noise contribution is calculated for four weather classes, which typically occur in Denmark. The frequency of weather classes in the calculations are included with a frequency as they occur in a Danish meteorology average year. The propagation model is based on geometrical ray theory computing the 1/3 octave band sound attenuation along the path from the source to the receiver, accounting for the properties of the terrain (shape, ground type, including impedance and roughness) and variations in weather conditions, appropriate when estimating yearly average noise levels. Various weather conditions have been predefined and respective noise levels computed. The long-term noise levels, as the yearly average noise contributions, are then determined by weighting the occurrence of the different weather conditions obtained from weather statistics. The Nord2000 method has been validated by more than 500 propagation cases, 9 of them involving residential road traffic noise [35], and validation of the method has furthermore been conducted for noise originating from higher sources, e.g. wind turbines [36]. However, validation is not possible for historical values, and it is reasonable to assume that estimation of noise further back in time is less precise that that more recent. Annual average levels of residential road traffic noise were estimated for each nurse at each of her

residential addresses between 1970 and 2013, as the equivalent continuous A-weighted sound pressure level (LA_{eq}) at the most exposed façade of the dwelling for the day (L_d, 0700–1900 h), evening (L_e, 1900–2200 h) and night (L_n, 2200–0700 h), and expressed as L_{den} (the overall noise level during the day, evening and night, calculated as the weighted 24-h noise level, with a 5 dB penalty for the noise levels in the evening hours, and a 10 dB penalty for the night time noise levels.). Our main noise exposure variable was the 24-year running mean of L_{den} from 1970 (oldest available) to 1993 or 1999, the beginning of study follow up. Additionally, we defined 10-year and 1-year running mean preceding diagnoses, and 1-year mean at the cohort baseline, to explore the effect of different exposure windows to residential road traffic noise. L_{den} was used also as a categorical variable with three levels, representing low (< 48 dB, 25th percentile of L_{den}), medium (48–58 dB) and high (≥ 58 dB, 75th percentile of L_{den}) residential road traffic exposure, for each time window. Finally, we explore the effect of LA_{eq}, L_d, L_e, and L_n, to explore whether day, evening, night, or overall exposure to residential road traffic noise was relevant for the risk of BC.

Statistical analyses

We used an extended Cox proportional hazards regression model, with age as the underlying time scale, to examine the association between residential road traffic noise and incidence of overall BC in two steps: in a crude model adjusted for age (age as the underlying time scale), and in a fully adjusted model, where we additionally adjusted for birth cohort (1990–1934; 1935–1944; 1945–1949; 1950–1955), body mass index (BMI) (< 18.5 kg/m^2; 18.5–25 kg/m^2; 25–30 kg/m^2; ≥ 30 kg/m^2), alcohol use (none; moderate: 1–14 drinks/week; heavy: > 15 drinks/week), leisure time physical activity (low; medium; high), smoking status (never; former; current), age at menarche (years), parity (yes; no), number of children, age at first birth (years), menopausal status (yes; no), HT use (never; ever), and oral contraceptive (OC) use (never; ever). The start of follow up was age at the cohort baseline (1 April 1993 or 1st April 1999) and end of follow up was age at the time of BC diagnoses (event) diagnoses, other cancer diagnoses (except non-melanoma skin cancer), death, emigration, or 31 December 2012, whichever came first. We evaluated the effect of the residential road traffic noise as time-varying exposure, with 24-year, 10-year, and 1-year means calculated as geometric means, and modeled in separate models.

Sensitivity analyses were included using LA_{eq}, L_d, L_e, and L_n, and with checks for adherence to the proportional hazards assumption for all noise proxies and confounders based on scaled Schoenfeld residuals. The effect modification of an association between residential road traffic noise and

BC by menopausal status, obesity, HT use, night shift work (yes - nurses those who were in work force at the cohort baseline and who reported typically working night shifts; no - nurses working at the cohort baseline and who typically work day, evening, or rotating shifts), and urbanicity (defined by population density at the municipality of residence at the cohort baseline in 1993 or 1999: rural areas - population density < 180 persons/km^2; provincial areas with 180–5220 persons/km^2; and urban areas with > 5220 persons/km^2) was evaluated by introducing interaction terms into the Cox model, and was tested by the Wald test. Separate analyses were performed for subtypes of BC according to ER status (ER+ and ER-) PR status (PR+ and PR-) and ER status combined with PR status (ER+/PR+, ER+/PR-, ER-/PR- and ER-/PR+). Additional sensitivity analyses included analyses of association between 24-year mean L_{den} and overall BC with additional adjustment for the baseline year (year of recruitment 1993 or 1999), mean income at the municipality of residence at the cohort baseline, as a proxy of neighborhood socio-economic level, and air pollution, in terms of particulate matter (PM) less than 2.5 nm, (PM$_{2.5}$) and nitrogen oxide (NO$_x$) at the baseline year We did not adjust for air pollution in the main model, since air pollution is still not recognized as a risk factor for BC, and since we have previously found no association between air pollution and BC in this cohort [37]. Results were presented as hazard ratios (HRs) and 95% confidence intervals (CI). Analyses were performed using Stata 11.2.

Results

Of the total 28,731 nurses in the Danish Nurse Cohort, we excluded 9 due to inactive (emigrated) vital status prior to study entry, 2556 with a cancer diagnosis before cohort baseline, 229 due to missing noise exposure, and 3471 with missing information on one or more covariates (see Additional file 1: Figure S1). Of the 22,466 nurses in the main analyses, 1193 developed BC during the mean follow up of 15.7 years or 353,775 person-years, with an incidence rate of 337 per 100,000 person-years. Of 1193 BC cases, information on ER status was available in 1061 cases and of these 884 (83.3%) were ER+ and 177 (16.7%) ER-. Of 1193 BC cases, information on both PR and ER status was available on 611 as follows: 393 (64.3%) were PR + and 218 (35.7%) PR- and 494 (80.9%) were ER+ and 117 (19.1%) ER-. Among the 611 the combination of ER and PR status was that 384 (62.8%) were ER+/PR+, 110 (18.0%) ER+/PR-, 9 (1.5%) ER-/PR+, and 108 (17.8%) ER-/PR-.

The mean age at baseline was 53.0 years, mean BMI 23.7 kg/m^2, 49.3% of the women were postmenopausal, 34.1% current smokers, 27.0% highly physically active, 22.8% heavy alcohol drinkers, 27.1% ever HT users, 58.9 ever OC users, and 14.1% were nulliparous and the mean age at 1st childbirth in parous women was 25.9 years

(Table 1 compares baseline characteristics of non BC cases to all 1193 BC cases in the cohort, and Additional file 1: Table S1 compares baseline characteristics of non BC cases to 611 BC cases with complete date on ER and PR status). Compared with women who remained free of BC by the end of 2012, those who developed the cancer were more likely to be obese, current smokers, heavy alcohol drinkers, nulliparous, postmenopausal, older than 12 years at menarche, and HT users, but were less likely to be highly physically active and use OC. Mean level of residential road traffic noise at the year of the cohort baseline (1993 or 1999) was 48.6 dB and was slightly higher for women who developed BC and ranged from 5 dB to 79.6 dB as depicted in the geographical variation of residential road traffic noise in Fig. 1. As expected higher levels of traffic noise are found around major cities and roads.

In the fully adjusted models, we found a positive and statistically significant association between each 10 dB increase in residential road traffic noise levels at the residence (24-year mean noise levels preceding diagnosis) and incidence of BC, ranging from a 10% (HR; 95% CI, 1.10; 1.00–1.20) increase in total BC incidence ($N = 1193$), to a 17% (HR; 95% CI, 1.17; 1.02–1.33) increase in incidence based on the 611 BC cases with ER and PR information (Table 2). Figure 2 shows increasing HR with increase in time-weighted 24-year running mean preceding diagnosis based on the fully adjusted model and indicates a dose-response association. This dose response is also reflected in the fully adjusted models in Table 2; compared to women living in areas with low residential road traffic noise levels (< 48 dB), the highest HRs were observed in the fully adjusted models for women exposed to the highest noise levels (> 58 dB) (HR; 95% CI, 1.30; 1.07–1.60 in 1193 of all BC cases and 1.42; 1.06–1.89 in 611 BC cases with full ER and PR hormone receptor status); and smaller HRs in women exposed to medium noise levels (48–58 dB) (HR; 95% CI: 1.24; 1.04–1.47 in 1193 cases and 1.28; 0.99–1.65 in 611 cases). Similar results were observed with alternative categorization of L_{den} by quartiles of noise exposure (see Additional file 1: Table S8). The same trends, albeit weaker, were found with 10-year and 1-year mean noise levels preceding diagnosis. The weakest association was found with the 1-year mean levels at the cohort baseline (Table 2). All associations were statistically significant in analyses with the 611 BC cases with full information on estrogen and progesterone hormone status. Associations per 10 dB of the 24-year mean preceding diagnosis for LA_{eq}, L_d, L_e, and L_n were almost identical to those with L_{den} (see Additional file 1: Table S2).

We found a positive and statistically significant association between residential road traffic noise (for each 10 dB increase in 24-year mean noise levels preceding diagnosis) and ER+ (1.23; 1.06–1.43, $N = 494$) and none with ER- (HR; 95% CI, 0.93; 0.70–1.25, $N = 117$) BCs (Table 3). The

Table 1 Descriptive statistics at the cohort baseline (1993 or 1999) among 22,466 female nurses from the Danish Nurse Cohort by breast cancer status at the end of follow up

	Total	Breast cancer	No breast cancer
	N = 22,466	N = 1193	N = 21,273
Age, mean (SD)	53.0 ± 7.9	53.6 ± 7.5	53.0 ± 7.9
Birth cohort			
< 1935, n (%)	5067 (22.6)	290 (24.3)	4777 (22.5)
1935–1944, n (%)	6878 (30.6)	446 (37.4)	6432 (30.2)
1945–1949, n (%)	4738 (21.1)	250 (21.0)	4488 (21.1)
≥ 1950, n (%)	5783 (25.7)	207 (17.4)	5576 (26.2)
Body mass index (BMI), mean (SD)	23.7 ± 3.5	23.8 ± 3.5	23.7 ± 3.5
BMI < 18.5 kg/m^2, n (%)	544 (2.4)	24 (2.0)	520 (2.4)
BMI 18.5–24.9 kg/m^2, n (%)	15,463 (68.8)	845 (70.8)	14,618 (68.7)
BMI 25–29.9 kg/m^2, n (%)	5161 (23.0)	247 (20.7)	4914 (23.1)
BMI > 30 kg/m^2, n (%)	1298 (5.8)	77 (6.5)	1221 (5.7)
Physical activity			
Low, n (%)	1466 (6.5)	79 (6.6)	1387 (6.5)
Medium, n (%)	14,944 (66.5)	806 (67.6)	14,138 (66.5)
High, n (%)	6056 (27.0)	308 (25.8)	5748 (27.0)
Smoking status			
Never, n (%)	7907 (35.2)	372 (31.2)	7535 (35.4)
Previous, n (%)	6901 (30.7)	356 (29.8)	6545 (30.8)
Current, n (%)	7658 (34.1)	465 (39.0)	7193 (33.8)
Alcohol consumption, mean (SD)	114.6 ± 128.1	123.2 ± 125.1	114.1 ± 128.2
Does not drink alcohol, n (%)	3444 (15.3)	189 (15.8)	3255 ± 15.3
Moderate drinker (1–14 drinks/week), n (%)	13,909 (61.9)	689 (57.8)	13,220 (62.1)
Heavy drinker (> 14 drinks/week), n (%)	5113 (22.8)	315 (26.4)	4798 (22.6)
Age at menarche			
≥ 12, n (%)	5431 (24.2)	301 (25.2)	5130 (24.1)
< 12, n (%)	17,035 (75.8)	892 (74.7)	16,143 (75.9)
Parity			
Nulliparous, n (%)	3165 (14.1)	192 (16.1)	2973 (14.0)
Parous, n (%)	19,301 (85.9)	1001 (83.9)	18,300 (86.0)
Number of births in parous women, mean (SD)	2.34 ± 0.88	2.31 ± 0.88	2.34 ± 0.88
Age at first birth, mean (SD)	25.9 ± 3.96	26.2 ± 4.11	25.9 ± 3.95
Menopausal status			
Premenopausal, n (%)	11,388 (50.7)	596 (50.0)	10,792 (50.7)
Post-menopausal, n (%)	11,078 (49.3)	597 (50.0)	10,481 (49.3)
Use of hormone therapy			
Never, n (%)	16,389 (73.0)	774 (64.9)	15,615 (73.4)
Previous, n (%)	2193 (9.8)	109 (9.1)	2084 (9.8)
Current, n (%)	3884 (17.3)	310 (26.0)	3574 (16.8)
Night work*			
Yes, n (%)	947 (5.4)	47 (5.1)	900 (5.4)
No, n (%)	16,598 (94.6)	873 (94.9)	15,725 (94.6)

Table 1 Descriptive statistics at the cohort baseline (1993 or 1999) among 22,466 female nurses from the Danish Nurse Cohort by breast cancer status at the end of follow up *(Continued)*

	Total	Breast cancer	No breast cancer
	$N = 22,466$	$N = 1193$	$N = 21,273$
Use of oral contraceptives			
Never, n (%)	9244 (41.1)	510 (42.7)	8734 (41.1)
Previous or current, n (%)	13,222 (58.9)	683 (57.3)	12,539 (58.9)
Residential area			
Urban, n (%)	3367 (15.0)	173 (14.5)	3194 (15.0)
Provincial, n (%)	9711 (43.2)	549 (46.0)	9162 (43.1)
Rural, n (%)	9388 (41.8)	471 (39.5)	8917 (41.9)
Road traffic noise levels at baseline residence			
L_{den}, mean (SD)	52.7 ± 8.2	53.0 ± 8.1	52.7 ± 8.2
LA_{24h}, mean (SD)	48.6 ± 8.2	48.9 ± 8.1	48.6 ± 8.2
L_d, mean (SD)	50.4 ± 8.2	50.7 ± 8.2	50.4 ± 8.2
L_e, mean (SD)	48.1 ± 8.1	48.4 ± 8.1	48.1 ± 8.1
L_n, mean (SD)	44.6 ± 8.0	44.8 ± 8.0	44.5 ± 8.0

*Only available for 17,545 nurses

association with PR+ BC was positive and statistically significant (HR; 95% CI, 1.21; 1.02–1.42, $N = 393$), and the association with PR- BC (HR; 95% CI, 1.10; 0.89–1.37, $N = 218$) was positive, albeit statistically non-significant. Compared to women exposed to noise levels < 48 dB, women exposed to noise levels > 58 dB had 59% (HR; 95% CI, 1.59; 1.14–2.20) and 66% (HR; 95% CI, 1.66; 1.14–2.40) higher risk of developing ER+ and PR+ BC, respectively. Results were consistent in a sample of 1061 BC cases with data on ER status, but not PR status (see Additional file 1: Table S3).

When considering BC per combined estrogen and progesterone status, we found the strongest associations between residential road traffic noise (for each 10 dB increase in 24-year mean noise levels preceding diagnosis) and ER+/PR+ (HR; 95% CI, 1.22; 1.02–1.42, $N = 384$) and ER+/PR- (HR; 95% CI, 1.33; 0.97–1.82, $N = 110$), and none with ER-/PR+ ($N = 9$) or ER-/PR- ($N = 108$) BCs (Table 4). Descriptive statistics for nurses by combination of ER and PR status are given in Additional file 1: Table S4.

There was no effect modification of association between residential road traffic noise and BC in which estrogen and progesterone hormone receptor status was available ($N = 611$), in ER+, PR+, or ER/PR+ BCs by menopausal status, HT use, obesity, or residential area. (Table 5). Results were similar for the 1193 BC cases (Additional file 1: Table S5). We did, however, find a statistically significantly (*p* value for interaction = 0.05) stronger association between residential road traffic noise (for each 10 dB increase in 24-year mean noise levels) and ER+ BC in nurses working night shifts (HR; 95% CI, 3.36; 1.48–7.63) than in those not working at night (HR; 95% CI, 1.21; 1.02–1.43) (Table 5).

We found that our results were robust to additional adjustment for the baseline year (1993 or 1999) and mean municipality income (Additional file 1: Table S6). Similarly, the main results were unchanged when adjusting for air pollution (Additional file 1: Table S7).

Discussion

We detected an association between road traffic noise levels at residences and BC incidence. The association was strongest for ER+ and PR+ BCs, and no association was found for ER- or PR- BCs. Nurses working at night may be more susceptible to the adverse effects of noise.

We present a novel finding of association between residential road traffic noise and BC overall, as well with ER+ and PR+ BC subtypes, in contrast to findings from two existing studies [5, 7]. Sørensen et al. linked road traffic and railway noise levels at residences to the postmenopausal BC incidence in 29,875 women from Danish Diet, Cancer and Health cohort, recruited between 1993 and 1997 (age 50–65 years) and found no association with total (HR; 95% CI, 1.02; 0.93–1.11) or with ER+ (HR; 95% CI, 0.99: 0.90–1.10) BCs, for each increase of 10 dB in 10-year mean noise levels, the longest available exposure window in that study [5]. However, the authors found 28%, 23% and 20% increases in ER- BC incidence per 10 dB increase in 1-year-, 5-year, and 10-year mean residential road traffic noise levels, respectively, suggesting the recent noise levels to be more relevant than the accumulated levels over many years [5]. In the Danish Nurse Cohort we found that the long-term exposure over 24 years was most relevant for the risk of BC, and that this association was strongest for the ER+ BCs (Table 3 and Table 4). Interestingly, although we found

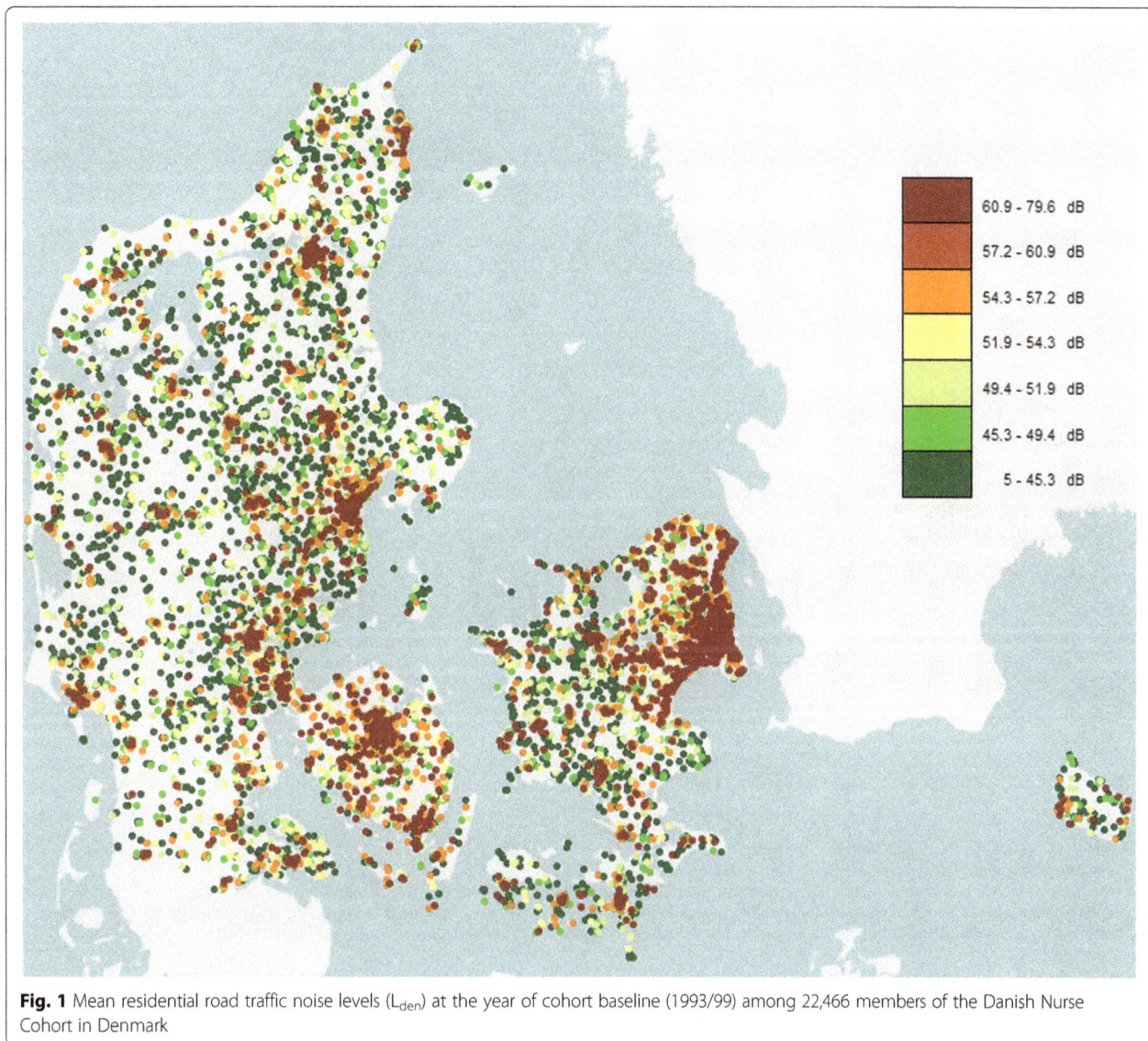

Fig. 1 Mean residential road traffic noise levels (L_{den}) at the year of cohort baseline (1993/99) among 22,466 members of the Danish Nurse Cohort in Denmark

no association between long-term noise exposure and ER- BC incidence, a positive, association was found with the most recent 1-year exposure window (HR; 95% CI, 1.10; 0.85–1.42) (Table 3). These results could suggest that early life and historical, long-term exposures to noise are most relevant for ER+ BC, while the more recent exposure to noise may be important for ER- BCs.

Several factors may explain discrepancies in results between the two Danish studies. First, the population age varied; while we included all BCs in women age > 44 years, including premenopausal and postmenopausal cancers, Sørensen et al. focused on an older population of postmenopausal women, age > 55 years [5]. Second, the geographical location of the residences differs between the cohorts, as the Sørensen et al. study included women only from highly urban areas (Copenhagen and Aarhus)

whereas the present study included nurses from the whole of Denmark, residing primarily in rural (42%) and provincial (43%) areas (Fig. 1). These factors seem not to explain the differences between two studies, as we found no evidence of effect modification by menopausal status or urbanicity (Table 5 and Additional file 1: Table S5). Third, the method of modeling residential road traffic noise and the number of years of follow up varied between the two studies; in the present study we used a state-of-the art Nord200 noise model providing annual mean estimates of residential road traffic noise at the nurses' addresses, allowing modeling of time-varying effects of noise exposure going back as far as 24 years, the longest exposure window to date. This model is considered superior to the Soundplan model used in the Sørensen et al. study, which estimates residential road traffic noise data at a lower resolution as 5-year

Table 2 Association between road traffic noise L$_{den}$ and incidence of overall breast cancer in 22,466 nurses from Danish Nurse Cohort

Road traffic noise	All breast cancers N = 1193			Breast cancer with ER and PR status N = 611		
	Number of cases	Crude model[a] HR (95% CI)	Adjusted model[b] HR (95% CI)	Number of cases	Crude model[a] HR (95% CI)	Adjusted model[b] HR (95% CI)
L$_{den}$ 24 years preceding diagnoses						
Linear per 10 dB	1193	1.11 (1.02–1.21)*	1.10 (1.00–1.20)*	611	1.17 (1.04–1.31)*	1.17 (1.02–1.33)*
Low: < 48 dB	166	1.00	1.00	80	1.00	1.00
Medium 48–58 dB	675	1.24 (1.04–1.47)*	1.19 (1.00–1.42)*	352	1.35 (1.06–1.73)*	1.28 (0.99–1.65)
High > 58 dB	352	1.35 (1.12–1.62)*	1.30 (1.07–1.60)*	179	1.45 (1.11–1.89)*	1.42 (1.06–1.89)*
L$_{den}$ 10 year preceding diagnoses						
Linear per 10 dB	1193	1.08 (1.00–1.16)*	1.06 (0.97–1.15)	611	1.16 (1.04–1.29)*	1.17 (1.04–1.32)*
Low < 48 dB	195	1.00	1.00	87	1.00	1.00
Medium 48–58 dB	646	1.19 (1.02–1.40)*	1.16 (0.98–1.37)	343	1.43 (1.13–1.81)*	1.38 (1.08–1.76)*
High > 58 dB	352	1.25 (1.05–1.49)*	1.21 (1.00–1.46)*	181	1.45 (1.13–1.88)*	1.45 (1.10–1.91)*
L$_{den}$ 1 year at the year of diagnoses						
Linear per 10 dB	1192	1.08 (1.01–1.17)*	1.07 (0.99–1.16)	610	1.15 (1.04–1.27)*	1.16 (1.04–1.30)*
Low < 48 dB	202	1.00	1.00	98	1.00	1.00
Medium 48–58 dB	644	1.25 (1.06–1.46)*	1.22 (1.03–1.43)*	333	1.34 (1.07–1.68)*	1.29 (1.03–1.63)*
High > 58 dB	346	1.29 (1.09–1.54)*	1.26 (1.04–1.52)*	179	1.39 (1.09–1.78)*	1.39 (1.07–1.81)*
L$_{den}$ 1 year at the baseline (1993/99)						
Linear per 10 dB	1193	1.05 (.98–1.13)	1.04 (0.96–1.12)	611	1.11 (1.01–1.23)*	1.12 (1.00–1.26)*
Low < 48 dB	235	1.00	1.00	110	1.00	1.00
Medium 48–58 dB	648	1.17 (1.01–1.36)*	1.13 (0.97–1.33)	347	1.34 (1.08–1.67)*	1.29 (1.03–1.62)*
High > 58 dB	310	1.20 (1.01–1.42)*	1.17 0.97–1.41)	154	1.29 (1.01–1.64)*	1.29 (0.98–1.69)

Abbreviations: ER Estrogen receptor, PR Progesterone receptor
[a]Crude model with age as underlying time scale
[b]Model adjusted for birth cohort, urbanization (urban, provincial, rural), body mass index (underweight, normal, overweight, obese), leisure time physical activity (low, medium, high), alcohol consumption (low, moderate, heavy), age at menarche (≤ 12 years of age, > 12 years of age), parity (nulliparous, parous), number of births, age at first birth, menopausal status (premenopausal, postmenopausal), use of hormone therapy (never, past, current), use of oral contraceptives (never, ever), and smoking status
*p-value<0.05

averages, and was only available at 10 years prior to BC diagnoses in the study of Sørensen et al. [5]. Thus, varying ability of the available noise data to better capture early exposure to residential road traffic noise, which may be more relevant for ER+ BCs, may explain the differences in our results compared to those of Sørensen et al. [5].

Hegewald et al., in a case-control (6643 cases and 471,596 controls) study of women older than 40 years and living close to Frankfurt airport between 2006 and 2010, linked residential road traffic noise data from 2005 to BC incidence, in total, and by ER status [7]. They found no association between residential road traffic noise (for each 10 dB increase) and total BC risk (odds ratio (OR); 85% CI, 0.99; 0.96–1.02), ER+ (OR; 95% CI, 0.98; 0.95–1.02), or ER- (OR; 95% CI 1.01; 0.96–1.07) [7]. Residential road traffic noise levels and geographical distribution of that cohort were comparable to ours ranging from < 40 dB to 85.7 dB, but the noise level was

estimated for 2005 only, thus representing only recent exposure. Furthermore, Hegewald et al. used prescriptions of anti-estrogens or aromatase inhibitors as indicators of ER+ tumors, by which they have likely underestimated the number of ER+ BCs (69.9%) and overestimated the number of ER- (30.1%) BCs. Both Danish studies used clinical data on ER and PR status. These inconsistencies in the literature call for more studies on residential road traffic noise and BC incidence.

We present novel finding of increased susceptibility to residential road traffic noise in nurses who work at night, as compared to those who typically work day, evening or rotating shifts (Table 5). This may be explained by smaller exposure misclassification, as nurses who work at night are at home in the daytime, when residential road traffic noise levels are highest, and when their day sleep or daily activities are more likely to be disrupted by noise, and result in annoyance and health effects. Disruptions to circadian rhythms due to

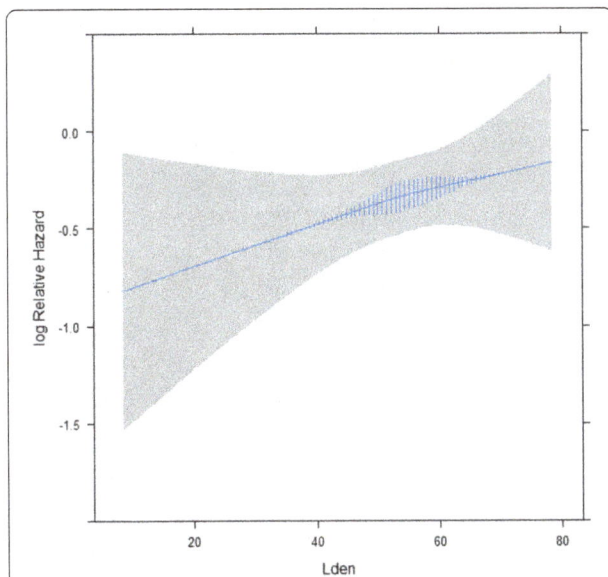

Fig. 2 Association between residential exposure to road traffic noise level (L$_{den}$) over 24 years and breast cancer (N = 1193) among 22,466 members of the Danish Nurse Cohort. Analyses adjusted for birth cohort, urbanization, body mass index, leisure time physical activity, alcohol consumption, age at menarche, parity, number of births, age at first birth, menopausal status, use of hormone therapy, use of oral contraceptives, and smoking status

night shift work have been shown to contribute to endocrine-dependent diseases, including breast carcinogenesis, by negatively impacting neuroendocrine and neuroimmune cells [38]. Our finding thus may suggest that women with circadian rhythm disruptions may be more susceptible to effects of noise than those without. Another possible explanation is that night shift workers represent a sensitive group, as they already have increased risk of poor sleep, sleep disturbance, lack of sleep, work-related stress, fatigue, etc. Sensitivity appears to play a key part in the health effects of environmental noise, as a specific type and level of noise may interact with sensitivity, causing some degree of annoyance and physiological response [4]. Although data on susceptibility to noise effects related to BC are sparse, studies with other health outcomes have suggested that the health effects of noise are enhanced and possibly limited to those who are annoyed by noise or susceptible to the effects of noise. For example, the association between aircraft or residential road traffic noise and increased hypertension has been limited only to those who reported annoyance by noise [2]. Similarly, a study found an association between residential road traffic noise and depressive symptoms only in those who suffer from insomnia [39], and an association between residential road traffic noise and

Table 3 Association[a] between road traffic noise L$_{den}$ and incidence of breast cancer by ER and PR status in 22,466 nurses with estrogen and progesterone hormone receptor status from the Danish Nurse Cohort

	Breast cancer type by ER status				Breast cancer type by PR status			
	Number of cases	ER+ HR (95% CI)	Number of cases	ER- HR (95% CI)	Number of cases	PR+ HR (95% CI)	Number of cases	PR- HR (95% CI)
24 years preceding diagnosis								
Linear per 10 dB	494	1.23 (1.06–1.43)*	117	0.93 (0.70–1.25)	393	1.21 (1.02–1.42)*	218	1.10 (0.89–1.37)
Low < 48 dB	58	1.00	22	1.00	45	1.00	35	1.00
Medium 48–58 dB	290	1.48 (1.10–1.98)*	62	0.77 (0.46–1.28)	231	1.51 (1.08–2.10)*	121	0.99 (0.67–1.47)
High > 58 dB	146	1.59 (1.14–2.20)*	33	0.97 (0.54–1.75)	117	1.66 (1.14–2.40)*	62	1.11 (0.70–1.75)
10 years preceding diagnosis								
Linear per 10 dB	494	1.22 (1.07–1.40)*	117	1.00 (0.76–1.30)	393	1.20 (1.03–1.40)*	218	1.13 (0.92–1.37)
Low < 48 dB	64	1.00	23	1.00	51	1.00	36	1.00
Medium 48–58 dB	279	1.55 (1.17–2.05)*	64	0.90 (0.54–1.48)	223	1.55 (1.13–2.12)*	120	1.13 (0.77–1.67)
High > 58 dB	151	1.65 (1.20–2.26)*	30	0.89 (0.49–1.61)	119	1.65 (1.16–2.35)*	62	1.16 (0.74–1.81)
1 year at the year of diagnosis								
Linear per 10 dB	494	1.18 (1.04–1.33)*	116	1.10 (0.85–1.42)	392	1.21 (1.05–1.39)*	218	1.08 (0.90–1.31)
Low < 48 dB	77	1.00	21	1.00	59	1.00	39	1.00
Medium 48–58 dB	268	1.34 (1.03–1.74)*	65	1.13 (0.68–1.89)	216	1.42 (1.05–1.91)*	117	1.11 (0.76–1.62)
High > 58 dB	149	1.47 (1.09–1.98)*	30	1.12 (0.61–2.03)	117	1.53 (1.09–2.15)*	62	1.18 (0.76–1.82)

Abbreviations: *ER* Estrogen receptor, *PR* Progesterone receptor

[a]Model adjusted for birth cohort, urbanization (urban, provincial, rural), body mass index (underweight, normal, overweight, obese), leisure time physical activity (low, medium, high), alcohol consumption (low, moderate, heavy), age at menarche (≤ 12 years of age, > 12 years of age), parity (nulliparous, parous), number of births, age at first birth, menopausal status (premenopausal, postmenopausal), use of hormone therapy (never, past, current), use of oral contraceptives (never, ever) and smoking status

*p value <0.05

Table 4 Association[a] between road traffic noise L_{den} and incidence of breast cancer by combination of estrogen and progesterone receptor status in 22,466 nurses from Danish Nurse Cohort

	ER+/PR+		ER+/PR-		ER-/PR+		ER-/PR-	
	Number of cases	HR (95% CI)	Number of cases	HR (95% CI)	Number of cases	HR (95% CI)	Number of cases	HR (95% CI)
24 years preceding diagnosis								
Linear per 10 dB	384	1.21 (1.02–1.42)*	110	1.33 (0.97–1.82)	9	1.14 (0.33–3.87)	108	0.92 (0.68–1.25)
Low < 48 dB	45	1.00	13	1.00	0	1.00	22	1.00
Medium 48–58 dB	226	1.49 (1.07–2.07)*	64	1.45 (0.78–2.69)	5	–	57	0.73 (0.43–1.22)
High > 58 dB	113	1.61 (1.11–2.34)*	33	1.51 (0.75–3.03)	4	–	29	0.88 (0.48–1.62)
10 years preceding diagnosis								
Linear per 10 dB	384	1.20 (1.03–1.40)*	110	1.30 (0.98–1.74)	9	1.22 (0.40–3.72)	108	0.98 (0.74–1.29)
Low < 48 dB	51	1.00	13	1.00	0	1.00	23	1.00
Medium 48–58 dB	218	1.53 (1.11–2.09)*	61	1.65 (0.89–3.06)	5	–	59	0.85 (0.51–1.40)
High > 58 dB	115	1.61 (1.13–2.29)*	36	1.83 (0.92–3.62)	4	–	26	0.79 (0.43–1.46)
1 year preceding diagnosis								
Linear per 10 dB	384	1.21 (1.05–1.39)*	110	1.07 (0.83–1.40)	8	1.15 (0.39–3.40)	108	1.10 (0.84–1.43)
Low < 48 dB	58	1.00	19	1.00	1	1.00	20	1.00
Medium 48–58 dB	212	1.42 (1.05–1.92)*	56	1.09 (0.64–1.87)	4	1.02 (0.11–9.59)	61	1.14 (0.67–1.92)
High > 58 dB	114	1.53 (1.09–2.15)*	35	1.27 (0.69–2.34)	3	1.35 (0.13–14.4)	27	1.09 (0.59–2.03)

Abbreviations: *ER* Estrogen receptor, *PR* Progesterone receptor

[a]Model adjusted for birth cohort, urbanization (urban, provincial, rural), body mass index (underweight, normal, overweight, obese), leisure time physical activity (low, medium, high), alcohol consumption (low, moderate, heavy), age at menarche (≤ years of age, > 12 years of age), parity (nulliparous, parous), number of births, age at first birth, menopausal status (premenopausal, postmenopausal), use of hormone therapy (never, past, current), use of oral contraceptives (never, ever) and smoking status

*p value <0.05

markers of obesity have been detected only in highly noise-sensitive women [25].

We present novel findings of the relevance of residential road traffic noise in ER+ but not in ER- BCs. Our finding are similar to the findings of the recent study, suggesting that the oxidative stress pathway promoting BC development and progression [12] was most relevant in ER+ BC [15]. Residential road traffic noise has been linked to increased risk of weight gain [24] and obesity [25] and BMI has been positively associated with risk of ER+ postmenopausal BC, but not with ER- BC [40]. It has been also suggested that lack of melatonin, due to sleep disturbance and light exposure at night, may be related to increased risk of ER+ breast cancer, although reports in the literature are not completely consistent [41].

The strength of this study include having data from a large, prospective nationwide cohort of 22,466 women residing in rural, provincial, and urban areas, providing for large contrasts in residential road traffic noise levels (Fig. 1). We benefited from having access to data from well-established Danish clinical cancer registers with detailed and validated information on BC incidence and subtypes by ER status, and for the first time, by PR status. We benefited from well-defined information on all relevant risk factors for BC, and associations

between BC and established risk factors, such as alcohol use [42], smoking [43], and HT [44, 45] have been documented earlier in this cohort. The cohort consists of a rather homogenous population of female nurses, with similar education, occupation, and socioeconomic status, minimizing the possibility of residual confounding by these factors. Danish nurses have been found to have a generally healthier lifestyle than a representative sample of Danish women, as they smoked less and had higher physical activity levels, but consumed more alcohol [30]. There are no large differences between Danish nurses and Danish women in general in the use of health care and in disease occurrence [30]. It is therefore reasonable to generalize the findings based on the Danish Nurses Cohort to Danish, and other, women in general.

We also benefited from having information on air pollution exposure in this cohort, an important confounder since air pollution and road traffic noise share the same major source (traffic) and are highly correlated. We have, however, found that additional adjustment for air pollution did not affect reported associations between road traffic noise and BC, which is line with our previous study in this cohort where we found no association between air pollution and BC [37]. We benefitted from a state-of-the art Nord200 noise

Table 5 Modifications of association[a] between 24-year mean road traffic noise L$_{den}$ (per 10 dB) and incidence of breast cancer by menopausal status, HT use, obesity, night work, and residential area in 22,466 nurses from the Danish Nurse Cohort

	Breast cancer with receptor status N = 611		ER+ N = 494		PR+ N = 393		ER+/PR+ N = 384	
	Number of cases	HR (95% CI)	Number of cases	HR (95% CI)	Number of cases	HR (95% CI)	Number of cases	HR (95% CI)
Menopausal status								
Premenopausal	334	1.16 (0.97–1.38)	272	1.25 (1.02–1.52)	231	1.17 (0.95–1.45)	226	1.19 (0.96–1.48)
Postmenopausal	277	1.18 (0.97–1.43)	222	1.21 (0.97–1.51)	162	1.26 (0.97–1.63)	158	1.23 (0.94–1.59)
p value for interaction[**]		0.9069		0.7135		0.6767		0.8909
HT use								
Never	390	1.16 (0.99–1.36)	319	1.21 (1.01–1.45)	256	1.18 (0.97–1.44)	254	1.19 (0.97–1.45)
Previous	57	0.98 (0.64–1.50)	44	1.12 (0.68–1.85)	33	1.03 (0.58–1.84)	31	0.99 (0.55–1.80)
Current	164	1.26 (0.96–1.65)	131	1.33 (0.99–1.80)	104	1.34 (0.96–1.88)	99	1.34 (0.95–1.89)
p value for interaction[**]		0.4685		0.6047		0.5697		0.6012
Obesity (BMI > 30 kg/m^2)								
No	572	1.18 (1.03–1.35)	459	1.25 (1.07–1.45)	367	1.22 (1.03–1.45)	358	1.22 (1.03–1.46)
Yes	39	1.03 (0.65–1.65)	35	1.04 (0.63–1.71)	26	1.03 (0.59–1.78)	26	1.03 (0.59–1.78)
p value for interaction[**]		0.9805		0.9489		0.7553		0.7704
Night work*								
No	473	1.16 (1.00–1.35)	386	1.21 (1.02–1.43)	317	1.22 (1.02–1.47)		1.23 (1.02–1.48)
Yes	24	1.86 (0.97–3.57)	17	3.36 (1.48–7.63)	9	1.88 (0.59–6.00)	310	3.04 (0.80–11.60)
p value for interaction[**]		0.3754		0.0477*		0.3000	8	0.1585
Residential area								
Urban	77	1.30 (0.81–2.10)	67	1.24 (0.74–2.07)	50	0.95 (0.52–1.75)	49	0.96 (0.52–1.77)
Provincial	299	1.21 (0.98–1.51)	234	1.43 (1.12–1.83)	192	1.57 (1.19–2.06)	185	1.57 (1.19–2.08)
Rural	235	1.12 (0.94–1.33)	193	1.12 (0.92–1.35)	151	1.06 (0.85–1.31)	150	1.06 (0.86–1.32)
p value for interaction[**]		0.6460		0.2610		0.0811		0.0893

[a]Model adjusted for birth cohort, urbanization (urban, provincial, rural), body mass index (underweight, normal, overweight, obese), leisure time physical activity (low, medium, high), alcohol consumption (low, moderate, heavy), age at menarche (≤ 12 years of age, > 12 years of age), parity (nulliparous, parous), number of births, age at first birth, menopausal status (premenopausal, postmenopausal), use of hormone therapy (never, past, current), use of oral contraceptives (never, ever) and smoking status

Traffic noise was entered as a continuous variable in all models as the 24-year running mean preceding diagnosis. Model adjusted for birth cohort, urbanization (urban, provincial, rural), body mass index (underweight, normal, overweight, obese), leisure time physical activity (low, medium, high), alcohol consumption (low, moderate, heavy), age at menarche (≤ years of age, > 12 years of age), parity (nulliparous, parous), number of births, age at first birth, menopausal status (premenopausal, postmenopausal), use of hormone therapy (never, past, current), use of oral contraceptives (never, ever) and smoking status. However, there was no adjustment for the stratification variable

HT hormone therapy, BMI body mass index, ER estrogen receptor, PR progesterone receptor

*Only available for 17,545 nurses

**Test of the null hypothesis that the linear trends are identical, for Wald's test for interaction

model providing historical annual mean estimates of residential road traffic noise at the nurses' addresses, allowing for modeling of time-varying effects of noise exposure going back as far as 24 years and providing the longest exposure window to date. The weakness of the study is lack of information on annoyance from noise, noise from neighbors, social noise, hearing impairment, noise exposure at work, time-activity patterns and time spent at home, placement of the bedroom, and window opening habits, etc. Modeled levels of noise at the most exposed façade at home are thus inherently associated with a certain levels of exposure misclassification and deviation from real personal exposures to noise. However, if this misclassification is non-differential, and effect estimates are likely biased towards zero.

Conclusions

In this large cohort of Danish female nurses older than 44 years, we found a positive association between residential road traffic noise and risk of BC. We present two novel findings: the association seemed limited to ER+ BCs, and nurses working at night may be especially susceptible to the adverse effects of noise. Our findings are in contrast to earlier finding of an association between road traffic noise and ER- BC [5], calling urgently for more data on noise and BC.

Additional file

Additional file 1: Table S1. Descriptive statistics at the cohort baseline (1993 or 1999) among 22,466 female nurses from the Danish Nurse Cohort by BC status at the end of follow up. Table S2. Association between 24-year mean road traffic noise L_{den}, LA_{eq}, L_d, L_e, and L_n, and incidence of overall BC and BC in women with receptor status available, among 22,466 nurses from the Danish Nurse Cohort. Table S3. Association between road traffic noise L_{den} and incidence of BC by ER and PR status in 22,466 nurses from the Danish Nurse Cohort. Table S4. Descriptive statistics at the year of cohort baseline (1993 or 1999) among 21,884 members of the Danish Nurse Cohort, by estrogen and progesterone BC receptor status. Table S5. Modifications of association[a] between 24-year mean road traffic noise L_{den} (per 10 dB) and incidence of BC by menopausal status, hormone therapy (HT) use, obesity, night work, and residential area in 22,466 nurses from the Danish Nurse Cohort. Table S6. Association between road traffic noise L_{den} (24 years preceding diagnosis) and incidence of overall BC in nurses from the Danish Nurse Cohort with additional adjustments for year of cohort inclusion (1993 or 1999) and average municipality income. Table S7. Association between road traffic noise L_{den} (24 years preceding diagnosis) and incidence of overall BC in nurses from the Danish Nurse Cohort with additional adjustments for air pollutants. Table S8. Association between road traffic noise L_{den} and incidence of overall BC in nurses from the Danish Nurse Cohort with additional noise categories, defined from quartiles of residential road traffic noise exposure at the year of cohort inclusion. Table S9. Descriptive statistics at the cohort baseline (1993 or 1999) among 1193 female nurses from the Danish Nurse Cohort with BC status at the end of follow up. Figure S1. Flow chart of inclusion criteria and the study population. (DOCX 101 kb)

Abbreviations

BC: Breast cancer; BMI: Body mass index; CI: Confidence interval; dB: Decibel; ER: Estrogen receptor; HR: Hazard ratio; HT: Hormone therapy; IARC: International Agency for Research on Cancer; LA_{eq}: A-weighted sound pressure level; L_d: A-weighted sound pressure level during the day 0700–1900 h; L_{den}: Overall A-weighted sound pressure level during the day, evening, and night; L_e: A-weighted sound pressure level during the evening 1900–2200 h; L_n: A-weighted sound pressure level during the night 2200–0700 h; OC: Oral contraceptives; PR: Progesterone receptor

Acknowledgements

We thank Mette Sørensen and Nina Roswall for good discussions on statistical analyses of road traffic noise data.

Funding

This study was supported by the Danish Council for Independent Research grant 'HEalth Risks associated with exposure to road traffic Noise' (HypERION), grant number: DFF-4183-00353.

Authors' contributions

All authors made substantial contributions to conception and design, analysis, and interpretation of data, and critical review of the manuscript. ZJA contributed with an idea and design for the study, secured funding, and drafted the manuscript. JTJ performed the statistical analyses and contributed revising of the manuscript. EL helped with the epidemiological design of the study and was involved in drafting the manuscript. SNL helped with the data merging and management and provided guidance on statistical analyses. CB, JEL, and THP provided road traffic noise data and consulted on the use of these data, interpretation of the results on the noise data, and contributed to drafting the part of the manuscript describing the noise models. LO has contributed with statistical analyses, epidemiological analyses, interpretation of results and drafting the manuscript. EVB and MKS have been involved in revising the manuscript critically for important intellectual content. All authors read and approved the final manuscript.

Competing interests

The authors declare that they have no competing interests.

Author details

[1]Section of Environmental Health, Department of Public Health, University of Copenhagen, Øster Farimagsgade 5, 1014 Copenhagen, Denmark. [2]Nykøbing F Hospital, University of Copenhagen, Ejegodvej 63, 4800 Nykøbing F, Denmark. [3]DELTA Acoustics, Venlighedsvej 4, 2970 Hørsholm, Denmark. [4]Diakonissestiftelsen and Parker Institute, Frederiksberg Hospital, Peter Bangsvej 1, 2000 Frederiksberg, Denmark. [5]Juliane Marie Center, Department of Growth and Reproduction, Capital Region of Denmark, Rigshospitalet, Blegdamsvej 9, 2100 Copenhagen, Denmark.

References

1. WHO. Burden of disease from environmental noise. Quantification of healthy life years lost in Europe. WHO Eur cent environ heal Bonn off WHO Reg off Eur. 2011.
2. Münzel T, Gori T, Babisch W, Basner M. Cardiovascular effects of environmental noise exposure. Eur Heart J. 2014;35:829–36.
3. Münzel T, Sørensen M, Gori T, Schmidt FP, Rao X, Brook J, et al. Environmental stressors and cardio-metabolic disease: part I–epidemiologic evidence supporting a role for noise and air pollution and effects of mitigation strategies. Eur Heart J. 2016;38:ehw269.
4. Recio A, Linares C, Banegas JR, Díaz J. Road traffic noise effects on cardiovascular, respiratory, and metabolic health: an integrative model of biological mechanisms. Environ Res. 2016;146:359–70.
5. Sørensen M, Ketzel M, Overvad K, Tjønneland A, Raaschou-Nielsen O. Exposure to road traffic and railway noise and postmenopausal breast cancer: a cohort study. Int J Cancer. 2014;134:2691–8.
6. Roswall N, Bidstrup PE, Raaschou-Nielsen O, Jensen SS, Olsen A, Sørensen M. Residential road traffic noise exposure and survival after breast cancer - a cohort study. Environ Res. 2016;151:814–20.
7. Hegewald J, Schubert M, Wagner M, Dröge P, Prote U, Swart E, et al. Breast cancer and exposure to aircraft, road, and railway-noise: a case–control study based on health insurance records. Scand J Work Environ Health. 2017;43(6):509–18.
8. Basner M, Babisch W, Davis A, Brink M, Clark C, Janssen S, et al. Auditory and non-auditory effects of noise on health. Lancet. 2014;383:1325–32.
9. Antonova L, Aronson K, Mueller CR. Stress and breast cancer: from epidemiology to molecular biology. Breast Cancer Res. 2011;13:208.
10. Flint MS, Bovbjerg DH. DNA damage as a result of psychological stress: implications for breast cancer. Breast Cancer Res. 2012;14:320.
11. Volden PA, Conzen SD. The influence of glucocorticoid signaling on tumor progression. Brain Behav Immun. 2013;30:S26–31.
12. Hemmingsen JG, Møller P, Jantzen K, Jönsson BAG, Albin M, Wierzbicka A, et al. Controlled exposure to diesel exhaust and traffic noise – effects on oxidative stress and activation in mononuclear blood cells. Mutat Res Mol Mech Mutagen. 2015;775:66–71.
13. Masruri B, Ashtarinezhad A, Yekzamani P. Data on the effect of lead concomitant noise on oxidative stress in rats. Data Br. 2018;18:1117–21.

14. Nourazarian AR, Kangari P, Salmaninejad A. Roles of oxidative stress in the development and progression of breast cancer. Asian Pac J Cancer Prev. 2014;15:4745–51.

15. Madeddu C, Gramignano G, Floris C, Murenu G, Sollai G, Macciò A. Role of inflammation and oxidative stress in post-menopausal oestrogen-dependent breast cancer. J Cell Mol Med. 2014;18:2519–29.

16. Halonen JI, Vahtera J, Stansfeld S, Yli-Tuomi T, Salo P, Pentti J, et al. Associations between nighttime traffic noise and sleep: the Finnish public sector study. Environ Health Perspect. 2012;120:1391–6.

17. Miedema HME, Vos H. Associations between self-reported sleep disturbance and environmental noise based on reanalyses of pooled data from 24 studies. Behav Sleep Med. 2007;5:1–20.

18. Erren TC, Morfeld P, Stork J, Knauth P, von Mülmann MJA, Breitstadt R, et al. Shift work, chronodisruption and cancer?--the IARC 2007 challenge for research and prevention and 10 theses from the cologne colloquium 2008. Scand J Work Environ Health. 2009;35:74–9.

19. Lin X, Chen W, Wei F, Ying M, Wei W, Xie X. Night-shift work increases morbidity of breast cancer and all-cause mortality: a meta-analysis of 16 prospective cohort studies. Sleep Med. 2015;16:1381–7.

20. Kamdar BB, Tergas AI, Mateen FJ, Bhayani NH, Oh J. Night-shift work and risk of breast cancer: a systematic review and meta-analysis. Breast Cancer Res Treat. 2013;138:291–301.

21. Travis RC, Balkwill A, Fensom GK, Appleby PN, Reeves GK, Wang X-S, et al. Night shift work and breast Cancer incidence: three prospective studies and meta-analysis of published studies. J Natl Cancer Inst. 2016;108:djw169.

22. Qin Y, Zhou Y, Zhang X, Wei X, He J. Sleep duration and breast cancer risk: a meta-analysis of observational studies. Int J Cancer. 2014;134:1166–73.

23. Qian X, Brinton LA, Schairer C, Matthews CE. Sleep duration and breast cancer risk in the breast cancer detection demonstration project follow-up cohort. Br J Cancer. 2015;112:567–71.

24. Christensen JS, Raaschou-Nielsen O, Tjønneland A, Nordsborg RB, Jensen SS, Sørensen TIAA, et al. Long-term exposure to residential traffic noise and changes in body weight and waist circumference: a cohort study. Environ Res. 2015;143:154–61.

25. Oftedal B, Krog NH, Pyko A, Eriksson C, Graff-Iversen S, Haugen M, et al. Road traffic noise and markers of obesity - a population-based study. Environ Res. 2015;138:144–53.

26. Pyko A, Eriksson C, Oftedal B, Hilding A, Östenson C-G, Krog NH, et al. Exposure to traffic noise and markers of obesity. Occup Environ Med. 2015;72:594–601.

27. Sorensen M, Andersen ZJ, Nordsborg RB, Becker T, Tjonneland A, Overvad K, et al. Long-term exposure to road traffic noise and incident diabetes: a cohort study. Env Heal Perspect. 2013;121:217–22.

28. La Vecchia C, Giordano SH, Hortobagyi GN, Chabner B. Overweight, obesity, diabetes, and risk of breast cancer: interlocking pieces of the puzzle. Oncologist. 2011;16:726–9.

29. Xia X, Chen W, Li J, Chen X, Rui R, Liu C, et al. Body mass index and risk of breast cancer: a nonlinear dose-response meta-analysis of prospective studies. Sci Rep. 2015;4:7480.

30. Hundrup YA, Simonsen MK, Jørgensen T, Obel EB, Jørgensen T, Obel EB. Cohort profile: the Danish Nurse Cohort. Int J Epidemiol. 2012;41:1241–7.

31. Pedersen CB. The Danish civil registration system. Scand J Public Health. 2011;39:22–5.

32. Gjerstorff ML. The Danish Cancer Registry. - NB - ei hinda andmekvaliteeti. Scand J Public Health. 2011;39:42–5.

33. Møller S, Jensen M, Ejlertsen B, Bjerre KD, Hansen HB, Christiansen P, et al. The clinical database and the treatment guidelines of the Danish Breast Cancer Cooperative Group (DBCG); its 30-years experience and future promise 2009;

34. DELTA. Nordic environmental noise prediction methods, Nord2000 summary report. 2001.

35. DELTA Acoustics & Electronics. Nord 2000. Validation of the propagation model. 2006.

36. DELTA Acoustics. Validation of the Nord2000 propagation model for use on wind turbine noise. 2009.

37. Andersen ZJ, Ravnskjaer L, Andersen KK, Loft S, Brandt J, Becker T, et al. Long-term exposure to fine particulate matter and breast cancer incidence in the Danish Nurse Cohort study. Cancer Epidemiol Biomark Prev. 2016: cebp 0578.2016.

38. Ball LJ, Palesh O, Kriegsfeld LJ. The pathophysiologic role of disrupted circadian and neuroendocrine rhythms in breast carcinogenesis. Endocr Rev. 2016;37:450–66.

39. Orban E, McDonald K, Sutcliffe R, Hoffmann B, Fuks KB, Dragano N, et al. Residential road traffic noise and high depressive symptoms after five years of follow-up: results from the Heinz Nixdorf recall study. Environ Health Perspect. 2016;124:578–85.

40. Munsell MF, Sprague BL, Berry DA, Chisholm G, Trentham-Dietz A. Body mass index and breast cancer risk according to postmenopausal estrogen-progestin use and hormone receptor status. Epidemiol Rev. 2014;36:114–36.

41. Hill SM, Belancio VP, Dauchy RT, Xiang S, Brimer S, Mao L, et al. Melatonin: an inhibitor of breast cancer. Endocr Relat Cancer. 2015;22:R183–204.

42. Mørch LS, Johansen D, Thygesen LC, Tjønneland A, Løkkegaard E, Stahlberg C, et al. Alcohol drinking, consumption patterns and breast cancer among Danish nurses: a cohort study. Eur J Pub Health. 2007;17:624–9.

43. Andersen ZJ, Jørgensen JT, Grøn R, Brauner EV, Lynge E. Active smoking and risk of breast cancer in a Danish nurse cohort study. BMC Cancer. 2017; 17(1):556.

44. Stahlberg C, Pedersen ATAT, Lynge E, Andersen ZJZJ, Keiding N, Hundrup YAYA, et al. Increased risk of breast cancer following different regimens of hormone replacement therapy frequently used in Europe. Int J Cancer. 2004;109:721–7.

45. Stahlberg C, Pedersen ATT, Andersen ZJJ, Keiding N, YA a H, Obel EBB, et al. Breast cancer with different prognostic characteristics developing in Danish women using hormone replacement therapy. Br J Cancer. 2004;91:644–50.

20

NR2F1 stratifies dormant disseminated tumor cells in breast cancer patients

Elin Borgen[1†], Maria C. Rypdal[1†], Maria Soledad Sosa[2,3†], Anne Renolen[1], Ellen Schlichting[4], Per E. Lønning[5,6], Marit Synnestvedt[7], Julio A. Aguirre-Ghiso[3*†] and Bjørn Naume[7,8*†]

Abstract

Background: The presence of disseminated tumor cells (DTCs) in bone marrow (BM) is an independent prognostic factor in early breast cancer but does not uniformly predict outcome. Tumor cells can persist in a quiescent state over time, but clinical studies of markers predicting the awakening potential of DTCs are lacking. Recently, experiments have shown that NR2F1 (COUP-TF1) plays a key role in dormancy signaling.

Methods: We analyzed the NR2F1 expression in DTCs by double immunofluorescence (DIF) staining of extra cytospins prepared from 114 BM samples from 86 selected DTC-positive breast cancer patients. Samples collected at two or more time points were available for 24 patients. Fifteen samples were also analyzed for the proliferation marker Ki67.

Results: Of the patients with detectable DTCs by DIF, 27% had ≥ 50% NR2F1[high] DTCs, chosen a priori as the cut-off for "dormant profile" classification. All patients with systemic relapse within 12 months after BM aspiration carried ≤ 1% NR2F1[high] DTCs, including patients who transitioned from having NR2F1[high]-expressing DTCs in previous BM samples. Of the patients with serial samples, half of those with no relapse at follow-up had ≥ 50% NR2F1[high] DTCs in the last BM aspiration analyzed. Among the 18 relapse-free patients at the time of the last DTC-positive BM aspiration with no subsequent BM analysis performed, distant disease-free intervals were favorable for patients carrying ≥ 50% NR2F1[high] DTCs compared with those with predominantly NR2F1[low] DTCs ($p = 0.007$, log-rank). No survival difference was observed by classification according to Ki67-expressing DTCs ($p = 0.520$).

Conclusions: Our study translates findings from basic biological analysis of DTC dormancy to the clinical situation and supports further clinical studies of NR2F1 as a marker of dormancy.

Keywords: Disseminated tumor cells, DTC, Dormancy, NR2F1, Bone marrow, Breast cancer, Occult disease, Micrometastasis

Background

Breast cancer patients may experience relapse and subsequent death from the disease many years after primary treatment. This indicates an ability of occult cancer cells to survive in a non- or slow-proliferating state, retaining a potential for progression and proliferation at a later time point [1, 2]. The window of time represented by such minimal residual disease (MRD) represents a possibility for therapeutic intervention to prevent development of future metastasis rather than treat overt metastasis. However, the biology of the population of residual disseminated tumor cells (DTCs) is poorly understood. Large studies have shown the presence of DTCs in bone marrow (BM) to be a strong predictor of recurrence over the next 5 years [3, 4]. However, about 60% of the DTC-positive patients remained relapse-free until the end of the follow-up period. Consequently, there is an urgent need for markers to disclose the functional state of DTCs and evaluate their progression potential. Such markers may help us to understand the biology of dormant DTCs in patients and as decision-making tools for current and new therapies.

* Correspondence: julio.aguirre-ghiso@mssm.edu; BNA@ous-hf.no
Elin Borgen, Maria C. Rypdal and Maria Soledad Sosa contributed equally as first authors, and Julio A. Aguirre-Ghiso and Bjørn Naume contributed equally as last authors to this work.
[3]Division of Hematology and Oncology, Department of Medicine, Department of Otolaryngology, Tisch Cancer Institute, Black Family Stem Cell Institute, Icahn School of Medicine at Mount Sinai, New York, NY 10029, USA
[7]Department of Oncology, Oslo University Hospital, Oslo, Norway
Full list of author information is available at the end of the article

Our experimental model studies of DTC dormancy revealed that NR2F1, an orphan nuclear receptor of the retinoic acid receptor family, is commonly downregulated in human cancer and metastatic tissues [5–7]. In contrast, in a PDX model of squamous carcinoma, NR2F1 was upregulated in the DTCs that entered spontaneous dormancy [6], and additional results suggested that NR2F1 may pinpoint dormant DTCs in different cancer types [6]. DTC analysis in the experimental models indicated that when 40–50% of DTCs displayed nuclear NR2F1, this correlated with quiescence markers, other dormancy markers such as DEC2 and SOX9, and lack of proliferation [6, 8]. In addition, a frequency of less than 20% of DTCs positive for NR2F1 correlated with a lack of expression of the above markers of dormancy, quiescence, and proliferation. Metastatic and local recurrence samples in head and neck squamous cell carcinoma that clearly escaped dormancy showed less than 5% of tumor cells positive for NR2F1 (supplementing data in [6]). Furthermore, dormant DTCs upregulated genes linked to NR2F1 signaling, including several retinoic acid-regulated genes [6]. In prostate cancer samples, we found that 43–47% of DTCs from patients with no evidence of disease after many years of relapse-free follow-up showed NR2F1 mRNA upregulation, compared with 10% of the DTCs in advanced prostate cancer [6]. Altogether, these results support further testing of NR2F1 as a dormancy marker in solitary DTCs from clinical samples, including assessment

of cut-off values to classify patients according to NR2F1 expression.

Three Norwegian early breast cancer cohorts were previously analyzed for DTCs in the BM [9–14] using the standard immunocytochemical method (standard ICC) [15, 16]. Clinical follow-up identified the presence of DTCs to be a significant, independent predictor of unfavorable outcome [9–12]. To explore the functional state of the DTCs, we optimized double immunofluorescence (DIF) protocols for detection of NR2F1 and Ki67 on DTCs and analyzed selected BM samples from these three breast cancer cohorts with comparison to clinical parameters. Our study is the first to translate findings from basic biological mechanism analysis of DTC dormancy to the clinical situation.

Materials and methods
Breast cancer patient cohorts
The patient material includes cytospins with BM mononuclear cells (MNCs) from breast cancer patients included in one of three different Norwegian studies in the period from 1995 to 2008. An overview of the studies and included patients is presented in Fig. 1, and below.

The NeoTax study enrolled 260 patients with stage III/IV breast cancer between 1997 and 2003 and randomly allocated them to treatment with paclitaxel or epirubicin, with a crossover between treatment arms if there was no response [9, 13, 14]. Stage IV patients were included only if they harbored a locally advanced disease (T3/T4 and/or

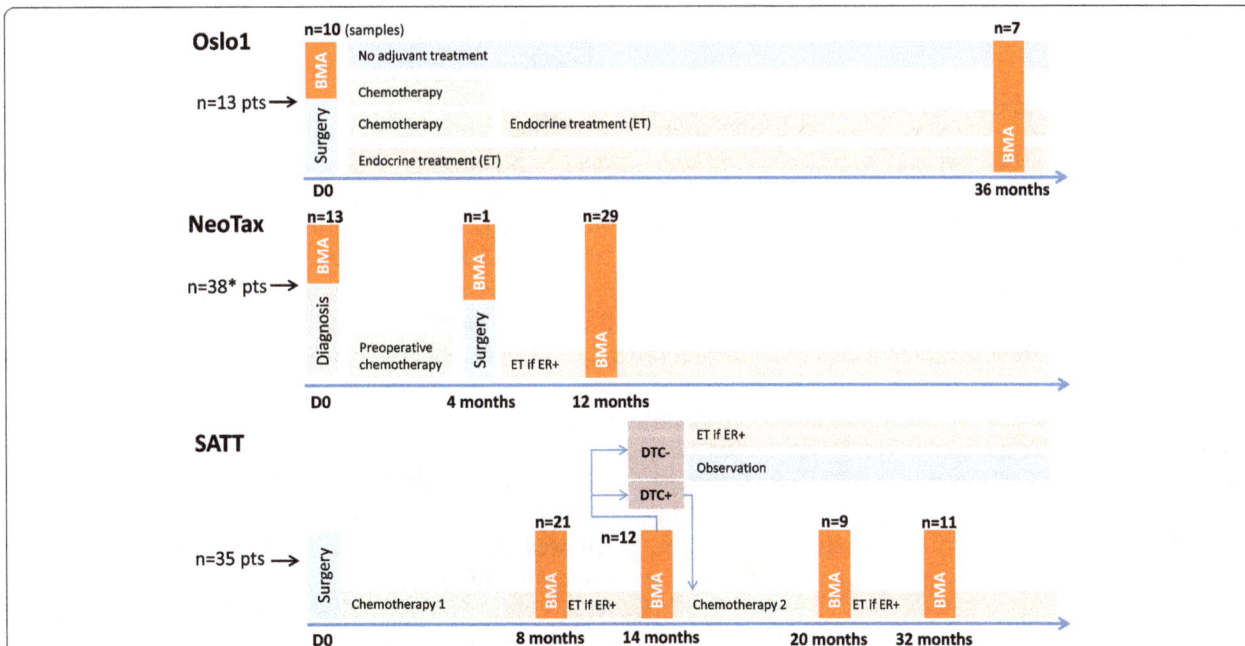

Fig. 1 Clinical studies overview. Overview of the clinical studies, number of patients, and number of samples analyzed by DIF in the present study. Bone marrow aspiration (BMA) time points are indicated, as well as therapy administered. *One patient had a BMA performed at an unknown time point; however not harboring any disseminated tumor cells (DTC) by DIF. ER estrogen receptor

N2/N3) with limited distant metastases. After chemotherapy, mastectomy with axillary clearance was performed, followed by radiotherapy and antihormonal therapy when estrogen receptor (ER)-positive. BM aspirations for DTC analysis were performed prior to the start of chemotherapy (BM1), at surgery (BM2), and 12 months after randomization (BM3).

The Oslo1 observational study enrolled 920 patients with stage I/II breast cancer between 1995 and 1998, and submitted them to standard adjuvant therapy, antihormonal therapy, and radiotherapy according to Norwegian guidelines at the time of the study. BM aspirations for DTC analysis were performed at surgery (BM1), and after 3 years of follow-up (for about one-third of the patients; BM2) [10, 11].

The SATT study [12, 17] enrolled 1121 patients with operable breast cancer between 2003 and 2008. In addition to chemotherapy, patients received antihormonal therapy, radiotherapy, and from 2005 also herceptin if HER2-positive, according to Norwegian guidelines at the time of the study. Patients who had completed six cycles of standard adjuvant fluorouracil, epirubicin, and cyclophosphamide (FEC) chemotherapy underwent BM aspiration 2 to 3 months (BM1) and 8 to 9 months (BM2) after FEC. The presence of DTCs in BM was determined by immunocytochemistry. If one or more DTCs were present at BM2, six cycles of docetaxel (100 mg/m^2, once every 3 weeks) were administered, followed by DTC analysis 1 and 13 months after the last docetaxel infusion (BM3 and BM4).

Preparation of bone marrow mononuclear cell samples and cytospins
Bone marrow was aspirated in heparin (1000 IE/ml; 0.5 ml per 10 ml BM) from iliac crests bilaterally under local anesthesia (5–10 ml per site) and pooled into one tube. The samples were stored at room temperature until processing within 24 h. The aspirates were diluted 1:1 in phosphate-buffered saline (PBS; Gibco, Life Technologies) and separated by density centrifugation using Lymphoprep (Axis-Shield, Oslo, Norway). Mononuclear cells were collected from the interphase layer, washed in 1% fetal calf serum in PBS (Gibco), and resuspended to 1×10^6 cells/mL. Cytospins were prepared by centrifugation of the BM MNCs down to poly-L-lysine-coated glass slides (5×10^5 MNCs/slide) in a Hettich cytocentrifuge (Tutlingen, Germany), air-dried at room temperature overnight, and stored at −80 °C until immunostaining.

Patient material
For all the studies, the large majority of DTC-positive samples had only one detectable DTC in the original standard ICC analysis. A minority of the original samples contained ≥ 2–5 up to several thousand DTCs. For

the present study, stored frozen cytospins prepared in parallel to the cytospins used for the initial (original) analysis were used when available. For some samples, viable BM MNCs stored in liquid nitrogen were thawed and new cytospins were prepared. To increase the chance of detecting DTCs in the study samples, we primarily selected patients having ≥ 3 DTCs per 2×10^6 BM MNCs by the original DTC analysis. However, patients with 0–2 DTCs were also included. When available, we prioritized BM from patients where successive samples over time were available. For some patients, no more spare BM was available for the present analysis. Normally, two cytospins containing in total 1×10^6 BM MNCs with adequate staining quality were analyzed for NR2F1 and for Ki67. The staining of samples and scoring of Ki67 and NR2F1 were performed by EB and MCR without access to the clinical database for the trials or information about time to relapse.

Based on this, the present study included cytospins of BM MNCs from a total of 86 patients categorized as DTC-positive by the original "gold standard" DTC analysis performed prospectively within the original studies (DTC-positivity in at least one original sample if more than one BM aspiration was performed; ICC APAAP technique, four cytospins, 2×10^6 BM MNCs analyzed) [15, 16], of which 13 were included in Oslo1, 38 in the NeoTax study, and 35 in the SATT study (Fig. 1). For 24 of these patients, successive analyses from two or three time points were analyzed (20 at two time points and 4 at three time points). Samples from 11 patients with no detectable DTCs by the original DTC analysis were also included. In total, 127 samples were analyzed (all presented in Additional file 1: Table S1).

NR2F1/Ki67 and AE1AE3 double immunofluorescence staining protocol
Double immunofluorescence was performed using the broad-specter anticytokeratin (anti-CK) monoclonal antibodies (mAbs) AE1/AE3 combined with anti-COUP TF1/NR2F1 for expression of dormancy. From a selection of the samples, parallel (additional) cytospins were available and DIF was performed using anti-CK mAbs AE1/AE3 combined with the marker Ki67 for proliferation expression. Cytospins (0.5×10^6 MNCs/slide) were fixed for 12 min in methanol/acetone (1:1) at room temperature and briefly air-dried, permeabilized in Triton X-100 (0.1% in PBS (DPBS Gibco-CaCl$_2$/MgCl$_2$)) for 7 min, followed by a wash in PBS. The slides were then incubated for 45 min with one of the following mAbs: NR2F1 Anti-COUP TF1 (Abcam Ab 41,858; 10 µg/mL) or anti-Ki67 clone MIB-1 (DAKO M7240; 1.15 µg/mL). They were subsequently labelled with Alexa Fluor 488 goat anti-mouse IgG (H + L) (Molecular Probes 11029; 4 µg/mL) and incubated for 45 min. To block for

cross-reactions (Ki67) the slides were then incubated with a mouse mAb MOPC21 (Sigma-Aldrich M9269; 20 μg/mL) for 20 min. Finally, a combination of the two anti-CK mAbs AE1 and AE3 (Chemicon Millipore mAbs 1611/1612) were added, fluorescently labelled by Zenon 555 (2 μg of the AE1/AE3 combination per slide was labeled by the Zenon 555 mouse IgG labeling kit (Life technologies Molecular Probes, Z25005) diluted to 20 μg/mL), and the slides were incubated for 45 min. Slides were washed 2 × 5 min in PBS, then sealed with ProLong Gold antifade reagent with DAPI (Life technologies P36931) and cover-slipped. Throughout the protocol, the slides were washed 2 × 5 min in PBS after each antibody incubation step. All antibodies were diluted in PBS/ 0.5% Tween20/ 5% normal goat serum. Cytospins ($0.5 × 10^6$ MNCs/slide) spiked with 1% MCF7 or SKBR3 breast cancer cell line cells were used as positive controls for the anti-CK staining and for optimization of the DIF protocols. Among the normal BM cells in the patient cytospins there were both Ki67-positive cells and cells with 0–5 small NR2F1 signals (see a more detailed description below), serving as internal positive controls for the NR2F1 staining.

Scoring of individual DTCs and NR2F1/Ki67 expression

Stained cells were identified by manual screening in a Leica Microsystems DMI6000B fluorescence microscope, using 20×, 40×, and 63× objectives. Only AE1/AE3-positive cells with a morphology compatible with tumor cells were scored as DTCs [15, 16].

The definitions of DTC as either NR2F1[low] or NR2F1[high] used in this study were determined prior to starting the screening of the patient samples. When optimizing the AE1AE3/NR2F1 DIF protocol we observed that a large majority (> 99%) of normal blood and BM MNCs showed from zero up to two small NR2F1 nuclear localization signals (Additional file 2: Figure S1), and only occasionally did normal BM cells harbor up to five small signals. In contrast, in MCF7 and SKBR3 breast cancer cell line cells, and in test patient samples harboring many DTCs, a range from zero up to many, often large, irregular NR2F1 nuclear localization signals were observed, often with an appearance compatible with localization in the nucleoli (Additional file 2: Figure S1); in some DTCs cytoplasmic signals could also be observed. From our previous immunofluorescence experience in experimental models and cell lines in vivo [6, 8] we have defined NR2F1[high] cells as cells with a strong NR2F1 signal detected in all the nuclear area (Fig. 2a, first row) or deposited as dotted or large irregular nucleolar-like signals (Fig. 2a, second row). In proliferative human and experimental tumors, the NR2F1 signal is either negative (no signal at all) or a weak speckled signal, except in certain areas that are hypoxic [8]. Based on these data from both experimental studies and testing on MCF7 and SKBR3-spiked normal MNCs, we defined as NR2F1[low] a range of NR2F1 immunostaining from entirely negative up to five small signals as seen in normal MNCs (Additional files 2 and 3: Figures S1 and S2). A NR2F1 staining > 5 small signals and/or large signals (≥ 1), and/or the presence of signal clusters defined DTCs as NR2F1[high] (Fig. 2, Additional files 2 and 7: Figures S1 and S2).

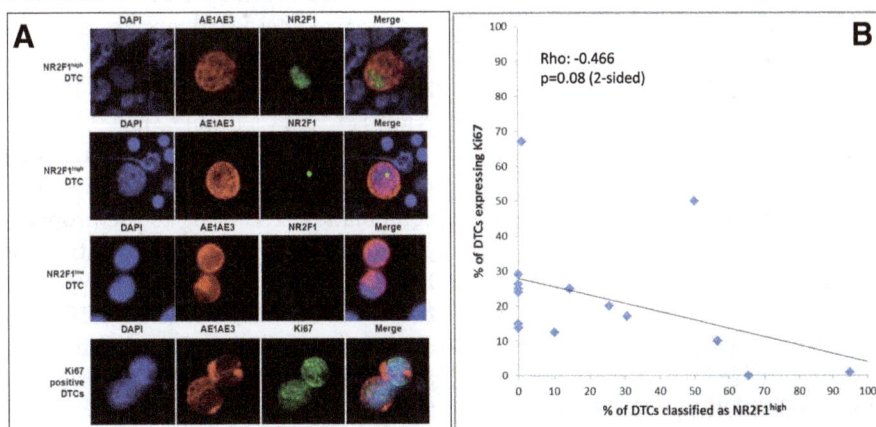

Fig. 2 Images of disseminated tumor cells (DTCs) stained by double immunofluorescence (AE1AE3/NR2F1 and AE1AE3/Ki67) and correlation between Ki67 and NR2F1 expression. **a** DTCs from the BM of study patients analyzed by DIF. The strong and irregular cytoplasmic cytokeratin staining (AE1AE3 antibody, in red fluorescence) identifies these cells as DTCs among the normal BM MNCs (AE1AE3-negative). The two upper rows show NR2F1[high] DTCs with the presence of nuclear NR2F1 signal clusters (in green fluorescence; first row) or one large size NR2F1 signal (i.e., larger than the size range observed in normal BM MNCs; second row). Third row shows two DTCs classified as NR2F1[low] containing only two (lower cell) or three (upper cell) small NR2F1 signals, i.e., expression not exceeding what may be observed in normal BM MNCs. The bottom row shows two DTCs positive for Ki67 (in green). **b** Comparison of the expression on DTC of NR2F1 versus the proliferation marker Ki67. Results from DIF analysis of Ki67/AE1AE3 versus NR2F1/AE1AE3, respectively, on 15 of the BM samples presented in Table 1, where additional cytospins were available for both analyses

In accordance with the preclinical study data presented above, we chose to classify, a priori, samples with ≥ 50% NR2F1^{high} DTCs as "dormant" and samples with < 50% NR2F1^{high} DTCs as "non-dormant".

One of the patients with DTC-negative status according to the original DTC analysis had one detectable DTC by the DIF analysis and was not classified according to "dormant" versus "non-dormant" status.

A Ki67-expressing DTC was defined as a cell exhibiting nuclear immunostaining of Ki67.

Statistics

The association between DTC status/characteristics and distant disease-free interval (DFI) was analyzed. Distant DFI was defined as survival without distant breast cancer recurrence or breast cancer death, and was constructed using Kaplan-Meier curves with accompanied P values obtained from a log-rank test. SPSS software was used for statistical analysis.

Results

Bone marrow cytospins from 86 DTC-positive patients identified by the original DTC staining procedure were analyzed by DIF for cytokeratin (AE1/AE3) and NR2F1 expression as described in Materials and methods. An overview of the BM aspiration (BMA) time points for the included patients is presented in Fig. 1. From 24 of these patients, BM samples at ≥ 2 time points were available for DIF analysis.

Cytokeratin-positive cells were classified as either NR2F1^{high} or NR2F1^{low} according to the level and pattern of expression (see Materials and methods, Fig. 2, and Additional files 2 and 3: Figures S1 and S2).

Expression of Ki67 was analyzed in parallel with the NR2F1 analyses on additional available cytospins from 15 DTC-positive patients (Table 1 and Fig. 2b). Of the total 103 samples found to be DTC-positive (i.e., ≥ 1 detectable DTC) by the original DTC staining procedure (of 2×10^6 BM MNCs), 32 (31%) had cytokeratin-detectable DTCs in the DIF analysis (of 1×10^6 BM MNCs) (Additional file 4: Table S2), in accordance with an expected lower sensitivity of this analysis. Twenty-four samples submitted to DIF had been concluded as DTC-negative by the original DTC analysis. These included 13 samples from 11 patients with no original detectable DTCs. One of the samples had one detectable DTC by DIF, and the remaining 23 were DTC-negative (Additional file 4: Table S2). Data on the original DTC-positive patients with DIF-positive results and available clinicopathological characteristics are presented in Table 1.

The DIF analysis revealed that most of the analyzed patients (24 out of 26) with CK-positive DTCs had ≥ 3 detectable cells and 16 had ≥ 10 DTCs in at least one BM sample, representing a patient group with high risk

of metastasis (Table 1, Additional file 5: Table S3). Indeed, 81% of the DTC-positive patients developed metastasis after the BMA ($n = 17$) or had metastasis at time of the BM aspiration ($n = 4$) (Table 1). Half ($n = 13$) of the patients had > 1% of NR2F1^{high} DTCs in at least one BM sample and 26.9% ($n = 7$) had ≥ 50% NR2F1^{high} DTCs. The latter parameter (≥ 50% NR2F1^{high} DTCs) was chosen as the a priori cut-off for classifying the patient as having a "dormant profile" in accordance with previous experimental studies [6, 8]. Of the samples with detectable NR2F1^{high} DTCs, the median proportion of NR2F1^{high} DTCs was 50%.

To explore changes in the expression of NR2F1 over time and during treatment, DIF analysis was performed on the 24 cases classified as DTC-positive in the original DTC staining procedure and with available samples from BM aspiration at two time points (see Additional file 6: Figure S3 for the original DTC staining results). Of the cases analyzed, 16 received chemotherapy (± endocrine treatment), 5 endocrine treatment only, and 3 no systemic treatment between the BM aspirations (Additional file 7: Table S4). The number of DIF-detected CK-positive DTCs and proportion of NR2F1^{high} DTCs are presented in Fig. 3. The results showed different patterns of change and did not appear to be related to the type of adjuvant treatment (Fig. 3). Three of the six patients with ≥ 50% NR2F1^{high} DTCs at the last BM analysis did not experience relapse. In contrast, 7 of 8 patients with ≤ 1% NR2F1^{high} DTCs at the last BM analysis had systemic relapse or breast cancer death within 12 months (i.e., < 8 months) (Fig. 3b, c). Additional information on the original DTC status, NR2F1 expression, and Ki67 expression of these patients are presented in Additional file 8 (Table S5). All patients with systemic relapse or breast cancer death within 12 months had ≤ 1% NR2F1^{high} DTCs (Table 1).

Table 2 presents the systemic relapse status among the patients with 1 and ≥ 2 BM aspiration time points in combination, according to the proportion of NR2F1-expressing cells in the DTC-positive cases (last positive BM aspiration time point if > 1 performed). Of the patients with predominantly NR2F1^{low} DTCs, 90% had, or experienced, systemic relapse or breast cancer death and 67% were recorded with bone metastasis. Similar figures were observed for those with ≤ 1 NR2F1^{high} DTCs. In contrast, in those patients with ≥ 50% NR2F1^{high} expressing DTCs, 57% had, or experienced, systemic relapse and 29% were recorded with bone metastasis. Survival analysis of all nonmetastatic patients at the time of last DIF DTC-positive BM aspiration revealed a difference in distant DFI (Fig. 4a; $p = 0.023$). Excluding patients analyzed for DIF-positive DTCs (with a negative result) at a subsequent BMA time point ($n = 18$), 93% experienced

Table 1 Overview of all originally disseminated tumor cell (DTC)-positive patients with detectable DTCs by double immunofluorescence technique and clinicopathological parameters

Patient identifier	Study	BMA time points[a]	NR2F1/AE1AE3 DIF analysis		Ki67/AE1AE3 DIF analysis		HR	HER2	T status	N status	Time (months) from BMA to systemic relapse or BC death	Relapse status or BC death (if not recorded relapse)	Time (months) from BMA to last observation if no relapse	Comment
			No. of DTCs	% NR2F1^high DTCs	No. of DTCs	% Ki67+ DTCs								
20	N	(BM1)-BM3	35	0	7	28.6	pos	nd	3	2	0.30	Bone and visceral		
74	S	(BM1-BM3)-BM4	3	0	nd	nd	pos	neg	1	1	1.09	Bone		
5	O	(BM1)/BM2	1000	0	1000	15.0	pos	pos	1	1	1.15	Bone		
60	S	(BM2)-BM3	1000	0[b]	84	26.2	pos	neg	2	1	1.84	Bone		
27	N	(BM1)-BM2	5	0[c]	nd	nd	neg	nd	3	0	5.69	Visceral		
62	S	BM2	40,000	0	nd	nd	pos	neg	2	0	5.79	Bone and visceral		Chemo after BMA
4	O	(BM1)-BM2	9	0	23	21.7	pos	neg	3	1	7.50	Bone and visceral		
3	O	BM1	11	0	nd	nd	pos	neg	2	1	11.22	Visceral		
78	S	(BM1)-BM2-(BM3)	26	0	29	13.8	pos	neg	2	3	13.19	Bone and visceral		Chemo after BMA
13	O	BM1	79	0	nd	Nd	neg	pos	1	1	13.22	Bone		Chemo after BMA
17	N	BM3	5	0	4	25.0	pos	nd	3	1	17.57	Bone and visceral		
34	N	BM1-(BM2)	2	0	nd	nd	pos	neg	3	1	47.43	Visceral		Chemo after BMA
12	O	BM2	16	0	nd	nd	pos	neg	2	1		No relapse	57.73	
66	S	BM1-(BM4)	3	0	nd	nd	pos	neg	1	2		No relapse	87.50	Chemo after BMA
11	O	(BM1)-BM2	500	1.0	87	66.7	neg	pos	3	1	3.72	BC death		
23	N	BM3	50	10.0	16	12.5	pos	pos	3	0	13.55	BC death		
35	N	(BM1)-BM3	7	14.3	12	25.0	pos	nd	3	2	N/A	[d]		Met. before BMA
48		(BM1)-BM3	17	25.5	10	20.0	pos	nd	3	0	12.24	Bone		
41	N	BM3	111	30.6	82	17.1	pos	nd	4	1	N/A	[d]		Met. before BMA
36	N	(BM1)-BM3	6	50.0	4	50.0	pos	nd	3	1	25.33	Bone		
84	S	(BM1)-BM2	2	50.0	nd	nd	pos	neg	2	2		No relapse	55.53	Chemo after BMA

Table 1 Overview of all originally disseminated tumor cell (DTC)-positive patients with detectable DTCs by double immunofluorescence technique and clinicopathological parameters (Continued)

Patient identifier	Study	BMA time points[a]	NR2F1/AE1AE3 DIF analysis		Ki67/AE1AE3 DIF analysis		HR	HER2	T status	N status	Time (months) from BMA to systemic relapse or BC death	Relapse status or BC death (if not recorded relapse)	Time (months) from BMA to last observation if no relapse	Comment
			No. of DTCs	% NR2F1[high] DTCs	No. of DTCs	% Ki67+ DTCs								
9	O	**BM1**	48	56.3	nd	Nd	neg	neg	2	1	N/A	Bone[d]		Met. at BMA
85	S	(BM1)-**BM2**	106	56.6	70	10.0	pos	neg	2	2		No relapse	56.02	Chemo after BMA
69	S	(BM1)-**BM2**-(BM3)	52	65.4	35	0	pos	neg	2	2	15.10	Visceral		Chemo after BMA
6	O	(BM1)-**BM2**	233	94.9	400	1.0	neg	pos	1	1	N/A	Visceral		Met. before BMA
57	S	(BM3)-**BM4**	6	100	nd	nd	neg	nd	2	0		No relapse	59.93	

BC breast cancer, *Chemo* chemotherapy, *DIF* double immunofluorescence, *HR* hormone receptor, *Met.* metastasis, *N* Neotax, *N* metastasis, *N/A* not applicable, *nd* not determined, *neg* negative, *O* Oslo1, *pos* positive, *S* SATT

[a] The bone marrow aspiration (BMA) time points for each patient are noted. In this table, the DTC results are only presented for the BMAs highlighted in bold (last positive sample); results from the other BMA time points are available in Additional file 1 (Table S1) and partly in Fig 3

[b] In the first bone marrow (BM) sample, 46.3% of the DTCs were NR2F1[high]

[c] In the first BM sample, 33.3% of the DTCs were NR2F1[high]

[d] Metastasis before BMA

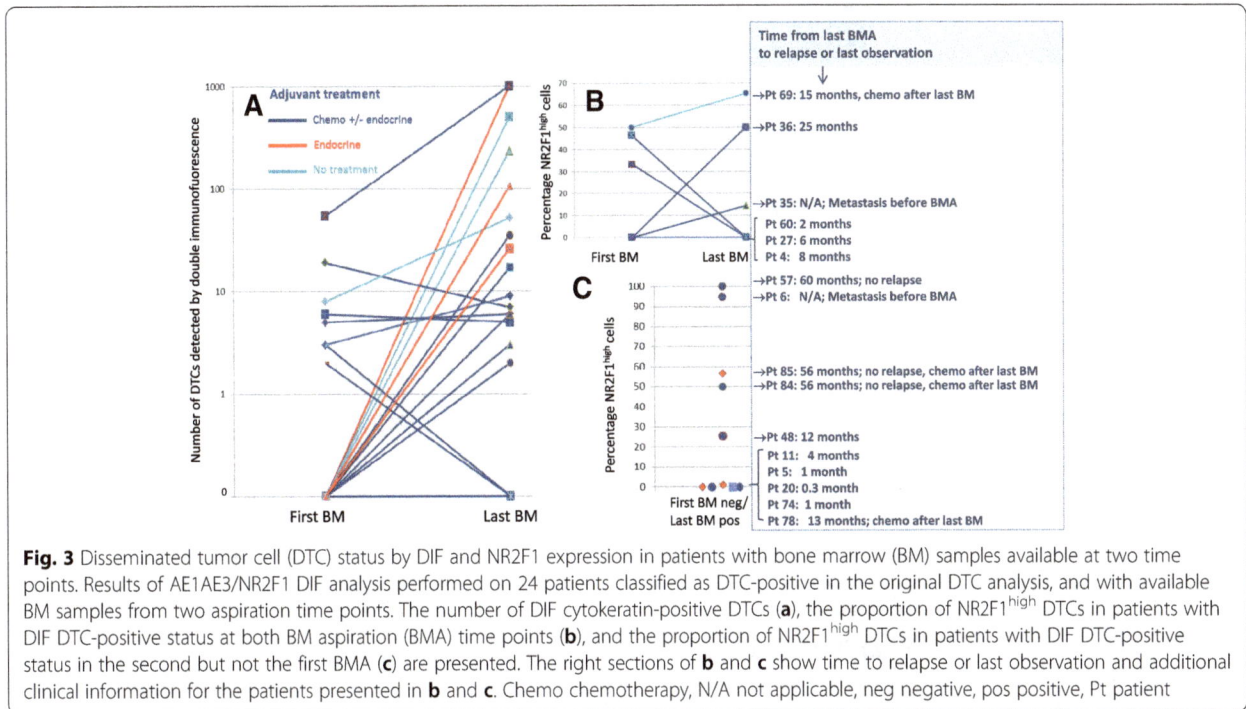

Fig. 3 Disseminated tumor cell (DTC) status by DIF and NR2F1 expression in patients with bone marrow (BM) samples available at two time points. Results of AE1AE3/NR2F1 DIF analysis performed on 24 patients classified as DTC-positive in the original DTC analysis, and with available BM samples from two aspiration time points. The number of DIF cytokeratin-positive DTCs (**a**), the proportion of NR2F1^{high} DTCs in patients with DIF DTC-positive status at both BM aspiration (BMA) time points (**b**), and the proportion of NR2F1^{high} DTCs in patients with DIF DTC-positive status in the second but not the first BMA (**c**) are presented. The right sections of **b** and **c** show time to relapse or last observation and additional clinical information for the patients presented in **b** and **c**. Chemo chemotherapy, N/A not applicable, neg negative, pos positive, Pt patient

systemic relapse/breast cancer death and 75% bone metastasis among the patients with a "non-dormant" DTC classification. One of the four patients with ≥ 50% NR2F1^{high} DTCs (a "dormant" DTC classification) experienced bone metastasis. Analysis of distant DFI among these 18 patients indicated a survival difference between the patients classified by DTCs as having < 50% versus ≥ 50% NR2F1^{high} expressing cells (Fig. 4c; $p = 0.007$). A few patients had exceptionally high DTC numbers. A survival analysis without the patients with ≥ 500 DTCs gave similar results ($p = 0.014$; Additional file 9: Figure S4A). The

patients included in the NeoTax study had higher stages (all with locally advanced disease) than the two other cohorts. Excluding these patients from the survival analysis did not change the results ($p = 0.022$; Additional file 9: Figure S4B).

Limiting the analysis to only those with no chemotherapy after the last BMA revealed similar results, although the interpretation is restricted by the low number of patients with ≥ 50% NR2F1^{high} DTCs ($n = 2$) (Table 2 and Additional file 10: Figure S5; $p = 0.091$).

Table 2 NR2F1 expression and clinical outcome

	Fraction of DTCs categorized as NR2F1^{high}		Distant metastasis (all) or death from breast cancer (%)	Bone metastasis[b] (%)
All patients[a] ($n = 26$)	< 50%	0 to < 50% NR2F1^{high}	17/19 (89.5)	10/15 (66.7)
		0–1% NR2F1^{high}	13/15 (86.7)	9/14 (64.3)
	50–100%		4/7 (57.1)	2/7 (28.6)
Patients without metastasis prior to last DTC-positive BMA and no negative DTC status at subsequent BMA ($n = 18$)	< 50%	0 to < 50% NR2F1^{high}	13/14 (92.9)	9/12 (75.0)
		0–1% NR2F1^{high}	11/12 (91.7)	8/11 (72.7)
	50–100%		1/4 (25.0)	1/4 (25.0)
Patients with no metastasis at time point for last DTC-positive BMA, no negative DTC status at subsequent BMA, and no chemotherapy after the BM analysis ($n = 14$)	< 50%	0 to < 50% NR2F1^{high}	11/12 (91.7)	7/10 (70.0)
		0–1% NR2F1^{high}	9/10 (90.0)	6/9 (66.7)
	50–100%		1/2 (50.0)	1/2 (50.0)

If analysis was performed at more than one time point, the last disseminated tumor cell (DTC)-positive sample is included

BMA bone marrow aspirate

[a]Includes results from 4 patients with metastases detected before bone marrow (BM) analysis and 8 patients receiving chemotherapy after the BM analysis

[b]No information on bone metastasis status was available from four patients in total

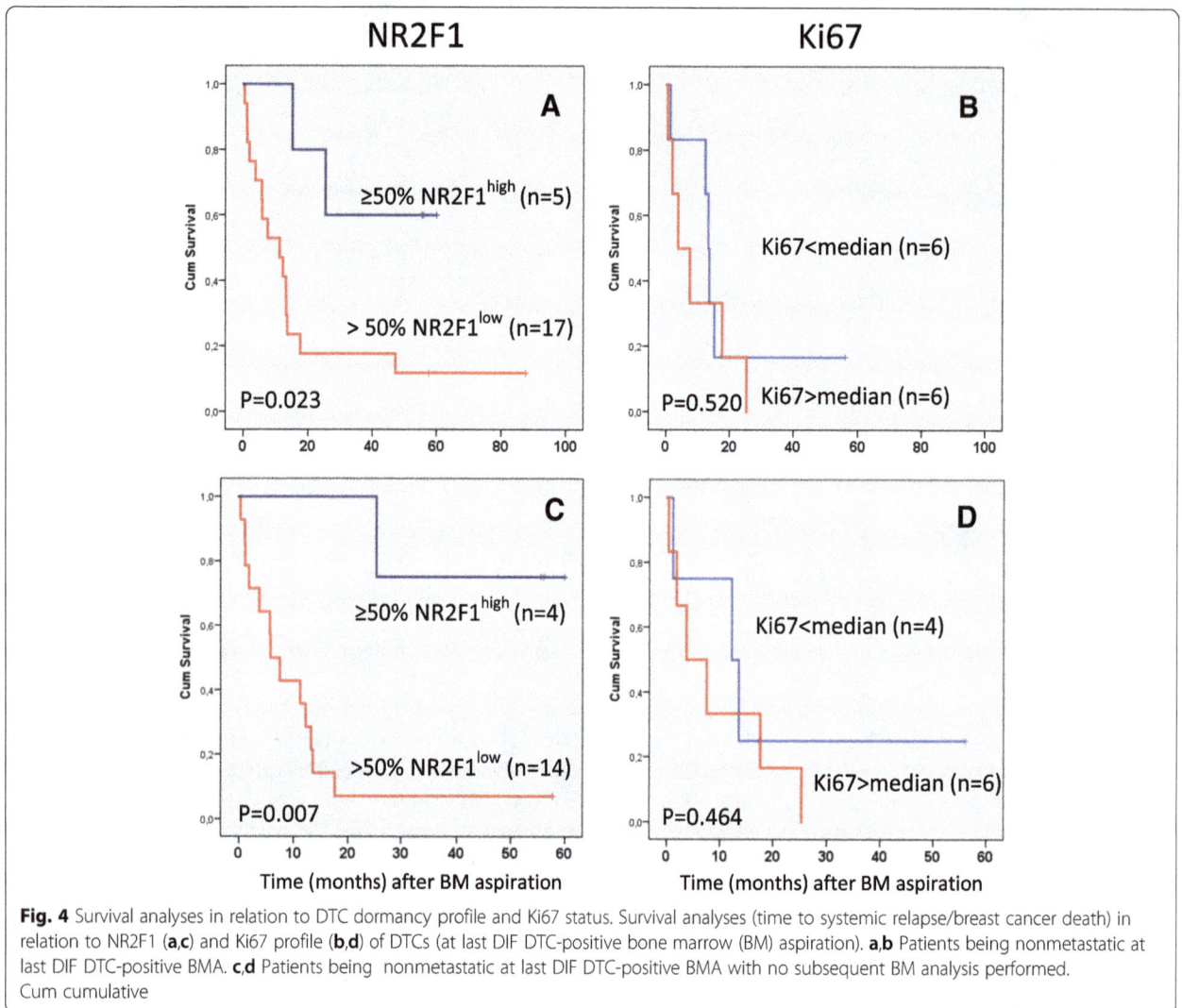

Fig. 4 Survival analyses in relation to DTC dormancy profile and Ki67 status. Survival analyses (time to systemic relapse/breast cancer death) in relation to NR2F1 (**a,c**) and Ki67 profile (**b,d**) of DTCs (at last DIF DTC-positive bone marrow (BM) aspiration). **a,b** Patients being nonmetastatic at last DIF DTC-positive BMA. **c,d** Patients being nonmetastatic at last DIF DTC-positive BMA with no subsequent BM analysis performed. Cum cumulative

To compare the expression of NR2F1 and the proliferation marker Ki67, 1–2 additional cytospins from 15 of the BM samples presented in Table 1 were analyzed by Ki67/pan-cytokeratin DIF. NR2F1 and Ki67 expression were not examined in the same DTCs (cytospins), and therefore the combined expression pattern at the single DTC level could not be addressed. The results showed that the proportion of Ki67-positive DTCs was weakly negatively correlated with the proportion of NR2F1^{high} DTCs ($\rho = -0.466$; $p = 0.08$; Fig. 2b), bearing in mind the low number of cases analyzed for both Ki67 and NR2F1. Survival was not different for patients classified into subgroups by Ki67 expression in DTCs using median dichotomization (Fig. 4b, $p = 0.520$; Fig. 4d, $p = 0.464$), or by the same cut-off value as for NR2F1 ($p = 0.753$, data not shown). The survival difference between patients with NR2F1^{high} and NR2F1^{low} expressing DTCs were similar if the analysis was restricted to only the patients with samples analyzed for Ki67 (Additional file 11:

Figure S6; $p = 0.019$ and $p = 0.026$ for the same patient categories as presented in Fig. 4).

Discussion

To further improve curative treatment of breast cancer, we need to identify patients with MRD and characterize the potential for MRD progression. To the best of our knowledge, this is the first report exploring dormancy marker profiling in DTCs in breast cancer patients. The analysis of NR2F1 expression, a critical node in tumor dormancy induction, can potentially differentiate between active occult tumor cells giving a risk for early metastasis development and more long-term quiescent DTCs. Such information may potentially contribute to future clinical decisions based on minimal residual cancer detection and its state of activation.

We observed that the samples from patients with very early systemic relapse (within 12 months) carried only NR2F1^{low} (non-dormant) DTCs in the last BM sample

($\leq 1\%$ NR2F1^{high} DTCs). This included patients that transitioned from having NR2F1^{high} expressing DTCs to a NR2F1^{low} DTC state in consecutive samples (Fig. 3). Likewise, longer disease-free interval/no detectable metastases were indicated among patients with a presence of predominantly NR2F1^{high} DTCs. This was further supported by the result from survival analysis of nonmetastatic patients showing a difference in metastasis-free interval in subgroups according to NR2F1^{high} expression (Fig. 4a). However, the results should be interpreted with caution due to the restricted number of patients analyzed and the heterogeneity in patient population and treatment. Nevertheless, the data provide clinical support to the abundant previous experimental and some clinical data (mRNA measurements) identifying NR2F1 as a candidate marker for clinically relevant characterization of MRD [6], and that NR2F1 may serve to identify DTC long-term dormancy candidates even among patients harboring larger number of DTCs. Indeed, the patients studied were not selected to be obvious DTC dormancy candidates by a long (many years) relapse-free follow-up period. Most of the BM samples were collected ≤ 3 years after diagnosis and were enriched for cases with ≥ 5 DTCs, a known poor prognostic feature [3, 4, 9–12]. Moreover, although the DTC Ki67 expression showed a weak negative correlation with NR2F1^{high} DTCs (Fig. 2b), no significant association with clinical outcome was observed. This indicates that a proliferation marker such as Ki67 is insufficient to characterize the MRD cell population.

Since Ki67 detects all phases of the cell cycle, except G0, it is possible that it may not accurately pinpoint true dormant cells. In our experience, retinoblastoma protein (pRb) and P-H3-negative, p27-positive cells are better indicators of a quiescent NR2F1-positive DTC [6, 8, 18, 19]. The Ki67 result may place into the proliferative population bin, cells that are in a G0/G1 boundary and arrested or slow cycling. Furthermore, it may classify nonarrested cells transiting through G0 as nonproliferative. In contrast, NR2F1 expression is remarkably stable, epigenetically controlled, and associated with a repressive chromatin state observed in terminally senescent or differentiated cells [6]. These data suggest that NR2F1 marks a durable, more long-lived phenotype of growth arrest. The presented data and results from our experimental models also suggest that NR2F1 is associated with cellular dormancy (quiescence) and not tumor mass dormancy (representing a small cancer cell mass that cannot surpass a certain size) characterized by a balance between proliferation and apoptosis where arrest is never observed. [20]. In our experience and that of other investigators, the latter phenomenon is not observed in solitary DTC dormancy [6, 8, 18, 19, 21, 22]. Published data also suggest that the mechanisms driving solitary DTCs share a significant overlap with those

regulating adult stem cell quiescence [6, 20, 23], which is a cellular dormancy mechanism. These mechanisms may explain the divergence between Ki67 and NR2F1, although additional validation is needed because these markers were not analyzed for in the same DTCs. Nevertheless, results presented in this study and prior results strongly support the concept [20] that lack of proliferation is not the same as dormancy, but rather that proliferative arrest is one characteristic of the dormancy program. This underpins the need for markers that can identify the biological key mechanisms for dormancy-associated quiescence that are different from the absence of cell cycle phase markers.

Improved techniques to assess the MRD population and their dormant or reactivating state will be key to identifying the risk of future metastasis despite undergoing standard treatment. This opens the way for testing new treatments that prevent metastasis by inducing/enforcing dormancy, and/or to eradicate MRD [2, 6]. Dormant cancer cells can evade chemotherapy and also express pluripotency genes that keep them in a long-term reawakening probability state [6]. Retinoic acid and 5-azacitidine are examples of dormancy-inducing/sustaining treatment strategies, showing the ability to reprogram malignant cells into dormancy and enforce dormancy programs in already quiescent tumor cells [6, 7]. These drugs will be tested in a clinical trial of prostate cancer patients at risk of developing metastasis (Mount Sinai IRB no. 18–00226; ClinicalTrials.gov identifier, NCT03572387).

Sustaining a dormancy phenotype could have life-saving consequences. In line with this, patients with NR2F1 expression in a few DTCs appeared to have longer disease-free survival in our study. This may suggest that those few DTCs are indicative of at least two parameters that need to be further investigated: first, that residual DTCs not detected in the test clearly share the same phenotype as those detected, and second, that the test seems to also inform on patients that may have niches that are pro-dormant and thus support dormancy of the residual DTCs for longer time periods. The first possibility is supported by abundant experimental evidence for a role of NR2F1 in DTC dormancy through a microenvironmental and epigenetic program of regulation [6]. The second is less explored, but it is possible that some patients may be better producers of dormancy-inducing cues as these are commonly signals involved in adult stem cell quiescence. Furthermore, androgen deprivation treatment in prostate cancer has been linked to upregulation of NR2F1 [24], suggesting that certain commonly used therapies may induce dormancy and cooperate in a long-term response by affecting the DTCs and the host to enter a pro-dormancy state. In breast cancer, response to tamoxifen was reported to be associated with the presence of transforming growth factor (TGF)β2, a dormancy-inducing factor [25, 26].

Furthermore, a reduced androgen receptor signaling resulted in TGFβ2 upregulation in the prostate and seminal gland tissue [27]. Thus, future studies may not only focus on detection of dormant DTCs, but also investigation of whether the host is producing pro-dormancy cues.

Among all the patients included in the studies used as the source for the current project [9–12] the majority of those identified as DTC-positive had only one or two detectable DTCs across the BMA time points (based on the original analysis; NeoTax ≥ 75%, Oslo1 ≥ 87%, SATT ≥ 75%). The group of patients with such low numbers of DTCs has the most favorable survival among the DTC-positive cases [9, 28] and would also be expected to be enriched in cases with quiescent DTCs. We attempted to include both patients with originally high and low numbers of DTCs in our analysis. However, in the majority of the samples, no DTCs were detectable by DIF from patients with low DTC burden. In addition to the Poisson distribution effect, this may be for several reasons. Firstly, a reduced sensitivity of the DIF technique compared with the standard (original) APAAP ICC technique can be expected due to a stronger amplification of the signals by the APAAP (three layers) than the direct Xenon-labeling of the anti-CK antibody used in the DIF protocol. Secondly, half the number of BM MNCs (1×10^6) were available for the DIF analysis. Thirdly, some of the DIF samples were prepared from liquid nitrogen-frozen MNC suspensions, which in our experience results in loss of tumor cells in some patients compared with cytospins prepared from fresh BM. Further assessment and characterization of dormancy in patients with very infrequent DTCs (i.e., below the detection level for our analysis) requires analysis of larger BM volumes in future studies, preferably using enrichment techniques [29] or automated scanning systems (http://rarecyte.com) combined with multi-marker analysis. In parallel with DTC analysis, capturing functional characteristics of circulating tumor cells (CTCs) from high volumes of peripheral blood, for instance by a multitube CellSearch analysis (https://www.cellsearchctc.com/), leukapheresis-related techniques [30], or intravascular capturing devices [31, 32], would clarify whether assessment of CTCs may be used for future dormancy studies.

Conclusions

Overall, we conclude that NR2F1 detection in BM DTCs may be a promising tool to determine the phenotype of DTCs and the prognosis of breast cancer patients. For decades, DTC biology has been relegated primarily to the area of enumeration and subsequent prognosis. Our bench-to-bedside work reveals the first potential dormancy marker that informs on the behavior of DTCs and suggests that enumeration should be followed by phenotype information. Markers such as NR2F1 coupled to

DTC genetics and other host-derived indicators may provide a breakthrough in the management of MRD and metastasis prevention.

Additional files

Additional file 1: Table S1. Descriptive data from all tested patients. (XLSX 15 kb)

Additional file 2: Figure S1. AE1AE3/NR2F1 DIF staining on normal MNCs spiked with breast cancer cell line cells. The first row shows normal MNCs (AE1AE2-negative) and one breast cancer cell line cell (MCF7; AE1AE3-positive). The MNCs contain 0–3 small/weak NR2F1 signals per nucleus and the cancer cell two similarly small signals. These cells are all defined as being NR2F1^{low} cells in the present study. Occasionally, normal BM cells harbored up to 5 small signals (not shown in the figure). The second row shows MNCs with a cluster of four breast cancer cell line cells (SKBR3), of which the lower left cell does not contain any NR2F1 signals and is therefore defined as NR2F1^{low}. The third cell from the left contains 7–8 small signals, with a tendency to signal clustering, and satisfies the criteria for an NR2F1^{high} cell. In cell numbers 2 and 4 from the left, 4–5 small signals are seen. Although the signals of these cells tend to melt together in clusters/larger signals they still represent expressions below the cut-off for NR2F1^{high} classification, but are approaching the cut-off level. The cells in the second row of this figure therefore illustrate the a priori defined cut-off between NR2F1-positive and -negative cells. (NR2F1 signals in MNCs in the second row are out of focus and therefore not visible on the images). For illustration of the NR2F1 classification of DTCs within the study, see Fig. 2a and Additional file 7: Figure S2. (PDF 684 kb)

Additional file 3: Figure S2. Illustration of the classification system for NR2F1 expression of DTC prospectively chosen for the present study. NR2F1^{low} DTC (A–C). (A) Cluster of three DTCs identified by AE1AE3 in red fluorescence and a morphology compatible with tumor cells. Two of the DTCs have no NR2F1 signals and one has one small NR2F1 signal. Surrounding BM MNCs have 0–1 NR2F1 signals of a similar size. (B, C) One DTC with 2–3 small NR2F1 signals. Adjacent normal BM MNCs with 0–1 small NR2F1 signals. NR2F1^{high} DTC (D, E): (D) Cluster of two DTCs with coarse, partly confluent NR2F1 signals of varying sizes (signals in BM MNCs not visualized because of not being in focus). (E) Cluster of 5 DTCs, three of them defined as NR2F1^{high} because of > 5 NR2F1 signals, partly of large signal size. The remaining two DTCs, with no NR2F1 signals, are assigned NR2F1^{low}, as well as the adjacent normal BM MNCs with 0–1 small NR2F1 signals. (PDF 337 kb)

Additional file 4: Table S2. Overview of patient material and DTC results. (DOCX 34 kb)

Additional file 5: Table S3. Characteristics of the DTC-positive cases by double immunofluorescence (DIF). (DOCX 33 kb)

Additional file 6: Figure S3. Serial BM samples: number of DTCs detected in the original DTC analysis (APAAP-ICC technique). (PPTX 128 kb)

Additional file 7: Table S4. Overview of received treatment between the two BM aspiration time points for the patients presented in Fig. 3. (DOCX 33 kb)

Additional file 8: Table S5. Additional results from the serial DTC analyses on samples presented in Fig. 3b and c (in the same order). (DOCX 39 kb)

Additional file 9: Figure S4. (A) Survival analyses (time to systemic relapse/breast cancer death) in relation to NR2F1 profile of DTCs for patients being nonmetastatic at the time point of last DIF DTC-positive BMA and having no subsequent BM analyzed; patients harboring ≥ 500 DTC excluded. (B) Survival analyses (time to systemic relapse/breast cancer death) in relation to NR2F1 profile of DTCs for patients being nonmetastatic at time point of last DIF DTC-positive BMA and having no subsequent BM analyzed; NeoTax study patients excluded. (PPTX 114 kb)

Additional file 10: Figure S5. Survival analyses according to NR2F1 and Ki67 DTC profiles of patients being nonmetastatic at the time of last DIF DTC-positive BMA, having no subsequent BM analyzed, and no chemotherapy after last BMA. (PPTX 120 kb)

Additional file 11: Figure S6. (A) Survival analyses (time to systemic relapse/breast cancer death) in relation to NR2F1 profile at last DIF DTC-positive BMA, restricted to those with Ki67 DTC analysis available (only patients being nonmetastatic at last DIF DTC-positive BMA included). (B) As A, but analysis restricted to patients having no subsequent BMA analyzed. (PPTX 68 kb)

Abbreviations
APAAP: Alkaline phosphatase–anti-alkaline phosphatase; BM: Bone marrow; BMA: Bone marrow aspiration; CK: Cytokeratin; Coup TF1: Chicken ovalbumin upstream promoter transcription factor 1; CTC: Circulating tumor cell; DFI: Disease-free interval; DIF: Double immunofluorescence; DTC: Disseminated tumor cell; ER: Estrogen receptor; FEC: Fluorouracil, epirubicin, and cyclophosphamide; ICC: Immunocytochemical; mAb: Monoclonal antibody; MNC: Mononuclear cell; MRD: Minimal residual disease; NR2F1: Nuclear receptor subfamily 2, group F, member 1; PBS: Phosphate-buffered saline; pRb: Retinoblastoma protein; TGF: Transforming growth factor

Acknowledgements
We thank the patients who have participated in the studies.

Funding
Funding was provided to BN by the Research Council of Norway, South-Eastern Norway Regional Health Authority, and the Norwegian Cancer Society. Funding was provided to JAA-G by the National Cancer Institute (US), US Department of Defense, and the Samuel Waxman Cancer Research Foundation. Funding was provided to MSS by the Melanoma Research Alliance, Susan G. Komen (US), and the National Cancer Institute (US).

Authors' contributions
Initiation and planning of the study: BN and JAA-G. Writing and revision of the manuscript and analyses of results: BN, JAA-G, MCR, MSS, and EB. Revision of the manuscript, patient inclusion and patient management: BN, PEL, MS, and ES. Double immunofluorescence staining and screening of samples: MCR. Laboratory administration and supervision: AR. All authors read and approved the final manuscript.

Competing interests
The authors declare that they have no competing interests.

Author details
[1]Department of Pathology, Oslo University Hospital, Oslo, Norway. [2]Department of Pharmacological Sciences, Icahn School of Medicine at Mount Sinai, New York, NY 10029, USA. [3]Division of Hematology and Oncology, Department of Medicine, Department of Otolaryngology, Tisch Cancer Institute, Black Family Stem Cell Institute, Icahn School of Medicine at Mount Sinai, New York, NY 10029, USA. [4]Department of Surgery, Oslo University Hospital, Oslo, Norway. [5]Department of Oncology, Haukeland University Hospital, Bergen, Norway. [6]Department of Clinical Science, Faculty of Medicine, University of Bergen, Bergen, Norway. [7]Department of Oncology, Oslo University Hospital, Oslo, Norway. [8]Institute of Clinical Medicine, University of Oslo, Oslo, Norway.

References
1. Linde N, Fluegen G, Aguirre-Ghiso JA. The relationship between dormant cancer cells and their microenvironment. Adv Cancer Res. 2016;132:45–71.
2. Aguirre-Ghiso JA, Bragado P, Sosa MS. Metastasis awakening: targeting dormant cancer. Nat Med. 2013;19(3):276–7.
3. Braun S, Vogl FD, Naume B, Janni W, Osborne MP, Coombes RC, Schlimok G, Diel IJ, Gerber B, Gebauer G, et al. A pooled analysis of bone marrow micrometastasis in breast cancer. N Engl J Med. 2005;353(8):793–802.
4. Janni W, Vogl FD, Wiedswang G, Synnestvedt M, Fehm T, Juckstock J, Borgen E, Rack B, Braun S, Sommer H, et al. Persistence of disseminated tumor cells in the bone marrow of breast cancer patients predicts increased risk for relapse—a European pooled analysis. Clin Cancer Res. 2011;17(9):2967–76.
5. Adam AP, George A, Schewe D, Bragado P, Iglesias BV, Ranganathan AC, Kourtidis A, Conklin DS, Aguirre-Ghiso JA. Computational identification of a p38SAPK-regulated transcription factor network required for tumor cell quiescence. Cancer Res. 2009;69(14):5664–72.
6. Sosa MS, Parikh F, Maia AG, Estrada Y, Bosch A, Bragado P, Ekpin E, George A, Zheng Y, Lam HM, et al. NR2F1 controls tumour cell dormancy via SOX9- and RARbeta-driven quiescence programmes. Nat Commun. 2015;6:6170.
7. Sosa MS. Dormancy programs as emerging antimetastasis therapeutic alternatives. Mol Cell Oncol. 2016;3(1):e1029062.
8. Fluegen G, Avivar-Valderas A, Wang Y, Padgen MR, Williams JK, Nobre AR, Calvo V, Cheung JF, Bravo-Cordero JJ, Entenberg D, et al. Phenotypic heterogeneity of disseminated tumour cells is preset by primary tumour hypoxic microenvironments. Nat Cell Biol. 2017;19(2):120–32.
9. Mathiesen RR, Borgen E, Renolen A, Lokkevik E, Nesland JM, Anker G, Ostenstad B, Lundgren S, Risberg T, Mjaaland I, et al. Persistence of disseminated tumor cells after neoadjuvant treatment for locally advanced breast cancer predicts poor survival. Breast Cancer Res. 2012;14(4):R117.
10. Wiedswang G, Borgen E, Karesen R, Kvalheim G, Nesland JM, Qvist H, Schlichting E, Sauer T, Janbu J, Harbitz T, et al. Detection of isolated tumor cells in bone marrow is an independent prognostic factor in breast cancer. J Clin Oncol. 2003;21(18):3469–78.
11. Wiedswang G, Borgen E, Karesen R, Qvist H, Janbu J, Kvalheim G, Nesland JM, Naume B. Isolated tumor cells in bone marrow three years after diagnosis in disease-free breast cancer patients predict unfavorable clinical outcome. Clin Cancer Res. 2004;10(16):5342–8.
12. Naume B, Synnestvedt M, Falk RS, Wiedswang G, Weyde K, Risberg T, Kersten C, Mjaaland I, Vindi L, Sommer HH, et al. Clinical outcome with correlation to disseminated tumor cell (DTC) status after DTC-guided secondary adjuvant treatment with docetaxel in early breast cancer. J Clin Oncol. 2014;32(34):3848–57.
13. Chrisanthar R, Knappskog S, Lokkevik E, Anker G, Ostenstad B, Lundgren S, Berge EO, Risberg T, Mjaaland I, Maehle L, et al. CHEK2 mutations affecting kinase activity together with mutations in TP53 indicate a functional pathway associated with resistance to epirubicin in primary breast cancer. PLoS One. 2008;3(8):e3062.
14. Chrisanthar R, Knappskog S, Lokkevik E, Anker G, Ostenstad B, Lundgren S, Risberg T, Mjaaland I, Skjonsberg G, Aas T, et al. Predictive and prognostic impact of TP53 mutations and MDM2 promoter genotype in primary breast cancer patients treated with epirubicin or paclitaxel. PLoS One. 2011;6(4):e19249.
15. Borgen E, Naume B, Nesland JM, Kvalheim G, Beiske K, Fodstad O, Diel I, Solomayer EF, Theocharous P, Coombes RC, et al. Standardization of the immunocytochemical detection of cancer cells in BM and blood: I. Establishment of objective criteria for the evaluation of immunostained cells. Cytotherapy. 1999;1(5):377–88.
16. Fehm T, Braun S, Muller V, Janni W, Gebauer G, Marth C, Schindlbeck C, Wallwiener D, Borgen E, Naume B, et al. A concept for the standardized detection of disseminated tumor cells in bone marrow from patients with primary breast cancer and its clinical implementation. Cancer. 2006;107(5):885–92.
17. Synnestvedt M, Borgen E, Wist E, Wiedswang G, Weyde K, Risberg T, Kersten C, Mjaaland I, Vindi L, Schirmer C, et al. Disseminated tumor cells as selection marker and monitoring tool for secondary adjuvant treatment in early breast cancer. Descriptive results from an intervention study. BMC Cancer. 2012;12:616.

18. Bragado P, Estrada Y, Parikh F, Krause S, Capobianco C, Farina HG, Schewe DM, Aguirre-Ghiso JA. TGF-beta2 dictates disseminated tumour cell fate in target organs through TGF-beta-RIII and p38alpha/beta signalling. Nat Cell Biol. 2013;15(11):1351–61.

19. Harper KL, Sosa MS, Entenberg D, Hosseini H, Cheung JF, Nobre R, Avivar-Valderas A, Nagi C, Girnius N, Davis RJ, et al. Mechanism of early dissemination and metastasis in Her2+ mammary cancer. Nature. 2016. https://doi.org/10.1038/nature20609.

20. Sosa MS, Bragado P, Aguirre-Ghiso JA. Mechanisms of disseminated cancer cell dormancy: an awakening field. Nat Rev Cancer. 2014;14(9):611–22.

21. Malladi S, Macalinao DG, Jin X, He L, Basnet H, Zou Y, de Stanchina E, Massague J. Metastatic latency and immune evasion through autocrine inhibition of WNT. Cell. 2016;165(1):45–60.

22. Gao H, Chakraborty G, Lee-Lim AP, Mo Q, Decker M, Vonica A, Shen R, Brogi E, Brivanlou AH, Giancotti FG. The BMP inhibitor Coco reactivates breast cancer cells at lung metastatic sites. Cell. 2012;150(4):764–79.

23. Cabezas-Wallscheid N, Buettner F, Sommerkamp P, Klimmeck D, Ladel L, Thalheimer FB, Pastor-Flores D, Roma LP, Renders S, Zeisberger P, et al. Vitamin A-retinoic acid signaling regulates hematopoietic stem cell dormancy. Cell. 2017;169(5):807–823.e819.

24. Thompson VC, Day TK, Bianco-Miotto T, Selth LA, Han G, Thomas M, Buchanan G, Scher HI, Nelson CC, Greenberg NM, et al. A gene signature identified using a mouse model of androgen receptor-dependent prostate cancer predicts biochemical relapse in human disease. Int J Cancer. 2012; 131(3):662–72.

25. Kopp A, Jonat W, Schmahl M, Knabbe C. Transforming growth factor beta 2 (TGF-beta 2) levels in plasma of patients with metastatic breast cancer treated with tamoxifen. Cancer Res. 1995;55(20):4512–5.

26. Buck MB, Coller JK, Murdter TE, Eichelbaum M, Knabbe C. TGFbeta2 and TbetaRII are valid molecular biomarkers for the antiproliferative effects of tamoxifen and tamoxifen metabolites in breast cancer cells. Breast Cancer Res Treat. 2008;107(1):15–24.

27. Lucia MS, Sporn MB, Roberts AB, Stewart LV, Danielpour D. The role of transforming growth factor-beta1, -beta2, and -beta3 in androgen-responsive growth of NRP-152 rat prostatic epithelial cells. J Cell Physiol. 1998;175(2):184–92.

28. Naume B, Wiedswang G, Borgen E, Kvalheim G, Karesen R, Qvist H, Janbu J, Harbitz T, Nesland JM. The prognostic value of isolated tumor cells in bone marrow in breast cancer patients: evaluation of morphological categories and the number of clinically significant cells. Clin Cancer Res. 2004;10(9): 3091–7.

29. Naume B, Borgen E, Nesland JM, Beiske K, Gilen E, Renolen A, Ravnas G, Qvist H, Karesen R, Kvalheim G. Increased sensitivity for detection of micrometastases in bone-marrow/peripheral-blood stem-cell products from breast-cancer patients by negative immunomagnetic separation. Int J Cancer. 1998;78(5):556–60.

30. Stoecklein NH, Fischer JC, Niederacher D, Terstappen LW. Challenges for CTC-based liquid biopsies: low CTC frequency and diagnostic leukapheresis as a potential solution. Expert Rev Mol Diagn. 2016;16(2):147–64.

31. Theil G, Fischer K, Weber E, Medek R, Hoda R, Lucke K, Fornara P. The use of a new cell collector to isolate circulating tumor cells from the blood of patients with different stages of prostate cancer and clinical outcomes—a proof-of-concept study. PLoS One. 2016;11(8):e0158354.

32. Gorges TM, Penkalla N, Schalk T, Joosse SA, Riethdorf S, Tucholski J, Lucke K, Wikman H, Jackson S, Brychta N, et al. Enumeration and molecular characterization of tumor cells in lung cancer patients using a novel in vivo device for capturing circulating tumor cells. Clin Cancer Res. 2016;22(9): 2197–206.

21

Ribociclib for the first-line treatment of advanced hormone receptor-positive breast cancer: a review of subgroup analyses from the MONALEESA-2 trial

Gabriel N. Hortobagyi

Abstract: Endocrine therapy is recommended for patients with hormone receptor-positive (HR$^+$) advanced and metastatic breast cancer without visceral crisis (symptomatic visceral disease). However, many patients experience disease progression during treatment, and most patients eventually develop endocrine resistance. Therefore, it is important to identify treatment options that prolong the effectiveness of first-line endocrine therapies. Ribociclib is an orally bioavailable cyclin-dependent kinase (CDK) 4/6 inhibitor that has been approved for use in combination with an aromatase inhibitor for the treatment of HR$^+$, human epidermal growth factor receptor 2-negative (HER2$^-$) advanced breast cancer. This approval is based on findings from the MONALEESA-2 study, a double-blind, placebo-controlled, randomized phase 3 trial (NCT01958021) in which first-line therapy with ribociclib + letrozole significantly improved progression-free survival (PFS) compared with placebo + letrozole in patients with HR$^+$/HER2$^-$ advanced breast cancer. This review will discuss the overall findings from the MONALEESA-2 study and will provide a summarized analysis of results from the available subgroups in the study by age, visceral metastases, bone-only disease, de novo disease, and prior therapy. On the basis of these data, ribociclib has established itself as a beneficial treatment option for these different populations.

Keywords: CDK4/6 inhibitor, Ribociclib, Endocrine therapy, Hormone receptor-positive, HR$^+$/HER2$^-$ breast cancer, MONALEESA-2

Background

Breast cancer accounts for 30% (252,710) of the new cancer cases and 14% (40,610) of cancer deaths in women in the US, according to statistics from 2017 [1]. Except in cases of visceral crisis, the standard of care in advanced hormone receptor-positive (HR$^+$) breast cancer includes endocrine therapy (ET) alone or in combination with a targeted therapy [2]. However, many patients with newly diagnosed advanced breast cancer progress within a year of treatment with single-agent aromatase inhibitors [3], and the majority eventually develop endocrine resistance [4]. Therefore, identifying optimal first-line treatment options that delay disease progression in patients with locally advanced or metastatic cancer is critical [4].

Available first-line options

The classification of trials as "first-line" is often unclear, as both patients with previous exposure to (neo)adjuvant ET and patients naive to ET are considered as receiving first-line treatment for advanced breast cancer [5]. However, factors such as differences in tumor biology, treatment approaches, and initiation and duration of prior treatment (if any) are significant considerations that inform treatment decisions [5]. To delay endocrine resistance, several therapies targeting the cyclin D1/cyclin-dependent kinase (CDK) pathway have been developed, including mammalian target of rapamycin (mTOR) inhibitors, phosphatidylinositol-3-kinase (PI3K) inhibitors/protein kinase B (AKT) inhibitors, and CDK inhibitors [6].

Correspondence: ghortoba@mdanderson.org
Department of Breast Medical Oncology, Division of Cancer Medicine, The University of Texas MD Anderson Cancer Center, 1515 Holcombe Boulevard, Houston, TX 77030, USA

Targeting the CDK4/6 pathway through treatment with CDK4/6 inhibitors in combination with letrozole has led to significant improvement in progression-free survival (PFS) compared with that achieved with single-agent ET in first-line HR$^+$ breast cancer [7, 8].

Currently, three CDK4/6 inhibitors, palbociclib, ribociclib, and abemaciclib, are approved by the US Food and Drug Administration (FDA) for use as first-line combination therapy with an aromatase inhibitor in the treatment of HR$^+$/human epidermal growth factor receptor 2-negative (HER2$^-$) advanced or metastatic breast cancer. These CDK4/6 inhibitors have been shown to significantly improve median PFS compared with endocrine monotherapy and/or placebo in randomized trials [7–9]. Ribociclib is an orally bioavailable small molecule that selectively inhibits CDK4/6, thereby inhibiting the phosphorylation of retinoblastoma protein, which prevents cell-cycle progression and arrests the cell cycle in the G_1 phase [8]. In 2017 [10], ribociclib was approved by the US FDA on the basis of results from the phase 3 MONALEESA-2 trial of 668 patients with advanced breast cancer (ClinicalTrials.gov number, NCT01958021), in which treatment with ribociclib + letrozole met the PFS endpoint (hazard ratio (HR) = 0.56; 95% confidence interval (CI) 0.43–0.72) [8]. Initial US FDA approval of palbociclib was based on results from the phase 2 PALOMA-1 trial (NCT00721409), in which treatment with palbociclib + letrozole doubled the PFS compared with single-agent letrozole (20.2 vs 10.2 months, HR = 0.488, 95% CI 0.319–0.748, $P = 0.0004$) [11]. In the randomized (2:1 ratio) phase 3 PALOMA-2 study (NCT01740427), PFS in patients treated with palbociclib + letrozole was 24.8 months (95% CI 22.1 to not estimable) compared with 14.5 months (95% CI 12.9–17.1) in the placebo + letrozole group (HR = 0.58; 95% CI 0.46–0.72; $P < 0.001$), and the clinical benefit rate (CBR) was 84.9% vs 70.3% in the two groups, respectively [7]. First-line approval of abemaciclib + aromatase inhibitor was based on the randomized phase 3 MONARCH 3 trial (NCT02246621) in which abemaciclib + aromatase inhibitor significantly prolonged PFS vs placebo + aromatase inhibitor (median PFS: not reached vs 14.7 months; HR = 0.54; 95% CI 0.41–0.72; $P = 0.000021$) [9]. The CBR was 78.0% in the abemaciclib group vs 71.5% in the placebo group. Another available first-line treatment option for HR$^+$ advanced breast cancer includes full-dose fulvestrant, a selective estrogen-receptor degrader [12]. In the randomized, double-blind phase 3 FALCON trial in patients with HR$^+$ breast cancer, PFS was significantly prolonged with first-line fulvestrant 500 mg treatment ($n = 230$) compared with anastrozole ($n = 232$) (HR = 0.797; 95% CI 0.637–0.999; $P = 0.0486$), with a median PFS of 16.6 months vs 13.8 months, respectively [12].

Overall results from MONALEESA-2

MONALEESA-2 was an international, randomized, double-blind, placebo-controlled, phase 3 trial that has been described in detail previously [8]. The MONALEESA-2 trial was conducted in accordance with the Good Clinical Practice guidelines and the provisions of the Declaration of Helsinki. A total of 668 patients, from whom written informed consent had been obtained, were randomly assigned 1:1 to orally receive either ribociclib + letrozole or placebo + letrozole and were stratified by disease site (presence or absence of liver and/or lung metastases) [8]. Postmenopausal women with locally advanced or metastatic HR$^+$/HER2$^-$ breast cancer with ≥ 1 measurable lesion (Response Evaluation Criteria in Solid Tumors (RECIST) v1.1) or ≥ 1 predominantly lytic bone lesion and an Eastern Cooperative Oncology Group (ECOG) status of ≤ 1 were included [8]. Patients with any prior systemic therapy for advanced breast cancer (including ET or chemotherapy), inflammatory breast cancer, or active cardiac disease or history of cardiac dysfunction (corrected QT interval with Fridericia's formula (QTcF) > 450 ms) were excluded [8]. At the initial interim analysis (data cut-off date, 29 January 2016), the trial met the primary endpoint of PFS. Patients in the ribociclib treatment group had a 44% lower relative risk of progression ($P = 3.29 \times 10^{-6}$) vs those in the placebo group. In the ribociclib treatment group, 195 patients (58%) remained on treatment vs 154 patients (46%) in the placebo group. Median PFS occurred at 14.7 months in the placebo group but was not reached in the ribociclib group due to continued treatment. The CBRs were 79.6% in the ribociclib group and 72.8% in the placebo group in the intention-to-treat population and 80.1% and 71.8%, respectively, in patients with measurable disease ($P = 0.02$ for both populations). The most common adverse events (AEs) occurring in ≥ 20% of the study population were neutropenia, nausea, infections, fatigue, diarrhea, alopecia, leukopenia, vomiting, arthralgia, constipation, headache, and hot flushes. The most common grade 3/4 AEs (> 3%) were neutropenia, leukopenia, abnormal liver function tests, infections, and vomiting. AEs leading to dose reductions of ribociclib occurred in 50.6% of patients receiving ribociclib + letrozole compared with 4.2% in patients receiving placebo + letrozole, and permanent discontinuation of ribociclib + letrozole due to AEs occurred in 7.5% of patients. The AE most frequently leading to dose reduction was neutropenia ($n = 104/169$ patients with dose reduction due to AE in the ribociclib group vs no patients in the placebo group). On-treatment deaths, regardless of causality, were reported in three patients (0.9%) treated with ribociclib + letrozole vs one patient (0.3%) treated with placebo + letrozole. Causes of death in patients taking ribociclib + letrozole were progressive disease, death (cause unknown), and sudden death (in the setting of grade 3 hypokalemia and grade 2 QT prolongation). The demographics of the populations included in the subgroup analyses of MONALEESA-2 were well-balanced, and median duration of the study in all subsets was ≥ 12 months. Median PFS and CBR results favored the ribociclib group across all predefined subgroups. The safety profile of ribociclib + letrozole was similar across all subsets (Table 1). Results from a second overall survival interim analysis (data cut-off, 2 January 2017) of MONALEESA-2 showed that the PFS benefit was maintained for ribociclib at 25.3 months vs 16.0 months for the placebo group (HR = 0.568; 95% CI 0.457–0.704; $P = 9.63 \times 10^{-8}$), with a consistent PFS benefit across patient subgroups (Hortobagyi GN et al. Updated results from MONALEESA-2, a Phase III trial of first-line ribociclib + letrozole in hormone receptor-positive, HER2-negative advanced breast cancer. Poster presented at the American Society of Clinical Oncology Annual Meeting, Chicago, IL, USA; 2–6 June 2017) (Fig. 1). However, this review will discuss results from the interim PFS data cut-off (29 January 2016) unless otherwise indicated.

Elderly patients
It is estimated that more than 40% of patients with breast cancer are aged ≥ 65 years [13, 14]. Compared with younger women, breast cancer in elderly women (≥ 65 years old) has been associated with a less aggressive disease course, higher incidence of comorbidities, higher avoidance of surgery, and lower trial enrollment due to exclusion criteria or treatment toxicity [15, 16]. These factors, in addition to age-related functional capability and quality of life, influence treatment decisions.

In MONALEESA-2, 295 patients (44%) were ≥ 65 years of age, of which 150 patients were randomized to receive ribociclib + letrozole; the remaining patients received placebo + letrozole. In patients < 65 years of age, 184 were randomized to the ribociclib group and 186 were randomized to the placebo group. Overall, the baseline characteristics were balanced between patients ≥ 65 and < 65 years of age, except for a higher proportion of ECOG performance status scores of 1 among elderly patients. The combination of ribociclib + letrozole significantly improved PFS compared with placebo + letrozole both in patients ≥ 65 years old (HR = 0.608, 95% CI 0.394–0.937) and in patients < 65 years old (HR = 0.523, 95% CI 0.378–0.723; Fig. 2a, 1b) [17]. In patients ≥ 65 years of age, median PFS was 18.4 months in the placebo + letrozole group vs 13.0 months in patients < 65 years old. Median PFS was not reached in the subsets of patients aged ≥ 65 years and < 65 years in the ribociclib + letrozole group. In patients ≥ 65 years of age, the overall response rate (ORR) in the ribociclib group vs placebo group was 37% vs 31%, compared with 44% vs 25% in patients < 65 years of age.

The safety profile of ribociclib + letrozole in patients ≥ 65 years old was similar to that observed in patients < 65 years old and was consistent with the safety profile of the full population (Table 1) [17]. Grade 3/4 AEs in ≥ 20% of patients in either arm (ribociclib vs placebo) were

neutropenia (≥ 65 years, 60% vs 0%; < 65 years, 59% vs 2%) and leukopenia (≥ 65 years, 21% vs 1%; < 65 years, 21% vs 1%); grade 3/4 liver enzyme elevation was reported in 9% vs 2% of patients ≥ 65 years of age and 10% vs 3% of patients < 65 years of age. Treatment discontinuation due to AEs in the ribociclib + letrozole group occurred in 13% and 12% of patients ≥ 65 and < 65 years, respectively. Dose interruptions due to AEs in the ribociclib group occurred in 71% of patients aged ≥ 65 years and in 66% of patients aged < 65 years. Dose reductions due to AEs in the ribociclib + letrozole group occurred in 53% and 49% of patients ≥ 65 and < 65 years, respectively. Neutropenia was the most common AE that led to dose interruptions or reductions in either group. The dose intensity of ribociclib was 86% in patients ≥ 65 years of age and 90% in patients < 65 years of age. In the ribociclib group, 1 patient aged ≥ 65 years experienced grade 3 prolonged QTcF (> 500 ms). Robust PFS data and a low rate of dose reductions and discontinuations suggest that ribociclib + letrozole is an effective first-line treatment option regardless of age.

Visceral disease
In MONALEESA-2, 393 patients (59%) had visceral metastases (including liver, lung, and/or other metastatic sites) (Burris HA et al. First-line ribociclib + letrozole in patients with HR⁺/HER2⁻ advanced breast cancer presenting with visceral metastases or bone-only disease: a subgroup analysis of the MONALEESA-2 trial. Poster presented at San Antonio Breast Cancer Symposium, San Antonio, TX, USA; 6–10 December 2016). The primary reason for treatment discontinuation in both patient subgroups was disease progression in 28% vs 47% of patients with visceral disease (ribociclib vs placebo group). Treatment benefit with ribociclib + letrozole was observed in patients with visceral metastases (Burris HA et al. First-line ribociclib + letrozole in patients with HR⁺/HER2⁻ advanced breast cancer presenting with visceral metastases or bone-only disease: a subgroup analysis of the MONALEESA-2 trial. Poster presented at San Antonio Breast Cancer Symposium, San Antonio, TX, USA; 6–10 December 2016) (Fig. 2c). Median PFS was not reached (95% CI 19.3 to not reached) in the ribociclib group and was 13.0 months (95% CI 12.6–16.5) in the placebo group (HR = 0.535; 95% CI 0.385–0.742). In patients with ≥ 3 metastases (high disease burden; Fig. 2d), comparable results were observed (Verma S et al. Ribociclib + letrozole vs placebo + letrozole in postmenopausal women with HR⁺/HER2⁻ advanced breast cancer and a high disease burden. Poster presented at the IMPAKT Breast Cancer Conference, Brussels, Belgium; May 4–6 May 2017). Median PFS was 19.3 months (95% CI 17.1 to not reached) in the ribociclib + letrozole group vs 12.8 months (95% CI 9.8–16.5) in the

Table 1 MONALEESA-2 safety profile: all-grade adverse events across studies (≥ 30% of patients in any group)

AE, n (%)	Age <65 years (n = 370) [17]		Age ≥ 65 years[a] (n = 294) [17]		Visceral metastases (n = 393) (Burris et al., 2016)		Bone-only disease (n = 146) (Burris et al., 2016)		De novo disease (n = 226) [21]		Prior CT (n = 289) (Conte et al., 2017)		No prior CT (n = 375) (Conte et al., 2017)		Prior ET (n = 344) (Conte et al., 2017)		No prior ET (n = 320) (Conte et al., 2017)	
	Ribo + L (n = 184)	Pbo + L (n = 186)[b]	Ribo + L (n = 150)	Pbo + L (n = 144)[b]	Ribo + L (n = 197)	Pbo + L (n = 196)	Ribo + L (n = 69)	Pbo + L (n = 77)	Ribo + L (n = 114)	Pbo + L (n = 112)[c]	Ribo + L (n = 146)	Pbo + L (n = 143)	Ribo + L (n = 188)	Pbo + L (n = 187)	Ribo + L (n = 175)	Pbo + L (n = 169)	Ribo + L (n = 159)	Pbo + L (n = 161)
Neutropenia[d]	137 (75)	10 (5)	111 (74)	7 (5)	156 (79.2)	10 (5.1)	44 (63.8)	4 (5.2)	80 (70)	5 (4)	115 (79)	8 (6)	133 (71)	9 (5)	137 (78)	11 (7)	111 (70)	6 (4)
Nausea	92 (50)	52 (28)	80 (53)	42 (29)	111 (56.3)	54 (27.6)	32 (46.4)	23 (29.9)	55 (48)	29 (26)	79 (54)	42 (29)	93 (50)	52 (28)	97 (55)	41 (24)	75 (47)	53 (33)
Fatigue	67 (36)	64 (34)	55 (37)	35 (24)	71 (36.0)	62 (31.6)	27 (39.1)	21 (27.3)	48 (42)	30 (27)	43 (30)	48 (34)	79 (42)	51 (27)	56 (32)	48 (28)	66 (42)	51 (32)
Leukopenia[e]	64 (35)	8 (4)	46 (31)	5 (4)	70 (35.5)	9 (4.6)	21 (30.4)	2 (2.6)	36 (32)	0	53 (36)	9 (6)	57 (30)	4 (2)	65 (37)	11 (7)	–	–
Alopecia	62 (34)	26 (14)	49 (33)	25 (17)	62 (31.5)	31 (15.8)	31 (44.9)	7 (9.1)	45 (39)	17 (15)	46 (32)	24 (17)	65 (35)	27 (14)	52 (30)	25 (15)	59 (37)	26 (16)
Diarrhea	56 (30)	36 (19)	61 (41)	37 (26)	66 (33.5)	40 (20.4)	28 (40.6)	22 (28.6)	32 (28)	24 (21)	48 (33)	27 (19)	69 (37)	46 (25)	70 (40)	31 (18)	47 (30)	42 (26)
Arthralgia	54 (29)	55 (30)	37 (25)	40 (28)	–	–	17 (24.6)	24 (31.2)	25 (22)	37 (33)	–	–	50 (27)	61 (33)	–	–	41 (26)	55 (34)
Vomiting	45 (29)	24 (13)	53 (35)	27 (19)	–	–	–	–	29 (25)	17 (15)	49 (34)	24 (17)	–	–	58 (33)	24 (14)	–	–

AE adverse event, *CT* chemotherapy, *ET* endocrine therapy, *L* letrozole, *Pbo* placebo, *Ribo* ribociclib

[a]Additional AEs (≥ 15% in either group) in patients ≥ 65 years of age (ribociclib group vs placebo group): anemia (26% vs 6%), constipation (25% vs 16%), decreased appetite (23% vs 17%), cough (19% vs 19%), peripheral edema (19% vs 12%), hypertension (19% vs 19%), rash (19% vs 19%), urinary tract infection (19% vs 10%), headache (18% vs 15%), liver enzyme elevation (17% vs 6%), asthenia (17% vs15%), back pain (15% vs 21%), and hot flush (15% vs 19%)

[b]Four patients in the Pbo + L group did not receive study treatment

[c]One patient in the Pbo + L arm was randomized but did not receive study treatment

[d]Neutropenia also includes "neutrophil count decreased" and "granulocytopenia"

[e]Leukopenia also includes "white blood cell count decreased"

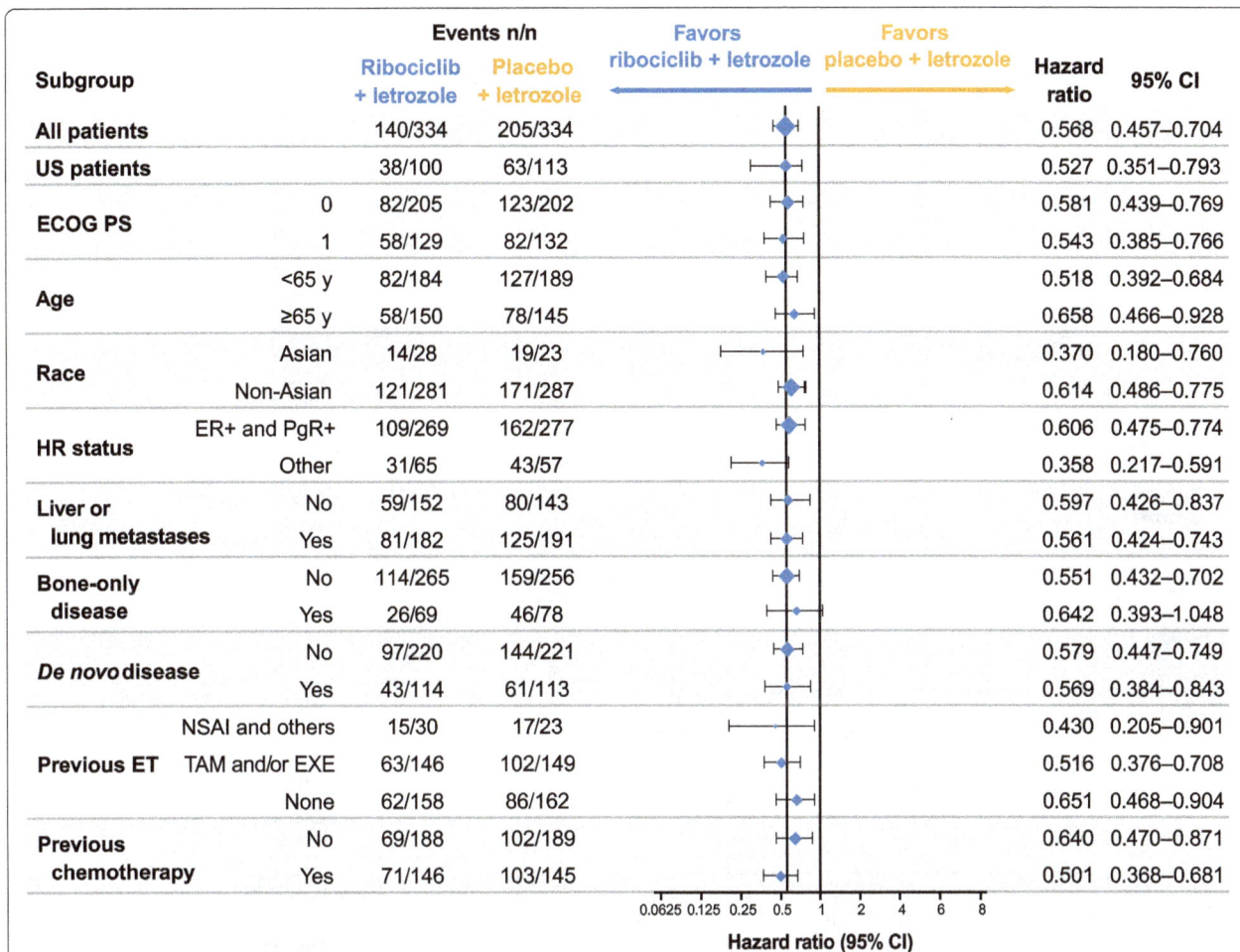

Subgroup		Events n/n Ribociclib + letrozole	Events n/n Placebo + letrozole	Favors ribociclib + letrozole / Favors placebo + letrozole	Hazard ratio	95% CI
All patients		140/334	205/334		0.568	0.457–0.704
US patients		38/100	63/113		0.527	0.351–0.793
ECOG PS	0	82/205	123/202		0.581	0.439–0.769
	1	58/129	82/132		0.543	0.385–0.766
Age	<65 y	82/184	127/189		0.518	0.392–0.684
	≥65 y	58/150	78/145		0.658	0.466–0.928
Race	Asian	14/28	19/23		0.370	0.180–0.760
	Non-Asian	121/281	171/287		0.614	0.486–0.775
HR status	ER+ and PgR+	109/269	162/277		0.606	0.475–0.774
	Other	31/65	43/57		0.358	0.217–0.591
Liver or lung metastases	No	59/152	80/143		0.597	0.426–0.837
	Yes	81/182	125/191		0.561	0.424–0.743
Bone-only disease	No	114/265	159/256		0.551	0.432–0.702
	Yes	26/69	46/78		0.642	0.393–1.048
De novo disease	No	97/220	144/221		0.579	0.447–0.749
	Yes	43/114	61/113		0.569	0.384–0.843
Previous ET	NSAI and others	15/30	17/23		0.430	0.205–0.901
	TAM and/or EXE	63/146	102/149		0.516	0.376–0.708
	None	62/158	86/162		0.651	0.468–0.904
Previous chemotherapy	No	69/188	102/189		0.640	0.470–0.871
	Yes	71/146	103/145		0.501	0.368–0.681

Hazard ratio (95% CI)
0.0625 0.125 0.25 0.5 1 2 4 6 8

Fig. 1 MONALEESA-2 subgroup analysis of locally assessed PFS. Data cut-off, 2 January 2017 (Hortobagyi GN et al. Updated results from MONALEESA-2, a Phase III trial of first-line ribociclib + letrozole in hormone receptor-positive, HER2-negative advanced breast cancer. Poster presented at the American Society of Clinical Oncology Annual Meeting, Chicago, IL, USA; 2–6 June 2017). CI confidence interval, ECOG PS Eastern Cooperative Oncology Group performance status, ER estrogen receptor, ET endocrine therapy, EXE exemestane, HR hormone receptor, NSAI nonsteroidal aromatase inhibitor, PFS progression-free survival, PgR progesterone receptor, TAM tamoxifen

placebo + letrozole group (HR = 0.456; 95% CI 0.298–0.700). The 12-month PFS rate was 71.5% in the ribociclib + letrozole group vs 53.5% in the placebo + letrozole group. An analysis of best overall response (BOR) per RECIST v1.1 showed that 45% of patients in the ribociclib + letrozole group vs 35% in the placebo + letrozole group had a BOR of complete or partial response.

Ribociclib + letrozole treatment in patients with visceral metastases exhibited a similar safety profile to that observed in the full population, irrespective of disease burden (Burris HA et al. First-line ribociclib + letrozole in patients with HR+/HER2− advanced breast cancer presenting with visceral metastases or bone-only disease: a subgroup analysis of the MONALEESA-2 trial. Poster presented at San Antonio Breast Cancer Symposium, San Antonio, TX, USA; 6–10 December 2016; Verma S et al. Ribociclib + letrozole vs placebo + letrozole in postmenopausal women with HR+/HER2− advanced breast cancer

and a high disease burden. Poster presented at the IMPAKT Breast Cancer Conference, Brussels, Belgium; May 4–6 May 2017) (Table 1). In patients with low disease burden, dose interruptions and reductions for ribociclib (in the ribociclib + letrozole group) were required in 153 (77.7%) and 109 (55.3%) patients, respectively; for placebo (in the placebo + letrozole group), dose interruptions and reductions were required in 79 (40.3%) and 12 (6.1%) patients, respectively (Burris HA et al. First-line ribociclib + letrozole in patients with HR+/HER2− advanced breast cancer presenting with visceral metastases or bone-only disease: a subgroup analysis of the MONALEESA-2 trial. Poster presented at San Antonio Breast Cancer Symposium, San Antonio, TX, USA; 6–10 December 2016). Treatment discontinuations were reported in 83 patients (42%) in the ribociclib group, and 111 patients (57%) in the placebo group, of which 8% in the ribociclib group and 2% in the placebo group were related to AEs. The most

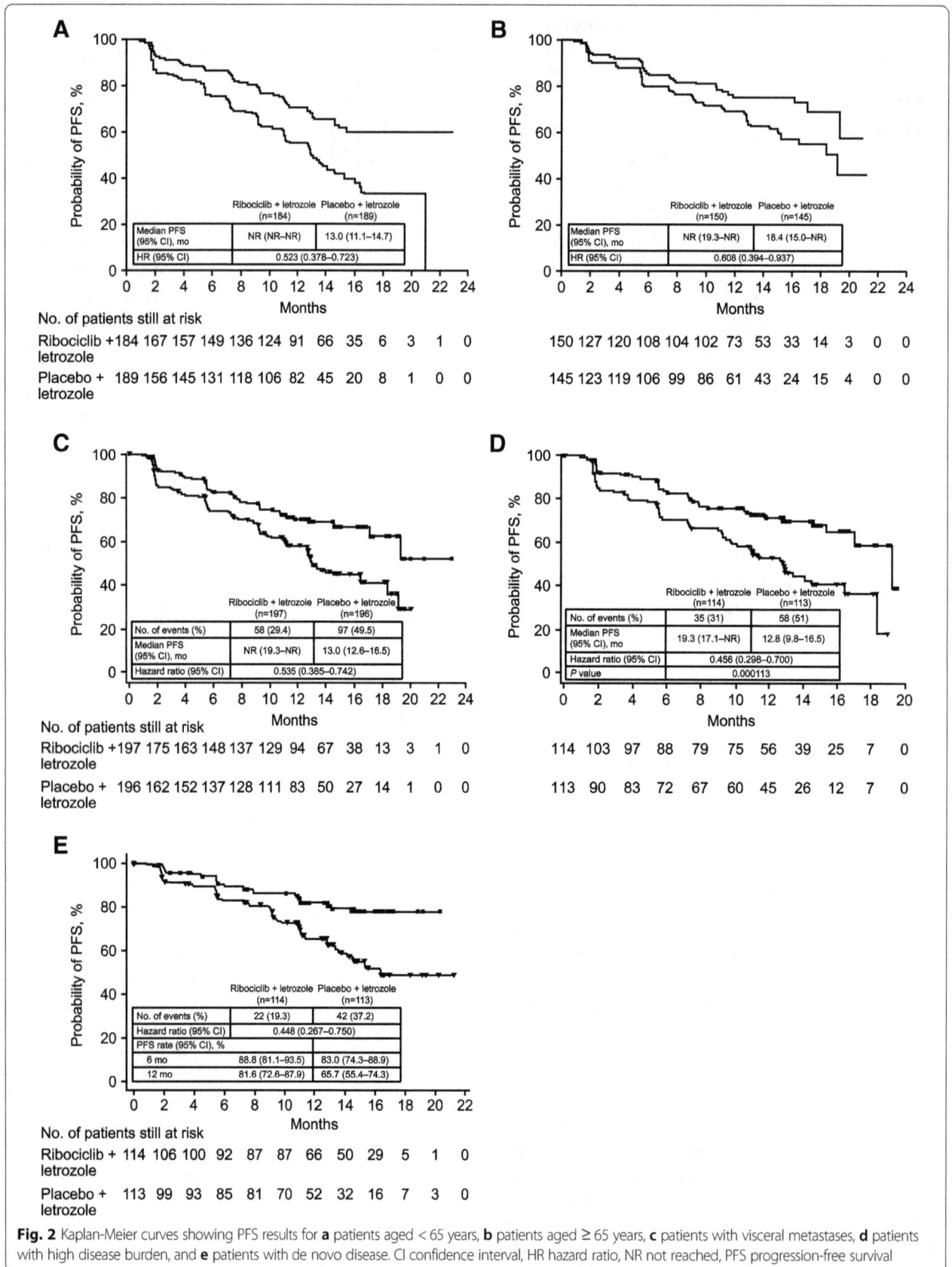

Fig. 2 Kaplan-Meier curves showing PFS results for **a** patients aged < 65 years, **b** patients aged ≥ 65 years, **c** patients with visceral metastases, **d** patients with high disease burden, and **e** patients with de novo disease. CI confidence interval, HR hazard ratio, NR not reached, PFS progression-free survival

common AEs leading to discontinuation in the ribociclib group were elevated alanine transaminase (ALT; 4.6%), vomiting (4.1%), elevated aspartate transaminase (AST; 2.5%), and nausea (1.5%). In the high-disease burden subgroup, AEs were the cause of ribociclib dose reductions in 50% of patients (vs 4% with placebo) and were the cause of dose interruptions in 74% and 11% of patients in the ribociclib group and placebo group, respectively (Verma S et al. Ribociclib + letrozole vs placebo + letrozole in postmenopausal women with HR$^+$/HER2$^-$ advanced breast cancer and a high disease burden. Poster presented at the IMPAKT Breast Cancer Conference, Brussels, Belgium; May 4–6 May 2017). Common AEs in the visceral metastases subset are shown in Table 1. Neutropenia and leukopenia were the most common grade 3/4 AEs irrespective of disease burden. This subanalysis highlights that ribociclib + letrozole can provide significant clinical benefit for patients with visceral metastases.

Bone-only disease

Breast cancer may adversely affect the bone health of patients. It is estimated that breast cancer metastasized to the bone in approximately 65% to 85% of patients during the disease course [18, 19]. Bone also represents the first site of metastasis for 26% to 50% of patients with metastatic breast cancer [19], and approximately 70% of patients with advanced or metastatic breast cancer exhibit metastatic bone disease [20]. In the MONALEESA-2 study, results from the bone-only disease subset (ribociclib group, $n = 69$; placebo group, $n = 78$) were similar to those in the overall population (Burris HA et al. First-line ribociclib + letrozole in patients with HR$^+$/HER2$^-$ advanced breast cancer presenting with visceral metastases or bone-only disease: a subgroup analysis of the MONALEESA-2 trial. Poster presented at San Antonio Breast Cancer Symposium, San Antonio, TX, USA; 6–10 December 2016). The number of PFS events was 18 vs 32 in the ribociclib + letrozole group vs the placebo + letrozole group. The median PFS in patients with bone-only disease was not reached vs 15.3 months in the ribociclib + letrozole group vs placebo + letrozole group, respectively (HR = 0.690; 95% CI 0.381–1.249). A BOR of complete or partial response was observed in 10% of patients in the ribociclib + letrozole group and 4% in the placebo + letrozole group.

Ribociclib + letrozole in patients with bone-only disease had a safety profile consistent with that observed in the full population (Burris HA et al. First-line ribociclib + letrozole in patients with HR$^+$/HER2$^-$ advanced breast cancer presenting with visceral metastases or bone-only disease: a subgroup analysis of the MONALEESA-2 trial. Poster presented at San Antonio Breast Cancer Symposium, San Antonio, TX, USA; 6–10 December 2016) (Table 1). The most frequent grade 3/4 AEs in the ribociclib + letrozole group ($\geq 20\%$ of

patients) were neutropenia and leukopenia. Discontinuations due to AEs in the ribociclib + letrozole group were reported in one patient for each of the following AEs: elevated ALT, elevated AST, hepatocellular injury, hepatotoxicity, joint stiffness, depression, and interstitial lung disease. Dose interruptions and reductions were required in the ribociclib + letrozole group in 54 (78.3%) and 35 (50.7%) patients and in the placebo + letrozole group in 30 (39.0%) and 3 (3.9%) patients, respectively. Results from MONALEESA-2 suggest that combination therapy with ribociclib and letrozole may help reduce disease progression in the bone; however, these observations are in a small sample size and need further confirmation in larger subgroups.

De novo disease

Patients are classified as having de novo advanced breast cancer if they present with advanced breast cancer but have not been previously diagnosed with an earlier stage of breast cancer, nor have they received prior therapy and relapsed. The benefit of ribociclib + letrozole treatment was maintained in 227 patients (34%) who had de novo advanced breast cancer in the MONALEESA-2 study [21]. Treatment was discontinued in 30% vs 43% of patients with de novo advanced breast cancer in the ribociclib vs placebo groups. In patients with de novo advanced breast cancer, the median relative dose intensity for placebo + letrozole was 100%; the relative dose intensity of ribociclib + letrozole was maintained at 88% despite dose adjustments.

Progression-free survival was prolonged in patients with de novo advanced breast cancer in the ribociclib group vs the placebo group (HR = 0.45; 95% CI 0.27–0.75) (Fig. 2e). Median PFS was not reached in the ribociclib group vs 16.4 months in the placebo group. The 12-month PFS rate in patients with de novo advanced breast cancer was 82% in the ribociclib group vs 66% in the placebo group. In all patients with de novo advanced breast cancer, the ORR (ribociclib vs placebo) was 47% vs 34% and the CBR was 83% vs 77%. Among patients with de novo advanced breast cancer who had measurable disease at baseline, the ORR (ribociclib vs placebo) was 56% vs 45% and the CBR was 82% vs 77% [21].

Ribociclib + letrozole in patients with de novo advanced breast cancer had a similar safety profile to that observed in the full population (Table 1) [21]. The most common grade 3/4 AEs ($\geq 20\%$ of patients with de novo advanced breast cancer; ribociclib vs placebo) were neutropenia (55% vs 1%) and leukopenia (21% vs 0); grade 3/4 elevated AST occurred in 6% of patients in the ribociclib group and none in the placebo group. The incidence of elevated ALT events was not reported. Adverse events caused dose reductions in 48% and 5% of patients and caused dose interruptions in 66% and 15% of patients in the ribociclib and placebo treatment groups, respectively. Neutropenia was the most frequent AE leading to dose interruption or reduction (49% of patients in the ribociclib group). Data from MONALEESA-2 suggest that ribociclib provides substantial clinical benefit in the de novo subset, with a safety profile similar to that of the overall population.

Prior therapy

It is estimated that approximately 20% to 40% of patients who present with nonmetastatic breast cancer at initial diagnosis will eventually relapse and receive subsequent treatment for recurrent disease [22]. However, the effect of prior (neo)adjuvant treatment on the response to subsequent therapy is unknown [23, 24]. In MONALEESA-2, 220 patients (66%) in the ribociclib + letrozole group and 221 patients (66%) in the placebo + letrozole group had recurrent breast cancer. Overall, a PFS benefit of ribociclib + letrozole vs placebo + letrozole was observed among patients with recurrent breast cancer (HR = 0.60; 95% CI 0.45–0.81) [8]. Furthermore, in an analysis conducted in the updated dataset (data cut-off, 2 January 2017), the PFS benefit of ribociclib treatment was maintained irrespective of the treatment-free interval (TFI) duration (Blackwell KL et al. Subsequent treatment for postmenopausal women with hormone receptor-positive, HER2-negative advanced breast cancer who received ribociclib + letrozole vs placebo + letrozole in the Phase III MONALEESA-2 study. Poster presented at the San Antonio Breast Cancer Symposium, San Antonio, TX, USA; 5–9 December 2017). Ribociclib + letrozole improved PFS vs placebo + letrozole in patients with TFI ≤ 24 months (ribociclib, $n = 64$; placebo, $n = 72$; HR = 0.455; 95% CI 0.296–0.701) and TFI > 24 months (ribociclib, $n = 85$; placebo, $n = 77$; HR = 0.455; 95% CI 0.287–0.720). In patients with TFI ≤ 36 months (ribociclib, $n = 84$; placebo, $n = 86$) and TFI > 36 months (ribociclib, $n = 65$; placebo, $n = 63$), HR (95% CI) was 0.422 (0.284–0.627) and 0.507 (0.303–0.851), respectively. In patients with TFI ≤ 48 months (ribociclib, $n = 95$; placebo, $n = 100$) and TFI > 48 months (ribociclib, $n = 54$; placebo, $n = 49$), HR (95% CI) was 0.449 (0.310–0.650) and 0.496 (0.274–0.898), respectively.

Progression-free survival was also analyzed according to the type of prior therapy received in the (neo)adjuvant settings (interim PFS cut-off). In the ribociclib group, 146 patients (44%) had prior (neo)adjuvant chemotherapy and 175 patients (52%) had prior (neo)adjuvant ET (Conte P et al. First-line ribociclib + letrozole in patients with HR$^+$/HER2$^-$ advanced breast cancer who received prior (neo)adjuvant therapy: a subgroup analysis of the MONALEESA-2 trial. Poster presented at the St. Gallen International Breast Cancer Conference, Vienna, Austria; 15–18 March 2017). In the placebo group, 145 (43%) and 171 (51%) patients had prior (neo)adjuvant chemotherapy and (neo)adjuvant ET, respectively. There were 74 patients (37 in each

treatment group) who had received a short duration (≤ 14 days) of letrozole or anastrozole for advanced breast cancer prior to enrollment; 36 of these patients had also received prior (neo)adjuvant ET (ribociclib group, $n = 19$; placebo, $n = 17$). Ribociclib significantly increased PFS vs placebo in patients who had received prior (neo)adjuvant chemotherapy (HR = 0.548; 95% CI 0.384–0.780) or ET (HR = 0.538; 95% CI 0.384–0.754) and in patients without prior (neo)adjuvant chemotherapy (HR = 0.548; 95% CI 0.373–0.806) or ET (HR = 0.570; 95% CI 0.380–0.854) (Conte P et al. First-line ribociclib + letrozole in patients with HR$^+$/HER2$^-$ advanced breast cancer who received prior (neo)adjuvant therapy: a subgroup analysis of the MONALEESA-2 trial. Poster presented at the St. Gallen International Breast Cancer Conference, Vienna, Austria; 15–18 March 2017) (Figs. 3a, b). In patients with prior (neo)adjuvant chemotherapy or ET, median PFS (ribociclib vs placebo) was 19.3 months vs 13.0 months for each of these subgroups. For patients who had not received prior (neo)adjuvant chemotherapy or ET, the median PFS was not reached in the ribociclib group and was 19.2 months for the placebo subgroups. Prior therapy did not appear to influence the response to ribociclib and letrozole based on similarities in HRs of patients with and without previous exposure to the treatment regimen. In patients with prior (neo)adjuvant chemotherapy, the ORR was 38% in the ribociclib group vs 24% in the placebo group; the ORR was 43% and 30% in the ribociclib and placebo group, respectively, in patients with no prior (neo)adjuvant chemotherapy. In patients with prior (neo)adjuvant ET, the ORR was 38% in the ribociclib group and 26% in the placebo group; the ORR was 43% and 29% in the ribociclib and placebo group, respectively, in patients with no prior (neo)adjuvant ET.

The safety profile of ribociclib was consistent with that of other subgroups (Conte P et al. First-line ribociclib + letrozole in patients with HR$^+$/HER2$^-$ advanced breast cancer who received prior (neo)adjuvant therapy: a subgroup analysis of the MONALEESA-2 trial. Poster presented at the St. Gallen International Breast Cancer Conference, Vienna, Austria; 15–18 March 2017). Dose discontinuations caused by adverse events occurred in 4% and 2% of patients in the ribociclib or placebo group, respectively, who had received prior chemotherapy and 10% and 2% of patients who did not receive prior chemotherapy. Adverse events led to treatment discontinuation in 9% vs 2% of patients with prior ET and 6% vs 3% of patients without prior ET in the ribociclib group vs the placebo group, respectively. Overall, findings from the patient subset with prior therapy suggest that ribociclib is equally effective in patients who received prior therapy for advanced breast cancer and in those who did not. The findings also provide further support for first-line therapy with ribociclib in combination with letrozole for disease recurrence during or after chemotherapy or ET.

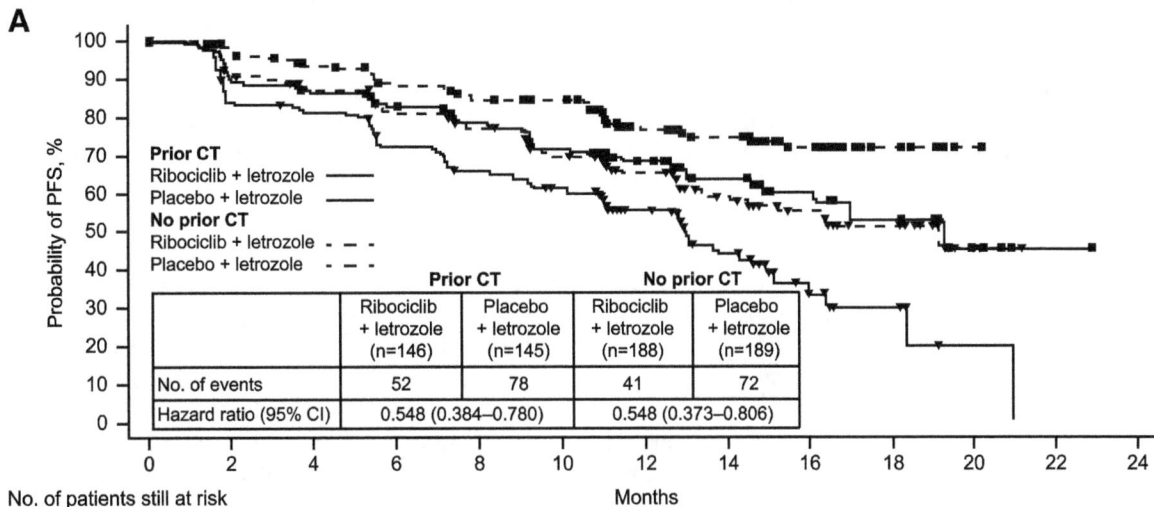

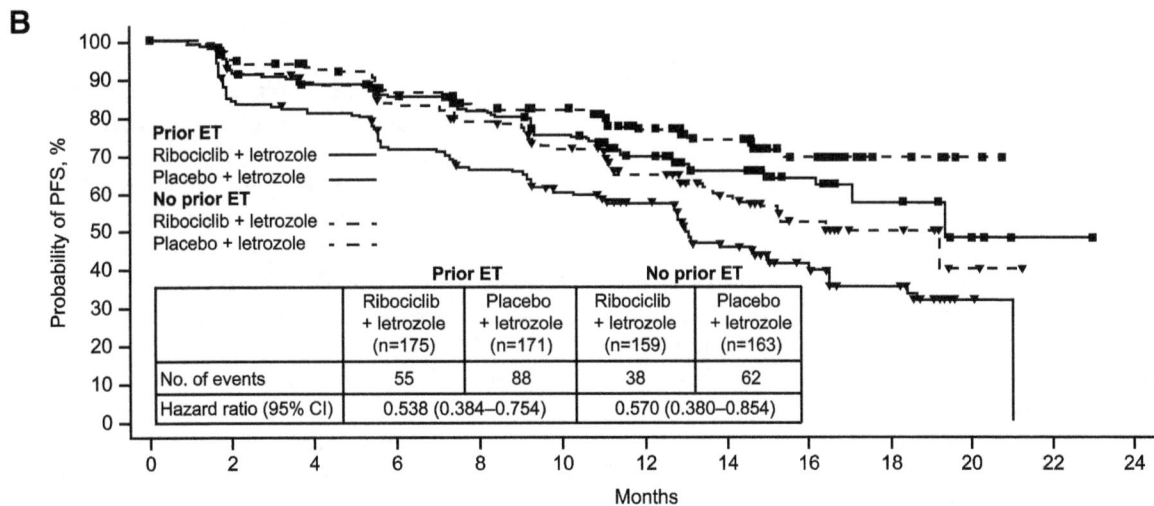

Fig. 3 Kaplan-Meier curves showing PFS results for **a** patients with or without prior CT, and **b** patients with or without prior ET in MONALEESA-2. CI confidence interval, CT chemotherapy, ET endocrine therapy, HR hazard ratio, NR not reached, PFS progression-free survival

Subgroup analyses in trials of other CDK4/6 inhibitors and fulvestrant

Direct comparisons of efficacy findings across trials should be generally avoided because of differences in study design that may confound interpretation. Limited data are available from trials of the CDK4/6 inhibitors palbociclib and abemaciclib, as well as fulvestrant, in patients with HR$^+$/HER2$^-$ advanced breast cancer. Subgroup analyses of PALOMA-1 showed that palbociclib + letrozole also improved median PFS vs letrozole alone across various subgroups such as elderly patients (patients ≥ 65 years), patients with ductal and lobular carcinoma, and patients with metastasis in bone only or in visceral or other sites [25, 26]. However, the overall sample size of the study was much smaller ($n = 165$) than MONALEESA-2, making the inference of any meaningful comparisons challenging. Data regarding efficacy of the different subsets in PALOMA-2 with palbociclib + letrozole treatment are limited and mostly align with the overall efficacy of the trial [7]. Data from subgroup analyses in MONARCH 3 show clinical benefit of abemaciclib + nonsteroidal aromatase inhibitor in most patient subgroups (Goetz MP et al. The benefit of abemaciclib in prognostic subgroups: an exploratory analysis of combined data from the MONARCH 2 and 3 studies. Oral presentation at San Antonio Breast Cancer Symposium, San Antonio, TX, USA; December 5–9 December 2017). Of note, in these exploratory subgroup analyses no PFS benefit with the addition of abemaciclib was found in patients with TFI ≥ 36 months (HR = 0.833; 95% CI 0.457–1.517); in comparison, patients with a TFI > 36 months in MONALEESA-2 did have a PFS benefit with ribociclib + letrozole (Blackwell KL et al. Subsequent treatment for postmenopausal women with hormone receptor-positive, HER2-negative advanced breast cancer who received ribociclib + letrozole vs placebo + letrozole in the Phase III MONALEESA-2 study. Poster presented at the San Antonio Breast Cancer Symposium, San Antonio, TX, USA; 5–9 December 2017). Although efficacy data obtained with most subsets in the FALCON trial were consistent with the overall population and demonstrated superiority of fulvestrant, no PFS benefit of fulvestrant vs anastrozole was observed in patients with visceral metastases (HR = 0.99; 95% CI 0.74–1.33), and the median PFS was shorter in the fulvestrant group (13.8 months vs 15.9 months; $P = 0.0092$) [12]. Thus, future trial outcomes of ribociclib in combination with fulvestrant will be of interest to deduce whether the combination can alter these results.

Conclusions

The MONALEESA-2 trial demonstrated a clinically meaningful improvement in PFS with ribociclib + letrozole therapy in patients with HR$^+$/HER2$^-$ advanced breast cancer,

and the consistency of the efficacy and safety results was demonstrated across all assessed subgroups. Most of the AEs observed were consistent with the class and were manageable. The incidence of hematologic AEs in the ribociclib + letrozole group was similar across all subgroups. QTc interval prolongation occurred in 3.3% of patients treated at the 600-mg dose of ribociclib, generally within the first 4 weeks of treatment [8]. The study protocol excluded patients at elevated risk for QT interval prolongation; careful monitoring, adequate dose reduction, and dose interruption were implemented as needed [8].

Overall, a retrospective head-to-head comparison of subgroup analyses across trials can be challenging because of differences in trial designs, enrolled patient populations, and unintended patient biases. A key limitation of the MONALEESA-2 trial is the inadequate understanding of the effects of ribociclib over longer periods of time. As the trial is still ongoing, insufficient information currently exists to determine the effect of ribociclib on long-term tolerability and overall survival. Furthermore, based on published literature, there have been fewer clinical trials so far than for palbociclib and, as a consequence, fewer patients have received ribociclib as first-line treatment. However, these shortcomings broadly apply to all the recent advances in first-line therapy of advanced breast cancer.

To address the current limitations and to gain better understanding of the role of ribociclib in different combinations, patient types, and treatment settings, further analysis of the clinical program is required. In the MONALEESA-7 trial (NCT02278120) premenopausal patients were randomized to receive the gonadotropin-releasing hormone agonist goserelin, in combination with a nonsteroidal aromatase inhibitor (letrozole or anastrozole), or tamoxifen, with or without ribociclib, in the first-line setting. The primary endpoint was met, with a median PFS of 23.8 months vs 13.0 months in the ribociclib vs placebo group (HR = 0.553; 95% CI 0.441–0.694; $P = 9.83 \times 10^{-8}$) (Tripathy D et al. First-line ribociclib or placebo combined with goserelin and tamoxifen or a non-steroidal aromatase inhibitor in premenopausal women with hormone receptor-positive, HER2-negative advanced breast cancer: results from the randomized Phase III MONALEESA-7 trial. Oral presentation at San Antonio Breast Cancer Symposium, San Antonio, TX, USA; 5–9 December 2017). In another ongoing phase 3 trial, MONALEESA-3 (NCT02422615), postmenopausal patients with advanced HR$^+$/HER2$^-$ breast cancer are randomized to receive fulvestrant with or without ribociclib in the first- or second-line setting. To expand information on the efficacy and safety of ribociclib, a phase 3b open-label, single-arm, multicenter study, CompLEEment-1, will examine efficacy and safety of ribociclib + letrozole in a larger and broader population than MONALEESA-2 (estimated enrollment = 3000 patients).

Overall, the clinically relevant results obtained from the MONALEESA-2 trial suggest that ribociclib in combination with other aromatase inhibitors such as letrozole can be successfully used in the treatment of advanced HR$^+$/HER2$^-$ breast cancer in a broad population.

Abbreviations

AE: Adverse event; AKT: Protein kinase B; ALT: Alanine transaminase; AST: Aspartate aminotransferase; BOR: Best overall response; CBR: Clinical benefit rate; CDK: Cyclin-dependent kinase; CI: Confidence interval; ECOG: Eastern Cooperative Oncology Group; ET: Endocrine therapy; FDA: Food and Drug Administration; HER2$^-$: Human epidermal growth factor receptor 2-negative; HR$^+$: Hormone receptor-positive; HR: Hazard ratio; mTOR: Mammalian target of rapamycin; ORR: Overall response rate; PFS: Progression-free survival; PI3K: Phosphatidylinositol-3-kinase; QTcF: Corrected QT interval (Fridericia's formula); TFI: Treatment-free interval

Acknowledgements

Medical writing and editorial assistance were provided under the direction of the author by Rajni Parthasarathy, PhD, and David Boffa, ELS, at MedThink SciCom and funded by Novartis Pharmaceuticals.

Funding

The study reviewed in this article was supported by Novartis Pharmaceuticals.

Authors' contributions

GNH contributed to the design of this review article, reviewed and revised it critically for important intellectual content, and approved the final version to be published.

Competing interests

GNH reports receiving personal fees from Novartis during the conduct of the study, and personal fees from Peregrine Pharmaceuticals, personal fees from Lilly, personal fees from Roche, and personal fees from Agendia outside of the submitted work.

References

1. Siegel RL, Miller KD, Jemal A. Cancer statistics, 2017. CA Cancer J Clin. 2017;67:7–30.
2. Referenced with permission from the NCCN Clinical Practice Guidelines in Oncology (NCCN Guidelines®) for Breast Cancer V.2.2016. © National Comprehensive Cancer Network, Inc. 2016. All rights reserved. Accessed 23 June 23, 2017. To view the most recent and complete version of the guidelines, go online to NCCN.org.
3. Reinert T, Barrios CH. Optimal management of hormone receptor positive metastatic breast cancer in 2016. Ther Adv Med Oncol. 2015;7:304–20.
4. Murphy CG, Dickler MN. Endocrine resistance in hormone-responsive breast cancer: mechanisms and therapeutic strategies. Endocr Relat Cancer. 2016; 23:R337–52.
5. Reinert T, Barrios CH. Definition of first-line endocrine therapy for hormone receptor-positive advanced breast cancer. J Clin Oncol. 2016;34:1959–60.
6. Yamamoto-Ibusuki M, Arnedos M, Andre F. Targeted therapies for ER +/HER2- metastatic breast cancer. BMC Med. 2015;13:137.
7. Finn RS, Martin M, Rugo HS, Jones S, Im SA, Gelmon K, et al. Palbociclib and letrozole in advanced breast cancer. N Engl J Med. 2016;375:1925–36.
8. Hortobagyi GN, Stemmer SM, Burris HA, Yap YS, Sonke GS, Paluch-Shimon S, et al. Ribociclib as first-line therapy for HR-positive, advanced breast cancer. N Engl J Med. 2016;375:1738–48.
9. Goetz MP, Toi M, Campone M, Sohn J, Paluch-Shimon S, Huober J, et al. MONARCH 3: abemaciclib as initial therapy for advanced breast cancer. J Clin Oncol. 2017;35:3638–46.
10. Kisqali [package insert]. East Hanover: Novartis Pharmaceuticals Corporation; 2017.
11. Finn RS, Crown JP, Lang I, Boer K, Bondarenko IM, Kulyk SO, et al. The cyclin-dependent kinase 4/6 inhibitor palbociclib in combination with letrozole versus letrozole alone as first-line treatment of oestrogen receptor-positive, HER2-negative, advanced breast cancer (PALOMA-1/TRIO-18): a randomised phase 2 study. Lancet Oncol. 2015;16:25–35.
12. Robertson JF, Bondarenko IM, Trishkina E, Dvorkin M, Panasci L, Manikhas A, et al. Fulvestrant 500 mg versus anastrozole 1 mg for hormone receptor-positive advanced breast cancer (FALCON): an international, randomised, double-blind, phase 3 trial. Lancet. 2016;388:2997–3005.
13. Howlader N, Noone AM, Krapcho M, Miller D, Bishop K, Kosary CL, et al, editors. SEER cancer statistics review, 1975-2014. National Cancer Institute. Updated Apr 2017. https://seer.cancer.gov/archive/csr/1975_2014/. Accessed 1 Feb 2018.
14. Molecular mechanisms of resistance and sensitivity to palbociclib re-challenge in ER+ mBC (BioPER). https://www.clinicaltrials.gov/ct2/show/NCT03184090. Accessed 22 May 2018.
15. Beadle BM, Woodward WA, Buchholz TA. The impact of age on outcome in early-stage breast cancer. Semin Radiat Oncol. 2011;21:26–34.
16. Bernardi D, Errante D, Gallligioni E, Crivellari D, Bianco A, Salvagno L, et al. Treatment of breast cancer in older women. Acta Oncol. 2008;47:187–98.
17. Sonke GS, Hart LL, Campone M, Erdkamp F, Janni W, Verma S, et al. Ribociclib with letrozole vs letrozole alone in elderly patients with hormone receptor-positive, HER2-negative breast cancer in the randomized MONALEESA-2 trial. Breat Cancer Res Treat. 2018;167:659–69.
18. Bendre M, Gaddy D, Nicholas RW, Suva LJ. Breast cancer metastasis to bone: it is not all about PTHrP. Clin Orthop Relat Res. 2003;415(suppl):S39–45.
19. Lipton A, Uzzo R, Amato RJ, Ellis GK, Hakimian B, Roodman GD, et al. The science and practice of bone health in oncology: managing bone loss and metastasis in patients with solid tumors. J Natl Compr Cancer Netw. 2009; 7(suppl 7):S1–29.
20. Coleman RE. Clinical features of metastatic bone disease and risk of skeletal morbidity. Clin Cancer Res. 2006;12:6243s–9s.
21. O'Shaughnessy J, Petrakova K, Sonke GS, Conte P, Arteaga CL, Cameron DA, et al. Ribociclib plus letrozole versus letrozole alone in patients with de novo HR+, HER2- advanced breast cancer in the randomized MONALEESA-2 trial. Breast Cancer Res Treat. 2018;168:127–34.
22. Zhang XH, Giuliano M, Trivedi MV, Schiff R, Osborne CK. Metastasis dormancy in estrogen receptor-positive breast cancer. Clin Cancer Res. 2013;19:6389–97.
23. Cardoso F, Costa A, Norton L, Senkus E, Aapro M, Andre F, et al. ESO-ESMO 2nd International Consensus guidelines for advanced breast cancer (ABC2). Ann Oncol. 2014;25:1871–88.
24. Dawood S, Broglio K, Ensor J, Hortobagyi GN, Giordano SH. Survival differences among women with de novo stage IV and relapsed breast cancer. Ann Oncol. 2010;21:2169–74.
25. Finn RS, Crown JP, Ettl J, Schmidt M, Bondarenko IM, Lang I, et al. Efficacy and safety of palbociclib in combination with letrozole as first-line treatment of ER-positive, HER2-negative, advanced breast cancer: expanded analyses of subgroups from the randomized pivotal trial PALOMA-1/TRIO-18. Breast Cancer Res. 2016;18:67.
26. Finn RS, Dering J, Conklin D, Kalous O, Cohen DJ, Desai AJ, et al. PD 0332991, a selective cyclin D kinase 4/6 inhibitor, preferentially inhibits proliferation of luminal estrogen receptor-positive human breast cancer cell lines in vitro. Breast Cancer Res. 2009;11:R77.

Permissions

The contributors of this book come from diverse backgrounds, making this book a truly international effort. This book will bring forth new frontiers with its revolutionizing research information and detailed analysis of the nascent developments around the world.

We would like to thank all the contributing authors for lending their expertise to make the book truly unique. They have played a crucial role in the development of this book. Without their invaluable contributions this book wouldn't have been possible. They have made vital efforts to compile up to date information on the varied aspects of this subject to make this book a valuable addition to the collection of many professionals and students.

This book was conceptualized with the vision of imparting up-to-date information and advanced data in this field. To ensure the same, a matchless editorial board was set up. Every individual on the board went through rigorous rounds of assessment to prove their worth. After which they invested a large part of their time researching and compiling the most relevant data for our readers.

The editorial board has been involved in producing this book since its inception. They have spent rigorous hours researching and exploring the diverse topics which have resulted in the successful publishing of this book. They have passed on their knowledge of decades through this book. To expedite this challenging task, the publisher supported the team at every step. A small team of assistant editors was also appointed to further simplify the editing procedure and attain best results for the readers.

Apart from the editorial board, the designing team has also invested a significant amount of their time in understanding the subject and creating the most relevant covers. They scrutinized every image to scout for the most suitable representation of the subject and create an appropriate cover for the book.

The publishing team has been an ardent support to the editorial, designing and production team. Their endless efforts to recruit the best for this project, has resulted in the accomplishment of this book. They are a veteran in the field of academics and their pool of knowledge is as vast as their experience in printing. Their expertise and guidance has proved useful at every step. Their uncompromising quality standards have made this book an exceptional effort. Their encouragement from time to time has been an inspiration for everyone.

The publisher and the editorial board hope that this book will prove to be a valuable piece of knowledge for researchers, students, practitioners and scholars across the globe.

Contributors

Bihong T. Chen, Taihao Jin and Ningrong Ye
Department of Diagnostic Radiology, City of Hope National Medical Center, Duarte, CA 91010, USA

Sean K. Sethi
The MRI Institute for Biomedical Research, Magnetic Resonance Innovations, Inc., Detroit, MI, USA

E. Mark Haacke
The MRI Institute for Biomedical Research, Magnetic Resonance Innovations, Inc., Detroit, MI, USA
Department of Biomedical Engineering, Wayne State University, Detroit, MI 48202, USA

Sunita K. Patel
Department of Population Science, City of Hope National Medical Center, Duarte, CA 91010, USA

Richard Yang, Heidi Tan, Vani Katheria, Rachel Morrison and Can-Lan Sun
Center for Cancer and Aging, City of Hope National Medical Center, Duarte, CA 91010, USA

Arti Hurria
Center for Cancer and Aging, City of Hope National Medical Center, Duarte, CA 91010, USA
Department of Medical Oncology, City of Hope National Medical Center, Duarte, CA 91010, USA

Russell C. Rockne
Division of Mathematical Oncology, City of Hope National Medical Center, Duarte, CA 91010, USA

James C. Root and Tim A. Ahles
Neurocognitive Research Lab, Memorial Sloan Kettering Cancer Center, 641 Lexington Avenue, 7th Floor, New York, NY 10022, USA

Andrew J. Saykin
Center for Neuroimaging, Indiana University School of Medicine, 355 West 16th Street, Indianapolis, IN 46202, USA

Andrei I. Holodny
Department of Radiology, Memorial Sloan-Kettering Cancer Center, 641 Lexington Avenue, 7th Floor, New York, NY 10022, USA

Neal Prakash
Division of Neurology, City of Hope National Medical Center, Duarte, CA 91010, USA

Joanne Mortimer, James Waisman, Yuan Yuan, George Somlo and Daneng Li
Department of Medical Oncology, City of Hope National Medical Center, Duarte, CA 91010, USA

Alexey A. Leontovich
Department of Biomedical Statistics and Informatics, Mayo Clinic College of Medicine, 200 First Street SW, Rochester, MN, USA

Mohammad Jalalirad, Jann Sarkaria, Liewei Wang, James N. Ingle, Minetta Liu, Tufia Haddad, Matthew Goetz, Candace Haddox, Mark Schroeder and Ann Tuma
Department of Medical Oncology, Mayo Clinic College of Medicine, 200 First Street SW, Rochester, MN, USA

Antonino B. D'Assoro
Department of Medical Oncology, Mayo Clinic College of Medicine, 200 First Street SW, Rochester, MN, USA
Department of Biochemistry and Molecular Biology, Mayo Clinic College of Medicine, 200 First Street SW, Rochester, MN, USA

Evanthia Galanis
Department of Medical Oncology, Mayo Clinic College of Medicine, 200 First Street SW, Rochester, MN, USA
Department of Molecular Medicine, Mayo Clinic College of Medicine, 200 First Street SW, Rochester, MN, USA

Jeffrey L. Salisbury and Mario W. Gambino
Department of Biochemistry and Molecular Biology, Mayo Clinic College of Medicine, 200 First Street SW, Rochester, MN, USA

Lisa Mills
Department of Molecular Medicine, Mayo Clinic College of Medicine, 200 First Street SW, Rochester, MN, USA

Maria E. Guicciardi
Department of Internal Medicine, Mayo Clinic College of Medicine, 200 First Street SW, Rochester, MN, USA

Luca Zammataro
Department of Obstetrics, Gynecology, and Reproductive Sciences, Yale University School of Medicine, New Haven, CT, USA

Angela Amato and Aldo Di Leonardo
Department of Cellular and Developmental Biology, University of Palermo, Palermo, Italy

James McCubrey
Department of Microbiology and Immunology, Brody School of Medicine, East Carolina University, Greenville, NC, USA

Carol A. Lange
Department of Medicine and Pharmacology, University of Minnesota, Minneapolis, MN, USA

Judy Boughey
Department of Surgery, Mayo Clinic College of Medicine, 200 First Street SW, Rochester, MN, USA

Johan Staaf and Mårten Fernö
Faculty of Medicine, Department of Clinical Sciences Lund, Oncology and Pathology, Lund University, Lund, Sweden

Martin Sjöström and Per Malmström
Faculty of Medicine, Department of Clinical Sciences Lund, Oncology and Pathology, Lund University, Lund, Sweden
Department of Haematology, Oncology and Radiation Physics, Skåne University Hospital, Lund, Sweden

Emma Niméus
Faculty of Medicine, Department of Clinical Sciences Lund, Oncology and Pathology, Lund University, Lund, Sweden
Faculty of Medicine, Department of Clinical Sciences Lund, Surgery, Lund University, Lund, Sweden
Department of Surgery, Skåne University Hospital, Lund, Sweden

Patrik Edén
Department of Theoretical Physics and Computational Biology, Lund University, Lund, Sweden

Fredrik Wärnberg
Department of Surgical Sciences, Uppsala University, Uppsala, Sweden

Jonas Bergh
Department of Oncology and Pathology, Cancer Center Karolinska, Karolinska Institutet, Stockholm, Sweden
Department of Oncology, Karolinska University Hospital, Radiumhemmet, Stockholm, Sweden

Irma Fredriksson
Department of Molecular Medicine and Surgery, Karolinska Institutet, Stockholm, Sweden
Department of Breast- and Endocrine Surgery, Karolinska University Hospital, Stockholm, Sweden

Colleen Chute, Xinhai Yang, Kristy Meyer, Ning Yang and Keelin O'Neil
Department of Pathology and Laboratory Medicine, University of Wisconsin-Madison, 6051 WIMR, MC-2275, 1111 Highland Avenue, Madison, WI 53705, USA

Andreas Friedl
Department of Pathology and Laboratory Medicine, University of Wisconsin-Madison, 6051 WIMR, MC-2275, 1111 Highland Avenue, Madison, WI 53705, USA
Pathology and Laboratory Medicine Service, William S. Middleton Memorial Veterans Hospital, Department of Veterans Affairs Medical Center, Madison, WI, USA
University of Wisconsin Carbone Cancer Center, Madison, WI, USA

Kevin Eliceiri
University of Wisconsin Carbone Cancer Center, Madison, WI, USA
Laboratory for Optical and Computational Instrumentation, University of Wisconsin-Madison, Madison, WI, USA
Morgridge Institute for Research, University of Wisconsin-Madison, Madison, WI, USA

Caroline Alexander
University of Wisconsin Carbone Cancer Center, Madison, WI, USA
Department of Oncology, University of Wisconsin-Madison, Madison, WI, USA

Ildiko Kasza
Department of Oncology, University of Wisconsin-Madison, Madison, WI, USA

Marta Smeda, Mateusz G. Adamski, Bartosz Proniewski, Magdalena Sternak, Tasnim Mohaissen, Kamil Przyborowski, Katarzyna Derszniak, Dawid Kaczor, Marta Stojak, Elzbieta Buczek and Agnieszka Jasztal
Jagiellonian Centre for Experimental Therapeutics (JCET), Jagiellonian University, Bobrzynskiego 14 St., 30-348 Krakow, Poland

Anna Kieronska and Stefan Chlopicki
Jagiellonian Centre for Experimental Therapeutics (JCET), Jagiellonian University, Bobrzynskiego 14 St., 30-348 Krakow, Poland
Department of Pharmacology, Jagiellonian University, Medical College, Grzegorzecka 16, 31-531 Krakow, Poland

Joanna Wietrzyk
Department of Experimental Oncology, Hirszfeld Institute of Immunology and Experimental Therapy, Polish Academy of Sciences, Rudolfa Weigla 4 St., 53-114 Wroclaw, Poland

Ken Tawara, Celeste Bolin, Jordan Koncinsky, Sujatha Kadaba, Hunter Covert, Caleb Sutherland, Laura Bond and Cheryl L. Jorcyk
Department of Biological Sciences, Biomolecular Sciences Program, Boise State University, 1910 University Drive, Boise, ID 83725, USA

Joseph Kronz
Mercy Medical Center, Nampa, ID, USA

Joel R. Garbow
Mallinckrodt Institute of Radiology, Washington University, St. Louis, MO 63110, USA

Mélanie Bousquenaud
Experimental and Translational Oncology Laboratory, Division of Pathology, Department of Oncology, Microbiology and Immunology, Faculty of Science and Medicine, University of Fribourg, Fribourg, Switzerland

Curzio Rüegg
Experimental and Translational Oncology Laboratory, Division of Pathology, Department of Oncology, Microbiology and Immunology, Faculty of Science and Medicine, University of Fribourg, Fribourg, Switzerland
Swiss Integrative Center for Human Health, Fribourg, Switzerland

Flavia Fico and Albert Santamaria-Martínez
Tumor Ecology Laboratory, Division of Pathology, Department of Oncology, Microbiology and Immunology, Faculty of Science and Medicine, University of Fribourg, Chemin du Musée 18, PER17, CH-1700 Fribourg, Switzerland

Giovanni Solinas
Department of Molecular and Clinical Medicine, The Wallenberg Laboratory, University of Gothenburg, Gothenburg, Sweden

Michael T. Barrett, Elizabeth Lenkiewicz, Smriti Malasi, Anamika Basu and Heidi E. Kosiorek
Division of Hematology and Medical Oncology, Mayo Clinic in Arizona, Scottsdale, AZ, USA

Jennifer Holmes Yearley and Lakshmanan Annamalai
Merck Research Laboratories, Palo Alto, CA, USA

Ann E. McCullough
Department of Pathology and Laboratory Medicine, Mayo Clinic in Arizona, Scottsdale, AZ, USA

Pooja Narang and Melissa A. Wilson Sayres
School of Life Sciences, Arizona State University, Tempe, AZ, USA

Meixuan Chen
Biodesign Institute, Arizona State University, Tempe, AZ, USA

Karen S. Anderson
Biodesign Institute, Arizona State University, Tempe, AZ, USA
Division of Hematology and Medical Oncology, Mayo Clinic in Arizona, Phoenix, AZ, USA

Barbara A. Pockaj
Division of General Surgery, Section of Surgical Oncology, Mayo Clinic in Arizona, Phoenix, AZ, USA

Nicholas A. Zumwalde and Jenny E. Gumperz
Department of Medical Microbiology and Immunology, University of Wisconsin School of Medicine and Public Health, Madison, WI, USA

Jill D. Haag and Michael N. Gould
McArdle Laboratory for Cancer Research, Department of Oncology, University of Wisconsin School of Medicine and Public Health, Madison, WI, USA

Kideok Jin
Department of Pharmaceutical Sciences, Albany College of Pharmacy and Health Sciences, Albany, NY 12208, USA

Niranjan B. Pandey
Department of Biomedical Engineering, Johns Hopkins University School of Medicine, Baltimore, MD 21205, USA

Aleksander S. Popel
Department of Biomedical Engineering, Johns Hopkins University School of Medicine, Baltimore, MD 21205, USA
Department of Oncology and Sidney Kimmel Comprehensive Cancer Center, Johns Hopkins University School of Medicine, Baltimore, MD, USA

A. N. Johnston
Translational Biology and Molecular Medicine, Baylor College of Medicine, Houston, TX 77030, USA
Lester and Sue Smith Breast Center, Baylor College of Medicine, Baylor College of Medicine, Houston, TX 77030, USA
Dan L. Duncan Cancer Center, Baylor College of Medicine, Houston, TX 77030, USA

J. Kapali
Lester and Sue Smith Breast Center, Baylor College of Medicine, Baylor College of Medicine, Houston, TX 77030, USA

L. Camacho, L. Xue, L. Qin and S. G. Hilsenbeck
Lester and Sue Smith Breast Center, Baylor College of Medicine, Baylor College of Medicine, Houston, TX 77030, USA
Dan L. Duncan Cancer Center, Baylor College of Medicine, Houston, TX 77030, USA

W. Bu and S. Hein
Lester and Sue Smith Breast Center, Baylor College of Medicine, Baylor College of Medicine, Houston, TX 77030, USA
Dan L. Duncan Cancer Center, Baylor College of Medicine, Houston, TX 77030, USA
Molecular and Cellular Biology, Baylor College of Medicine, Houston, TX 77030, USA

Y. Li
Translational Biology and Molecular Medicine, Baylor College of Medicine, Houston, TX 77030, USA
Lester and Sue Smith Breast Center, Baylor College of Medicine, Baylor College of Medicine, Houston, TX 77030, USA
Dan L. Duncan Cancer Center, Baylor College of Medicine, Houston, TX 77030, USA
Molecular and Cellular Biology, Baylor College of Medicine, Houston, TX 77030, USA
Molecular Virology and Microbiology, Baylor College of Medicine, One Baylor Plaza, Houston, TX 77030, USA

C. Nagi and J. Nangia
Dan L. Duncan Cancer Center, Baylor College of Medicine, Houston, TX 77030, USA

S. Garcia
SMART PREP Program, Baylor College of Medicine, One Baylor Plaza, Houston, TX 77030, USA

K. Podsypanina
Institut Curie, PSL Research University, CNRS, UMR3664, Equipe Labellisée Ligue contre le Cancer, F-75005 Paris, France

Sorbonne Universités, UPMC Université Paris 06, CNRS, UMR3664, F-75005 Paris, France

Roberto R. Rosato, Daniel Dávila-González, Dong Soon Choi, Wei Qian, Wen Chen, Anthony J. Kozielski, Helen Wong, Bhuvanesh Dave and Jenny C. Chang
Roberto R. Rosato and Daniel Dávila-González contributed equally to this work. Houston Methodist Cancer Center, Houston Methodist Hospital, Houston, TX 77030, USA

Clarice R. Weinberg
Biostatistics and Computational Biology Branch, National Institute of Environmental Health Sciences, National Institutes of Health, Research Triangle Park, NC 27709, USA

Katie M. O'Brien
Biostatistics and Computational Biology Branch, National Institute of Environmental Health Sciences, National Institutes of Health, Research Triangle Park, NC 27709, USA
Epidemiology Branch, National Institute of Environmental Health Sciences, National Institutes of Health, Research Triangle Park, NC 27709, USA

Dale P. Sandler, Zongli Xu and Jack A. Taylor
Epidemiology Branch, National Institute of Environmental Health Sciences, National Institutes of Health, Research Triangle Park, NC 27709, USA

H. Karimi Kinyamu
Chromatin and Gene Expression Section, Epigenetics and Stem Cell Biology Laboratory, National Institute of Environmental Health Sciences, National Institutes of Health, Research Triangle Park, NC 27709, USA

Quing Zhu
Biomedical Engineering and Radiology, Washington University in St Louis, One Brookings Drive, Mail Box 1097, Whitaker Hall 300D, St. Louis, MO 63130, USA

Susan Tannenbaum, Alex Merkulov, Poornima Hegde and Mark Kane
University of Connecticut Health Center, Farmington, CT 06030, USA

Scott H. Kurtzman and Kert Sabbath
Waterbury Hospital, Waterbury, CT 6708, USA

Patricia DeFusco and Andrew Ricci Jr
Hartford Hospital, Hartford, CT 06102, USA

Hamed Vavadi and Feifei Zhou
University of Connecticut, Storrs, CT 06269, USA

Chen Xu
New York City College of Technology, City University of New York (CUNY), New York, USA

Liqun Wang
Department of Statistics, University of Manitoba, 186 Dysart Road, Winnipeg, Manitoba R3T 2N2, Canada

Todd M. Pitts, Adrie van Bokhoven, Dara Aisner, Daniel L. Gustafson, Sharon Sams, Peter Kabos, Kathryn Zolman, Tiffany Colvin, Anthony D. Elias, Dexiang Gao, John J. Tentler and Virginia F. Borges
University of Colorado Cancer Center, Aurora, CO, USA

Jennifer R. Diamond
University of Colorado Cancer Center, Aurora, CO, USA
Division of Medical Oncology, University of Colorado Anschutz Medical Campus, University of Colorado Cancer Center, 12801 East 17th Avenue, Mailstop 8117, Aurora, CO 80045, USA

S. G. Eckhardt and Anna Capasso
Department of Oncology, University of Texas at Austin, Dell Medical School, Austin, TX, USA

Anna M. Storniolo, Bryan P. Schneider and Kathy D. Miller
Indiana University Melvin and Bren Simon Cancer Center, Indianapolis, IN, USA

Sara Jansson, Pär-Ola Bendahl, Charlotte Levin Tykjaer Jörgensen and Kristina Aaltonen
Department of Clinical Sciences Lund, Division of Oncology and Pathology, Lund University, Lund, Sweden

Anna-Maria Larsson, Lotta Lundgren and Niklas Loman
Department of Clinical Sciences Lund, Division of Oncology and Pathology, Lund University, Lund, Sweden
Department of Hematology, Oncology and Radiation Physics, Skåne University Hospital, Lund, Sweden

Cecilia Graffman
Department of Hematology, Oncology and Radiation Physics, Skåne University Hospital, Lund, Sweden

Lisa Rydén
Department of Clinical Sciences Lund, Division of Surgery, Lund University, Medicon Village, SE-223 81 Lund, Sweden
Department of Surgery and Gastroenterology, Skåne University Hospital, Malmö, Sweden

Stefanie Tiede and Gerhard Christofori
Department of Biomedicine, University of Basel, Mattenstrasse 28, 4058 Basel, Switzerland

Nathalie Meyer-Schaller
Department of Biomedicine, University of Basel, Mattenstrasse 28, 4058 Basel, Switzerland
Present address: Institute of Pathology, University Hospital of Basel, Basel, Switzerland

Chantal Heck
Department of Biomedicine, University of Basel, Mattenstrasse 28, 4058 Basel, Switzerland
Present address: Integra Biosciences AG, Zizers, Switzerland

Mahmut Yilmaz
Department of Biomedicine, University of Basel, Mattenstrasse 28, 4058 Basel, Switzerland

Present address: Roche Pharma, Basel, Switzerland

Cody Ramin, Betty J. May, Mikiaila M. Orellana, Brenna C. Hogan and Michelle S. McCullough
Department of Epidemiology, Johns Hopkins Bloomberg School of Public Health, Baltimore, MD 21205, USA

Kala Visvanathan
Department of Epidemiology, Johns Hopkins Bloomberg School of Public Health, Baltimore, MD 21205, USA
Johns Hopkins Sidney Kimmel Comprehensive Cancer Center, Baltimore, MD, USA
The Johns Hopkins School of Medicine, Baltimore, MD, USA

Richard B. S. Roden and Deborah K. Armstrong
Johns Hopkins Sidney Kimmel Comprehensive Cancer Center, Baltimore, MD, USA

Dana Petry
The Johns Hopkins School of Medicine, Baltimore, MD, USA

Jeanette Therming Jørgensen, Lea Elsborg and Søren Nymand Lophaven
Section of Environmental Health, Department of Public Health, University of Copenhagen, Øster Farimagsgade 5, 1014 Copenhagen, Denmark

Zorana Jovanovic Andersen
Section of Environmental Health, Department of Public Health, University of Copenhagen, Øster Farimagsgade 5, 1014 Copenhagen, Denmark
Nykøbing F Hospital, University of Copenhagen, Ejegodvej 63, 4800 Nykøbing F, Denmark

Elsebeth Lynge
Nykøbing F Hospital, University of Copenhagen, Ejegodvej 63, 4800 Nykøbing F, Denmark

Claus Backalarz, Jens Elgaard Laursen and Torben Holm Pedersen
DELTA Acoustics, Venlighedsvej 4, 2970 Hørsholm, Denmark

Mette Kildevæld Simonsen
Diakonissestiftelsen and Parker Institute, Frederiksberg Hospital, Peter Bangsvej 1, 2000 Frederiksberg, Denmark

Elvira Vaclavik Bräuner
Juliane Marie Center, Department of Growth and Reproduction, Capital Region of Denmark, Rigshospitalet, Blegdamsvej 9, 2100 Copenhagen, Denmark

Elin Borgen, Maria C. Rypdal and Anne Renolen
Department of Pathology, Oslo University Hospital, Oslo, Norway

Maria Soledad Sosa
Department of Pharmacological Sciences, Icahn School of Medicine at Mount Sinai, New York, NY 10029, USA
Division of Hematology and Oncology, Department of Medicine, Department of Otolaryngology, Tisch Cancer Institute, Black Family Stem Cell Institute, Icahn School of Medicine at Mount Sinai, New York, NY 10029, USA

Julio A. Aguirre-Ghiso
Division of Hematology and Oncology, Department of Medicine, Department of Otolaryngology, Tisch Cancer Institute, Black Family Stem Cell Institute, Icahn School of Medicine at Mount Sinai, New York, NY 10029, USA

Ellen Schlichting
Department of Surgery, Oslo University Hospital, Oslo, Norway

Per E. Lønning
Department of Oncology, Haukeland University Hospital, Bergen, Norway
Department of Clinical Science, Faculty of Medicine, University of Bergen, Bergen, Norway

Marit Synnestvedt
Department of Oncology, Oslo University Hospital, Oslo, Norway

Bjørn Naume
Department of Oncology, Oslo University Hospital, Oslo, Norway
Institute of Clinical Medicine, University of Oslo, Oslo, Norway

Gabriel N. Hortobagyi
Department of Breast Medical Oncology, Division of Cancer Medicine, The University of Texas MD Anderson Cancer Center, 1515 Holcombe Boulevard, Houston, TX 77030, USA

Index

www.ingramcontent.com/pod-product-compliance
Lightning Source LLC
Chambersburg PA
CBHW061329190326
41458CB00011B/3943